Case Management
in Health Care

www.elsevierhealth.com

Case Management in Health Care

Second Edition

Peggy A. Rossi, BSN, MPA, CCM, CPUR

Director of UM/CM/QM/Health Education and Pharmacy
Catholic Health West Medical Foundation
Sacramento, California

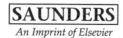

SAUNDERS

An Imprint of Elsevier

SAUNDERS
An Imprint of Elsevier

The Curtis Center
Independence Square West
Philadelphia, Pennsylvania 19106

CASE MANAGEMENT IN HEALTH CARE, SECOND EDITION   ISBN 0-7216-9558-2

Library of Congress Cataloging-in-Publication Data

Rossi, Peggy.
    Case management in health care / Peggy A. Rossi.—2nd ed.
      p. ; cm.
    Rev ed. of: Case management in healthcare, 1999.
    Includes bibliographical references and index.
    ISBN 0-7216-9558-2
     1. Community health services—Case studies. 2. Medical care —Case studies. I. Title.
    [DNLM: 1. Case Management. 2. Delivery of Health Care. W 84.7 R833ca 2002]
    RA427.R67 2002
362.1—dc21   2003040756

Executive Vice President, Nursing & Health Professions: Sally Schrefer
Acquisitions Editor: Yvonne Alexopoulos
Associate Developmental Editor: Danielle M. Frazier
Publishing Services Manager: Deborah L. Vogel
Project Manager: Deon Lee
Design Manager: Bill Drone
Cover Designer: Studio Montage

Printed in the United States of America.

Last digit is the print number: 9 8 7 6 5 4 3 2

To my husband of 41 years, Nick, and my sister, Pam. A few years ago Pam almost died and had horrific experiences with discharge planning, health care, and alternate funding systems in her state. However, she survived, and despite her disabilities she is a strong advocate for the disabled. She volunteers countless hours helping senior citizens and the disabled apply for programs for which they are entitled and spends countless other hours helping disabled artists have their artistic talents recognized.

Contributors

Elizabeth M. Akers, RN, BSN, PHN
Utilization Manager
Home Health Department
Kaiser Permanente
Sacramento, California

Pamela Blackmore, MHA, RN,C
Director
Transformation Services
The TriZetto Group, Inc.
Newport Beach, California

Anne P. Foster, RN, MSN, CPHQ
President
Care Review Resources
Huntington Beach, California

Patrice Hilgendorf, BSN, MHS
Quality Assurance/Utilization
  Management Coordinator
Home Health Department
Kaiser Permanente
Sacramento, California

Molly Kostlan, RNC
Patient Care Coordinator
Eldercare Department
Kaiser Permanente
Sacramento, California

Mindy S. Owen, RN, CRRN, CCM
Principal
Phoenix Healthcare Associates
Phoenix, Arizona

Gay Raney, RN, MSN
Pulmonary Care Manager
Care Management Department
Kaiser Permanente
Sacramento, California

Sharon M. Reichle, BS, MA, URQAP
President/Chief Executive Officer
Care Continuum, Inc.
Huntington Beach, California

Patricia Sweetland Roberts, RN, MS
Founder and President
PSR Consulting, Inc.
California

Marsha L. Scribner, RN, MSN, CPUR
Patient Care Coordinator - Emergency
  Department
Continuity of Care Department
Kaiser Permanente
Sacramento, California

Gregory Speicher, PharmD
Assistant Professor
School of Pharmacy
University of California, San Francisco
San Francisco, California
Clinical Pharmacist
Catholic Healthcare West MedClinic
  Medical Group
Sacramento, California

Marilyn R. Stebbins, PharmD
Associate Clinical Professor Step II
Clinical Pharmacy Department
School of Pharmacy
University of California, San Francisco
San Francisco, California
Pharmacy Utilization Manager
Catholic Healthcare West MedClinic
    Medical Group
Sacramento, California

Brad Stuart, MD
Medical Director
Sutter VNA and Hospice
Emeryville, California

Gary S. Wolfe, RN, CCM
Case Manager
Private Practice
Editor-in-Chief
Care Management
Salinas, California

Patricia Ann Zrelak, RN, MS, PhD
Managing Director of Stroke Research
Sutter Neuroscience Institute
Sacramento, California

Reviewers

Sherry L. Aliotta, RN, BSN, CCM
CEO
S.A. Squared, Inc.
Farmington Hills, Michigan

Joyce Brett, RN, MS, CRRN, CCM, CDMS
Team Manager
Zurich North America
Schaumburg, Illinois

Laurie Dazarow, MSN, RN,C
Director
Senior Services
Saginaw Cooperative Hospitals, Inc.
Saginaw, Michigan

Connie Gardner, BS, RN, CCM
Director of East Coast Operations
Care Products, Inc.
Northbrook, Illinois
National Treasurer
Case Management Society of America
Little Rock, Arkansas

Judy A. Harris, BSN, MS, MSN
Advanced Registered Nurse Practitioner
Nurse Practitioner Certified
Seniors First HealthCare
Tallahassee, Florida

Nancy Hudecek, RN, BS, CCM, MSIAM
President
Hudecek & Associates
Medford, Massachusetts

Ruthie Robinson, RN, MSN, CCRN, CEN
Faculty
Nursing Department
Lamar University
Beaumont, Texas

Preface

Even as I wrote the first edition of *Case Management in Health Care*, I realized a second edition would soon be needed. This is due to our rapidly changing health care environment—advancing technology, an aging population, and shrinking resources—as well as the demands placed on the system by consumers, policyholders, and regulators. I see this edition as almost a second volume. Whereas some chapters have merely been revised, almost an equal number are on new topics. Thus, readers who have both books will have a complete guide to handling cases and an idea of the many factors that affect case management processes, programs, and practices.

Laws have always shaped health care and the processes a discharge planner or case manager follows. However, during the past few years we have seen some additional laws that are equally as challenging and that will shape our health care environment as much the laws of the past have. For instance, a skilled case manager must now have knowledge of the Balanced Budget Act (BBA), Emergency Medical Treatment and Active Labor Act (EMTALA), Health Insurance Portability and Accountability Act (HIPAA), Patient Bill of Rights, and other such important legislation. With many of these new laws we have also seen tremendous shifts in reimbursement and, consequently, shrinking resources as agencies have closed or merged with others, placing new challenges on the case manager.

Much has changed in the world of health care in the short time since the first edition. Many of the changes are the result of multiple factors. However, possibly the two biggest factors are the BBA and the impact of technology and our aging population. The BBA of 1997 brought about many changes, including new requirements for reimbursement as well as a reimbursement methodology known as the Prospective Payment System (PPS). With technology, we are seeing a patient population that is older and has more chronic and disabling illness and conditions.

As I wrote the first edition, I saw a need for at least two additional chapters: one on the moral and ethical issues that health care professionals face almost daily, and one on quality. In my years in health care, I have seen both topics take on new and deeper meanings. For example, while we as health care professionals have had to deal with moral and ethical issues for years, technologic advances and our aging and more chronically ill populations have placed a new importance on making appropriate decisions and promoting well-being. Moral dilemmas often become litigious when technology advances but the procedures or drugs are still in the experimental stages. The payer often refuses to reimburse for experimental treatments, and yet the patient and family, hoping for a miracle, may demand them. A battle may ensue and leave the case manager caught in the middle, trying to be both a patient advocate and a loyal employee.

The Consumer Bill of Rights, the new emphasis of the National Committee for Quality Assurance (NCQA), and the Joint Commission for the Accreditation of Healthcare Organizations (JCAHO) have all played a large role in the demand for quality. The NCQA and JCAHO set the gold standard for health care organizations, creating new performance pressures and processes. With this comes the need to produce meaningful data and statistics that validate the quest for quality. Measuring quality often involves a cumbersome process called *auditing*. Every health care organization must endure audits of one sort or another during the course of any year. Therefore, it is vital to understand why audits are important and how to prepare for them. Audits can be performed by a private auditing firm for a policyholder or by the NCQA, JCAHO, Department of Health and Human Services (DHHS), or Centers for Medicare & Medicaid Services (CMS) (formerly the Health Care Financing Administration); all will ask for data, reports, and updated or new policies and procedures. Preparing for an audit often falls on the shoulders of a manager or director, so knowing what information is needed to pass one or to meet an accrediting body's standards is critical because it affects all staff within the department.

The writing of the second edition has again been a wonderful opportunity for which I am grateful to have had the ability and honor to undertake. As with the first edition, the intent of this text is not to be a cookbook on how to do case management but to be a resource to educate readers of some of the processes involved. More importantly, it is designed to give the reader an understanding of some of the factors that affect what we do, how it is done, and why things do not always go as planned. Little has changed since the first edition with regard to the conditions that require case management assistance and the voluminous resources these patients frequently consume. What has changed is our access to the Internet and the wealth of information that is now available to us and our patients. This edition concentrates on using the Internet for accessing information that we might need as we attempt to help the patients we serve.

This edition was written with the help of many experts in the field, who provide tips of the trade and information needed to perform case activities. Case management is evolving faster and in more directions than ever envisioned. These changes as well as those in the health care system in general have made it evident how important nursing case management is to the clients we serve. Regardless of the employer setting, nursing case management and the knowledge nursing expertise brings to the forefront allow for the levels of efficiency and effectiveness that produce superior health outcomes for patients in virtually any setting.

When I wrote the first edition, very little had been written about medical case management, and the few books that were available concentrated heavily on workers' compensation techniques and processes. Therefore, my intent was to help health professionals interested in case management learn to function in a world of managed care. This second edition will have even more of an impact than the first because it focuses on the many changes that have occurred and continue to occur in health care without signs of abatement. This edition again presents basic information on various topics that nurses and other health care professionals involved with case management need to understand if they are to become active advocates for their clients and to be able to activate health care resources and alternate funding when needed.

Perhaps the three biggest challenges facing case managers are related to the economics; financing; and health care policies, laws, and regulations that affect our day-to-day ability to function. No case manager today can function without a basic understanding of the everyday costs and knowledge of how finances influence every move we make with our clients. Although it often seems that case managers are the only ones facing major problems, every health care professional faces similar challenges with the growth of managed care and its many constraints, as well as the constraints and oftentimes the lack of public programs and community resources.

As with the first edition, this edition is designed for nurses and students of case management in all areas of medicine. As the health care system changes, often so do the types and processes of case management. Thus, the literature in this area continues to grow, making it difficult for those who are learning to identify the more important areas for study. This edition attempts to identify the key issues to help case managers keep their skills sharpened.

The concept driving case management is so basic and the results are so straightforward that it is hard to believe that we must still educate medical professionals, senior management, politicians, and others regarding its benefits rather than simply implementing its processes. I say this because, even today, many organizations do not recognize the benefits true case management has to offer. Also, many organizations continue to streamline operations by combining case management with utilization review or utilization review with discharge planning. They unwisely believe they should avoid having two people in the chart at the same time. The end result is often disastrous because it is impossible to do two jobs at once and still devote the time needed to each. Every job takes a different level of expertise, and one job *always* takes the backseat and therefore its outcome will suffer. As case

managers you must continually educate your superiors of the benefits of doing a job well and of the fact that only one job can be done at a time.

Because so much of case management is patient, insurer, or community specific, it is almost impossible to give examples of what will be useful for all readers. The information in this text is based on my own expertise and that of my colleague writers. The book draws from my background as a discharge planner, utilization reviewer, and health care payer case manager, as well as from my leadership abilities. As with the first edition, I have attempted to focus on the importance of all case managers working closely with each other for joint planning. I have included the health care payer case management perspective because it can offer valuable input into overall planning. Far too often case managers are left out of the picture because their role is confused with that of the health care payer's utilization review nurses.

This book is designed to give an overview of the key areas needed to do a job and do it well, rather than as a source of universally applicable examples for all case management situations or employer settings. To write a book that contained information on every topic and case example would be impossible. Therefore, I have attempted to give basic information and indicate where additional information can be located. Keep in mind that one of a case manager's best skills is the ability to network. Networking allows for not only friendship but an opportunity to expand one's knowledge base.

My thanks and gratitude to all who made this book possible. Thank you! Thank you!

Peggy A. Rossi

Acknowledgments

A special thanks to the following people for all their hard work:

Yvonne Alexopoulos and especially **Danielle Frazier** at Elsevier Science, who helped make this book possible

My daughter, Debbie, who spent thousands of hours typing and retyping all that I wrote

My sister, Pam, for all her work looking up websites for the community agencies listed in the text

My many colleagues who were contributing authors for the various chapters or sections within chapters of this edition

My colleagues at the LeMoore Naval Station, TRICARE Service Center, who sent me multiple flyers on the TRICARE programs during the time the CHAMPUS website was down due to the red worm virus

Judith Cherrie, RN, MSN, UM/CM Supervisor MedClinic Medical Group, for her editing of Chapter 14

Kian Rowhani, RN, BSN, Case Manager, Catholic Heath West Medical Foundation, for editing Chapter 1

Billie R. Rozell, DSN, Associate Professor Emeritus, The University of Alabama in Huntsville, for her encouragement to write this text book and further the education of case managers

Liz Valencia, RN, Manager Care Coordination (UM/DCP Unit), Kaiser Permanente Hospital South Sacramento Campus, for editing of the postacute care chapter

Nancy C. White, LCSW, Psychiatry, Kaiser Permanente Hospital South Sacramento Campus, for helping with the mental health section in Chapter 17

Brief Contents

Contents

CHAPTER 6
Medicare and Medicaid, 111
Peggy A. Rossi, BSN, MPA, CCM, CPUR

CHAPTER 7
Children's Health Coverage—Programs and Services, 162
Peggy A. Rossi, BSN, MPA, CCM, CPUR

CHAPTER 17
Case Management of the Mentally Ill Patient, 566
Peggy A. Rossi, BSN, MPA, CCM, CPUR

CHAPTER 18
Geriatric Considerations, 585
Molly Kostlan, RNC

CHAPTER 19
Pharmaceuticals and Enteral Therapy, 597
*Marilyn Stebbins, PharmD, and
Gregory Speicher, PharmD*

PART V
Postacute Care, 615

CHAPTER 20
Introduction to Postacute Care, 617
Peggy A. Rossi, BSN, MPA, CCM, CPUR

Changes and Tools of Case Management

Introduction to Changes and Tools for Case Management

Peggy A. Rossi, BSN, MPA, CCM, CPUR

OBJECTIVES

- To be able to list at least six of the major events that have helped shape the health care system of today
- To be able to list at least three of the incentives and priorities that have shifted health care from a discipline-driven model to a service model
- To be able to list the seven essential components for processes for case management
- To be able to list at least five of the reasons case management goals are not met

Many dramatic changes have occurred over the past 30 plus years, not only in the practice and delivery of health care but also in the role nursing case management plays in the medical field. These changes have had both a positive and a negative effect on the realities and complexities of the current health care system.

With these changes the U.S. health care system has also seen major shifts not only in the practice and delivery of health care but also in the proliferation of scientific and technologic services, government regulations, market competition, and economic constraints. These economic constraints are further heightened by a wave of health care mergers, reorganizations, and at times, actual failures of major health care corporations.

Consumers are better educated and very savvy about use of the Internet, and this allows them to make their voices heard, especially through the many demands they now make as they use the health care system. Although consumers have opted for managed care in an attempt to keep their out-of-pocket costs to a minimum, they continue to push for health care as it was under the fee-for-services plans of yesteryear.

Although little has changed when it comes to diagnoses and the multiplicity of needs, equipment, referrals, and services provided to patients by case managers, other areas of change that have affected not only case management but health care in general include the following:

- A health care system that is fraught with complications, constraints, and uncertainty.

- The impact technology advances have made on health care (both good and bad), and with it, greater demands placed on ethical dilemmas, increased patient expectations of a cure regardless of cost, and increased litigation when things do not go as planned or desired.
- The impact that the Balanced Budget Act (BBA) of 1997, prospective payment system, and the Health Insurance Portability and Accountability Act (HIPAA) have had on many areas of health care.
- More modalities for treating high-risk patients and populations have surfaced (e.g., disease management, demand management, care management, telemedicine), and case management is no longer limited to hospitals or insurers because it is offered by a variety of entities in the postacute-care arena (e.g., home health, disease-specific and other community-based providers and organizations, skilled nursing facilities, adult day-care centers, and durable medical equipment companies).
- Case management is now integrated into many federal and state policies associated with the delivery of health care and social support systems, as well as in Medicaid programs and many federally funded demonstration projects.
- The lack of postacute-care health care resources to effectively treat patients with ongoing care needs, especially those who require technologic support or complex treatment modalities and those with multiple complicated conditions, each demanding a variety of services.
- The time required to search for the appropriate levels of care and resources, or frequently, the scurry-

ing it takes to locate the payer source, if one exists.
- The multiple gaps and fragmentation found primarily in the post-acute-care arena, which often lead to dehumanized care as patients are shifted, dropped, or denied access to programs. This lack is often due to budgetary constraints that close or lock eligibility criteria, but in most cases it is due to lack of a funding or payer source for the care needed.
- The lack of nurses at all levels of care greatly affects the ability to move the patient smoothly through the continuum of care.
- Shorter inpatient stays caused by cost shifting, much of which can be attributed to the prospective payment system (PPS) and the growing number of uninsured patients.
- Increased awareness of ethics and ethical competencies demanded by purchasers, health care regulators, and the public as a whole.
- Increased mandates surrounding such issues as confidentiality, compliance, and the use of advanced directives.
- A myriad of chronic conditions, many with serious complications and any of which can be costly, requiring frequent treatments or encounters with the health care system.
- The increase in the population of persons with catastrophic and long-term disabilities (this is divided into two categories: those with young to midlife adult onset of disability—spinal cord injuries, traumatic brain injury, and rheumatoid arthritis; and those with developmental or early life onset of disability—cerebral palsy, mental retardation, muscular dystrophy).
- The increased use of the Internet by patients as they take more interest in

their own health, which in some cases has led to an additional layer of change—self-diagnosing or obtaining inaccurate information. This affects case managers, because they must now ensure that patients are receiving accurate information and using the information appropriately. On the flip side, case managers can now use the Internet as a resource for new information to support a request or as they educate patients and direct them to quality sites and services.

- An older population with a multitude of acute to chronic disabling conditions, for whom there are few financial resources for long-term ongoing care and for whom caregivers may be as old and debilitated as the patients.

Recent shifts in the nation's demographics are also causing substantial change in the way health care is delivered to Americans. Add to this the many mergers and unsuccessful attempts to "make it" in a very competitive marketplace, many health care organizations find themselves struggling with this transformation. These shifts can be attributed to any of the previously mentioned areas of change, but the primary drivers are the increasing elderly population, the AIDS epidemic, changes in consumer behavior, and most recently, the legislation enacted to provide protection of the civil rights and liberties of individuals with chronic illness. Any one of these events can be the impetus that prompts health care leaders to look for alternatives to the traditional approaches to acute care, and consequently, the growth of case management.

As a result of these changes, many health care organizations have begun to develop programs and services that will help increase patient access to resources and care and to then evaluate and monitor cost-effectiveness of such tactics. The final results will be used as organizations try to implement plans that encompass the long-range social, economic, and health care needs of the growing elderly population and persons with chronic medical conditions.

Through the years, health care has shifted from a discipline-driven model to a service model, and so have the incentives and priorities. Therefore it is common to see the following:

- Large employers or purchasers of health care benefits have cut their health care costs by changing benefit packages, eliminating specific coverage or making it available under specific benefit riders, insisting on use of specific drug formularies or providers, increasing copayments and deductibles, and other cost-containing tactics as these entities become the driving force for health care change.
- The managed health care market is price-driven, and quality must be redefined and agreed upon by all the stakeholders, not just the provider.
- The consumer of services is becoming a more sophisticated participant who is interested in outcomes, value, and costs.
- The value of a provider to a payer rests in the provider's ability to achieve the best outcome at the right time, in the right place, with the right team, and at the right cost.
- The focus of health care's leadership is to save and expand the business, and any professional discipline's future is directly related to the value it brings to the patient, payer, or organization.
- Although managed health care looks different from one market place to another, the basic cost-based principles do not dramatically change.

- Mature managed health care organizations are directing major resources toward prevention, early detection, and health maintenance opportunities.
- Industrial-strength solutions that include widespread downsizing and redesign without individualization of the institution's needs and identified use of specific talent required for future planning yield organizations that are stripped of the human resources needed for the change process.
- Managed care and therefore the business of health care will not be successful if, in addition to physicians, the people delivering and clinically managing the care are not fully involved in the development of the managed health care program.[1]

MANAGED CARE AND CASE MANAGEMENT

Title XVIII of the Social Security Act of 1965 created Medicare, and with it, came the mandates for discharge planning, which is a strong forerunner of today's case management. These mandates occurred before the emergence of managed care and today's convoluted insurance schemes that attempt to contain escalating health care costs. Likewise, this era predates the list of complexities now associated with health care and the movement of patients through the health care continuum.

These complexities are further magnified by (1) the many types of specialists required to treat today's patients, who are often faced with a laundry list of chronic medical conditions, each in its own right as complicated as the other, and many further complicated by dependency on technologic advances; (2) the ethical dilemmas brought forth by technology, the aging of our population, and the decreasing financial resources for such care; (3)

the lengthy list of health care professionals that comprise the multidisciplinary team and with whom interactions are needed; (4) the shift of care from an inpatient to outpatient setting or the rapidity of discharges from the hospital into another setting; and (5) increased consumer awareness, education, and access to the Internet, consumer interest groups, and legislation, which have increased consumer demands and expectations for care or the "right to care."

The continued development and proliferation of effective managed care and case management programs are imperative for any health care organization if it is to survive and compete in today's market. With this in mind, it is critical for case managers to understand the managed care process and how it affects the challenges they face in the practice of their profession and health care as a whole.

Managed care organizations that take a medical case management approach to their high-cost or high-frequency users of health care perform a variety of studies to evaluate the cost-effectiveness and quality of their programs. In most studies successful outcomes are the result of the following:

- Early identification and intervention, which ensures access to the most appropriate and least restrictive level of care as a patient's condition progresses or regresses
- Appropriate linkage and use of resources, whether from the insurer's provider network or community-based organizations
- Appropriate linkage to alternate funding programs when benefits are limited or excluded
- A cooperative and supportive patient, case manager, and provider/physician relationship
- A more compliant patient who assumes buy-in for self-management of his or her care

Challenges

Case management has evolved over the past 30 years from an insurance payer perspective to what it is today, and it is offered by a variety of methods and by almost every health care entity. One of the greatest challenges in developing a consistent approach has been the lack of training. Also, until recently, there were no formal training programs; and actually, until the mid to late 1990s, very little was actually written on processes for case management. Consistency in case management has been further hampered by almost no research and a lack of common definitions; the absence of a common set of training modalities; and a lack of standards for education, ethical behavior, and consequently, practice patterns.[2]

Another challenge is the one that arises when one attempts to be both a patient advocate and a gatekeeper for the cost of care and use of resources. It is this difficult balancing act that causes many case managers to walk a fine line as they attempt to meet two very different taskmasters—one that wants to provide the care needed by the patient and the other that often expects stringent allocation of the resources available to meet these needs.

Many of the issues faced by case managers center around ethical issues and have to do with the sorting out of rights and access to care in any given case. The case manager is often required and contractually expected to administer access to services within policy or dollar limits or any number of contractual constraints or restrictions to authorization or reimbursement. Thus the case manager, often seen as both patient advocate and gatekeeper, is charged according to the standards of case management to promote autonomy, beneficence, and justice.

Unfortunately, the many ambiguous areas in which case managers are asked to practice, coupled with the failure of the medical model to address many issues, presents ongoing ethical dilemmas and challenges for practicing case managers. Because of the complexities of most situations in case management, each case manager should be grounded in a value system that allows ethical decision making. To deal with the ethical dilemmas common to the job, case managers must bring to their workplace a well-developed sense of personal ethics, philosophy, and values. Similarly, managers of case management units must work with their staff to come to a consensus about what a reasonable case manager should do when confronted with various ethical dilemmas.

Still another challenge is to be knowledgeable about the many caveats to managed care and the reimbursement methodologies dominating health care. As the managed care environment has tightened, strategies have changed. Multiple strategies now dominate managed care, and many are discussed briefly in the managed care section of this text. Strategies for care have also changed, and we now have a system that provides care in an outpatient setting, which only a few years ago, was provided only in a hospital. As managed care has taken a dominant role in health care, we are also faced with new strategies for authorization of and payment for care.

Case management, and with it the need for nurses in the role of case manager, has evolved over the years. As such, it is a strong component of managed care and it fits well with the "shared-risk model" of true managed care. As outlined in the managed care section of this text, in a shared risk model all participants (payer, provider, and patient) are at risk if the process of health care delivery is not carried out with technical efficiency and fairness.

The shared risk model brings with it the rationale that presupposes the provider will practice ethically and not withhold or deny care when it is required. It also brings with it assumptions that the patient has no hidden agendas or secondary gains from the disease and that the managed care organization's policies and procedures are consistent, fair, and honest in conception and practice. The end result will be that patients who are involved in case management will be engaged in a system that requires them to play an active part in formulating their plan of care. This structural control technique enables the plan of care to be appropriate to the goals of the patient, and consequently, all parties have an incentive to keep the plan of care on track to ensure that quality of care is the final outcome.

As we know, if done right, case management is the essence of quality improvement. To reach this goal, case management systems must act like well-functioning human beings and stay focused on the task at hand, interact without duplicity, learn and respond to new situations and information in a positive way, and always strive to be honest and forthright in all communications. Although well-functioning case managers and case management systems may not always do everything right, they must also strive to do the right thing, thus influencing others in the system to also act with integrity and take advantage of the opportunity to provide quality, cost-effective health care.[2]

NURSING CASE MANAGEMENT

Although case management is by no means limited to the field of nursing, nursing over the past 30 some years has moved to the forefront as the primary professional discipline that assumes the role. The changing health care environment and the nature of health care economics have forced many hospitals and health care organizations to view nursing as the discipline of case management and case management as an alternative to the delivery of direct care services.

Like health care in general, case management has also undergone many changes. It is now a service provided not only by insurers and hospitals but also by any number of organizations that supply health care benefits in the postacute-care arena. Thus the definition of case management varies and is dependent on the personnel employed and their duties, the staff mix, the setting in which the model operates, the entity that employs it, and more importantly, the professional discipline that provides it (e.g., nursing or social work).

Nursing case management is often described as occurring within the walls (WTW) where the emphasis is on acute-care hospital case management activities. It is also associated with the term, *beyond the walls* (BYW), which describes those models that function in an outpatient or community-based setting, as well as those case management programs that operate within a managed care organization (MCO) or health maintenance organization (HMO) and are often referred to as *medical case management programs*. Regardless of the model, the primary focus is to balance the cost and quality components of care, services, and patient outcomes. Case management is therefore evolving into a professional model that is both sensitive and responsive to America's ever-changing health care environment and demands.

Through the years, many hospital-based case management programs have engaged registered nurses as the primary providers of case management. It is through their involvement in case management that nurses are allowed to influence and direct the delivery and ultimately the quality of care a patient receives. Nurse case management, although often believed to be hospital-based, is not confined to this area alone. It can also be seen in the many medical case management models associated with managed care or those offered by community-based organizations.

Because there are so many models of case management in existence today, it is literally impossible to cover them in a text of this sort. Fortunately, one of the benefits of the growth of case management is the variety of literature now available that describes the various case management programs in detail (e.g., New England Medical Center in Boston, Hermann Hospital in Houston, Carondelet St. Mary's Health Center in Tucson, Jackson Memorial Healthcare System in Miami, St. Joseph's Mercy Hospital's Pontiac and Port Huron projects, St. Joseph's Medical Center in Wichita, Sioux Valley Hospital in South Dakota, and St. Michael Hospital in Milwaukee). It is also important to read about other successful case management models—especially those offered by the Department of Defense/TRICARE Case Management programs, the Shanti Project, and many of the other community-based case management models used by large cities such as San Francisco and New York—in the development and implementation of programs to assist the homeless; persons without insurance; and persons with immune disorders, mental illness, and communicable diseases.

A review of the literature on the history of case management also indicates that some of the past and current nursing practice approaches and delivery models of care have been incorporated into the development of case management. Although the intent is to show the correlation between hospital nursing and hospital-based nursing case management and how it draws from the philosophy and collaborative practice strategies of both the primary and team nursing processes, nursing case management is no longer limited to the hospital setting. However, as nursing case management evolves, it is through these nursing processes that many of the

professional practice demands, initiatives, and characteristics of alternative patient care delivery models are integrated. It is also through the emphasis on patient-centered care that the nursing case management approach embraces business techniques and the view of the patient as a customer who has the right to demand the best in health care.

Placing the patient at the core of nursing's power base authorizes the profession to reconfirm its commitment to society. Nursing case management then incorporates a way of looking at the relationships among cost, quality, and nursing care. It emphasizes the autonomy, authority, and accountability of professional nursing practice by promoting an open system of care in which information is shared by all disciplines.[1]

Bedside Nurses as Case Managers

Unfortunately, with health care changing so rapidly, many nurses are leaving the bedside and looking at case management as a way to escape the labor-intensive duties associated with institution-based health care. The downside of this is that few want to accept that they have little if any of the insurance or community skills needed to perform the job. Likewise, few want to accept a low starting salary, vague job descriptions, vague or unestablished policies and procedures, and the lack of training and support in many organizations coupled with the demands of one person performing multiple tasks. Many find it difficult to give up the hands-on care they traditionally performed as hospital and bedside nurses. At times, such individuals cannot relinquish their previous mode of practice in which they were led by concrete documents (i.e., pathways or traditional procedural methods) and have difficulty assuming a role in which they might need to determine what needs to be done. Thus they have a hard time with developing innovative ways to assist patients when they are given permission to think outside the box.

When interviewing potential candidates for case management, I have a standard question for nurses who are leaving the bedside environment: "Can you give up your nursing cap and traditional role duties and assume a business hat?" Other interview questions center on situations in which candidates must be creative in their responses. Also, to emphasize that case management requires not only a patient-centered but also a business approach, at many staff meetings when serious business issues must be discussed, staff members wear cheap black men's fedoras (purchased from a novelty store) as "business" is discussed and their responses or ideas are solicited.

COMMON CASE MANAGEMENT THREADS IN HEALTH CARE

Case management roles and responsibilities vary according to the organization represented, the population served, the level of physician involvement, the culture of the organization, the client mix, the case managers' education and training, and the type of case management offered. Although nursing case management is often the modality used by many organizations, case management is by no means limited to this professional discipline. In today's health care arena, case management is offered by a variety of organizations in a variety of ways (e.g., medical social models, medical models, long-term care, disease management, telemedicine), and each job carries with it its own set of priorities and variations to the role. For example, an adult day-care center's case manager's role, priorities, and responsibilities will be totally different from those of a hospital-based case manager, a case manager assigned to an insurer, an independent case manager, or a case manager employed by a home health agency or skilled nursing facility.

Consequently, roles and responsibilities vary because virtually every category of client served will have its own needs, and these needs will dictate the scope and depth of case management required.

The model for case management may be hospital-driven or primary therapist–driven (mental health), offered with a generalist approach, or offered to a specific group of clients (e.g., geriatric or those with a specific disease). However, most have the same essential components. The common and essential components are processes for the following:

- *Identification* of appropriate clients
- *Assessment* of clients for the services they require
- *Coordination, planning, and identification* of the level of care and then the level of services and scope of resources required to meet patient care needs
- *Implementation, coordination, and linkage* of clients expeditiously to the resources they require
- *Direction, oversight, and monitoring* of the distribution of services clients require and ensuring that appropriate and effective services have been established as clients move through the continuum of care
- *Advocacy and the ability to act on behalf of clients* to ensure that needed interventions are obtained and clients are progressing as anticipated
- *Evaluation and continuous monitoring* to ensure the usefulness and effectiveness of the case management plan and that outcomes and goals are reached

Regardless of the type of clients served or the practice setting for case management, common characteristics of case managers include the following:

- Educational level
- Experience and expertise in the practice specialty to be case-managed and the total professional experience

- Ability to have a holistic perspective and see the patient as a whole person
- Knowledge of protocols and systems and how to procure resources to accomplish care goals
- Communication skills and the ability to effectively interact with the patient and health care team
- Ability to problem-solve and overcome hurdles and obstacles
- Ability to be creative and innovative
- Ability to be self-directed, because there is often no role model to follow
- Personal vision of the role

The case manager role has three dimensions. The first is the clinical role, which requires collaboration with the interdisciplinary team and involves the development of protocols that list the key tasks or events that must be accomplished for assisting patients. Case managers then use these protocols to direct, monitor, and evaluate patient treatment and the outcomes or responses to treatment. The second dimension is the managerial role, and this refers to the scope of managerial responsibilities it takes to coordinate the care of patients. The third dimension involves the financial aspect of planning, and this involves access to information about diagnosis-related groups, the cost of each diagnosis, and information on allocated lengths of stay or the number of treatments or procedures that will be allowed. To be effective, case managers must have access to information on case-mix index, cost of resources, and consumption; and they must be familiar with the prospective payment system and other current methods of reimbursement.[1]

One of the features that makes case management models appealing is that the structure must be extremely flexible. The design of the program can be modified to fit the needs and budgetary constraints of any health care setting. Therefore the case management theme can have many variations, and there is no right or wrong way to design a case management unit. The key to the success of the unit will be the roles and scope of functions the staff members are allowed to perform.

GENERALIST ROLE

Certainly, there are no set criteria as to who will do well in case management, but one must keep in mind that case management is a model of care. It is through this model that the primary goal of providing quality patient care in the most cost-effective manner must flow. Goals and designated time frames must be established to achieve successful patient outcomes. Because all care in today's health care arena is very time-sensitive, many models use a multidisciplinary collaborative approach so that "many hands are helping to do the tasks of one."

The multidisciplinary team approach is often used in case management because many medical organizations and even some hospital programs use a nurse case manager who is a "generalist." The generalist case manager has the expertise to handle most cases, but because of the variety of cases handled, he or she is not an expert in all areas or is not able to handle all the tasks required, especially with the rapid movement of patients through the health care system. Thus, although the generalist case manager model is structured to provide direct services, the generalist's role should be viewed as the one that serves to coordinate and implement the plan and then monitor the patient's progress toward specific goals.

To function appropriately, the generalist case manager relies heavily on the sharing of information from other professionals such as physicians, social workers, other nurses, and mental health and other rehabilitation therapists as the case management plan is developed. Information sharing and education are fundamental components in developing and implementing a collaborative case management program. Information must be obtained and shared with all parties and at all levels to expedite the reception and understanding of the anticipated plans and actions.

EVALUATIONS

Once a collaborative case management program is established, the focus must change to ensure that the program is maintained and to ensure that changes are made as issues are identified. A process such as this ensures that the program will remain viable. For a program to remain viable, it must include ways to do the following:

- Ensure that direction, commitment, and support from senior leadership continues
- Develop and initiate a formal networking program for the case management staff
- Develop, encourage, and ensure professional growth opportunities for staff members
- Develop a method of capturing details to ensure regular reporting of case management activity
- Develop a method whereby staff can measure quality assurance through routine self or peer auditing of case events
- Ensure that program goals, objectives, and achievements are communicated to the leaders and other interested parties
- Ensure that staff members can share ideas and have input in refinement of the program
- Celebrate and recognize accomplishments of individual case management staff members and the program as a whole
- Implement a quality improvement process by which issues and oppor-

tunities for improvement can be identified
- Provide feedback to the staff on achievements and improvements that have contributed to the success of the program
- Ensure that program evaluations occur on an annual basis, at a minimum

Evaluation is an important and intrinsic component of case management, whether this is from individual case monitoring or monitoring of the unit or program as a whole. Program evaluation can help to determine whether there has been any impact and the degree to which the impact affected the organization or the populations served. An evaluation process that is both sound and valid produces an objective picture of the strengths and weaknesses of a program and helps to identify any potential or real problems. More important, it helps to provide the evidence with which to justify the program's existence and expansion if and when it is needed.

The methods selected to evaluate the program must be such that the data collected can be analyzed and decision making about the program's effectiveness can occur. To be totally effective, evaluation methods must be well thought out and planned before program implementation, because this will provide a baseline from which one can measure progress. Evaluation methods selected must therefore do the following:

- Match the program components to be measured
- Have the methodology determined before the program is implemented
- Have a baseline from which comparisons and improvements can be made
- Have the tools designed to capture and collect relevant data that will allow one to know whether the program and its interventions have

been successful and which ones need revision

- Identify any variables that affect the final results
- Identify how the data will be presented and to what audience

Tools used to evaluate success often include the use of satisfaction surveys of the patients, providers, and staff or data that allow comparison of before and after encounters (e.g., number of visits, number of readmissions, number of emergency department visits, or length of stay all captured before and after case management) for specific populations or diagnoses. This includes processes related to the collection, analysis, and final dissemination of not only the statistical data but also any anecdotal data collected. The use of data is perhaps the best way to obtain and gain support of the organization's leaders.

Organization-Wide Commitment to Collaborative Case Management

As the demand for cost-effective high quality health care continues to grow, all organizations must explore innovative approaches to improving delivery of patient care. Developing an effective case management program is one way, but this requires a framework of total organizational commitment. Most often, this commitment must extend to the restructuring of programs that can meet the needs of today's health care system and the patient populations served. This requires a shared organization-wide mandate and commitment, as well as a vision of what role case management will play. It also requires accessible and reliable data of sufficient scope from which outcomes, whether good or bad, can be captured and improvements made. Likewise, it should include an appropriate organizational structure that must be seen as a core function in which all members of the team participate using well-defined guidelines and in which incentives are aligned to ensure develop-

ment of true partnerships, collaboration, and achievement of goals.

Although many case management goals will not be met as a result of non-compliance by the patient or family or the lack of a payer source for the needed care and services, unmet goals are often the result of factors such as the following:

- Lack of understanding of the complexities of the case management processes on the part of senior management
- Lack of a formal (and at times informal) training program for the organization's case managers
- Lack of job descriptions or ones that are vague
- Lack of the tools needed to do a job—policies and procedures, a computer system that can capture and report details and outcomes
- Lack of strong leadership or leadership that micromanages
- Caseloads that are so high that nothing other than crisis intervention or the putting out of fires as events occur can be achieved
- Lack of an understanding by all participants in the organization of the principles of case management and the need to be flexible and creative
- Lack of cooperation by physicians when specific requests are made
- Lack of understanding by the case management staff of managed care and its requirements, processes, modalities of reimbursement, and risk arrangements
- Inadequate staffing by social services to support the multiplicity of psychosocial aspects for care needed by the clients in a case management program
- Lack of providers or trained providers to offer the level and type of care required, often resulting in fragmented care; delays in services

or lack of care all together; expensive or inappropriate levels of care; unnecessary readmissions or increased lengths of stay; unnecessary or increased dependence on emergency department use; suboptimal use of health care resources, leading either to overutilization or underutilization; patient and family dissatisfaction with care and possible increased likelihood of lawsuits; increased quality-of-care issues; and increased complications caused by ineffective care

QUALITY AND CASE MANAGEMENT

Because the terms *managed care* and *case management* are frequently used interchangeably, there is much confusion as to the differences between the two concepts. Managed care and medical case management are both effective approaches that can be used as the demand for cost-effective high-quality health care continues to grow. These two modalities will provide the basis for exploration of new and innovative approaches to improving patient care delivery systems and outcomes. The primary focus of medical case management found in managed care is to improve patient outcomes and control costs through the coordination of health care services to meet patient needs. Medical case management has become an effective way for private insurers and providers to maintain control over the use and costs of health care resources. It is also a way to offer continuous quality improvement (CQI).

CQI and case management go hand in hand. Both focus on the processes used to achieve goals. These processes can be clinical, financial, or operational issues. Each step in the process must be analyzed; then, a plan for improvement must be tested and refined. The three leaders in the CQI process are Deming, Juran, and Crosby.

Each has made unique contributions toward improving the quality of work performed in the industrial setting, and now their concepts are being applied to health care. Under the CQI premise, case management is linked in philosophy and process, and the first step is to identify problems that appear to be more than isolated events; then all of the issues that may affect the outcomes must be identified.[1]

Through the use of case management and the CQI processes, procedures that are excessively used, extended lengths of stay, and health care delivery systems that lack coordination or promote duplication or fragmentation can be identified, analyzed, and trended for opportunities in which corrective actions and improvements can occur. Also, through the use of efficient medical case management controls, both the demand for and the supply of health care can be measured. This is accomplished by identifying potential high-cost cases and then coordinating and channeling the delivery of health care among providers by managing the patient's existing benefit plan for the level, type, and scope of care needed. To identify issues and come up with solutions, the case manager should do the following:

- Audit medical records to determine whether unnecessary tests, treatments, or procedures are being performed and whether other factors are contributing to increased costs, lengths of stay, or use of resources.
- Review complaints and incident reports, as well as other documents that identify issues, to determine whether opportunities for improvement exist.
- Interview key staff, including the medical staff, to solicit their input and identify areas for improvement.
- Review and analyze patient records to identify which costs can be eliminated or which processes can be improved.

- Evaluate current data to ensure that the information obtained is indeed needed, and if not, what information is needed to evaluate the areas that require change.
- Evaluate patient, physician, and staff satisfaction surveys to determine issues and identify areas that require change.

In contrast, poor quality often equates to the following:

- Additional costs associated with the wrong medications or treatments or placement of the patient at the wrong level of care
- Increased costs related to misuse of personnel or products or resources
- Delays in services and consequently added costs as a result of increased lengths of stay or additional treatments
- Loss of personnel because of dissatisfaction with their jobs or the belief that they are not bringing value to the workplace
- Loss of sales or customers (e.g., large health care purchasers select another insurer or entity with whom to do business; patients switch to other insurers; quality providers drop their contractual arrangements)

Regardless of what is studied or the tools and data used to study issues, the key to quality improvement is to have a process in place that measures the before and after events and to take the steps necessary to make change and then monitor the changes to ensure they are effective. If the changes are not effective, the process should be reexamined and started again.

Only through the use of a computerized and integrated information system and interpretable and standardized reporting mechanisms can continuous data monitoring and analysis occur and program objectives, health care delivery systems, and final outcomes be compared

and validated. Goals and successful outcomes can only be reached if they are offered within a framework of total organizational commitment in which the restructuring of care to meet the needs of today's health care provider and patient population can occur. By ensuring that appropriate outcomes are achieved, both managed care and case management provide a framework for continuous and refined planning of nursing and multidisciplinary care and ensure appropriate and cost-effective use of health care resources. Both models also contribute to the foundation of total quality improvement and ensure continued delivery of high-quality patient care.

TOOLS OF THE TRADE

With all the changes in health care as one moves into case management or advances in the field, it is important to understand the tools essential for the trade. These tools vary from human skills and expertise to actual manuals and the processes needed to accomplish the job. Also, in this day and age of computer technology, no case management unit should be paper-driven.

As one evaluates the tools, it is important to examine the qualities necessary to perform case management because case management is not for the weak at heart. It also requires skills far above the clinical skills needed by the general hospital floor duty nurse or even the nurse in an intensive care unit.

Documentation

A key tool in the field of case management is a consistent approach to capture and document case events. This requires expertise on the part of management to develop the tools needed to ensure that documentation occurs and includes the periodicity or frequency expected for case events.

The importance of documenting the facts cannot be understated. Documentation is what is used to protect oneself in the event of litigation. Keep in mind the two following quotes: "Keep it simple," and as the old saying goes, "If it is not documented, it did not occur."

Job Descriptions

Workplace job descriptions, if vague, are meaningless. As Mr. Wolfe stated in his chapter on credentialing, careful thought should be given to the development of a job description, and if it is well developed, as it should be, it should be used not only in the recruitment process but also as evaluations for performance are given. He goes on to say that generally, job descriptions have a history of being necessary documents, but little time has been given to their development. Consequently, organizations do not have good job descriptions. A well-developed job description will assist in the credentialing process, as well as in facilitating good performance from an employee because the employee will know what is expected in his or her performance.

To be effective, a job description should be clear and delineate the responsibilities and functions of the case manager, as well as reflect the expectations and level of educational background expected.

Other Tools—The Strength of the Case Manager

Although the listing of strengths needed by case managers is fairly lengthy, even the most advanced of case managers may have some weak areas because not everyone is strong in all of the competencies required for case management. According to the literature, a case manager must be the following:

- Astute in the area of clinical expertise, and consequently, the identification of the resources necessary to manage the type(s) and level(s) of care required
- An educator

- Able to exhibit excellent assessment, communication, organizational, and management skills
- Assertive and diplomatic
- Able to develop and retain interpersonal relationships
- Knowledgeable about age, cultural, and linguistic competencies
- Able to prioritize
- Flexible, creative, and able to adapt
- Able to assist patients, families, and other interested parties and professional disciplines to identify and coordinate the activities needed to put the case management plan into operation
- Astute and savvy about insurance and managed care and the many caveats to each
- Knowledgeable about community resources and patient entitlement to services
- Knowledgeable about alternate funding sources or other coverage sources for medical benefit payments or ways to stretch the health benefit dollars allowed by the insurer (including patient entitlement to eligibility and ultimately payment for services)
- Knowledgeable about managed care and its many caveats for authorization, provider use, and ultimately reimbursement
- Knowledgeable about legalities of care, quality of care, and standards for care
- A protector of privacy and confidentiality of information
- An advocate for both the patient and the organization

As a result of frequent mergers and downsizing in the health care system, many nurses, and sometimes social workers, are thrown into positions for which they are ill-equipped because of lack of training and/or management support to handle the new job responsibilities. Consequently, if this occurs, one must be prepared to negotiate for the training and equipment needed to perform the job.

TECHNOLOGY SUPPORT FOR CASE MANAGEMENT

Although many case managers prefer today's computerized systems and integrated software solutions, many programs continue to rely on the use of manual processes and volumes of paper. As stated in Ms. Blackmore's section on technology, one cannot view a software program as a means to reduce the volumes of paper. One must view it as allowing an integrated system to retrieve information that is not always available when a manual process is used. In today's organization one or more software applications or "programs" support most business processes, and the same must be true for case management.

Unfortunately, in most cases as case management systems are established, they are not started from scratch but built by using whatever processes are already in place. Although this has its good and bad points, the bad points often dominate, since old habits and bad images are hard to break. Consequently, it is often better to start from scratch rather than try to fix a broken ineffective, inefficient system. So, what might the case manager need to do in situations such as these?

- Work closely with senior leadership and key physicians to create a joint organization-wide approach to case management (key physicians are those respected by their colleagues in the community).
- Invest aggressively not only in data support systems but also in other systems that will technologically support the case management model and processes.

- "Blow up" or get rid of inefficient old systems and processes—again, use key physicians to evaluate and implement ways to make positive changes.
- Aggressively create and implement new guidelines, championing such efforts with physician leaders as a start.
- Track and trend progress and outcomes against defined goals and then disseminate the information through a variety of forums (e.g., newsletters, informal and formal clinical sessions, and various committees).

SUMMARY

Case management is built on the premise of prevention. Case management focuses on partnerships between providers and patients and sets new delivery-of-care arrangements that make health care services a more interactive and vital part of individual and community life. Case management ensures that health services are appropriate, effective, cost-efficient, and focused on patient needs.

Thus case managers, regardless of their practice setting, are the ideal professionals to oversee and assist with the process and ensure that patients, treatment plans, and providers are linked together to achieve goals favorable for patient outcomes, controlled costs, and satisfaction at all levels. By ensuring that appropriate outcomes are achieved, case management provides a framework for continuous and refined planning of nursing and multidisciplinary care and ensures appropriate and cost-effective use of health care resources. Through its various models, case management can contribute to the foundation of total quality improvement and ensure continued delivery of high-quality patient care.

Chapter Exercises

1. In a group, discuss the events that have affected health care over the past 10 years and list at least six of the major events.
2. In the same group, discuss the many reasons that health care has shifted from a discipline-driven model to one of service and list at least three of the incentives and priorities.
3. List the seven essential components for any case management process.
4. Review the organizational commitment section and list at least five reasons case management goals are not met. Add to this any goals you know cannot be met because of organizational or other issues.

Suggested Websites and Resources

www.milliman.com—Milliman and Robertson website

www.urac.org—American Accreditation Healthcare Commission for Utilization Review

www.NCQA.org—National Committee for Quality Assurance

www.aahp.org—American Association of Health Plans (AAHP)

www.interqual.com—InterQual website

www.jcaho.org—Joint Commission on the Accreditation of Healthcare Organizations website

REFERENCES

1. Cohen EL, Cesta TG: *Nursing case management from concept to evaluation*, St Louis, 1993, Mosby.
2. Newell M: *Using nursing case management to improve health outcomes*, Gaithersburg, Md, 1996, Aspen.

BIBLIOGRAPHY

Cohen EL: Nursing case management: Does it pay? *J Nursing Administration* 21(4):20-24, 1991.

Cohen EL, Cesta TG: *Nursing case management from essentials to advanced practice applications*, ed 3, St Louis, 2001, Mosby.

Cohen EL, DeBack V: *The outcomes mandate: case management in healthcare today*, St Louis, 1999, Mosby.

Del Togna-Armanasco V, Hopkin LA, Harter S: *Collaborative nursing case management: a handbook for development and implementation*, New York, 1993, Springer.

Ethridge P, Lamb G: Professional nursing case management improves quality, access and costs, *Nursing Management* 20(3):30-35, 1990.

Zander K: *History and rationale and clarification of acute care case management*, Paper presented at the meeting of the Individual Case Management Association, Orlando, Fla, September 1993.

Changes in Case Management

Mindy S. Owen, RN, CRRN, CCM

OBJECTIVES

- To be able to recognize the increase in the number of case management models and describe at least two models
- To identify "new competencies" required in the practice of case management
- To identify the differences between the case manager's role of advocacy and financial management and oversight

The health care delivery system is constantly evolving. As changes in technology and funding mechanisms occur, case managers remain vital links and valued team members who ensure that the patients' best interests are always central to every care plan and ultimately that patients receive all the appropriate services to which they are entitled. Despite what some might call the "good and bad" inside the practice of case management, case managers bring clarity, clinical experience, and health care knowledge, along with resources, to many individuals and families coping with complex needs.

HOSPITAL-BASED MANAGEMENT

In the past several years, hospital-based case management has emerged as a model focused on the patient who requires complex, acute care and multiple services and resources provided by or coordinated within the facility. The term *nurse case manager* (NCM) has been the title given to many professional nurses functioning in the role of case manager in the hospital setting. "To date hospitals have developed their own job descriptions, recognizing the NCM in ways that fit their needs, standards, policies and procedures, and financial positions."[1]

In 1997 Toni Cesta wrote that "one key definition of Nursing Case Management (NCM) is an approach that focuses on the coordination, integration, and direct delivery of patient services and places internal controls on the resources used for care. It is a nursing care delivery system that supports cost-effective, patient outcome oriented care."[2] This definition suggests that the NCM may be responsible for meeting customer (third-party payers, providers, patients/families) needs and juggling cost and quality care issues while designing and implementing an individualized plan of care.

In today's health care arena, this is an emerging role. Many times, NCMs function in muddy waters, with several masters to serve. A hospital-based NCM must have a knowledge base that includes understanding the *case mix index*, the cost of resources, and the utilization picture, as well as third-party reimbursement procedures. The hospital (one master) expectation is that the NCM will most effectively determine which resources are most appropriate for which group of patients and how to best allocate those resources in the most efficient manner.

To meet this expectation, NCMs must provide care planning, facilitate communication, collaborate with all team members, teach patients and families care management techniques, supervise the appropriate level of care, act as patient advocates, and review quality improvement audits to evaluate efficacy and outcomes and the impact that case management has on patient care.[2] The problem here is that the populations of patients receiving case management services in the hospital are complex and often have catastrophic or chronic illnesses. The hospital-based model continues to focus on the initial episode of acute care and struggles with the dilemma of how to serve these patients after discharge and through the continuum of care.

POSTACUTE-CARE MODELS

Hospitals, outpatient clinics, and home health care agencies have collaborated to provide innovative case management models throughout the continuum of care in specific practice settings. These models most often provide services for a high-risk population after an episode of acute care, including evaluation of future care needs and implementation of a plan. The goal in this case management process is to reduce the use of acute-care resources and main-tain the patient in the most appropriate level of care available, while maximizing the patient's overall health status. Examples of community-based models include the following.

Carondelet St. Mary's Health Center, Tucson, Arizona

Carondelet St. Mary's Health Center was initially designed as an acute-care model with the case manager responsible for management along the continuum of care. The population was stratified by risk and managed in neighborhood-accessible community health centers. This was the first funded, community nursing organization to provide case management services to a risk-adjusted, capitated, and ambulatory population. In 1989 Carondelet developed a community nursing organization to provide health care services to the elderly, chronically ill, or disabled within a Medicare senior plan contract.[3] Today, as a result of market-driven financial implications, this population is served through an acute-care model with case management responsible for leadership. The Carondelet model introduced an innovative approach to nursing case management. It was a nationally recognized program that was studied with respect to how it would enhance health care in partnership with managed-care disease management programs. Nursing case management, community-based programs, health systems, and managed care can all benefit from "lessons learned" from the development, implementation, and eventual closure of this program.

Mercy Hospital's Port Huron Project

Mercy Hospital's Port Huron Project incorporates case management through collaborative practice arrangements, providing preventive educational programs and outpatient services, as well as in-home care coordination including respite resources.[3]

Jackson Memorial Healthcare System, Miami, Florida

Abbe Bendell, RN, BSN, MBA, director of clinical resource management, indicates that Jackson Memorial Healthcare System (JMHS) uses both an acute-care/case management model and a community-based case management/disease management model in caring for patients in Miami-Dade County. As one of the nation's preeminent urban tertiary care facilities, it has been a leader in case management and disease management.

When the approach of a case manager's supporting clients over the continuum is used, the model expands beyond the walls of the hospital. All elective admissions are "case managed" before admission to the hospital, during hospitalization, and after discharge. Emergency admissions are case managed during the hospital stay, and case managers coordinate care for the immediate postdischarge period. Additional support is given through referrals to various health care systems and disease management programs for further support, education, and self-management skills.

JMHS's first disease management program was initiated in 1995 and is related to diabetes. This program expanded to cover employees. Other disease management programs for asthma, renal disease, and HIV/AIDS soon followed. Another innovative program developed by JMHS is the provider service network, which is a Medicaid look-alike of the Medicare Provider Service Organization. In this program, initiated in 1998, a provider-based system provides the administrative structure and oversight of Medicaid services and patients. This includes case management and disease management services.

The most recent innovative program in which JMHS is participating is the Florida: Healthy State Program, which provides disease management services for high-risk patients with any of four chronic diseases. This program's population management approach comes from the core of case management principles and standards.

DISEASE MANAGEMENT MODELS

Since the early 1990s, disease management models have been established to reduce the risk of managing populations with the most prevalent chronic disease states. The intent is to identify the high-risk populations, stratify those groups into levels of risk, and provide resources and services by using standardized treatment strategies across the continuum of care to maximize the individual's health and quality of life. Managed care organizations (MCOs) and other organizations that have established disease management models have determined that the most effective way to provide ongoing individual management is through a case management approach. The process of disease management is as follows:

- Establish the disease state and the comorbidities that will be included.
- Identify, through agreed-upon criteria, the at-risk population (by using claims and demographic, pharmacy, and utilization data).
- Stratify the population through a combination of severity program triggers and case management assessment (i.e., who will most likely benefit from the agreed-upon interventions, and in what projected time frame?).
- Design and coordinate the interventions into an overall health care plan (i.e., population-based interventions incorporating the comorbidities and reflecting severity level).
- Implement the interventions in an individualized health care plan with the consumer and family.

■ Evaluate clinical, financial, satisfaction, and quality outcomes by using predesigned tools in the disease management program.

Many case managers today find themselves working within these models of care and bring their clinical expertise, process-driven skill sets, and passion for providing patient education and advocacy to an at-risk, clinically compromised population. Having health care practitioners (case managers) at the center of these models only enhances the services provided and increases the trust level of the populations served.

At best, disease management is a collaborative approach to care, bringing providers, payers, consumers, government agencies, and other interested parties together in an effort to reduce acute-care risks and to improve the overall outcomes of these individuals. Case management has a significant role to play in building and implementing disease management models.

At worst, disease management is a stand-alone approach to care that will be unable to "prove" its value in a consumer-driven health care arena and will not be allowed the time necessary for analysis and presentation of its results.

DISABILITY MANAGEMENT

"*Disability Management* is the process of limiting a disabling event, providing immediate intervention once an injury or illness occurs, and returning the individual to work in a timely manner."[2] The basis of the process is the effectiveness of the return-to-work program in place. Today, many employers understand the benefit of incorporating disability management initiatives with workers' compensation, health care benefits, short-term disability, long-term disability, available state disability programs, union plans, medical leave of absence, sick leave, and Social Security dis-

ability income. These programs are commonly referred to as *24/7 benefit plans* because they include a broad spectrum of benefits.

The Case Manager's Role in Disability Management

Even though the components are the same as those of case management (assessment, planning, implementing, coordinating, and evaluating), the complexities inside of disability management are numerous. Examples include the following:

■ Developing a communication protocol
■ Selecting a software program specific to facilitating documentation regarding catastrophic injuries or illnesses and associated costs for both inside and outside company use (must comply with Health Insurance Portability and Accountability Act [HIPAA] regulations)
■ Implementing an early intervention program
■ Developing and maintaining a bank of modified, transitional, and routine job duties
■ Coordinating with a health care facility to provide wellness visits, preventative health care screenings, and interventions

The case manager is ultimately responsible for coordinating the return-to-work plan in collaboration with the individual's rehabilitation team and for communicating the plan within and outside of the workplace as appropriate. The case manager's accountability encompasses securing effective, quality health care services that will produce return-to-work outcomes. "The case manager has the responsibility to keep both the employee and business healthy."[4]

In disability management the goal has not changed, nor has the plan. However, today the corporate policies include HIPAA regulations, state and federal mandates, and corporate cultures struggling to maintain their place in the market. Case managers need to bring to the table their clinical, business, and advocacy skills to have an impact on the masters they serve in this model.

LIFE CARE PLANNING

Life care plans were first identified in the rehabilitation and legal literature as a part of rehabilitation evaluation. Their purpose was to predict the impact of catastrophic injury on an individual's future. Differentiated from discharge planning by specifications of costs of long-term needs, the most frequent use for life care plans was in litigation.

Today the definition and use of life care plans has expanded. The current nationally accepted definition is as follows:

A Life Care Plan is a dynamic document based upon published standards of practice, comprehensive assessment, data analysis and research, which provides an organized, concise plan for current and future needs with associated costs for individuals who have experienced catastrophic injury or have chronic health care needs (International Academy of Life Care Planners, 2000).[5]

Life care planning, according to this definition, may be applied in many case management settings. The document may be used by insurance or reinsurance companies to establish reserves and to chart an expected pathway for an insured individual with probable high-cost care needs. Life care plans are valuable in elder care management as a teaching tool and education resource. For facilities, life care plans offer a means for outcome measurement and a tool for discharge planning. Increasingly, families and individual patients request life care plans, as written guides, to maintain health.

As options for quality health care continue to evolve, life care plans provide a mechanism for documenting, monitoring, and evaluating health care delivery. Often considered an outcome of case management, the life care plan serves as a guide for patients, families, and teams of health care providers.

MANAGED CARE ORGANIZATIONS

An MCO is a delivery system of health care in which all aspects of patient care are coordinated to produce cost-effective, efficient, quality-focused care, incorporating utilization review, case management, credentialing, best practices/guidelines, formularies, disease management, and outcome analysis.

It has been suggested that inside of managed care there are two models of case management. One model emphasizes cost-effectiveness through intense financial oversight, beginning in the initial clinical decision-making period and including authorization. This model ties quality and cost together and may contribute to the reputation that managed care has developed. The purpose of managed care has always been to provide and ensure the highest quality of care. Case managers are at the frontlines of the process, representing the philosophy and mission of the MCO to a variety of stakeholders, and yet, they may be the "best kept secret" in the organization.[6]

The second model of case management in the managed care arena is the patient advocacy model, which emphasizes a more comprehensive coordination of services across the continuum of care and takes into consideration the individual's requests and preferences when possible. This model is patient-centered and consumer-focused.

Because health care plans are focusing on consumer-driven benefits, case managers are in an ideal position to blend these two models into one that maintains financial responsibility for high-cost, high-risk populations and presents an advocacy approach in delivering case management services to consumers. Today we are seeing the aging baby boomer population focusing on their own and their families' health care issues. MCOs see this as a challenge to provide value-added benefits to this population and demand that they maintain a financially responsible organization.

This has been a major component in MCOs' changing to patient-centered relationships among delivery systems, practitioners, health care providers, MCOs, and employers, based on shared knowledge and consensus on guidelines and quality care.

TELEHEALTH TECHNOLOGIES AND THE CASE MANAGER

Technology and Nursing Practice: Case Management

U.S. health care costs are projected to exceed $1 trillion in the first decade of this 21st century.[7] Yet with all the increased costs, the availability and quality of health information and services pose significant challenges to U.S. consumers, industry, all levels of government, and most directly, the providers of health care. Quality and access to care remain variable across the country. As "market" pressures force an in-depth reexamination of the health care system, the need for improved access to information at all levels in the system to facilitate accurate decision making, as well as the coordinated and improved delivery of more appropriate patient care, will become more evident.

The current U.S. health care delivery system is fragmented. It often relies on the patient as the information carrier and historian. The key element, appropriate and timely patient data, constitutes the most crucial part of the decision-making process for accurate and effective diagnosis, and treatment has yet to be digitally automated. Providers often spend more than 40% of their time processing paperwork and looking for fragmented pieces of critical patient information to enable diagnosis and treatment. Most health care diagnoses and decisions made today are still done without total access to real-time pieces of relevant patient information.

As the health care industry continues to evolve and explore new and innovative methods for managing larger populations more efficiently, technology will play a significantly greater role in the facilitation and coordination of care. Although often viewed as the scapegoat for rising health care costs, technology has shown itself to be a means of increasing productivity in the health care setting while reducing resource use in a variety of high-risk populations. The evolving application of information technology, coupled with rapidly expanding communication capability, has spawned a revolution in the health information infrastructure.

According to Marie Mann, RN, MPS, National Business Manager, Government Affairs Health Hero Network Inc.:

The critical foundation for health care system success, improving health access with real-time information access, is the first step in the process of inventing a proactive health care model that facilitates patient-oriented and cost-effective delivery of services. This model for technology integration allows providers to concentrate information and the delivery of primary health services where it makes the most sense...to households and individuals in convenient, familiar places, especially the patient's home.[8]

Rita Kobb ARNP, Director of Lake City Veterans Hospital (Lake City, Florida), explains:

Telemedicine is the exchange of health information and services across geographical, social, and cultural barriers. Telemedicine has been with us in health care for over thirty years. Until recently, telemedical applications of technology have focused only on physician-driven initiatives such as teleconsultation and telediagnostics that feature the use of high-quality audio-video conferencing.[8]

Ms. Mann further indicates:

Driven by advances in communication technology, telemedicine is expanding beyond the realm of the physician provider to include all health care providers, especially nursing, as well as affecting transactions for health purchasers, payors and government. Telemedicine has the potential to improve the delivery of health care in America by bringing a wider range of health services to underserved communities and individuals in both urban and rural areas. Additionally, telemedicine can provide ongoing training and collaboration to health care professionals in all areas, including case managers.[8]

When telemedicine is applied to the day-to-day management of patients through nursing case management, it encompasses much more than the physician-to-physician consultation. Models of case management in which telemedicine technology is part of the core infrastructure have the capability to identify problems in patients with chronic disease long before the problem progresses to the point of high cost, high levels of care, and hospitalization.

Telemedical appliances that provide communication between the patient and caregiver allow for timely transmission of relevant clinical data and, when used by case managers, allow for early detection of the clinical variations that may herald the onset of more serious disease symptoms. Proactive recognition and subsequent intervention on the part of case managers can effectively reduce fragmentation of services and result in improved patient outcomes and quality of life. Telemedicine gives the NCM the ability to educate patients about their health while promoting active participation in making decisions about health and problems. Telemedical education puts the focus of care on patients and encourages patients to take responsibility for the management of their course of care and for improving their quality of life.

Telemedicine projects and networks of today are just beginning to unleash the potential of telemedicine to deliver health care services safely and efficiently. What is known today about telemedicine represents only an initial snapshot of technology, which is changing and expanding daily. Other technologies in which disease and population management strategies are used to monitor high-risk populations such as the frail elderly are also making an impact on health care.

Technology, combined with effective nursing case management, has led to improved patient health and better access to health care. Nursing case management as a practice is in a unique position to use technologic advancements to convert a health care system that currently focuses on the costly treatment of illness to a system that emphasizes primary health care services and the promotion, restoration, and maintenance of health. The NCM's clinical judgment and strong commitment to patient advocacy, as well as to professional and patient education, put the NCM in the expanded role of "technology advisor" to the patient. Effective NCMs realize that technology deepens nurse-patient interactions and gives the patient a more unique support system.

Technology, when used in an infrastructure built on a patient-centric case management model, is supportive of the presence of nurses in the case management process. The appropriate use of technology, determined by patient needs, has enhanced the nurse-patient relationship by allowing nurses to spend more quality time with their patients.

If the potential of technology is to enhance health care while maintaining quality, its acceptance and use will require a commitment from nursing leadership and frontline medical providers, as well as from leaders in government, payers, and employer purchasers. Technology applications alone cannot solve the health care industry's problems. However, technology can uniquely empower health care providers who recognize, understand, and use these tools to improve practice outcomes.

Case management is built on the premise of prevention. Case management focuses on partnerships between providers and patients and sets new delivery-of-care arrangements that make health care services a more interactive and vital part of individual and community life. Case management ensures that health services are appropriate, effective, cost-efficient, and focused on patient needs.

If, in fact, health care providers accept this premise of case management, then technology, when used appropriately, can only enhance care and make case managers more efficient. As health care reform continues to shape the future, one key to success will be the ability of the NCM to recognize and take advantage of all the tools that are available to improve care and encourage healthier lifestyles.

ALTERNATIVE MEDICINE AND CASE MANAGEMENT

Complementary and alternative medicine (CAM) is not only big business, it is also beginning to be recognized by employers as employees demand CAM coverage. In 2000 consumers spent between $40 billion and $50 billion on alternative medicine.[9]

Today most alternative medicines and treatments are paid for "out of pocket," without regard to the type of coverage a consumer may have. This indicates that consumers are finding a benefit in CAM and will continue to explore the effectiveness of including these treatments in their overall health care plans. Despite this interest by consumers in nontraditional treatment modalities such as acupuncture, homeopathy, and naturopathy, most physicians will not ask patients about their use of these alternatives. Sensing physi-

cians' distrust and uneasiness with the topic, consumers have indicated that they do not disclose any information about such treatments to their physicians.[9] A case manager, as a patient advocate, has an obligation to complete a full assessment of the individual's health care profile and relay the information obtained with the individual's consent to the appropriate team members (i.e., primary care provider [PCP]). It is important for the case manager to build a milieu of trust with the consumer and the PCP so as to allow collaboration and an openness that will lead to an "integrative treatment plan." The term *integrative medicine* is recognized as encompassing alternative, complementary, and traditional treatment modalities.

Assessment Questions

The acceptance of alternative medicine and treatments certainly expands the number of assessment tools that a case manager may use and provides an opening for a dialogue that should include *all* forms of treatment in which an individual is participating. For example, assessment questions might include the following:

- Please share with me the names of all medicines you are currently taking. Include *all* over-the-counter (OTC) medications you have in your possession.
- Have you received any treatment or medication from anyone other than your primary care physician? Please list name and specialty. Include yoga, tai chi, smoking cessation, and massage in your answers.

The Plan

Some employers are encouraging the inclusion of integrative medicine in their employees' overall health care plans. For instance, in the case of a patient with chronic heart disease, the plan of care might include services from providers such as exercise physiologists, behavioral health specialists, and nutritionists. The plan of care might then include an aerobic exercise regimen, support groups that help the patient focus on psychologic and spiritual issues, and a special diet.

Many oncology programs are building "patient-centered models of care" and include stress management, spirituality, complementary medicines, and other alternative treatments in their models. The case manager's responsibility is to encourage the health care team to recognize the plan as the patient's; therefore, the patient has the right to include the treatments he or she believes to be most beneficial.

Outcomes

Employers are beginning to see significant outcomes when integrative medicine techniques are implemented. Higher productivity, happier employees, and a tight lid on the overall medical expenditures are just some of the positive outcomes that have been observed. Case managers should not only be a part of this process, they should be getting the word out as to the benefits (financial, satisfaction, health-related) for both the employer and employees.

COMPETENCIES FOR CASE MANAGERS

According to Susan Gilpin, JD, chief executive officer of the Commission for Case Manager Certification:

Case management is not a health care discipline, but rather a transdisciplinary advanced practice of health care professionals from a variety of disciplines. This makes case management very different from other health care practices. By applying the process of case management, the case management professional achieves client wellness and autonomy through advocacy, communication with patients, families, providers and payers, education, as well as identification of service resources and service facilitation.[10]

As the practice of case management has developed over the years, the expecta-

tions and competencies have risen to higher levels. Case managers must be proficient with skills beyond coordination, negotiation, communication, collaboration, and facilitation.

Today, we add to the list: personal computer (PC) proficiency, telephone triage, telehealth technology implementation, report design, data analysis, and other skills that were not apparent in the early evolution of case management.

THE BIG "Ts" FOR EFFECTIVE CASE MANAGEMENT: TOOLS, TECHNIQUES, TRACKING, AND TRAINING

Tools
PC Proficiency

Software programs have been developed to assist in the management of most populations of individuals. It is important that a case manager be familiar with the basics of PC use. However, most organizations have either designed their own program or have customized a program to fit the population and program they are delivering and therefore will train the case manager in their proprietary programs. These programs are designed to assist the case manager in providing an effective, orderly, consistent management record, and not take away the case manager's personal interaction with the patients in his or her caseload.

Internet Resources

A case manager today may find a wide spectrum of resources on the Internet, including guidelines for care, home health care in a particular area, rehabilitation services, community and support groups, pharmaceutical education, and more. Familiarity with the Internet as a tool and its ability to provide "good and bad" information is essential for the case manager in the 21st century. The stakeholders we work with many times "rely" on the Internet for the information they receive, and it is the case manager's responsibility to review and discuss the information presented.

Telehealth—Home Monitoring Devices

Many disease management programs rely on home monitoring devices for a selected population of the chronically ill. This tool is designed to provide the case manager with a clearer picture of a specific segment (criteria-based) of the population. It assists the case manager in prioritizing (triage) his or her responsibilities and focusing on the individuals in the population with the highest risk for requiring acute care. These devices are also beneficial to the case manager in determining the individual's health care educational needs and helping the case manager provide appropriate information and instruction. Interfacing the device, incorporating the case management software, and analyzing its benefits for the individuals served and the program in place bring a new dimension to the practice of case management.

Techniques
Critical Thinking Skills

Use of critical thinking skills is a purposeful, outcome-driven process that assists in making judgments based on facts and scientific principles.

An individual or population with whom a case manager works is many times overwhelmed by catastrophic or chronic illness. It is the case manager's responsibility to assist by objectively "putting order" to the situation. It has never been more necessary, with the potential for "information overload," that a case manager lead the individual and team in the problem-solving process using *critical thinking skills*.

Business Skills

Case managers are called upon to incorporate business skills in their everyday practice. These include leadership and supervisory ability, internal and external professional communication, internal and external negotiation, regulatory and legislative knowledge and its affect on the practice, marketing and sales strategies, corporate strategic planning, and outcome analysis from clinical, satisfaction, and financial perspectives. These skills have increased the value of the case manager, irrespective of the practice setting, and only enhance the worth of the case manager in the health care arena.

Tracking
Report Design and Analysis

Case managers have always been called upon to evaluate the care plans and strategies implemented through the case management process. By using assessment tools, quality indicators, and stratification data, case mangers can *track* the individuals they serve and analyze the process and next steps. The evaluation (i.e., outcome) of this process not only gives case managers the knowledge they need to provide professional services but also solidifies their roles as valued team members who make an invaluable contribution to the process. In addition to providing traditional reports, case managers have contributed to the development of stratification reports indicating high-, moderate-, and low-risk population groups; quality indicators by disease state (e.g., in diabetes: glycosylated hemoglobin level, yearly retinal and microalbumin examinations, and percent of population proficient in self-monitoring of blood glucose levels). In chronic heart failure, some indicators may include increased knowledge of risk factors, daily weight monitoring and rationale, and medication management to include OTC medications and their impact on the overall treatment plan from both clinical and financial perspectives.

Training

Depending on the practice setting, clinical and case management experience, job requirements, and desire for advancement, the training issues may vary. Several areas of training that have developed as the practice has evolved include PC training, regulatory and legislative training (HIPAA), cultural and diversity training by area or region, eldercare training, telephonic triage training, disease-specific clinical updates, Medicare and State Medicaid rules and regulations that may affect the practice, and business development and implementation. Local case management associations, community colleges and universities, medical centers, and pharmaceutical firms may provide various types of training.

Accountability

With case management being an *advanced* practice and case managers having the ability to practice independently, accountability to the stakeholders they serve is an imperative. Doing the right thing at the right time and for the right reason ensures the trust relationship that is the foundation of case management.

ACADEMICS: GETTING THE RIGHT CURRICULUM

"When an individual earns a bachelor's degree in social work or nursing, the public has a fairly clear understanding of the preparation that an individual has received for the role of social work or nurse," notes Susan Gilpin, JD, Chief Executive Officer of the Commission of Case Manager Certification. "However, because case management evolved as a transdisciplinary advanced practice without the benefit of a nationally recognized and standardized core curriculum, there is no similar clear understanding of what preparation an individual has for the role of case manager."[10]

Today most colleges and universities that offer a nursing or allied health care curriculum indicate that they have some courses in managed care and case management available at the undergraduate level. However, such courses are not always seen as requirements, but as electives, carrying less weight in the program curriculum. This presents a challenge in academic preparation for the practice of case management.

A handful of graduate level programs are available to students seeking a master's degree in case management. Established programs include the following:

- San Francisco State University
- Pace University–New York
- University of Arizona
- Florida Atlantic University–Boca Raton, Florida
- University of Kansas

The slow evolution of graduate level, academic programs may reflect the lack of demand for "master's prepared" case managers in the workplace.

However, certification provides the public with a nationally validated tool for determining that a case manager possesses the education, skills, and experience necessary to provide appropriate services based on sound case management principles. Until we see a widely accepted nationally standardized core curriculum for case management at the university level, available in more than a handful of settings, certification remains the best tool for establishing that an individual is qualified to practice case management.

At present there is no "best" certification. Each case manager must evaluate his or her professional goals, educational preparation, and clinical experience and then review the certification options available before choosing the certification process that best fits his or her needs.

Established certification programs include the following:

- Certified Case Manager (CCM)
- Nurse Case Manager (RN-NCM)
- Case Manager Certified (CMC)

- Certified Professional in Healthcare Quality (CPHQ)
- Case Manager Administrator, Certified (CMAC)
- Continuity of Care Certification, Advanced (A-CCC)
- Certified Disability Management Specialist (CDMS)
- Certified Rehabilitation Registered Nurse (CRRN)
- Certified Social Work Case Manager (CSWCM)
- Certified Managed Care Nurse (CMCN)
- Certified Occupational Health Nurse/Case Manager (COHN/CM)[10]

JOB MATCHING: GETTING THE RIGHT PERSON THE RIGHT JOB

With the variety of practice settings and case management models in place, it is sometimes difficult to determine the "best fit."

Questions to consider include the following:

1. What model (practice setting) am I most comfortable working in?
2. What clinical expertise do I bring to the program?
3. What type of caseload do I prefer?
   - Small caseload versus population-based caseload
   - One that consists of 40 to 70 patients or more with some on-site responsibility
   - One that consists of patients with a mixture of acute, catastrophic, and chronic illnesses
4. What are the key elements to my job satisfaction?
   - Telephonic approach versus telephonic and on-site mix
   - Working independently versus working in a group setting
   - Providing patient/client education versus coordinating patient education

- Comfort level with technology-based programs
5. Do I prefer to work in an entrepreneurial environment where I can assist in program development? Or am I more comfortable in a well-established model and program?
6. Do I agree with and support the organization's mission and philosophy in providing case management services to the stakeholders they serve?

With the continual evolution of case management and the changes being both good and bad, it is as important for the case manager to interview and evaluate the prospective employer as it is for the employer to interview the case manager. Today, more than ever, there is no "one size fits all" in case management; however, with an understanding of one's own values and talents, the opportunities are endless.

MASTERING THE ART OF NETWORKING

One way case managers may explore these endless opportunities, as well as increase their knowledge base, is to "network" with new and old colleagues and business associates. The case managers' network, whether formal or informal, may become a support group and provide an arena for educational offerings. It is through networking that case managers may find new resources for their stakeholders, educational offerings for themselves, and new friends in the case management practice. Therefore mastering the art of networking is not only important to survival, it also takes case managers to a new level in job enhancement, which benefits all stakeholders. Louis Feuer, MA, MSW, President of Dynamic Seminars and Consulting, Inc., states that "some case managers do the networking scene very well; while others just aren't sure how to play the room." Getting out of our own comfort zone is always difficult, and we may need a push, but it is the best way to explore the ever-changing world of case management.[12] Several tips that Mr. Feuer shares include the following:

1. Go to meetings by yourself and be open to meeting others.
2. Look for dinner or lunch partners you do not know and use this time for interaction and possibly undiscovered opportunities.
3. If you are at meeting with a speaker, introduce yourself to the speaker (after the presentation) and respond to the presentation. Exchange business cards.
4. Make the first move to engage colleagues in conversation. Ask questions and show interest in what they have to say.

The definition of *case management*, as adopted by the Case Management Society of America (CMSA) and the Commission of Case Manager Certification, begins with the statement, "Case Management is a collaborative process." Therefore it supports networking, and it is important for us to remember that collaboration is critical to the practice of case management. It is not only critical for our clients/patients and their families but for us as well, if we are to advance the practice of case management collectively and as individuals. Collaboration begins with effective networking.

SUMMARY

Despite the "good and bad" inside the practice of case management, case managers bring clarity, clinical experience, and health care knowledge, along with resources, to many individuals and families coping with complex needs.

Many times, the NCM functions in muddy waters, with several masters to serve. An NCM must have a knowledge base that includes understanding the *case mix index*, cost of resources, and the utilization picture, as well as third-party reim-

bursement procedures. Thus hospitals, outpatient clinics, and home health agencies have collaborated to provided innovative case management models throughout the continuum of care in specific practice settings. These models most often provide services for a high-risk population, after an episode of acute care, including evaluation of future care needs and implementation of a plan. The goal in this case management process is to reduce the use of acute-care resources and maintain the patient in the most appropriate level of care available, while maximizing the patients' overall health status.

Case management, as defined by the CMSA and the Commission of Case Manager Certification, is a collaborative process. Therefore it supports networking, and it is important for us to remember that collaboration is critical to the practice of case management.

Chapter Exercises

1. In a group setting, discuss the many changes that have occurred in case management and why case management models have increased in numbers over the past few years; describe in detail at least two of the models.
2. In a group setting, discuss the many "new competencies" required in the practice of case management and why each is important.
3. In a group setting, discuss the case manager's roles in patient advocacy and financial management and oversight; why each is important; how they differ; and why it is important to keep the roles separate.

Suggested Websites and Resources

www.cmsa.org—Case Management Society

www.acmaweb.org—American Case Management Association

www.ccmcertification.org—Commission of Case Manager Certification

www.lifecarecenter.com/helpful/html—National Center for Life Care Planning

www.shanti.org—Shanti Project in San Francisco

www.u.arizona.edu/ic/srl/stmarys.html—Carondelet St. Mary's Hospital, Tucson, Arizona

REFERENCES

1. Tahan H: The nurse case manager in the acute care settings; job description and function. *JONA* 23(10), 1993.
2. Powell S, Ignatavicius D: *Core curriculum for case management*, Philadelphia, 2001, Lippincott.
3. Powell. S: *Case management: a practical guide to success in managed care*, Philadelphia, 2000, Lippincott.
4. Flynn B: Benefits integration: 24 hour coverage, *Case Review* May/June:48
5. McCollom P: Personal communication, Nov 2001.
6. Mulahey K: Personal communication, Nov 2001.
7. United States Advisory Council on the Information Infrastructure, Article from Subcommittee. *A nation of opportunity: realizing the promise of the information superhighway:* p 10.
8. Mann M, Kobb R: Personal communication, Nov 2001.
9. Lippman H: Can complementary and conventional medicine learn to get along? *Business & Health* Oct:15, 2001.
10. Gilpin S: Personal communication, November 2001.
11. Hospital Case Management™ Special Report: Building a successful CM career. February 2001.
12. Feuer L: Very guarded secrets to strategic networking: notes from a friend who is watching you! *Case Manager* Nov/Dec:22, 2001.

Case Management and Technology

Pamela Blackmore, MHA, RN,C

OBJECTIVES

- To understand how the system life cycle is applied to case management software selection
- To understand the importance of reporting and decision support for case managers and what needs to occur to transform data into knowledge
- To be aware of the technology available to the case manager

The impressive skill set of the primary case manager has always included not only a great depth of comprehension of the health care system but also a compassionate understanding of both patient and provider needs. In addition to their caring approach to patients, successful case managers are also noted for their acute communication skills and effective negotiation abilities. However, in today's world of economic downturns and staff reductions, there is a critical skill that case managers must acknowledge and embrace in their career of multitasking.

Technology is often seen simply as an obstacle in an already multidimensional field. Although technology has proven in some situations to enhance process improvements and save valuable time, case managers must remember that technology is not always easy to use and may not meet all of their needs. Therefore case managers should be familiar with the technology available so that they can make informed decisions when technologic changes to current processes are necessary.

BUSINESS PROCESS IMPROVEMENT

Software implementation projects are an ideal modality to evaluate departmental process improvement opportunities. Business process improvement (BPI) is the process that is used to evaluate and redesign tasks with the goal of improving business processes (e.g., streamlining procedures and saving time/money). Ideally, these evaluations should occur before the implementation of a software program to maximize the benefits of the software and to correct problems such as duplication and unnecessary or outdated processes. Business process reviews may include attention to both the internal and external organization (customer) activities. A major component of the BPI process is the creation of business process workflows.

Workflows

A workflow is a narrative or graphic depicting the flow of a process from beginning to end, either within one department or through multiple departments (Figure 3-1). The purpose of the workflow is to seg- ment each step in a business process. Workflows are best understood when displayed graphically with a software program specifically designed for BPI purposes. Information and documents that are helpful in evaluating the current

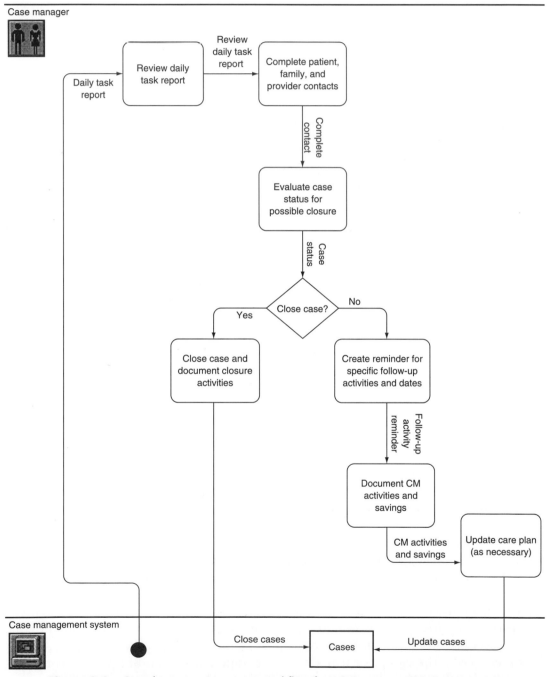

Figure 3-1 Sample case management workflow for existing cases. *CM*, Case manager.

process and creating workflows may include the following:

- Policies and procedures
- Interviews and meetings with staff
- Care plans
- Assessments or surveys
- Existing workflows
- Reports
- Benchmarking data or generally accepted benchmarks or industry standards (Joint Commission on Accreditation of Healthcare Organizations [JCAHO], National Committee for Quality Assurance [NCQA], American Accreditation HealthCare Commission [URAC], the Health Insurance Portability and Accountability Act of 1996 [HIPAA])
- Federal and state regulatory requirements
- Provider contracts and provider manual documents
- Required clinical criteria

Ideally, two workflows are created. The "as is" model describes the current business process, and the "to be" model describes the proposed business process in which improvements have been incorporated into the flow. Workflows can be simple or very detailed and can include task information or can be expanded to address time and cost requirements. Inclusion of staff, time, and cost requirements is helpful in comparing the "as is" and "to be" workflow models to identify efficiencies and cost-effectiveness. Workflows should be completed for every business process; that is, a workflow should be created for activities related to existing cases and evaluation of cases referred for case management.

SYSTEM LIFE CYCLE

Case managers prefer today's computerized systems and integrated software solutions to the manual processes still being used in many practices. Often, the only expected advantage of a software solution is a reduction of paper. However, case managers who have successfully implemented software also find an increased ability to retrieve information that is not always available when a manual process is used. In today's organization, one or more software applications or "programs" support most business processes. Those that interface with multiple departments result in a more complex business process. Therefore it is critical that the case management and information technology (IT) departments work together from the beginning to ensure the success of the project.

The system life cycle is defined as the multiple phases of a software solution, and it repeats itself once the software is replaced or is no longer needed (Figure 3-2). At some point, the system is retired, and the initial stages of the life cycle are repeated. To help users better understand the phases of the system life cycle in a business setting, the following section describes the five phases—system planning, system analysis, system design, system implementation, and maintenance/support—in more depth.

System Planning

System planning is the initial process that occurs when it has been determined that the current system (software application or manual system) no longer meets the case manager's needs. The current system may be a manual process that is no longer acceptable because of organizational growth, absence of or inaccurate reporting, or inefficiencies (paper); or the current software might not be tailored to meet the organization's needs. Nurses may not be using the current software because it is not user friendly and may be difficult to learn.

In the past few years, mergers and acquisitions among software companies have created situations in which multiple

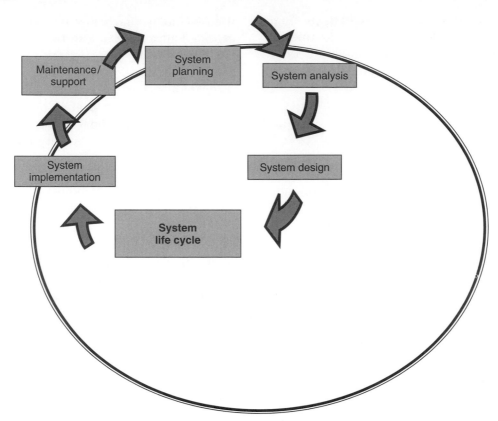

Figure 3-2   System life cycle.

software systems exist, causing IT problems with testing, upgrades, and internal support. Frequently, training becomes an issue for case managers when they must be proficient in multiple systems to do their jobs. When this happens, corporate aggregate reporting becomes almost impossible. It then becomes apparent that one system (existing or new) that best meets the combined needs of the organization and the case management department must be selected.

A successful systems planning team should include individuals from various departments who come together for the purposes of determining their software needs and selecting software that meets those needs. As the project moves into the analysis, design, implementation, and maintenance/support phases, input from additional staff members and software end

users may be needed. The organization's strategic plan and goals should be discussed and documented to assist in the anticipation of future application needs. Human resources should be evaluated to determine how the project would be supported while still meeting and maintaining operational needs.

System Analysis

System analysis is the phase in which organizational needs are defined and an approach is determined; the approach may include system selection, software creation, or a decision to remain with the current system or process.

Since case management, disease management, referral, and prior authorization modules are frequently included in case management applications, many departments may need to be included in the software analysis and selection process. Typically, selected users and departments, including IT, are asked to define their process and prioritize their needs and wants by preassigning a weight to allow scoring of each need and want. A need is described as a necessary function and would have more weight (points) than a want, which is functionality that is not considered necessary to the case management process but may increase efficiency or be considered an enhancement to the current process.

Each need and want will be categorized as a requirement, and the functions needed today and future business needs must be taken into account. Future business needs to be considered may include changes in the severity and complexity of cases that are targeted in the case management program based on client requests or internal cost-benefit analyses. Lists of these needs should be combined and included in the evaluation of various software products. By formalizing this process with weighted scores, the team can objectively justify its choice of vendor and the dollars allocated to the project. This will also be used as documentation to ensure that the product was methodically and objectively chosen to help prevent any vendor objections or potential management concerns. Figure 3-3 shows examples of functional, technical, and business requirements.

A feasibility study that outlines the organization's requirements and presents a proposal for potential solutions with a recommendation for the most desirable solution may be conducted. A feasibility study should include a complete analysis of the costs and resources required to complete the project (e.g., medical management, IT staff). The proposed solution may include modifications to the existing system, a turnkey system, a customized software package, or an internally developed or contracted software system. *Buy* (prepackaged)

and *build* (create) are the terms used to describe some of these options.

Buy or Build?

One thing to keep in mind is that, typically, there is no software that will meet all of an organization's needs. Creating a software system from scratch sounds attractive because it could be designed to meet every specific requirement. However, these types of projects are often canceled only after a lot of time and money have been spent and large quantities of staff resources have been used, leaving a host of internal issues unresolved. Examples of criteria that may be used by the organization to determine whether building software is more cost-effective than purchasing it may include the following:

- Less than 80% to 90% of needs are met by the software application—another example of the old "80/20 rule."
- The organization only needs a small component of a larger prepackaged application.
- Core business needs cannot be met by packaged software programs.
- Competitiveness can be enhanced by building software.
- Only one vendor has the desired product, and this vendor appears financially unstable or does not provide customer support.

During this phase, team members may gather software information by conducting Internet searches on case management software programs, ordering software vendor brochures, or attending case management conferences. The case manager may visit vendor booths at these conferences for software demonstrations and communicate directly with the vendor about the software features. The team members may also want to speak with other case managers to determine what system they are using, whether they are satisfied with their software, and how they "successfully"

Item	Functional Requirements	Need or Want	Weight	Score	Comments
1	Generates activity list including patient name, priority, due date, and specific activity (e.g., call physician)				
2	Generates standard reports listing and templates				
3	Enables nurse to create ad hoc reports (not requiring programming staff)				
4	Generates customizable care plan templates				
5	Contains flags that notify the user of other coverage, previous case management				
6	Tracks time and creates invoice for client billing				
7	Enables nurse to view current and past medications, including ordering physician				
8	Tracks case complexity				
9	Tracks case savings by activity and total				
10	Tracks providers involved in care and categorizes type of services delivered (primary care, endocrinologist, etc.)				
11	Allows for desktop and laptop technology in field case management				
12	Enables nurse to access clinical criteria directly through the application				
13	Allows patient to electronically enter daily weight, and if weight is outside of preestablished parameters, an electronic alert is sent to the case manager				
Item	Technical Requirements	Need or Want	Weight	Score	Comments
1	Compatibility with networks and existing databases				
2	Existing interfaces with other software (claims, utilization management)				
3	Time to implement				
4	IT staff resource requirements				
5	Transaction response time				
6	Availability of vendor staff to support project on a consultative basis				
7	Scalability: ability to add additional users and increased transactions without compromising performance				
Item	Business Requirements	Need or Want	Weight	Score	Comments
1	Budget including costs for the following: ■ Software application ■ Internal resources needed to implement (case management, IT) ■ Hardware (new or upgrade computers and servers) ■ Database costs ■ Network costs				
2	Change in future lines of business (e.g., adding workers' compensation)				
3	Consultant for software selection				

Figure 3-3   Sample functional, technical, and business requirements. *IT*, Information technology department.

improved their business processes and implemented new software packages.

Software Selection

A request for information (RFI) or a request for proposal (RFP) may be the chosen method for identifying a potential vendor. The RFI is a formal request for information about the vendor's product. After the responses to the RFI have been evaluated, an RFP may be sent to vendors being seriously considered by the software review team. The RFP reflects the organizational functional, technical, and business requirements identified during the analysis phase and requests information on how vendors believe their software packages can meet those requirements. Occasionally, a combined RFI/RFP will be released; vendor selection will be based on the responses to the RFI/RFP, a separate RFP will not be released.

The RFI or RFP outline must first be developed by the software team to ensure that the document reflects the organization's needs. The RFI/RFP must be released to all identified vendors on the same date with specified response dates clearly spelled out so that each vendor has the same time frame in which to respond. The case management organization's legal department may be requested to supply a sample contract for the RFI/RFP or to be available to review a sample contract provided by the vendor. If the organization is a government entity, vendor evaluation may be more structured and formal, and the final decision-making process may be more public.

Organizations may decide to evaluate only one vendor rather than assessing multiple vendors (Box 3-1). Frequently, this occurs because of a staff member's previous experience with a particular vendor in another organization. In this situation the staff member can provide valuable information related to the software's actual performance, which would not normally be available. Also, the RFI/RFP process may cause delays to the procurement of the software and has a cost associated with the staff time required to evaluate multiple vendors. Frequently, a consultant is engaged to help with this process, and those costs must also be included in the budget. An organization may consider using a consultant for many reasons, including the consultant's familiarity with the market and ability to assist in creating an objective environment for vendor selection. The consultant may also be engaged in implementing the selected software to bring his or her expertise to the organization, in addition to knowledge of the functional, business, and technical requirements that have been established and used for vendor evaluation.

The tool created during the system analysis phase may be used internally to score the vendors' proposals. In addition, the vendors may be asked to score themselves as part of the RFI/RFP requirements (see Figure 3-3). Scoring each proposal or response allows the department to objectively evaluate and compare vendors to identify the one that best meets the organization's requirements. A list of the highest scoring vendors is compiled, and an on-site demonstration by each vendor may be requested if a presentation was not initially included in the evaluation process.

Occasionally, when the evaluation and demonstrations have been completed, there may be a few remaining issues and the organization may not be prepared to make a decision. It may then be necessary

---

BOX 3-1
Vendor Evaluation Tools

Vendor corporate information
Planning requirements documents
Vendor proposals
Vendor demos
On-site visits to vendor and customers

to request a second demonstration for which case managers have provided information that would depict actual situations that case managers may encounter during their daily tasks. The vendor would then set up the demonstration with the information provided by the organization (e.g., sample care plans, workflows, daily work assignments). In this way, the vendor can demonstrate how the software might function in a live environment specific to the organization.

In addition to the functional, technical, and business requirements listed in the RFI/RFP, software review teams should consider requesting the following information from vendors:

- Vendor company description: number of employees, location, time zone (for possible customer service issues)
- Financial stability: an annual report or financial statements
- Specifications regarding hardware and software, including database or network requirements
- Sample contract (if not already provided)
- Availability of training
- Client demographics: types of organizations that have installed the software, number of clients, number of users
- Customer references: current clients who have chosen the vendor's software and who are similar in size and complexity
- Frequency of upgrades
- Customer relations summary, including implementation support, hours of support after go-live, response time, user groups, and customer input into future enhancements
- Product enhancements that are in the development process and any costs associated with the enhancements

- Annual software and maintenance costs
- Position with federal or state legislation or other industry standard requirements (HIPAA, URAC Case Management, or JCAHO: Management of Information Standards)
- Coordination of an on-site visit to an existing customer or the vendor's office to evaluate how the software is being used and to elicit comments about experience with implementation and customer service and how well the software meets organizational needs
- Availability of vendor consulting services for implementation or specific tasks to support the organization where necessary resources may not be present

Software review teams should request that vendors demonstrate their "out of the box" software packages. These are software programs that do not require any customization and are literally "ready to go" once installed in your system. "Out of the box" software is created after vendors have researched best industry practices and studied the processes most often used in a particular profession. Vendors will provide the opportunity to customize the software, but the team should be mindful that customizing a software package is very costly and can create programming problems for the organization. Programming dollars are added to every customized function, so the final software price can be substantially higher than the originally quoted price.

Multiple bids from various vendors may be required for government entities (e.g., must obtain three vendor bids). Obtaining multiple bids allows comparison of price, functionality, and customer support and adds to the ability to negotiate a more appropriate contract. A well-written RFP that addresses all issues and needs allows the organization to more easily evaluate the responses, make a decision, and present the team's software selection to executive management to request contracting approval and funding.

System Design

System design is the phase when business and technical needs are addressed to design the application to meet the case management department's needs. This assessment process begins after the software selection has been finalized. Depending on the vendor, an overview implementation meeting at the vendor or client site may be scheduled. Frequently, this is scheduled soon after the contract has been signed. It is also recommended that training be scheduled early for the "super user." A super user is a user who may be very involved in the design and implementation of the system and will be considered a resource for training end users or supporting the system after the go-live date. Vendor schedules are usually booked several months in advance, and scheduling a meeting as early as possible ensures training dates that meet the project schedule.

At this time the client should request the following copies of key documents from the vendor:

- Sample project schedules
- Sample test plans (used to test the software for volume, interfaces)
- Software manual (describes the user screens, security, and other functions)
- User training materials
- Implementation manual (including technical documents, data dictionary, and Erwin diagrams)

The documents provided by the vendor can be used as a reference for creating organization-specific documents including a project schedule, training materials, and test plans.

PROJECT MANAGEMENT OVERVIEW

The goal of project management is to successfully complete the project with suffi-

cient resources while remaining within budget and on schedule. The project schedule is one tool that is key to managing the tasks including resources (staff), task dependencies, and time frames. Typically, project management is directed by the IT department; however, as more case managers increase their technology and project management skills, more case managers may be equipped to lead projects.

The Project Management Institute (PMI) is a professional association for project management. This organization has created the *Guide to the Project Management Book of Knowledge*, or the PMBOK guide, which is the international standard for project management in fields ranging from construction to IT. After successfully completing an examination, individuals may become a PMI-certified Project Management Professional (PMP). For more information on project management, please refer to the Project Management Institute or PMI website at www.pmi.org.

Project Planning

Project planning is one of the first steps involved in project management (Box 3-2). Project planning involves identifying the executive sponsor, steering committee membership, project manager, and project team members who are essential to initiation of the project.

The executive sponsor supports the project from a high level and is updated on the project's status and issues and is responsible for executive decisions related

---

BOX 3-2
Project Team Composition

Executive sponsor
Steering committee
Project manager
Technical analysts
Business analysts

to the project. The executive sponsor is typically a member of the steering committee. The steering committee's function is to oversee the project and to make high-level decisions about the project from an organizational team perspective. For example, if the project scope has changed, requiring several staff members to be reassigned, the steering committee would address various options including delaying implementation or contracting with outside consultants and evaluating the business impacts of each of the options.

The project manager is the person responsible for the project and may be a member of the IT department or the medical department. The project manager uses several tools to manage the project including project management software that displays the projected schedule according to major tasks, staff resources, and time frames. In the schedule there may be many dependencies, meaning that a specific task may not be initiated until another task is completed. A project management software tool allows tracking of dependencies to determine the impact of delays on specific tasks, as well as on the entire project.

The project team will also include technical and business analysts. Based on experience, complexity of the project, and case management software, the project manager may also serve as an analyst.

The technical analyst is responsible for supporting technical components of the implementation, for example, participating in the interface mapping of software fields from one application to another, followed by interface programming and testing. Typical interfaces from other systems generally include transferring of data on members or patients and providers from claims or hospital patient databases into the case management system. Data conversion is defined as the transfer of data from a preexisting system into the new system, which normally requires significant programming. Most project delays are related

to difficulties with interfaces or data conversion, since programming and testing of the interfaces can be fairly complex. If the case management software does not need to interface with other applications, implementations can be relatively simple.

The business analyst primarily represents the users and may assist in mapping fields for interfaces, identifying report requirements, and configuring the software to meet the users' needs. Configuration may include setting up the security: specifying who has access and defining categories of users and the level of access that is assigned to them. For example, a supervisor may have "read," "write," and "delete" privileges; whereas a case manager may only have the read and write privileges but not the authorization to delete. In addition, configuration may also include defining pull-down table values or establishing business rules.

In some cases, business and technical analysts may also be involved as superusers who be looked to as resources for training the end users or supporting the system after go-live.

Other major tasks may include setting up hardware (personal computers, servers, and networks); testing; letter and report development; loading of care plans, case management surveys, and assessments; and configuration. These tasks may require the involvement of both the business analyst and the technical analyst. Table 3-1 describes types of databases (also called *environments*) that are recommended for every software application.

One item to keep in mind when the project schedule is being set up is evaluation of staff resources that are needed to complete the project. Frequently, staff members are responsible for their continued operational duties, as well as the tasks assigned to them for the project. This can cause a high level of frustration for the staff and affect the motivation necessary to stay involved in the project. Identification of

TABLE 3-1 Database/Environment Description	
Database	**Description**
Production	Used once the application is live (real transactions with real patients). Provider and member files are accessible for operations.
Testing	Used to test programming and upgrades before they are put into production and training. A testing environment is highly recommended to prevent interruption or loss of data in the production environment.
Training	Used to provide training and is set up with patients, providers, health care coverage plans, and employers that emulate the production environment.

events that could also have an impact on the timelines (e.g., JCAHO, URAC, NCQA, or federal or state site visits or audits) must be determined when the schedule is created.

Reports supplied by the vendor may not meet the needs of the organization, resulting in additional efforts by the organization to develop usable reports. During the BPI or system implementation phase, reports should be evaluated to determine which ones are mission-critical (required for board, client, or federal or state reports). Efforts should be made to minimize duplication and maintain only meaningful reports.

SYSTEM IMPLEMENTATION

System implementation activities include system hardware and software configuration, software installation, final testing, documentation, and end-user training in preparation for use of the system in a production environment. Ideally, all interface and conversion programming will have been completed and tested by the pro-

grammers before system implementation. In some cases workflows and policies and procedures may begin during the system design phases but are finalized during the system implementation phase. Figure 3-4 is a sample of a very high-level project schedule for software design and implementation.

User acceptance is testing in an environment that has been configured to have all the components of the production environment. Cases are entered as they would be during normal operations to evaluate software and interface performance. Testing is typically assigned to the super users, and if necessary, to other department staff as well. Patient, provider, and employer information is loaded into the testing or training environment, allowing the testers to work within the application, which is identical to the production or live environment.

Workflows and policy and procedure development can be completed while the software design phase is in process. The workflows created during the BPI phase will be the basis for any new workflows. Policies and procedures need to be updated or created to document the current process. End-user training dates (for case managers and their supervisors) need to be verified (if they were scheduled early in the system design phase). Depending on the situation, the vendor or organization may conduct "train the trainer" sessions for key staff members so that they may train other users. It is advisable to allow approximately 1 to 2 weeks between end-user training and the go-live date for positive training outcomes. After more than 2 weeks, users begin to forget key system functions and may not be as motivated to continue self-training. In addition, when training is scheduled, many organizations separate the trainees into two or more groups, so some staff members are still at their desks to continue operations (e.g., answering phone calls) while others are

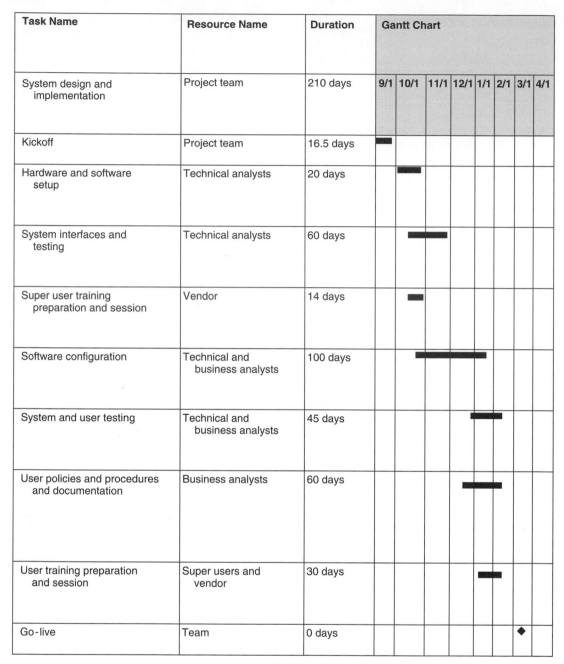

Task Name	Resource Name	Duration	Gantt Chart							
			9/1	10/1	11/1	12/1	1/1	2/1	3/1	4/1
System design and implementation	Project team	210 days								
Kickoff	Project team	16.5 days	▬							
Hardware and software setup	Technical analysts	20 days		▬						
System interfaces and testing	Technical analysts	60 days			▬					
Super user training preparation and session	Vendor	14 days		▬						
Software configuration	Technical and business analysts	100 days				▬				
System and user testing	Technical and business analysts	45 days						▬		
User policies and procedures and documentation	Business analysts	60 days						▬		
User training preparation and session	Super users and vendor	30 days						▬		
Go-live	Team	0 days							◆	

Figure 3-4   Example of high-level project schedule.

being trained. The case managers and IT staff who will support the software internally must be identified and trained before the go-live date.

Go-Live

Go-live is the date the production environment is activated and staff members are entering real data into the system. Most case management applications take from four to seven months from contracting to the go-live date. These time frames are dependent on the complexity of the application, support from the vendor, and the staff members available to work on the project.

Maintenance/Support

Maintenance/support is defined as the phase in which the system is live, and maintenance and support of the application are the primary tasks. Software support agreements vary among vendors, and some may allow unlimited customer support or may charge for support based on the number of hours used. It is suggested that a few super users be identified as the first contacts for issues or problems. This requires internal staff to become knowledgeable about the software. They would be responsible for contacting the vendor about problems they could not resolve and for identifying any remaining training needs or issues.

Once the system is live, users will quickly identify items that they would like to change, ranging from configuration to reports. Input from users should be collected, evaluated, and prioritized by focusing on the most critical and cost-effective suggestions. When changes are suggested, staff should evaluate them to anticipate their impact on the department, based on the change and when it would take place. For example, if the existing table values for case management case complexity are changed on April 16, the monthly (i.e., April), quarterly, or annual report would certainly be affected. In some cases this may be a critical report that may affect caseload assignments for case managers; it may also be a deliverable report released to clients on a monthly basis.

It is highly recommended that all three databases—production, testing, and training—be maintained on an ongoing basis (Box 3-3). It is easy to understand that the production environment is necessary; however, some discussion may be required to convince others of the need for a testing and training environment. If the vendor sends an upgrade, it is highly advisable that the upgrade be tested before moving into production. The upgrade may have problems that could cause the system to

> **BOX 3-3**
> **Maintenance/Support**
>
> Hardware/software maintenance
> Upgrades
> Enhancements
> User changes

function poorly or just shut down. Conducting tests in a separate environment prevents the risk of contaminating or losing data or shutting the system down. Training is an ongoing issue, and most programmers do not appreciate having trainees working in their database while they are programming or testing.

The software vendor will also release periodic upgrades that need to be added to the current application. Typically, the upgrades include software enhancements and the correction of identified "bugs" or problems by using a "patch." It is not advisable to load the software and "go-live" with the enhancement without first testing the upgrade or patch. Depending on the complexity of the enhancement, there may also be changes to the software that would involve the users, as well as the IT staff. For example, additional modules could require new configuration efforts: security or table changes or additions that make report changes necessary.

The application should have minimal downtime so that production is not adversely affected. Backups and disaster recovery plans should be in place in the event that the system crashes and data cannot be retrieved. Testing of backups is critical; just backing up the data without testing can prove to be a mistake. Frequently, backups are done incorrectly and data cannot be retrieved, affecting internal and customer reporting.

At some point the software may be retired because it no longer meets the department needs. The system life cycle then repeats itself.

Reporting and Decision Support

Health care is experiencing an explosion of data, and the increased availability of data is not necessarily a positive situation. For example, individuals everywhere are harvesting data from the Internet, and the harvesters (patients and providers) are proud of their catch. It is no longer uncommon for patients to walk into a physician's office with reams of paper, demanding that the physician read each and every page. Often patients collect information related to their disease process only to have unknowingly located invalid information in their search for "wisdom," and they are only too willing to share it with their information-inundated physician.

Often, monthly and quarterly reports are produced, collect dust, and are destroyed when the next reports arrive. These types of reports are a waste of valuable resources and energy that could be better spent creating more meaningful reports. If used appropriately, new technology can provide the key to decreasing administrative costs and assisting business executives in obtaining meaningful data and creating useful, reliable, and timely reports.

DATA VERSUS KNOWLEDGE

This section focuses on several approaches of simplifying informational needs into key elements to meet overall business needs. First, it is suggested that the following terms become familiar:

- Data
- Information
- Knowledge

Data are in a raw form and are not considered information, because information implies knowledge. This means information must be focused and available in a format that is timely, meaningful, and easily interpreted. Instead of evaluating the meaningfulness of information by its sheer weight, as illustrated by the patient with reams of paper, the focus should be on management reporting and transforming information into knowledge.

Data, information, and knowledge are necessary to effectively evaluate health care processes. However, first, measures must be taken to ensure that the data are accurate. Data collection includes evaluation and monitoring of databases, data integration, and data integrity. These processes are essential to building a foundation that allows an organization to access "good" information. The following are suggestions for attaining the goal of collecting useful data.

Data Collection

Today the methodology for data collection must be analyzed to prepare for the future. There are many different ways to collect data, ranging from paper to Internet-based applications. HIPAA definitely brings electronic transmissions into the 21st century. In the past few years, Internet-based products for case management have been increasing. This is a truly paperless process and is generally well received by patients who are computer literate or have received adequate training.

Reports are only as good as the data collected, and data elements that have not been collected certainly cannot be analyzed. Therefore it is necessary to carefully assess reporting needs to evaluate the strength of the existing database. Accordingly, the following questions must be asked:

- Will the database produce focused, driven information?
- Does the database reliably capture the critical elements necessary for output reporting?
- Should the data be integrated with multiple databases?

Data Integrity

Data are necessary for managing a successful health care business organization; however, the data must be factual. This section focuses on the presentation of factual data. When data are collected from internal sources, it is critical that mandatory data elements be identified. Reports will only be produced from data that have been collected and will be in the same format from which data were collected. Strategic decisions should never be made at an executive level without verification of the validity of the data. If the data are inaccurate, the outcome of decision making could be costly to the organization. The following questions should be asked:

- Has the integrity of the data been verified by using ongoing quality control measures (e.g., data entry error rate, incomplete fields, and accurate formulas)?
- Is the database reliable?

Factual Data

A successful organization must be committed to producing factual data; otherwise, there is no reliability for internal and external recipients of the data. Quality control measures to collect reliable data should be a planned, ongoing process with clear assignments for this responsibility. Case managers or support staff should be systematically monitored to ensure ongoing compliance with predetermined data entry standards. Data entry statistics (including error rate and incomplete fields) should be included in annual performance evaluations. Minimizing the error rate in a production environment prevents customer issues from arising and reduces overhead as well. Verification of correct formulas is also included in monitoring data integrity. If formulas are entered inaccurately, the data are of no real value. These types of errors can increase the potential for making inappropriate strategic decisions when organizations are implementing the business planning process.

The data source should also be rated for its reliability. Sometimes other reports from separate databases or from the same database can be created to compare results between reports.

Implementing a data warehouse requires a data cleansing process, and it is critical to the success of accurate reporting. If data cleansing is not accomplished in the early stages, reports will ultimately be rendered useless and unreliable. In some cases, according to the number of systems that are integrated, data cleansing can take up to a year. Inconsistencies in the data must be identified, and quality control mechanisms must be enacted to correct or prevent continued errors. In some organizations special data integrity teams have been created to monitor data integrity issues on an ongoing basis. To ensure the successful integration of data integrity measures, the team should be empowered to make changes in processes. Finally, focus should be directed toward data standardization whenever multiple systems are used, in an effort to eliminate errors by creating identical data entry requirements for similar fields.

Information and Knowledge

Applying business intelligence to an organization should result in the application of data analysis from multiple perspectives. This means that a report can be designed to display information by employee, employer, provider, diagnosis, procedure, and plan. Ideally, information from multiple sources (e.g., claims, medical management, and sales or marketing) can also be combined.

Organizations that maximize the use of their data will be better positioned to compete in the marketplace and meet customers' needs through more reliable forecasting. Providing meaningful, appropriate information to a customer is one way an organization can stand above the competition. Also, the more easily and quickly the information is delivered, the more responsive the organization is and the happier the clients will be.

Today's clients are now demanding outcome data. The federal government requirements and NCQA standards are driving much of the demand. Good health-care–related data are needed to evaluate treatment that results in the best outcome. Quality, utilization, and disease and case management are even more important in managed care companies as they continue to compete in the marketplace. In these programs there is a proactive approach to controlling costs, ensuring quality cost-effective care, and providing the best outcomes. This has created a need for quality, utilization, and case and disease management software programs that store and analyze data.

REPORT PLANNING, REPORT DESIGN, AND BENCHMARKING

Report Planning

What information is needed to strategically run the organization or department? Is statistical analysis necessary to correctly interpret data? How large is the sample size? When groups of patients are studied, are the data adjusted for severity? How is severity or case mix monitored?

All these questions and more need to be addressed so that meaningful reports can be created. Without preplanning, less than optimal reports may be produced, causing a need to create more reports. This increases the cost of report production and wastes valuable resources and time.

Routine reports should provide a snapshot of what is occurring in an organization and should be stored in a report library, making them easily accessible to each user. They should be run on a scheduled basis and include analysis such as trending information whenever possible. They should also be targeted to capture only information necessary to monitor organizational performance. Simplicity is crucial. Because the goal is to provide relevant information, reports should address

critical business issues. Excessive or irrelevant data can create confusion and prevent an organization from identifying and solving actual problems.

Keep It Simple

Ad hoc reports are used to drill down data to further analyze information from routine reports. They are run on an as-needed basis. The ideal situation would allow users to access the data reporting tools needed to create ad hoc reports. The less IT support is needed for report production, the less costly it is to produce reports and the more quickly the organization can respond to informational needs. The ideal reporting situation is one in which a case manager or supervisor can sit at his or her desk and view reports on demand.

Report Design

A user-friendly and consistent report format assists individuals in their review of data and helps them derive business conclusions. It should also alert the individual to request additional information through ad hoc reports. The format should be consistent in similar reports; for example, case management reports with the same data elements should have the same layout. This will make the reports familiar to the reader and decrease the amount of time spent trying to interpret what is displayed.

Reports in which graphic presentations are used can create a message that can be understood at a glance (Figure 3-5). They may also show conclusions that may not be easily seen when only a spreadsheet is used.

Case managers need reports so that they can quickly identify areas of concern. Organizational performance is better evaluated when data are displayed in a manner that assists the reader in evaluating key issues, developing corrective action plans, planning strategically, or requesting additional research.

Assigning specific staff to review detail reports can help identify issues, such as data integrity or data entry errors. For example, caseload reports should be reviewed by case management supervisors for caseload, case complexity, and accuracy of data entry by the staff. Since supervisors are actively involved in their assigned jurisdictions, they are better equipped to analyze data, evaluate issues, and create action plans for their staff based on information displayed in detail reports. Without this type of ongoing monitoring and cleanup, supervisors may have incomplete and inaccurate reports. The report design should meet internal and external informational needs, which may vary according to each organization's procedures.

Information can be a very powerful educational tool. For example, provider profiles have allowed physicians to see how they compare as individuals with their peers. In many situations this has successfully changed practice patterns to steer the physician toward the norm.

Benchmarking

Benchmarking is defined as information used to compare an organization's performance with that of outside organizations, industry standards, or its own previous performance. An organization may choose to access an external comparative database or to benchmark against its own history by using trended data.

Maintaining historical data is very useful and should be viewed as a requirement for organizational reporting. The value of using data trending in a graphic display is immeasurable. Trending alone can provide an organization with sufficient information to investigate, create action plans, and monitor those action plans for effectiveness. It is probably one of the most important components of data analysis.

A department that has implemented a new program will benefit from benchmarking the new program's results against historical data. The cost benefit of using data wisely and appropriately is key to

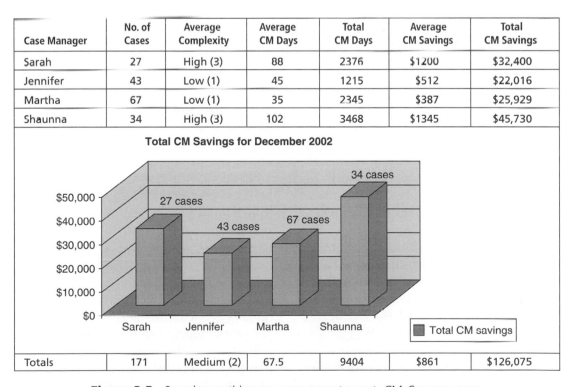

Case Manager	No. of Cases	Average Complexity	Average CM Days	Total CM Days	Average CM Savings	Total CM Savings
Sarah	27	High (3)	88	2376	$1200	$32,400
Jennifer	43	Low (1)	45	1215	$512	$22,016
Martha	67	Low (1)	35	2345	$387	$25,929
Shaunna	34	High (3)	102	3468	$1345	$45,730
Totals	171	Medium (2)	67.5	9404	$861	$126,075

Total CM Savings for December 2002

Figure 3-5 Sample monthly case management report. *CM,* Case manager.

focused program development or analysis of existing programs.

TECHNOLOGY

Case managers are increasingly exposed to new technology. Although technology is a necessary component of a health care organization, the use of technology in health care is still behind that in health care businesses. In the previous sections, software and decision support/reporting were discussed. This section provides a brief overview of the technology tools and resources now available to the case manager. Advances in technology have made communication and information instantly available to the case manager. Research is now a task that can easily take place in front of a computer.

Internet

As discussed in the reporting section, a plethora of clinical information is available on the Internet. The biggest issue today for professionals and consumers is whether the easily accessible information is accurate and reliable. One of the first efforts to deal with this particular issue is the URAC Health Web Site Standards. URAC is adhering to the Hi-Ethics Principles as the basis for the standards (see www.hi-ethics.org). In addition, Hi-Ethics and TRUSTe (www.truste.org) are developing an E-Health Seal for health websites. The URAC standards can be found on the URAC website at www.urac.org. URAC is a health care accreditation organization that has created standards for case management accreditation.

Organizations that may be seeking accreditation could include health maintenance organizations and insurance companies, health care providers, and health care information websites. Each organization must adhere to the standards to receive accreditation for consumer online health information, and their internal processes should ensure compliance with standards.

e-Health

"e-Health" or "electronic health" sites are electronically submitted services (including dial-up and web-based connections) that provide access to administrative and clinical functions and increase efficiency and timeliness of information transactions for organizations, providers, and patients.

Providers and payers are moving toward more interactive e-health websites. Currently, many organizations have websites that, with a log-in or user name and password, allow the following:

- Providers may check eligibility, benefits, or clinical criteria; request authorization; or check on the status of a claim.
- Enrollees or patients may sign up for health education classes, respond to surveys, and in some cases, log on to contact their case manager to provide information on their health care status.
- Hospitals allow their physicians access to medical records, including diagnostic studies.

Webcasts

Internet conference management is available through many different products. Webcasts provide video and audio conferencing live or archived for others to view at a later date. Since the technology of these types of products has improved tremendously in the past few years, use has increased. To minimize the costs of software demos, vendors frequently choose to provide a webcast demo as the first stage of the sales process. The use of webcasts can decrease the need for travel and subsequently reduce costs and still provide an acceptable method to communicate information by using multiple software programs (e.g., PowerPoint, vendor software programs, or video). Depending on the technology used, software may have to be loaded or individuals may be required to log on to the Internet and call in for the audio portion of the webcast. Prices for webcasting also vary by vendor.

NCQA has used webcast technology to broadcast their "State of Managed Care Quality" press conference (www.ncqa.org).

Home Monitoring

Patients can now have information on their weight, blood pressure, and blood sugar levels sent electronically to their case managers, thanks to technology. By combining the clinical information with the virtual case management "home visit" via video camera with images sent through the computer, a nurse can be more effective by focusing immediately on patient problems. Many vendors now provide these types of products; however, these "visits" have not yet become the standard of case management. Many studies are in process to evaluate outcomes of Internet monitoring programs, and early results indicate significant savings.

HIPAA SECURITY AND PRIVACY

The Health Insurance Portability and Accountability Act of 1996 (HIPAA) (August 21), Public Law 104-191, amended the Internal Revenue Service Code of 1986 and may also be referred to as the *Kennedy-Kassebaum Act*. The primary purpose of the Act is to improve the Medicare and Medicaid programs and the efficiency and effectiveness of the health care system.

The administrative simplification section of this act required that the U.S. Department of Health and Human Services mandate the use of standardized transaction and code sets, as well as security and privacy for protected health information. In addition, the HIPAA mandated creation of national identifiers for patients, providers, payers, and employers to assist in standardizing how health care business

is conducted. The cost of HIPAA implementation will be significant (in millions of dollars) and will affect how providers and payers conduct their businesses.

The requirements of the HIPAA will have implications for most of the topics addressed in this chapter. The transaction and codes set component of the rule will certainly streamline the process and subsequently reduce costs for providers, health plans, and government programs. The security and privacy component of the rule will have the biggest impact on case managers in such areas as transferring patient information on the Internet through e-mail or home monitoring information. Many technology products and health care organizations will need to provide assurance that protected health information cannot be inappropriately accessed either within or outside of the organization. One change that will be necessary is the encryption of e-mails that include patient information. As security and privacy policies are revised and finalized, accessibility of patient information will certainly affect how health care is delivered in the future.

The Workgroup for Electronic Data Interchange has created an HIPAA glossary that is accessible on the Internet at www.wedi.org under the resources section. This is an excellent resource to assist individuals in understanding many of the acronyms and terms that are used in the HIPAA rule. Several other resources are listed in the website listing section of this chapter.

EDUCATION

Professional Continuing Education Units

There are many sources for Internet continuing education unit (CEU) courses. For example, the *California Nurseweek* (www.nurseweek.com) monthly magazine has CEU courses that can be accessed on the Internet with online tests and immediate grading of the responses. In today's fast-paced world, instant CEUs are just another method of managing a busy case manager's schedule.

Nursing Informatics Educational and Certification Programs

The American Nursing Informatics Association (ANIA) was created to provide an organization for nursing informatics. The ANIA website (www.ania.org/ni/index.htm) includes a listing of conferences (including CEUs) to educate nurses about the field of informatics or to prepare nurses for certification in nursing informatics, as well as general information about the certificate program. The American Nurses Association (ANA) has now recognized nursing informatics as a specialty and offers nursing informatics certification through the American Nurses Credentialing Center (ANCC) at www.nursingworld.org/ancc/. The requirements for certification are included on the ANCC website.

The American Medical Informatics Association (AMIA) is a nonprofit organization for health care technology (www.amia.org). The AMIA has also created the Nursing Informatics Working Group (NIWG) (www.amia-niwg.org). The NIWG website offers information on membership and educational programs, job descriptions, a newsletter, and nursing informatics-specific conferences offered through AMIA.

■ SUMMARY

Case managers cannot escape the reality of technology in their daily tasks. With their busy schedules they need all the tools possible to complete their jobs in the most efficient way. Understanding technology and its impact on the case management department allows case managers to make informed decisions by minimizing tedious manual tasks or inefficient processes. Through understanding and application of technology, case managers are often able to focus more on their patients and the services they provide.

Chapter Exercises

1. Briefly describe the five phases of the system life cycle.
2. Describe the importance of data integrity in relationship to reporting/decision support outcomes.
3. Describe two methods of communication involving technology.

Suggested Websites and Resources

Informatics Websites

www.amia.org—American Medical Informatics Association (AMIA)

www.amia-niwg.org—Nursing Informatics Working Group of the AMIA

www.ania.org/ni/index.htm—American Nursing Informatics Association

www.nursingworld.org/ancc/—Nursing informatics certification through the American Nurses Credentialing Center (ANCC)

www.hi-ethics.org—Principles for ethical guidelines on privacy and confidentiality, quality of health information, advertising and commercial relationships, consumer relations and best practices

www.NCQA.org—National Committee for Quality Assurance

www.pmi.org—Project Management Institute. The Project Management Institute Book of Knowledge (PMBOK guide) is the standard for project management.

www.rnpalm.com—Articles, software listings, software reviews, listserv, search engine and links related to handheld devices in health care *www.truste.org*—Developing E-Health seal for health websites by using Hi-Ethics principles

www.urac.org—Health care accreditation organization

www.webopaedia.com—On-line technology dictionary

www.wedi.org—Workgroup for Electronic Data Interchange. Highly involved in HIPAA, website has HIPAA glossary

HIPAA Websites

www.aspe.os.dhhs.gov/admnsimp—U.S. Department of Health and Human Services: Government site; proposed and final rules, FAQs, and HIPAA Implementation Guides

www.computerworld.com—Articles on HIPAA

www.hipaadvisory.com—Latest HIPAA news

www.wedi.org—HIPAA glossary

BIBLIOGRAPHY

American Nurses Association: *Scope and standards of nursing informatics practice*, Washington, DC, 2001, American Nurses Publishing.

Ball M, Hannah K, Newbold S et al: *Nursing informatics: where caring and technology meet*, ed 3, New York, 2000, Springer-Verlag.

Cross MA: Home but not alone, *Internethealthcaremag. com (technologyinpractice.com)*. Accessed June 2001.

Dash J: Health groups urge feds not to delay changes to privacy rules, *Computerworld.com*. Accessed Aug 13, 2000.

Gillespie G: Hospital web sites face an unpredictable future, strategies are evolving as CIOs and Web site developers implement interactive applications, *Health Data Management* May 2001, available online at www.healthdatamanagement.com.

Hebda T, Czar P, Mascara C: *Handbook of informatics for nurses & health care professionals*, Menlo Park, Calif, 1998, Addison-Wesley.

Kelly B: Intranets succumb to irresistible pull of e-health, the Internet and the e-health boom are helping shape the future of providers' and payers' next generation Intranets, *Health Data Management* Dec 2000, available online at www.healthdatamanagement.com.

Lacher D, Nelson E, Bylsma W et al: ACP-ASIM survey. Computer use and needs of internists. Paper presented to the AMIA Annual Symposium in Los Angeles, *PR Newswire*, Nov 6, 2000.

LeGrow G, Metzger J: *E-disease management*, Oakland, Calif, November 2001, First Consulting Group, California HealthCare Foundation.

McDonald K, Case J, Metzger J: *E-encounters*, Oakland, Calif, November 2001, First Consulting Group, California HealthCare Foundation.

Proforma Corporation: *Enterprise application modeling, vision and strategy for the ongoing development of ProVision Workbench™*, Southfield, Mich, 2001, The Corporation.

Proforma Corporation: *Manage process change using ProVision Workbench™ (a technical white paper)*, Southfield, Mich, 2000, The Corporation.

4

Introduction to Funding

Peggy A. Rossi, BSN, MPA, CCM, CPUR

OBJECTIVES

- To have a better understanding of health care insurance and be able to describe the differences between fee-for-service insurance and health care coverage provided by employers who offer a health maintenance organization plan for their employees
- To be able to describe the importance of exploring alternate funding when working with persons who have long-term and chronic medical conditions
- To describe the basic differences between Medicaid and Medicare

Understanding the basics of health insurance and alternate funding programs and how services are paid is extremely important to case management. The case manager should be familiar with not only the person's primary health care insurance provider but also the providers with which that insurance company will coordinate benefits, if there is more than one insurer. Of equal importance is an understanding of how managed care works and of the funding programs to which patients might be entitled, if they meet eligibility requirements. As one works cases and coordinates benefits, it is common to deal with more than one insurer or payer source.

In today's health care arena, dual insurance coverage is a reality for many patients. This dual coverage can be from private health care insurance, Medicare, Medicaid, a Title V Children's Medical

Services program, the state's program for the developmentally disabled, TRICARE, or the Department of Veterans Affairs (VA), to mention the primary sources. If one is managing a case for an adult with a disabling condition, that person could be eligible for private insurance, as well as Medicare and Medicaid. If one is managing a case for a child, that child could have coverage from any one of the foregoing insurers, with the exception of the VA. This same child could also be eligible for some services from the local school district; or if the child is eligible for TRICARE (the old Civilian Health and Medical Program of the Uniformed Services [CHAMPUS]), he or she could have some limited coverage from TRICARE's exceptional family member program or its program that serves the disabled. A patient who is a veteran may have coverage through his or her VA benefits package, if the condition now needing coverage is related to a disability incurred during active duty. Unfortunately, at times a person will have no insurance or insurance that is limited, has exclusions, or is exhausted. Despite applications to different funding programs for which the person might be eligible, the person may not receive coverage because of the many variations in requirements for such programs.

With the exception of Medicare, TRI-CARE, and the VA, for which eligibility for coverage and benefits is consistent throughout the United States and its territories, eligibility for private health insurance and many of the other funding programs varies drastically. It varies from private health plan to private health plan, and for public programs, from state to state. To complicate matters even more, the public funding programs may even vary from county to county within a state. Variations occur not only in eligibility but also in the actual benefits allowed. For instance, although some Title V Children's Medical Services programs cover such services as acute care or care for patients with acquired immune deficiency syndrome, others do not.

With the foregoing in mind, case managers must become very familiar with the alternate funding programs for which patients might be eligible. This knowledge includes any county or state variations that apply for the various programs. More important, they must know the basic eligibility requirements and how and when to make referrals. This minimum knowledge is necessary because delays in the actual referral process can make a difference in the patient's qualification for the program, payments for services, and the appeals process. It is equally important for case managers to know which state agency regulates health plans and the role this agency plays in setting and enforcing standards and state statutes.

Because dual eligibility for insurance and public funding programs is a reality, as a case manager works with his or her patient load he or she must be very cognizant of which insurers are primary and which are secondary. The case manager must also be aware that many other insurance or funding programs will not pay for services if the patient's health care insurer denies payment simply because the services are not available within the primary health care insurer's network. The case manager must also be aware that if a public funding program does provide coverage for a specific service, it will do so only if benefits are truly limited or excluded by the person's primary insurer and the patient has met the public funding program's eligibility criteria. Because of the stigma associated with public funded programs or because patients or families believe they will not be eligible because they were told "no" on the phone, case managers must encourage families to apply for specific benefits to which they might be entitled and then ensure that any denial issued is done so in writing. This allows an avenue for recourse or appeal. Far too often patients and families, for whatever reason, take this verbal denial as gospel when they were eligible all along. They may not question a denial of coverage because they are frustrated by the whole system and having to "fight for everything" or because they are tired from the strains of care giving.

When benefits or dollars are limited, exhausted, or excluded, the case manager must continually search for alternate sources to pay for needed services or those that can augment the plan of care. The wise case manager stays abreast of his or her state's programs for which patients may be eligible. This knowledge is necessary if one is to help patients conserve their health care benefits. In many cases, viability of the case management plan rests on the patient's eligibility for other funding programs. Certainly, if the patient has other health insurance (regardless of type—auto, disability, Medicaid or Medicare), exploration and coordination of any benefits available from these plans are critical. Other ways to augment benefits are to use community resources and to teach all aspects of care to the patient and family whenever possible.

To ease the minds of the patient and family regarding finances, case managers must always encourage patients and families to explore eligibility for any and all private disability income policies, any unemployment benefits, and state disability programs. At times, this may also include application for a state's general assistance program. Similarly, if dealing with seniors, the case manager must have some basic knowledge about long-term care insurance. At a minimum, this includes knowledge of the processes for activation. With patients living longer and many requiring "custodial" care, long-term care insurance coverage can be a valuable asset for those persons who have been able to financially keep the premiums current. Although long-term care insurance is not an income policy, many plans will cover custodial care needs either at home or in a facility.

As one works with insurance, it is also necessary to have a general knowledge of the different types of coverage; what it means when one must use a network or participating provider; when one must obtain prior authorization before services are rendered, even when medical necessity is evident; what it means when the insurer says that only skilled care, and not custodial care, is covered; and what some of the common reimbursement mechanisms for health care are, and more important, what each means in terms of out-of-pocket expenses for the patient.

Of key importance while working as a case manager is at least a basic knowledge of Medicare and Medicaid, managed care, and utilization review. This knowledge is important because Medicare is often considered the "grandfather" of utilization review and benefit structures. Therefore most insurers use Medicare guidelines as they develop their benefit structures and utilization review programs. Most medical insurance programs now offer some form of managed care, and with it, come restrictions and constraints and a variety of utilization review mechanisms and processes and none covers long-term or custodial care. Although the original intent of Medicaid was to provide health care for the medically needy, Medicaid is now the key payer for long-term care.

Because it is important to maximize a person's health care coverage, another area in which at least basic knowledge is necessary is community resources. One must know what resources are available, how to locate them, and how and when to make a referral if one is to augment the case management plan and have overall success.

■ SUMMARY

A basic knowledge of insurances is key to successful case management regardless of the setting. For example, with the advent of many workers' compensation programs that follow a managed care process similar to those used by medical case managers, a basic knowledge of managed care is necessary, along with the many caveats this brings to arrangements for linkage of patients to care. Equally as important is a basic knowledge of alternate funding or public programs and their requirements for entitlement. This knowledge is vital if the patient's health care benefits are to be maximized and case management goals are to be reached.

Chapter Exercises

1. Briefly list the main differences between fee-for-service insurance coverage and that now offered by many health maintenance organizations.

2. Give at least two reasons that exploration of alternate funding for patients with long-term, chronic medical conditions is important.
3. List the key differences between the two federal programs Medicaid and Medicare.

Suggested Websites and Resources

www.healthfinder.gov/organizations—Website with links to multiple websites on health care and insurance

www.hhs.gov—U.S. Department of Health and Human Services

www.cms.hhs.gov—Centers for Medicare & Medicaid Services

www.nwica.org—National Special Supplemental Nutrition Program for Women, Infants, and Children (WIC) Association

www.ssa.gov—Social Security Administration

www.acf.dhhs.gov—Administration for Children and Families

www.acf.dhhs.gov/programs/add/—Administration on Developmental Disabilities

www.managedcareinfo.com—On-line information website on managed care

www.ahrq.gov—Agency for Healthcare Research and Quality

www.aahp.org—American Association of Healthcare Plans

www.cdc.gov/nchs/—National Center for Health Statistics

www.nih.gov—National Institutes of Health

www.odphp.osophs.dhhs.gov/—Office of Disease Prevention and Health Promotion

Managed Care

Peggy A. Rossi, BSN, MPA, CCM, CPUR

OBJECTIVES

- To identify three types of managed care organizations (MCOs) and describe how an MCO differs from an indemnity insurance plan
- To list the core benefits required by the federal government for MCOs under the HMO Act of 1973
- To list the methods used by MCOs to control costs

The insurance industry (commercial insurers and public funded programs) plays a vital role in the U.S. health care system. Private insurance funds nearly three quarters of all of health care. Thus if case managers are to maximize a patient's insurance benefits, basic knowledge of the insurance system, the main types of insurance, reimbursement mechanisms, and managed care is critical.

The main types of insurers that dominate the U.S. health care system are as follows:

- Indemnity plans
- Blue Cross and Blue Shield
- Public funded programs (e.g., Medicare, Medicaid, and Children's Medical Services)
- MCOs (e.g., health maintenance organizations [HMOs], exclusive provider organizations [EPOs], preferred provider organizations [PPOs], and point of service [POS] plans)

The primary mechanisms for reimbursement for health care include:

- **Capitation**—Pays a predetermined amount for all care related to resolving the problem. The focus is on coordination of care, reducing resource use, and offering only necessary services in the least number of days.[1]
- **Diagnosis-related groups (DRGs) or per hospital stay**—Pays a predetermined amount for hospital stay or aftercare. The incentive is to do only what is appropriate or necessary. Length of stay and use of resources or other services are minimized.
- **Indemnity**—Pays a specific amount for services regardless of the provider. Any balance between what is billed and what is paid is the responsibility of the patient.
- **Per diem rate**—Pays for various types of care but is commonly used for hospital care or services. The

incentive is to maximize days in the hospital and minimize the use of services and resources.

Unfortunately, statistical reports show that approximately 17.5% of all Americans are without health insurance. For a current report of the number of persons covered by insurance and managed care, as well as those not covered by health insurance at all, see the U.S. Census Bureau's website at www.census.gov/Press-Release/date.html. For further information, contact the Housing and Household Economic Statistics Division at 301-763-8576; their website is www.census.gov/ftp/ pub/hhes/ www/.

TYPES OF HEALTH CARE COVERAGE

Indemnity Insurance

Indemnity insurance is historically the oldest type of payment system for health care. Many persons do not favor an indemnity plan because only 70% to 80% of a person's actual health care expenses are reimbursed. Although the provider is paid on a fee-for-service basis (what is billed), the remainder of the charges is the responsibility of the consumer. In addition to higher out-of-pocket expenses, another downfall of an indemnity plan is that it does not cover some basic and preventive services, such as routine physical examinations, immunizations, and contraceptives.

When covered by indemnity insurance, the patient not only has an annual deductible but also the responsibility for paying any balance between what was billed and what was reimbursed (Box 5-1). Despite these downfalls, many patients favor indemnity insurance because it allows them the freedom to seek care from any provider without a referral or prior authorization.

With indemnity insurance, claims are paid retrospectively on a fee-for-service (FFS) basis. Additionally, a system called *usual, customary, and reasonable (UCR)* is used. Thus when a patient's insurance company is billed under the FFS system, the insurer applies UCR criteria to the claim before the final adjudication and payment of the claim. UCR takes into account the average charge for the service in a geographic region and the area providers' usual charges for the service.

The down side of the UCR system is that the patient must pay any uncovered portion of the bill plus any deductibles, copayment, or coinsurance fees. The FFS method gives providers strong financial incentives to perform more services, because the more services they perform, the more money they receive. Also because

---

BOX 5-1
Old Indemnity Insurance

Before managed care became so popular, a patient's health care expenses, if covered by an insurer, were paid through the traditional indemnity method. Other features of indemnity insurance include the following:

■ No restrictions on the choice of providers because the insurer pays for care regardless of the provider serving the patient.

■ Care that is not coordinated. Since patients may obtain care from any provider of their choosing, care can be fragmented or duplicated and treatments can interfere or interact with each other, because one provider may not know what the other has ordered.

■ Reimbursement is based on billed charges and paid through the FFS payment system. If the fee is more than what is reimbursed, the patient is responsible for not only the difference but also any copayments or deductibles associated with the health plan chosen. Thus in the end the provider is paid in full for services rendered.

■ FFS creates an environment and strong incentive to bill for greater numbers of services and more complex services and encourages high-tech illness-oriented treatment instead of prevention-oriented care.

preventive health care is not a covered benefit, patients often do not obtain services until they are sick. Furthermore, FFS providers know that if the insurer does not reimburse their costs, patients are held accountable for any or all costs.

Indemnity plans commonly use methods such as what are termed *experience rating* or *community rating* to set premiums. In the experience rating system, premiums are based on the claims experience of a group (e.g., claims for a specific group of insured are averaged by using both high and low costs of cases, resulting in wide premium variations from group to group). In the community rating system, the claims experience of the entire population served by the insurer is taken into consideration. Using a community rating system minimizes the impact of individual case costs on premiums, because even though both high and low claims costs are used, the actual premium is based on the average of the two.

Blue Cross/Blue Shield (The Blues)

Blue Cross and Blue Shield are among the oldest insurers. Unlike other insurers that may offer many products, the Blues have one product line only—health insurance. Founded in 1930 as service plans, each was organized and specialized in providing reimbursement for different categories of care. For example, Blue Cross pays for hospital care, whereas Blue Shield pays for care provided by physicians and other medical providers. At one point the Blues used indemnity practices including an FFS and UCR method for claims reimbursement. Over the past several years, they have added MCO options and have adopted many managed care techniques for services and payments.

Medicaid and Medicare
Medicare

Title XVIII of the Social Security Act of 1965 created Medicare. The original intent of Medicare was to provide health care coverage for persons older than 65 years, but it now covers disabled persons younger than 65 years if they meet the Social Security Administration's eligibility requirements. Since its inception, Medicare has undergone multiple changes, and over the years, eligibility requirements have changed. In recent years the most drastic changes to Medicare occurred and allowed what is called *Medicare + Choice*, with the biggest changes occurring in the payment methods now used by Medicare.

Medicare HMOs have been around since before the HMO Act of 1973. However, with the passage of the Balanced Budget Act of 1997, many changes in Medicare MCOs have occurred. For one, the MCO option is now referred to as a *Medicare + Choice plan*. Under the Medicare + Choice option, Medicare members sign up with a specific MCO if there is one in their geographic location. Their Medicare benefits are then administered by the HMO. Medicare managed care has many advantages over FFS Medicare. For example, in addition to receiving the benefits of regular Medicare, members receive enhanced benefits from the MCO. These benefits might include some medications, eye care, and preventive services not covered by traditional Medicare. When a Medicare beneficiary signs up to join a Medicare + Choice plan, the MCO is paid directly by the Centers for Medicare & Medicaid Services (CMS) because the HMO administers the members' Medicare benefits and assumes all responsibility for the management of the beneficiaries' care. One caveat to Medicare + Choice is that the MCO can enhance benefits but the traditional benefits allowed by FFS Medicare cannot be taken away. To join a Medicare + Choice plan, Medicare beneficiaries must be covered by both Part A and Part B Medicare. They are also required to pay a small premium (Part B monthly charge), as well as the copayments for services such as medications and physician and home health care visits established by the MCO.

Medicaid

Title XIX of the Social Security Act created Medicaid, a program that provides medical assistance for certain individuals and families with low incomes and resources. The program became law in 1965 and is a jointly funded cooperative venture between the federal and state governments. Medicaid is the largest insurance program that provides medical and health-related services to America's poorest people. The basic differences between Medicare and Medicaid are simple. Medicare is primarily available to persons older than 65 years and disabled persons younger than 65 years, regardless of income benefits, and criteria for eligibility are the same regardless of location in the United States. Medicaid, on the other hand, is available to persons of any age, and eligibility is based on financial need, but benefits and eligibility criteria vary from state to state. The biggest difference is that although both Medicare and Medicaid cover acute care, since its inception, Medicaid has been the major funding source for long-term care, covering more than half of all long-term custodial care costs.

In recent years, Medicaid has changed its programs, and Medicaid HMOs are now available to many low-income persons. Most states have mandatory enrollment requirements for specific categories of residents who are eligible for Medicaid. For example, in California there are several Medicaid HMO options, and these options may further vary from county to county. In Sacramento County the Medicaid managed care is called *geographic managed care (GME)*. With geographic managed care, recipients of Aid to Families with Dependent Children (AFDC) are mandated to make a choice and enroll in one of six health plans within the area. If AFDC recipients do not choose a health plan, the geographic managed care enrollment contractor chooses one for them. However, in neighboring counties enrollment in a Medicaid plan is voluntary.

Managed Care

Before the HMO Act of 1973, managed care was not a common household word. However, since 1973, managed care has become the dominant insurer of health care services. Now most health care insurers, including many public funding programs, use some form of managed care as they attempt to control health care costs. Three such programs are TRICARE, Medicaid, and Medicare.

For instance, in the mid 1980s the Department of Defense changed their insurance strategies with the awarding of the Civilian Health and Medical Program of the Uniformed Services (CHAMPUS) Reform Initiative Project to Foundation Health Systems Incorporated (now known as *Foundation Health Federal Services*, a division of HealthNet) in Sacramento, California. This was a four-year demonstration project that covered military dependents and retirees in California and Hawaii. Under this initiative, the military followed in the footsteps of many employers by allowing military beneficiaries a triple option choice (CHAMPUS Prime [HMO model], CHAMPUS Extra [PPO model], and CHAMPUS standard [indemnity insurance]). It was also at this time that case management services were required by their MCO contractors. The goal of the program was again to contain costs, especially for the catastrophically ill or injured.

The early 1990s saw a flurry of managed care activity for Medicare, as well as the various Medicaid programs. Under legislation, called *the Section 1115 Waivers to Medicaid*, states were allowed to expand their Medicaid programs. They could enter into contracts with MCOs and offer managed care to Medicaid beneficiaries. With the passage of the Balanced Budget Act of

1997, Medicare made a strong entrance into the managed care arena.

MANAGED CARE ORGANIZATIONS

HMOs, and more recently other types of MCOs, are basically organized health care systems that are responsible for both the financing and delivery of services. Why? Under traditional indemnity health insurance, the insurance company merely reimbursed providers for the cost of care and services rendered without any controls. In contrast, MCOs have the following primary responsibilities:

- Providing health care to members
- Ensuring that members have access to covered health care services
- Ensuring that services are appropriate and of quality
- Reimbursing providers for services rendered

Unlike indemnity insurance in which controls or requirements are not placed on the providers, MCOs use many of the following:

- Different financial incentives and management controls intended to direct patients to efficient and cost-effective providers
- A multitude of financial and other methods to add maximum value to health care purchasers by channeling volume to high-quality providers participating in HMOs, PPOs, or other point-of-purchase arrangements
- A complex system of financial incentives, penalties, and administrative procedures to redefine the doctor-patient relationship (Under the current reimbursement system, many managed care reimbursement policies are harmful to efficient providers: efficient providers are paid the same as inefficient, poorly motivated providers; thus the best providers subsidize the bad ones,

and the result is that many physicians are leaving managed care.)

MCOs have been created for a variety of reasons. Two primary reasons are that they offer better cost control and make health care more affordable and accessible. On the down side, most MCO models are organized to be for-profit and there is no clear definition of managed care. Boland[2] indicates that "managed care defies a commonly accepted definition because it means different things to different people depending on their professional affiliation, type of business, and experience in the field." Possibly the biggest down side of MCOs is the reimbursement modalities and other techniques used to gain the market share, increase patient volume, and maximize profit margins.

Because the term *managed care* is not necessarily synonymous with either HMOs or PPOs,[2] managed care is most successful when the following occur:

- Physicians, hospitals, financial incentives, and administrative services are fully integrated.
- Effective managed care delivery systems that control the quality and use of services available.
- Clinical and operational costs are controlled.

MCO Characteristics

MCOs have several characteristics that set them apart from traditional insurance. First and foremost is the lower out-of-pocket cost to the member and the fact that paperwork (submission of claims primarily) is reduced to nil. Other characteristics include those listed in Box 5-2.

EMPLOYERS, REGULATORS, TRADE ASSOCIATIONS, AND GOLD SEALS

The market for the increase in managed care has one primary driver—employer demands—because medical costs are the driving force behind premium price

BOX 5-2
Comparison of MCOs with Traditional Insurance

MCOs	Traditional Insurance
Care is prepaid (providers, especially primary care providers, are paid in advance for every member assigned to them and paid by the month—called *PMPM* or *per member per month*). Before, during the provision of the services, and during claims review, services are subject to utilization controls (e.g., primary physician gatekeeper roles, prior authorization, concurrent review, case management and retrospective review).	Claims are paid retrospectively with few if any utilization controls placed on the claim.
Lower out-of-pocket costs that start with lower premiums. May have some deductibles and copayments but copayments are generally fixed with many under $20. Provides a more comprehensive set of benefits.	Premiums are generally higher, and the patient is responsible for annual deductible copayments (could be 20% or higher), as well as any balance between what the insurer paid and what the provider billed.
Under the MCO, the financial risks are shared between the providers and the MCO through such contractual reimbursement systems as capitation, subcapitation, per diem, case rates, global rates, fee schedules, discounted fee-for-service, DRGs, shared risk pools or incentive pools.	With traditional insurance, the provider holds little risk, but it is shifted to the insurance company who in turn shifts it to the patient (i.e., higher copayments and deductibles) and employer (i.e., higher premiums if care for a group is too costly).
Members have no paperwork because the providers submit the claims and are paid directly. Member has no involvement with coordination of benefits (when more than one insurance company is involved) or for tracking of claims payments. In most cases the member never even sees a claim or bill, other than when copayments have not been paid.	The patient may be totally responsible for all claims submission and may be required to pay for services before services are rendered, submitting the paid bill for reimbursement. Reimbursement is then paid directly to the member. If more than one insurance company is used, the patient needs to keep track of what was paid and submitted; the patient is responsible for coordination of his or her own benefit payments.
Restrictions on members to only use the MCO's network or contacted providers. The emphasis is on using primary care physicians for routine care and if specialty services are required, referral from the primary care physician to a contracted provider, as well as prior authorization must occur before services can be rendered. Using contracted providers protects patients because it ensures the necessary care will be provided at the lowest possible rate. More importantly, the provider credentialing process used by MCOs ensures that qualified providers are made available to members.	No limit on providers or provider location. No guarantee to the consumer of the provider's credentials or controls on the costs for care.
Emphasis is on preventive medicine and services.	Emphasis is on illnesses and treatments. Many times this includes complex or costly treatment, since the more the provider orders, the more he or she is paid. There is little, if any, disincentive to not overtreat.
Rates are prenegotiated for services.	No rates are negotiated. Patient pays the provider's set rates, and there is little if any ability to negotiate rates.

Continued

BOX 5-2
Comparison of MCOs with Traditional Insurance—cont'd

Utilization and case management controls are in place to ensure the patient receives the right care, at the right location and level of care, at the right time, and at the right cost. Services are often reviewed by using national criteria such as InterQual to ensure the admission meets the severity of illness (SI) and intensity of service (IS) criteria. For continued stays, they must meet the intensity of service (IS), as well as discharge screens (DS). The incentive is to keep costs as low as possible.

Quality monitors—MCOs are under continued scrutiny by regulators and accrediting agencies to ensure quality health care is provided to patients. Quality monitors include the use of standardized review criteria and written policies and procedures. Additionally, quality processes include the use of provider credentialing programs, provider performance report cards, and quality studies. Studies are most often conducted to measure outcomes and identify opportunities for improvements. Another tool used out to measure quality is a satisfaction survey. This is often conducted with two different audiences—patients/members and providers. Here the audience selected is queried either in person, by telephone, or by a mailed survey about their satisfaction with a particular issue or process. From these findings actions are taken as appropriate to the responses received (e.g., if dissatisfaction with a particular issue or process is found, corrective action and steps are taken to correct the situation, with a built-in plan for monitoring to ensure compliance once corrected).

Depending on the insurer, some utilization review might be performed. However, in most cases, there are rarely any UR restrictions imposed. Thus there are no incentives to keep costs contained.

Because of the lack of contractual obligations, there are few quality controls that can occur or can be enforced.

increases. To control costs MCOs use a variety of techniques such as linkage of members to contracted providers, a variety of contractual reimbursement mechanisms, and incentives for members to use contracted providers (e.g., lower copayments and deductibles).

Although large employers are the primary purchasers of health care and select the benefit packages for their employees, many of which are managed care plans, federal guidelines outline the core structure or minimum standards for coverage. However, the state's statutes target and enforce compliance with any federal regulations or requirements. In most states MCOs are licensed and regulated by agencies such as the Department of Insurance and Department of Health Services, and in some states, the Department of Corporations or Department of Managed HealthCare. These agencies are charged with enforcement and monitoring of compliance with the state's statutes. The state's statutes are based on federal laws and are designed to do the following:

- Define the service area to be served by the HMO (an HMO can only market and enroll members within its licensed service area)

- Protect consumers from unethical advertising
- Ensure adequacy of staffing resources
- Ensure access to care and benefits
- Ensure financial viability and stability of the plan to further ensure that the plan can deliver the care it has committed to provide to policyholders

In the competitive environment of health care, the goal of many MCOs is to be a federally qualified HMO. Federal qualification is a voluntary application process; however, an MCO must meet the requirements of the CMS's Office of Managed Care. These requirements include accessibility to provider networks, financial stability, complaint resolution, management structure, and acceptability of membership materials. In addition, MCOs must offer a set of core benefits as outlined by the HMO Act of 1973. Core benefits that must be offered include the following:

- Complete range of physician services, including inpatient and outpatient coverage
- Inpatient hospital care, including acute-care inpatient rehabilitation
- Full range of ancillary services such as laboratory and radiologic services
- Durable medical equipment (DME)
- Emergency services both in and out of the area
- Mental health and chemical dependency programs (this is changing in many states with the enactment of mental health parity laws)
- Skilled nursing facility care
- Outpatient prescription drugs

To be competitive and retain their market share, many MCOs offer additional services such as preventive care and dental, vision, and limited prescription drug coverage. Until recently, the most restricted benefits were those related to psychiatric illness and chemical dependency. Fortunately, this is changing as more states recognize and implement mental health parity laws. According to mental health parity laws, mental health care benefits must be at the same level as those offered for medical and surgical care.

Another goal of MCOs is to be accredited by the National Committee on Quality Assurance (NCQA). Not only does this accreditation validate an organization's commitment to quality, it is also the standard sought by most large employer groups who are the primary purchasers of health benefits for employees.

Application for or renewal of accreditation is not automatic, and each plan must request the process. Once an application is submitted for accreditation, the MCO has more than a year to prepare for the review. To assist reviewers in the accreditation review process, the organization will have each department prepare a binder or series of binders describing its operational processes and how that department relates to the organization as a whole. During the actual review, the reviewer will focus on such areas as operations, finance, quality, the complaint and grievance process, utilization management, and the provider network. Final accreditation is based on the outcome of the review. If the plan fails the review in any one area, accreditation is denied.

In addition to being monitored and regulated by a state agency, the managed care industry is evaluated by trade associations at both the state and federal levels. The leading trade agency for national MCOs is known as the *American Association of Health Plans* (AAHP). AAHP is based in Washington, DC. Its website is www.aahp.org. AAHP represents all types of MCOs on national policy and legislative issues. AAHP is looked to for its educational programs, newsletters, research activities, standards, and plan-specific performance reports and demographic data.

HMO STRUCTURE

There are many titles and structures for HMOs. For example, an HMO may be classified as a staff model, group practice model, network model, or independent practice association (IPA). In most cases the overall MCO has one of two structures: (1) a mixed model HMO in which the provider network consists of a combination of delivery systems, without emphasizing any particular model or (2) a direct contract model HMO in which the physician network is built by using individual contracts with community physicians instead of through an IPA or other group model.

Staff Model HMOs

Staff model HMOs offer care through physicians who are employed by the HMO. Care is usually provided in a facility such as a clinic or medical center owned by the health plan. Physicians employed under this model receive a salary and bonus or incentive payments based on their performance. It is believed that the staff model HMO can offer lower premiums because greater control over the provision of health care and costs can be exercised. If a staff model HMO is to meet the needs of enrolled members, the HMO must employ physicians in all the common specialties. In addition to network hospitals and ancillary providers, the HMO must have contracts with selected specialists or subspecialists in the community for infrequently needed services.

Staff models can be referred to as *closed-panel HMOs*. In this model community physicians not enrolled with the HMO as a provider are not allowed to participate. A big advantage to a staff model HMO is that the organization has greater control over the practice patterns of the physicians. Unfortunately, there are the following disadvantages:

1. The HMO is more costly to develop and implement because of the larger salary expenses for physicians and staff.
2. The HMO frequently provides a limited choice of participating providers from which potential members may choose.
3. If the HMO must expand, it is costly to construct new clinics or facilities.

Group Model HMOs

Group model HMOs are formed around multispecialty medical groups that contract to provide physician services exclusively to the HMO. The physicians are employees of the group practice and not the HMO. Also, the physicians often share equipment, support staff, and medical records. In the group model physicians may see not only HMO patients but also patients with other insurance; however, their primary function is to serve HMO members. Services offered by group model HMOs are often comprehensive because they include primary and specialty physician care; ambulatory care; surgery suites, and laboratory, pharmacy, and radiology or imaging services. Many also provide hospital services in the same location. Group model HMOs have several disadvantages in common with staff model HMOs. The primary disadvantages are (1) a limited choice of participating physicians is provided, and (2) geographic accessibility to services may be restricted.

The most prominent example of a group model is the Kaiser Foundation Health Plan. Here physicians from The Permanente Medical Group provide physician services to Kaiser Foundation Health Plan members. The Kaiser Foundation Health Plan is the licensed entity responsible for marketing, enrollment, collection of premiums, and performing other HMO functions as outlined by laws and regulations.

Direct Contract Models

Direct contract models are, as the name implies, a contract directly between the

HMO and an individual physician. Direct contract models are very similar to IPAs in that the HMO attempts to recruit and contract with broad panels of community physicians (both primary care and specialist physicians). Like IPAs, direct contract models reimburse physicians on either a FFS or primary care capitation basis, with the latter being the more common practice. In contrast to IPAs in which the risk is shifted to the IPA providers, the direct contract model retains most of the financial risk. Two distinct disadvantages of direct contract models are: (1) recruiting physicians is more difficult and time-consuming, and (2) utilization management controls are more difficult to enforce because the contracts are with individual physicians. Thus there is little incentive to participate in the utilization management programs.

Independent Practice Associations

IPAs are plans that are built around a group of physicians (PCPs, internists, and some other specialists) who organize for the purpose of contracting with one or more HMOs or insurers. Although the group may have an exclusive relationship with the HMO, this relationship does not prevent the physicians in the group from seeing non-HMO members. Physician services are typically provided in the private offices of the participating physicians, with laboratory tests and x-ray examinations performed by community providers. Most MCOs are organized along the IPA structure. In this model a single contract links the HMO to all of the physicians in the group or association.

Other Models

An organized medical group might also be known as a *group practice* or *medical group*. In recent years, some physicians have organized into what is termed a *physician delivery system*.

Some of the more successful IPAs have further expanded and taken on a name and are now known as *medical service organizations (MSOs)*. Under the MSO structure, the medical group offers a variety of either individual or full administrative functions (e.g., office administration, claims processing, utilization review, case management, and provider credentialing) to other medical groups. Regardless of size, the strength and sophistication of a medical group lie in the group's ability and willingness to allow quality management controls, effectiveness in controlling costs, and the ability of the group's administration to motivate physicians to work efficiently as a coordinated network.

Once organized, physician groups are governed much like other organizations by having a board of directors. In most cases the board of directors is made up primarily of member physicians. In addition to the board of directors, the group will have a medical director. The number of physicians employed by an organization and the role and function of the medical director depend on the size of the organization. The size of the group often dictates the administrative capabilities of the group. Some small medical groups may have an outside MSO handle the administrative functions. Duties often contracted out by these smaller groups vary from all the administrative functions (e.g., utilization review, quality review, credentialing functions, claims processing, development of provider-specific and other medical group-specific printed manuals, training and educational programs for staff) to information technology support and the running of reports.

Should two or more IPAs or medical groups form a physician network, it might be referred to as a *network model HMO*. Network model HMOs are formed through contracts with more than one medical group practice. With a network model the MCO can offer a variety of physician services to its members. Groups may be broad-based, offering a variety of multispecialty services, as well as PCP services (e.g., family practice, internal medicine, and obstetrics and gynecology). The HMO traditionally compensates physicians on an all-inclusive capitation basis in exchange for the group assuming responsibility to provide all physician services to the HMO's members assigned to the group. Thus if referrals are made to other physicians, the group is financially responsible for reimbursements to those physicians. Network models may be closed-panel or open-panel plans. If a network is considered a closed-panel plan, the network HMO will contract with a limited number of medical groups. If it is considered an open-panel plan, participation is open to any physician who meets the HMO's and medical group's credentialing criteria. The resulting network allows an HMO to market its services in a broader geographic area than would be possible with a single physician group.

Like HMOs, medical groups may subcontract for some health care services. Almost any service can be subcontracted. This includes such services as specialized physician care, laboratory tests, anesthesia services, utilization review, and mental health or rehabilitation services. Subcontractors may be individual providers or other organized provider groups who are not part of the medical group or directly related to the medical group's contractual arrangements or controls. When a provider is subcontracted either to a medical group or HMO, the contractual arrangements are transparent to the patient.

OTHER MCO MODELS

Preferred Provider Organizations

PPOs, sometimes referred to as *preferred provider arrangements* (PPAs), are entities through which health insurers contract with selected providers (participating providers) to purchase health care services for members. Under a PPO contract, the participating providers agree to certain utilization management controls in exchange for the reimbursement structure and payment level agreed on in their contract. In contrast to HMOs, PPOs often limit the size of their provider panels. Members are allowed to use non-PPO providers in exchange for higher out-of-pocket copayments or deductibles. The common characteristics of PPOs are as follows:

- **Select provider panels**—Providers are selected to participate based on their cost efficiency, community reputation, and scope of services offered. A PPO's panel will also include hospitals, physicians, and other diagnostic or ancillary provider facilities.
- **Negotiated payment rates**—Contractual agreements with the provider require the participating provider to accept the PPO's payment as payment in full for services rendered (except for applicable copayments or deductibles). Under the contractual agreements, PPOs attempt to negotiate payment rates that provide a competitive cost advantage. These negotiated rates are usually in the form of discounts, all-inclusive per diem rates, or payments based on DRGs.
- **Rapid payment term**—In exchange for the provider's willingness to serve members, the MCOs are willing to include prompt payment features in the contract. For example, if a clean claim is submitted, the MCO will reimburse the provider within a specific time frame (often 15 days) in return for the rates agreed on in the contract.
- **Utilization management**—To assist in the control of costs and ensure appropriate utilization of services,

many PPOs use some methods of utilization management. In the more sophisticated PPOs, the utilization management programs are similar to those used by HMOs.

- **Consumer choice**—This is probably the most desirable area for consumers when they have a choice between an HMO and a PPO. Under a PPO the consumer has a choice of using participating providers or non-PPO providers and realizes that if a non-PPO provider is selected, the copayment will be higher. PPOs are often the plan of choice when one or more members reside outside the traditional service area for the PPO's participating provider panel.[3]

Exclusive Provider Organizations

Exclusive provider organizations (EPOs) are similar to PPOs in both organization and purpose. The primary difference is that an EPO limits its members to use of only its panel of providers for all health care services. If other providers are used, the EPO does not cover the services and the member must assume the cost of care. Like many MCO models, EPOs require the PCP to be the gatekeeper for any non-primary care services.

The primary difference between EPO and MCO models is that MCOs are governed according to HMO laws and regulations, whereas EPOs are governed according to insurance laws and regulations. Another difference is in how employers view EPOs. If an EPO is employer-driven, it is generally selected for the cost savings afforded to employers through reduction of premiums. In cases such as this, employers are less concerned about employee reaction to the EPO's severe restrictions because they are more concerned with their overall cost savings. Because of the severe restriction of

provider choice, few large employer groups are willing to convert their health benefit programs to an EPO format.[3]

Point of Service Plans

Over the past few years, another model of insurance, which has arisen from the consumer backlash in response to HMO, MCO, and PPO restrictions, is what is now termed *the point of service plan.* This model was introduced when the MCOs recognized that the inability to expand their market share was often due to the reluctance of consumers to forfeit completely their ability to use nonparticipating providers. As a result, many MCOs adopted an indemnity-type coverage model that also used utilization review controls. With a point of service plan, members have the ability to use providers outside the HMO's network in exchange for much higher copayments and deductibles. In other words, the consumer is allowed to make a choice at the point the services are required but knows that making this choice will include higher out-of-pocket expenses.

MANAGEMENT STRUCTURE

Board of Directors

Most MCOs have a board of directors. Although the makeup and functions of the board will vary and be influenced by many factors, the primary responsibility of any board is governance of operations. Legal requirements for boards are spelled out in each state's regulations and statutes. If the MCO is a federally qualified HMO, there are further requirements.

Board composition varies with it functions. It also varies according to whether the MCO is new or part of a national MCO, whether it is for-profit, and whether it is a provider-sponsored plan. Depending on the size of the MCO, the board may delegate specific functions to specific committees. These committees are as follows:

- **Executive**—Used when decisions must be made quickly
- **Compensation**—Used to set general compensation guidelines for the plan, chief executive officer (CEO), or other directors or to approve and issue stock options
- **Finance**—Used to review financial results, approve budgets, set and approve spending authorities, review annual audits, and review and approve outside funding
- **Quality**—Used to review all quality management documents, approve the annual quality program plan and quality reports, and make recommendations based on findings and activities

Because the function of a board is governance, basically everything rests with the board and its members' decisions. Most boards will have the final authority on such issues as the following:

- **Corporate bylaws**—The areas that govern the basic structure of power and control of not only the plan officers but also of the board itself
- **Fiduciary responsibility**—Oversight and approval of fiscal events, because it is the board's responsibility to protect the interest of stockholders
- **Legal responsibility**—This area includes review of all reports and documents before the final signing.
- **Policy responsibility**—This area includes the final approval of policies and procedures.
- **Oversight of the quality management program**—In many MCOs the board has a special responsibility to oversee all quality activities and to ensure that quality care is delivered to the members.

Organizational Structure

If the MCO assumes full responsibility for most operational areas, the list of senior officers includes the following:

- **Chief Executive Officer**—This is plan-specific, but for many plans, the CEO is responsible for all operational aspects, with key officers and directors reporting directly to the CEO and the CEO reporting to the board.
- **Marketing Director**—This person is responsible for the marketing of the plan's products. In most plans this position includes oversight of the marketing representatives, advertising, client relations (policyholders), and enrollment forecasting.
- **Finance Director**—This person is generally responsible for all financial and accounting operations. Depending on the size of the plan, this could include underwriting, as well as billing, accounting, fiscal reporting, enrollment, and budget preparation.
- **Medical Director**—Almost all managed care plans will have a medical director. The amount of time spent in this position depends on the size of the organization and the scope of responsibilities assigned to this position. In most plans the medical director is responsible for provider relations, quality management, utilization management, and medical policy. In other plans the medical director may assume the role of provider recruiting. The medical director may also act as a medical consultant or may be responsible for assistance with claims review, coverage determinations, or the approval of new physician applications. The person in this position might also assume responsibility for provider relations, as well as the recruiting and credentialing of providers. In larger organizations many plans will employ an associate medical director to perform the day-to-day tasks associated with utilization review or quality

management. The medical director is then afforded the time necessary to provide leadership and direction for critical areas such as utilization management, quality management, network operations, and medical policy.

- **Operations Director**—Common responsibilities include oversight of claims, information systems, member services, and enrollment services. Depending on the size of the organization, other tasks (e.g., provider relations or compliance) needed to ensure smooth operation of the plan might be assigned to this position. In some organizations this position might be responsible for such activities as governmental affairs, contractual negotiations with governmental agencies, or ensuring adequacy of the provider network.

Committees

Like the organizational makeup of a board, that of other committees will vary, and there is little consistency from plan to plan. Although some plans may have standing committees for specific tasks, others will have ad hoc committees that meet as issues arise and dissolve as soon as a decision is reached. If there are standing committees, many will be as follows:

- **Quality Management**—This committee is essential for oversight of all quality management activities for the plan. In most plans all committees will have reports and other key documents that flow through the quality committee to the board.
- **Medical Management/Utilization Management**—This committee reviews medical management issues. In some plans this committee reviews and issues the final coverage determination when the medical director or physician advi-

sor has been unable to reach a determination. This committee traditionally reviews utilization reports, trends, and patterns.

- **Credentialing Committee**—This committee reviews and issues the final determination in the credentialing process for new applicants or issues renewal of credentials to existing providers.
- **Medical Advisory Committee**—This committee reviews general medical management or provider contracting issues. In some plans this committee approves clinical practice guidelines, required by the organization of its providers.
- **Pharmacy and Therapeutics Committee**—This committee is key for plans with a pharmacy benefit. This committee is charged with the development of a plan's drug formulary and with reviewing, changing, and updating the formulary on a regular basis. This committee also reviews any pharmacy reports. It is also charged with reviewing abnormal prescription utilization patterns of providers.
- **Technology Assessment Committee**—This committee is generally found in larger MCOs. The committee is used to evaluate the effectiveness of new therapies, drugs, devices, and procedures. To expedite committee review, staff assigned to this committee will conduct literature or database searches on issues under review to determine suitability and efficacy and views of the medical and scientific community. Once information is available, it is compiled and presented to the committee for possible approval of its use and inclusion in the organization's treatment protocols and medical policies.

Departmental Structure

The departmental structure of MCOs varies and depends on the size of the organization, the number of enrollees and providers, and the environment or region served. In smaller MCOs, MSOs are often used to perform many of the specific duties that are key to operational functions. Functions assumed by an MSO might be administration, membership and enrollment, claims processing, utilization management, and case management. Common departments found within MCOs include the following:

- **Claims Department**—This department processes the medical claims submitted by providers. To assist with handling the volume of claims received, most organizations use an auto-adjudication computerized system, which allows the data that are entered from the claim to be searched in the preprogrammed database. As claims are processed, they are reviewed for member eligibility at the time of service, the quantity and types of services performed, whether services were performed by a network provider, and whether a required prior authorization is present. If all goes smoothly, the claim will move quickly through the system and will be paid. If for some reason the claim includes data that are not compatible with the claims-processing database (e.g., a nonnetwork provider was used, the member was not eligible, an authorization is missing, or an issue requires special review), the claim will be edited out and suspended for manual review. Most claims processing departments are organized into special handling units. These units are designed to handle a specific task or line of claims. For example, this could include in-plan providers when claims are reviewed against the contractual agreement; out-of-area claims when nonnetwork providers have been used; emergency claims; claims related to third-party liability (TPL) events; claims for which one or more insurance policies are in place and coordination of benefits (COB) must occur. In some claims units there is a special unit that handles only high-dollar claims, which must be tracked for reinsurance reporting.
- **Enrollment and Membership Accounting**—This is a key department charged with data entry of enrollment of new members or groups, new dependent additions, disenrollments, and terminations into the information system. This unit is also accountable for the issuance of membership cards and the mailing of both cards and membership materials.
- **Information Systems**—This is a critical department for MCO livelihood, because it is needed to ensure that insurance systems (IS) operations keep pace with the MCO's growth as new sites, staff, employer groups, and members are added. A properly functioning IS department is critical to the smooth processing of claims, prior authorizations, and member data that must be processed and maintained monthly. It is also necessary for the production of the various reports that must be programmed and generated (monthly, quarterly, or annually).
- **Sales and Marketing**—This is another key department. Basically, the sales department is the "the bread and butter" of an organization because it brings in new clients The size and tasks of this unit again vary with the size of the organization. In smaller organizations the

sales unit might assume all functions, whereas in larger organizations functions will be separated into various departments. Regardless of how the unit is aligned, the sales staff has the responsibility of selling the MCO's product lines, either directly or through brokers. In some organizations this same staff might be responsible for the provision of support to specific employer groups. They might assist the groups with open enrollment, billing, and coverage issues; or they might serve as a point of contact for employers when issues arise. Under the marketing umbrella, the staff is charged with development of new coverage products and riders, both of which are based on input from market feedback and strategic planning information maintained by the sales and marketing department.

- **Actuarial or Underwriting Unit**—This unit is responsible for the analytical expertise needed to set premiums, determine utilization rates, and assess risks as new groups are added. The unit often depends on case managers to assist with assessments of a new group's high-risk or high-cost patients. When these patients are known upfront, the goal is to ensure continuity of care as the plan is transitioned. Assessments allow realistic premium rate quotes for the new group. The actuarial unit is also charged with the analyses of provider contract rate negotiations, the development of rates for new or renewing groups, the analysis of the utilization characteristics of provider groups, the costs of new products or lines of business proposed by the sales and marketing staff, and forecasting specific costs.

- **Member Services**—This is a key department because it offers direct assistance to members. This department is the one to which members can direct complaints. Member service staff has two basic tasks: to provide members with information and to help them resolve problems. This department is key in providing information to members about benefits; explaining policies, procedures, and information from the member handbook; explaining copayments and deductibles; making address or PCP changes; and entering enrollment, disenrollment, or termination information on members. This department is often the first contact members use when they want to file a grievance or appeal.

- **Provider Relations/Contracting**—This department is key for provider relations and for the contracting of the required providers for the MCO network. Depending on the size of the organization, this department may be divided into two departments—provider relations and contracting. Like the member services department, this department is key for directly assisting providers with problems, issues, or complaints. Functions of this department include identification of any new providers that will enhance the network, contract negotiations, maintenance of the provider data bank and provider directories, maintaining the renewal process and contracts, and assisting the medical affairs staff or medical director when special rates are needed for nonnetwork providers. In smaller MCOs this department may also be charged with the credentialing and recredentialing of providers within the plan's network.

- **Medical Affairs**—This department, often headed by the medical director or at times a CEO or a vice president if the person is a licensed physician, is a multifunctional department. For example, it may handle such duties as implementation of the MCO's medical and clinical policies and procedures, oversight of all medical aspects of a plan's operations, and consultation as needed for complex cases. The person in this position may also assist or act as chairperson to the pharmacy and therapeutics committee.
- **Compliance or Government Affairs**—This unit serves as the liaison between governmental agencies, whether federal or state. Tasks include the monitoring of legislative and regulatory developments. The unit ensures compliance with laws: the staff makes sure that the plan can implement new requirements, and if not, what is needed to meet the requirements. The unit approves applications of regulators, prepares or oversees applications for expansion, oversees new employer or provider group contracts, coordinates and ensures preparation for any audits, and negotiates for governmental contracts and premium rates.
- **Finance**—This department monitors the organization's financial performance by tracking revenues and expenses. It is also charged with the monitoring of financial indicators. The finance department produces financial statements and reports of internal and external spending; administers the capitated provider contracts each month, determines the number of members covered by capitation, and calculates payments due from providers; prepares revenue and expense projections; oversees the annual budget; and manages the organization's taxes and other monetary transactions. This department may also be involved with reinsurance reporting to ensure the organization is reporting reinsurance cases. It is this department's charge to track cases and capture repayments by the reinsurer.
- **Quality Management**—This is another key department. This department is charged with the development and administration of the organization's quality improvement program. This department designs and conducts studies that are representative of the organization's activities. Studies are designed to ensure conformance to standards and determine outcomes for comparison with regional or national norms. If the plan participates with NCQA on Healthplan Employer Data and Information Sets (HEDIS) reporting, the quality department assumes primary responsibility for the collection and reporting of such data. This department is also responsible for tracking and trending quality events. Quality events are often referred to as *potential quality indicators*. If a quality or potential quality event is suspected, it is reported to the quality staff for further investigation, reporting, tracking, and then monitoring, to ensure that any corrective action plan implemented is working
- **Health Education**—This department varies drastically from organization to organization. If it is a functional department, the staff is charged with the development or promotion of health education programs and literature for the organization. If written information is produced, it is designed for

individual members with specific diagnoses or for various purposes such as the use of preventive services. The information may be disseminated by means of a newsletter or other published materials or direct mailings to members and providers. Many larger organizations offer full-scale health education centers. Members can browse the literature, watch videos on the topic, or have access to the Internet for their own literature searches. In larger MCOs this department may also provide on-site classes for members or employers. Some also provide on-site workshop consultations (e.g., ergonomic assessments or stress management classes).

- **Utilization Management**—This department is responsible for ensuring that the MCO's utilization programs are enforced. This includes prior authorization, concurrent review, retrospective review, and case management. Depending on the size of the MCO, the utilization management staff may assist with retrospective review of claims. The utilization management department frequently interacts with other key departments within the MCO such as member services, sales, finance, contracting, quality management, and claims. Interactions are needed for validation of eligibility, benefits, and employer benefit packages; reporting of potential reinsurance cases or TPL cases; clarification of any contracting-specific questions; or clarification of COB or Consolidated Omnibus Reconciliation Act (COBRA) issues. Additionally, utilization management works closely with the quality management department in reporting any quality indicators or potential quality indicators or as complaints

and appeals are researched and resolved.

ELIGIBILITY AND ENROLLMENT

Although individuals may elect an MCO for their health care coverage (usually because of lower out-of-pocket expenses), many have difficulty following MCO's rules. For example, on joining an MCO, patients must seek routine care from their elected or assigned PCP, and they are no longer able to seek specialty care without a referral from their PCP. Following the rules may also require members to use a call center for the scheduling of appointments. In these cases the caller is screened by a nurse for symptoms and for the urgency of the situation. Once this assessment is completed, either an appointment is scheduled or directions for care are given based on the responses (e.g., home care or direction to seek emergency care).

Possibly the hardest rule to follow is the one that requires a referral from a person's PCP before services from a specialist can be received. The actual referral often rests on the opinion of the PCP and is granted only *if* the PCP agrees that specialty care is required. With specialty care, appointments and appointment setting differ from PCP to PCP practice. For example, some PCPs will give the patient a formal referral form and it is up to the patient to book his or her own appointment. In other cases the PCP's staff will make the appointment and relay the information to the patient. In any event, the specialist used is often chosen by the PCP from the MCO's network of providers, and the member rarely has a choice in the matter.

OPEN ENROLLMENT

When it comes to health insurance, large employer groups are required to offer their employees a variety of health insurance options. These often include an MCO

BOX 5-3
Key Points of Open Enrollment

- The open enrollment period is generally limited to one month each year at a specific time. Consequently, if an employee wants to make changes to another health plan during the course of the year, he or she must wait until the next enrollment period.
- During open enrollment, the employees and their dependents are allowed to choose any plan offered by the employer. It is during this period that dependents often join a new plan or make changes.
- Large employers are required to ensure continued coverage for preexisting conditions. However, small group employers may not allow this same protection, should any of their employees have a preexisting condition at the time of enrollment.
- If insurance is provided through an employer plan, most employer insurance is obtained or changed during an employer's open enrollment period or after the probationary period for a new employee.
- On occasion, larger employers may offer additional benefits (e.g., prescription coverage, rehabilitation services, durable medical equipment, or additional psychiatric services) through what are called *riders*.
- When additional benefits are offered, the large employer pays the additional premiums. In contrast, smaller employers may have extreme limits on coverage and offer no additional benefits.

---

option, choice of an indemnity plan, or a PPO. In contrast, small groups may offer only a single option. Therefore if insurance is obtained from an employer, the subscriber and dependents are limited to the health plans selected by the employer. In contrast to members being allowed to change their PCPs monthly if desired, changes from one health plan to another can only occur during the employer's annual *open enrollment season*. Key points of open enrollment are listed in Box 5-3.

Enrollment Process

At the time of enrollment, the prospective subscriber (employee, or if an individual policy, the one obtaining the insurance) must complete an enrollment form for each dependent to be covered. The actual coverage date for services does not start until the enrollment application is processed and the benefit period starts (which could be several months from the date of enrollment [e.g., open enrollment might be in October but benefit coverage will not start until January of the next year]).

In most cases the enrollment date occurs on the first month after the plan's receipt of the application. If the enrollment application and premium are sub-

mitted after a cutoff date established by the plan (e.g., fifteenth of month), the subscriber and dependents may not be covered until the first of the next full month (e.g., premium submitted on June 18 but patient eligibility for services does not start until August 1) (Box 5-4).

At the time of enrollment, the subscriber and dependents must select a PCP. If one is not selected, the MCO will select one from its panel of PCPs that show openings.

Depending on the MCO, PCP choice may be limited to the same PCP for all members. Other plans may allow the subscriber and any of the dependents to select a different PCP for each member. This

---

BOX 5-4
Important Note About Member Coverage

Case managers must be cognizant of the fact that members are only covered for services during the period in which they are actually enrolled. This becomes an issue when a patient is terminated or loses insurance as a result of nonpayment of premiums. The real confusion often starts when a patient elects COBRA but does not make the premium payments within the specified time frame.

latter capability is extremely important in case management provided for children with special needs. It is important because not all PCPs have the training or expertise to treat many of the conditions or deal with the special issues that frequently arise with this category of patients. Consequently, a pediatrician best serves children with special needs.

Membership Packets

Once the enrollment applications are processed, the subscriber and dependents will receive their "new member enrollment packet" within approximately 30 days. This packet includes a certificate of coverage, often referred to as the *EOC* or *evidence of coverage*; the member handbook, which is key for case-managed cases because it describes coverage limitations and exclusions; identification cards (one for each member enrolled); and a provider directory listing all providers within the MCO's network.

PREMIUMS

If the insurance is obtained through an employer, the employer generally pays all or part of the premiums due. The amount of the premiums paid by the employer, who can be covered, and what extent of benefits will be afforded to those covered often depend on the size of the employer group. Consequently, the employer may pay all the premiums for the subscriber (employee) and for all the subscriber's dependents; in other cases, the employer may pay full premiums for the employee and partial premiums for dependents. If the employee is required to pay a portion of the insurance, the portion taken from his or her paycheck is called *employee contribution*.

DEPENDENT CHILDREN

A subscriber's dependent children are typically covered through the age of 19 years.

However, many plans do cover full-time students until the age of 23 years if there is proof of full-time schooling on file with the MCO. If the employee has a dependent child with special needs and the child is dependent on the parent for all care, most plans will cover the dependent indefinitely regardless of age for as long as the subscriber remains eligible for insurance benefits. In most plans new dependents are covered if they are enrolled within the first 30 days of life or adoption.

In the case of newborns, services are provided and approved by using the mother's enrollment data; and if the newborn is discharged at the same time as the mother, there are often few claims issues. It is when the child remains in the hospital after the mother's discharge that issues can arise. For example, if an infant is premature or born with a catastrophic condition or has an illness or other condition that requires a continued stay, the case manager must work closely with the family to ensure that enrollment of the infant occurs as quickly as possible. At this time the child's medical needs must be evaluated for possible enrollment in a state's children's medical services program, developmental disabilities program, or Medicaid.

If the subscriber's dependent child gives birth to a baby, the baby is only covered under the dependent's insurance until discharge. After discharge, if the baby needs ongoing care or services, the subscriber or dependent must ensure that the baby is enrolled into insurance in his or her own name. In most cases this will be the state's Medicaid program.

MENTAL HEALTH PARITY

Although not recognized by all states, mental health parity rights have been signed into law by many states. According to mental health parity laws, a person's mental health care can no longer be limited, either by the number of visits or days or by dollar amount. In essence, the law requires parity of mental health benefits with what is allowed for any medical or surgical benefits afforded by group health coverage. Because many cases referred for case management will have dual diagnoses, case managers must have a general knowledge of their state's laws as they relate to mental health parity and coverage and how these laws interface with the medical benefits portion of the plan. As of this writing, 32 states have mental health parity laws. For a current listing of states that do, see the National Association of Mental Illness website at www.nami.org/campaign/statepar.htm.

MCO QUALITY IMPROVEMENT SYSTEMS

Although quality is covered in this text in a separate chapter, it is important for a case manager to understand some of the processes used by organizations as they investigate, act on, and report quality issues and findings. This is necessary because the cases followed by case management are complex. In these cases one can uncover quality-of-care issues, as well as member dissatisfaction with processes or providers.

The U.S. health care system has developed various programs to ensure the quality of health care services. These external programs operate independently of MCOs and include the following:

- Physician licensing and board certification
- Facility certification
- Accreditation from agencies such as Joint Commission on Accreditation of Healthcare Organizations (JCAHO) or NCQA and Medicare
- Formal and informal state and federal regulatory authorities, medical boards, and trade associations such as the American Medical Association (AMA)

Additionally, the MCO may have large employer groups as policyholders or state contracts for managed care for Medicaid or a federal contract to serve as a Medicare + Choice plan; these employer groups hire independent auditing firms whose primary function is to audit the MCO's operations as they relate to enforcing quality-of-care standards. Thus anyone using an MCO and its health system is a beneficiary of the impacts and effectiveness of these external programs.[4]

Although quality programs will vary and depend on the size of the organization and the populations they serve, some of the quality processes used by HMOs and MCOs include the following:

- **Grievance and appeal system—** This is the process required by federal regulations and state laws that allow members to file a grievance, appeal a decision, make a complaint, and voice concerns. Grievances and appeals most often occur when a member disagrees with a plan's or medical group's decision on an issue or when there is a concern about claims administrative issues or the quality of care from a specific provider.

  The process for any grievance or appeal is a formal process in which the MCO must record the issue, and the recording and actions taken must be on file with the member services department. When members complain, there is often no record of the issue and no indication of whether the issue was resolved. Unfortunately, if the member is not directed to member services and a more formal process for resolution does not ensue, the member's complaint may remain unresolved, and the issue will not be included in any reporting done by the organization. If complaints are received, it is important to have the member file a formal complaint with the organization's member services department to ensure that the issue is handled according to regulations and laws.

Most MCOs take responsibility for all quality issues including all levels of appeal. However, this process varies among states and organizations. The processes used may vary by employer groups such as the Federal Employees Health Benefits Plan, Medicare, and Medicaid. Enrollees in these groups have their own processes for appeals. Most appeals use the following processes:

- **First-level appeal**—The member submits the issue, a re-review is conducted, and another determination is made on the topic at hand. In some organizations the medical director conducts the re-review and determination and uses a committee only when he or she cannot make a determination or when he or she issued the original coverage determination. In other organizations only a committee may handle the final determination on appeals. In any event, the final decision rests on new information submitted. If a decision is made to reverse the original denial, the organization must ensure the services are provided or paid for as originally requested. If a decision is made to uphold the original denial, the member will be given instructions on what processes he or she can follow to take the issue to the next level.
- **Second level**—This level is always at the plan level, and in most cases a committee issues the final determination. If the issue progresses to this level, most plans allow the member to be present to discuss the case. As with the first level, if the decision is

made to reverse the original denial, the plan must provide or pay for the services originally requested. If a decision is made to uphold the original denial, the member is notified of the next level of review, which is generally arbitration.

- **Arbitration**—This level is conducted as an independent hearing. At the hearing both the member and MCO have an opportunity to present their sides of the case before a judge or arbitrator. Arbitration decisions are usually considered binding, and the MCO must follow the decisions rendered on the case. Although many plans require several steps be taken before a member can file for arbitration and not sue an organization, this process may change if the Patient Bill of Rights (McCain-Kennedy-Edwards Bill) is passed. If passed, this bill will give patients the right to sue their MCO. Under the current grievance and appeal system, if an issue is in dispute and the member is not satisfied with the decision, the member has the right to take the issue from grievance to appeal and then to arbitration.
- **Third-party or outside review**—This level of review is used for requests for coverage of treatment deemed experimental or treatment not considered to be efficacious or a standard of care. It might also be used when the issue at hand requires an independent third party's expertise. Prudent organizations frequently use this level of review before a coverage determination is issued. In other organizations this level is used only after coverage is denied and the member appeals.

For Medicare beneficiaries, although the processes can be as described previously, the plan must go an additional step if they uphold the denial wholly or partially. In the case of any Medicare denial, the case must be forwarded to CMS's Center for Healthcare Resolution and Dispute (CHDR) following very rigid time lines for the final ruling.

Medicaid beneficiaries have the right to file their appeal directly with the state's fair hearing office. Often they may bypass the health plan's complaint, grievance, or appeal processes and file their appeal directly with their state's department of health services designee office. Technically, they should follow their MCO's rules on the filing of grievances and appeals.

- **Member satisfaction surveys**— Most health plans use this quality modality to learn how members feel about their services. In most organizations surveys such as these are conducted annually either by phone or mail (if mailed most health plans know statistically the return rate is very low, even when the survey is accompanied with postage-paid return envelopes). The intent of the survey is to solicit information about services received and the members' perceptions of events and treatment. With these findings, the organization can take steps to improve the processes. Results are shared with providers and members through newsletters and other communication tools used by the organization.
- **Treatment protocols/clinical practice guidelines**—These are the standards of care or best practices established by an MCO for treating common medical conditions. Basically, treatment protocols are based on current knowledge of practitioners and their best practices.

These best practices describe the recommended sequence for diagnosing and treating a condition. Although the MCO can adopt treatment protocols based on its own research, many rely on those already proven and adopted by external and national authorities. Once a treatment protocol is chosen, the organization works closely with its providers to ensure acceptance and implementation. Treatment protocols and the resultant clinical policy are products of the quality management process. Quality is enhanced when an organization's providers use treatment protocols. Thus both the MCO and the members benefit because providers are ordering tests and services that yield the best diagnostic information and treatment in the most economical way with the least inconvenience and cost to the member.

- **Provider satisfaction surveys**—Like member satisfaction surveys, these surveys are conducted by the organization to see how their contracted providers view processes. As with the member satisfaction surveys, the intent is to ascertain the provider's perception of the MCO and its various departments. The provider survey results are most often shared internally through newsletters or other communication tools.
- **Provider credentialing**—This is a process used to validate a provider's licensure and qualifications. This is a very rigid and time-sensitive process. As such, it is often assigned to a specific department. This process starts at the time a provider submits an application to the health plan for inclusion in the network. Before the finalization of any contract for inclusion as a network provider, a provider's credentials are

verified. In this process a multitude of credentialing and licensure verification entities, as well as regulatory criteria, are used. If the provider is credentialed, a re-review is conducted biannually thereafter. As part of the credentialing process, the credentialing staff review (1) past litigation sanctions against the provider, (2) documents maintained on the provider by member services and documents from the grievance appeal process, (3) medical office and chart reviews of a provider, and (4) provider files and reviews conducted by the quality staff if a quality issue was researched.

- **Quality improvement studies**— This is a means of providing objective data on various issues. In most cases quality improvement (QI) studies are conducted retrospectively, and many focus on specific areas of concern. The study results are compared with the MCO's own goals or external standards or norms. Results are used for a variety of purposes: (1) for increasing awareness of a standard and performance, (2) for refining policies and procedures, or (3) for participation in outside reporting to regulatory bodies or as contractually required with purchasers, or if a medical group, with the HMO.
- **Provider profiling**—This is a process used by MCOs to analyze provider practice patterns, especially those of physicians. In most cases the following areas are profiled: utilization rates, referral rates, cost of care to members, lengths of stay, hospital admission and readmission rates, emergency department (ED) use by patients, and any quality concerns (e.g., member complaints or lawsuits). Although

provider profiling can have a down side if all factors are considered, it can be a useful tool with which to identify efficient providers when the MCO is trending and suggesting areas of improvement for others.

- **Report cards**—These reports are similar to provider profiling, but in this case the report centers on the organization's performance in terms of quality measures. Report cards target MCO members and their employers and are useful tools that validate the organization's claims of "quality of services." Probably one of the most rigid report cards is the one used to report HEDIS. HEDIS is a registered trademark of NCQA and is considered to be the gold standard for quality reporting. HEDIS reports not only clinical and preventive indicators but also financial and member satisfaction data for the MCO. To report HEDIS data, an MCO must follow detailed standards if it is to collect data as required and then categorize the data according to HEDIS standards and format for the final reporting. To collect the data required, most organizations use a combination of data gathering techniques such as chart review or administrative data (e.g., claims or other encounter data).

FEE STRUCTURES

In managed care there are a variety of techniques used to reimburse, finance, and control utilization of health care services. Fee structures are derived from actuarial methods and statistical data commonly used by MCOs. As stated earlier, indemnity insurance holds no risk to the provider because risk is shared by the insurer and the patient.

Rates and fee structures used by MCOs vary. Many rate reimbursement or fee structure methods are linked to varying degrees of risk for either the provider or the MCO. Many MCOs use fee structures in some of the following ways:

- To remove a provider's incentive to overtreat by transferring some of the financial risk for care to the actual provider
- To improve efficiency of referrals for specialty services and diagnostic and therapeutic modalities
- For adjustments to the intensity of services for the type of patient or case
- As a response to results from patient satisfaction surveys

MCOs and providers are becoming more sophisticated and realistic about negotiating agreements with one another. Although negotiation styles still run the gamut, there is a growing consensus that the traditional adversarial or "us versus them" approach no longer works because it does not produce a business trust. When negotiating health care rates, providers and purchasers usually focus on at least four broad contract negotiation categories:

- **Provider network**—Provide high-quality physicians (primary care and specialty), hospitals, and ancillary services but limit the size of the network so that there is a guarantee of volume to the provider, as well as ensured access for members.
- **Reimbursement**—Negotiating competitive rates, giving each side a stake in the process while establishing a viable framework for future relationships. Each side must be able to live with the terms of the agreement and not feel taken advantage of because of inexperience, misrepresentation, or intimidation.
- **Cooperation**—Establish a framework for an ongoing partnership while following utilization and quality controls.

- **Contract agreement**—This is key because it requires adherence to contract specifications and performance standards. For the provider it prohibits balance billing, and for the purchaser it allows a clause to terminate inefficient providers or those who repeatedly provide medically unnecessary or inappropriate care. It also allows for binding arbitration to resolve disputes.

Typical rate reimbursements or fee structures for MCOs include the following:

- **Capitation**—This is used in contracting with medical groups, especially when primary care services are needed. Capitation is a form of prospective payment system that is based on a flat rate of reimbursement per person. It is paid on a monthly basis for a specific range of services for all persons enrolled with the specific provider. Capitation is commonly used for the reimbursement of laboratory, radiology, and other ancillary services.

  Capitation is successful as a form of prospective payment because the provider is paid a set fee on a monthly basis for each member. This is referred to as *per member per month* or *PMPM*. This set fee is paid to the provider regardless of the fact that some members for whom he or she will be paid may not use any services within the month. Therefore if the provider's claims for the month are lower than the capitation reimbursement, the provider makes a profit. If not, the provider loses money.

  If the HMO is contracting with a medical group to provide services, the HMO may view capitation with an attitude that if quality-of-care issues are transferred to the medical group, it will the medical group that must respond when quality issues arise. This is true in part. However, it is the HMO that is held more accountable for the quality of services provided to their members. Two main stakeholders hold HMOs accountable: (1) employers who continue to want complete and accurate utilization and quality data and (2) regulators who are under extreme pressure by consumer groups to hold and make HMOs accountable. To ensure that medical groups share equally, many HMOs require, as part of the contract, that the medical group submit utilization and financial data to them within a specific time frame. Also, if the medical group subcontracts with other providers, this process should be seamless, and the medical group should have mechanisms built in for oversight of processes and quality from these subcontracted providers.

In addition to flat-rate capitation or per member per month, there are other variations to capitation such as age and sex adjustments in which provider payments are adjusted according the age and sex of the plan's members. In other cases capitation could be by benefit plan capitation. In this model, rates are adjusted for differences in the cost of providing care for the variety and richness of benefit packages sold. Percentage of premium capitation is another form of capitation. With this methodology, the MCO pays the provider a percentage of all premiums for members in the provider's panel. Capitation is also pared with risk or incentive pool arrangements. This modality gives contracted providers an additional incentive to control costs or meet utilization targets. A more detailed descrip-

tion of the other forms of capitation is as follows:

- **Capitated primary care**—Under this model, if the physician is a PCP, reimbursement is made with a capitation method of payment. Capitation is basically a fixed amount of money paid to the PCP monthly for each member enrolled with the PCP.
- **Capitated preferred providers**—Although capitation is often the reimbursement method for primary care, it is also used with other medical services such as laboratory or hospital services or some specialty care. This modality for reimbursement allows the MCO an avenue for transfer of some financial risk to the provider. As with PCP capitations, if these providers do not treat or see the members, the provider is paid the same set fee as is paid for another member who might have had one or more encounters with the provider during the same given month. In essence, capitation can be a two-edged sword. If the provider is successful in keeping claims to a minimum, a profit can be made. In contrast, if claims are in excess of the capitation due members having multiple encounters in the month, the provider loses money. The overall goals of capitation of preferred providers are that costs among enrollees will average out over time and the provider will make money. Therefore it is clearly in the provider's interest to ensure members assigned or enrolled remain healthy. The major down side of capitation is that providers may undertreat members to maximize their profits.
- **Age/sex adjustment capitation**—Another method of capitation is termed *age/sex adjusted*. With this

type of reimbursement, the provider's payments are adjusted based on projected differences in utilization based on age and sex of enrollees. According to the age/sex adjustment theory, payment rates vary according to age and sex of members to reflect the expected differences in utilization. For example, a person older than 65 years will use more services than a healthy minor child. Similarly, a woman of childbearing years will consume more health care services than a healthy man of the same age.

- **Benefit plan capitation**—Benefit plan capitation adjusts the differences in the cost of providing various benefit plans sold by the MCO. Richer benefit plans cost more to provide (e.g., those with lower copayments or unlimited visits) versus those rich plans that offer higher copayments or limits on visits. Benefit plan capitation compensates for those differences by varying the capitation payment according to the richness of a member's benefit plan or package.[4]

- **Percentage of premium capitation**—With this method of payment, the provider's reimbursement is based on premium revenue, regardless of age or benefit mix. Instead of being paid a fixed per-member-per-month fee, the provider agrees to accept a fixed percentage of the premium revenues for the members enrolled with the provider. The provider shares in the risk and rewards of care on the same basis as the MCO. However, the provider relies on the MCO's ability to set premiums that adequately and accurately capture the age and sex mix and benefit options for enrollees.[4]

Other Rate Methodologies

Other rates used or negotiated by the MCO industry include the following:

- **Per diem rates**—This is a flat rate payment per day that covers all services agreed on in the rate. Per diem rates are prenegotiated and vary by contract. Some contracts go even further and include varying levels of per diem rates for different levels of care. This type of rate methodology is often used for institutional care such as that provided in acute-care hospitals or skilled nursing facilities. Under per diem rates, many contracts include an outlier clause. This allows protection to providers when high-cost cases are encountered. Per diem rate negotiation is a common method used by case mangers, as they negotiate rates for services for specific clients in their caseload.

- **Diagnosis-related groups**—DRGs are the basis of payment for Medicare and TRICARE and are used for reimbursement of hospital services. In this system patients are categorized by diagnoses. Rates are then assigned to the various diagnoses based on the resources traditionally used to treat a specific diagnosis. The DRG rate is the amount the hospital receives regardless of the amount of time a patient remains as an inpatient or the amount of resources the patient uses during the hospitalization. If the patient requires a longer length of stay and the stay qualifies as an outlier, additional payments can be allowed.

- **Case rates or global rates**—Rates under this methodology differ from per diem rates in that a set or specific rate is used for a specific procedure. Case rates are prenegotiated.

Unfortunately, if an outlier agreement is not prenegotiated, the rate contractually agreed on would be the rate paid regardless of the length of stay or intensity of services performed. Therefore if case rates are used, it is imperative to include all anticipated services within the rate structure. This methodology is frequently used for transplants, open-heart surgery, and obstetric services.

- **Fee schedules**—This is a simple method of listing specific services and assigning a price to each. Fee schedules are commonly used for procedures and services that can be represented by service codes or CPT codes (i.e., Common Procedural Terminology, a coding system used to bill professional services and procedures) or RBRVS codes (i.e., Resource Based Relative Value Scale, a coding system used primarily by Medicare for billing physician services).

- **Risk or incentive or shared risk pools**—Risk or incentive pools are common methods used by MCOs to reward providers. Use of pools such as these rewards provider performances when budget or utilization expectations of the MCO are met. Unfortunately, many risk arrangements do not address the problems associated with creative provider billing practices, especially that of unbundling.

    With a risk pool, the HMO withholds a portion of the medical group's prospective payment. If the group performs below expected and budgeted levels, a portion of the withheld money is returned. If an incentive pool is used, individual providers are given bonuses.

    Another type of pool is termed a *shared risk pool*. Shared risk pools are used more commonly with hospitals or specialty provider groups but can be set up for any type of service. According to a shared risk pool agreement, the degree of risk or reward is directly linked to performance that is based on budgeted expenses or utilization rate targets.

    Although there are many caveats to the following example and it does not begin to address all the issues, a good example of a shared risk plan is one used by Western Health Advantage (WHA), a provider-owned HMO in Sacramento. WHA and its owner groups (University of California Davis Medical Center at Sacramento, Catholic Health West of Sacramento, and North Valley Medical Center) set up a network that spanned a three-county area for coverage. Under this arrangement a shared risk pool was established by WHA for what it calls its *advantage referral program*. This program was developed in an attempt to stall MCO backlash. As it is set up, it allows members the ability to choose any provider within the WHA network for specialty care when the PCP believes specialty care is needed. If hospitalization is required as a result of the specialty referral, the member has the ability to use that specialist's hospital network. The same is true if the member is hospitalized in any WHA network hospital and the admission is linked to emergency services performed at that facility. All claims associated with any specialty referrals or emergency admissions associated with the advantage referral program are paid from the shared risk pool.

Although there are a variety of reasons that providers may want to share in the risk of offering managed care to members, the following are common means used by providers to minimize their risk:

- **Outliers**—This is a technique used by providers to protect themselves against high-cost cases. An outlier clause allows the provider to set a maximum dollar amount per case. When the limit is exceeded, the payment changes to another payment system agreed on in the contract. Many MCOs, including Medicare, recognize two types of outliers: day outliers and cost outliers. Day outliers are used when the normal length of stay is exceeded, and cost outliers are used when costs exceed normal costs for the diagnosis or procedure. When outliers are used, the MCO loses its price protection, but the individual provider is protected against unpredictable higher costs associated with the more complex cases.

- **Discounted fee-for-service rates**— This is a method preferred by providers because it exposes them to a minimum amount of financial risk. More important, it is similar to the old FFS methodology to which many are accustomed. This methodology offers the MCO a discount in exchange for something desired by the provider. For example, this could mean guaranteed patient referrals or expedited claims processing. If discounted fees are used, case managers must be careful to ensure that extra strings are not attached to the final negotiations, since in the end, the cost of services could be greater than anticipated. For example, if the case rate is established by using this method and the case manager agrees to the provider's demands that retrospective review of the claims will not occur, when the claims do come and they are reviewed and unbundling or other billing tactics are found and the claims are higher than they would

have been under normal circumstances, there is nothing that can be done but pay the claims as per the agreed-on terms.

- **Underreferral**—This is a serious consequence of capitation and probably the biggest reason for managed care backlash. Underreferral occurs when the capitated physicians try to provide all care and minimize referrals to specialists and referrals for testing as a way to enhance their own revenues. Underreferral also occurs when there are very restrictive prior authorization requirements that impede access to specialty services (even when medically necessary) but the PCP or referring physician does not wish to cooperate or be pressured for the information (e.g., what has been tried or done to date, as well as the patient's responses to treatments).

- **Stop-loss or reinsurance**—To protect itself from unexpected catastrophic expenses, the provider or MCO may purchase what is termed *reinsurance*. Reinsurance is purchased from a reinsurance company, a specialized insurance company. This insurance is an indemnity-type insurance that carries with it a large deductible or stop-loss (e.g., for institutional care a $50,000-$500,000 deductible, which is based on a per case or per member per year). Before submitting claims to the reinsurance carrier, the MCO or provider must meet the predetermined deductible as outlined in the policy. Claims are then reimbursed according to the reinsurance contract (e.g., the reinsurer will pay approximately 80% after the deductible has been met). Since many cases under case management will be in the reinsurance category, it is imperative that case managers working for an MCO or provider that pays for reinsurance be familiar with the reinsurer's policies, procedures, and expectations. This is necessary to assist in reducing losses; in addition, the reporting of such cases is often a contractual requirement of the reinsurer. If the case is not reported, the party covered by the reinsurance might be required to withstand the entire brunt of the claims losses.

- **Carve-outs**—This is a special arrangement that is made for specific diagnoses, procedures, or conditions for which there are wide variations in cost. With this method, the carved-out condition is paid on a different fee basis. If specific conditions are carved out, they are specified and negotiated as part of the provider's contract with the MCO. Carve-outs traditionally include transplants and mental health services. In the case of Medicaid managed care, children who have a condition covered by a state's Children's Medical Services program will have that eligible condition carved out. Thus coordination of care and prior authorizations must be obtained from another entity.

- **Subcapitation**—This is a method used by some capitated providers when they wish to pass on some portion of their capitated services to other providers. Mental health, home health, DME, and laboratory and radiology services are good examples of this methodology. Under this arrangement, the initial provider is capitated to the MCO but in turn capitates to other specific entity for portions of services. This method is used when the other provider has more expertise, can

accommodate the volume, or can provide the services in a more cost-effective manner.

- **Fee maximization**—This is a common technique used by providers to increase their reimbursements. However, if the MCO has a sophisticated claims software system, the following can be detected and prevent payment when the provider tries to:
  - **Upcode**—Process used when several procedures are performed but the procedure code that results in the higher payment is the one used for billing purposes.
  - **Unbundle**—Process used when several procedures are performed and billed as one (e.g., chemistry panel). If a test within a panel is requested separately, it is billed at a higher rate. However, when that same test is included in a panel (or "bundled"), the panel is billed as one test. When panels are unbundled, the provider separates the tests, billing individually for each, often at a higher rate.
  - **DRG creep**—Results when a provider manipulates the patient's primary, secondary, and additional diagnoses and codes them separately. The order in which the codes are billed affects the patient's assigned DRG and payment.

MANAGED CARE CONTROLS

National trends indicate that patient days are on a decline, whereas lengths of stay are climbing. This incline in the lengths of stay is believed to be due largely to increased severity or complexity of illness and morbidity of hospitalized patients, many of whom are older or have a multiplicity of chronic medical conditions. The other drivers of health care costs include the following:

- High-priced technology
- Inflation
- Rising expectations of consumers (and the belief that health care is a right)
- Continued focus on illness rather than prevention
- Malpractice rates and the resultant defensive medical practices
- Antitrust regulations
- Aging population with more complex care and socioeconomic issues
- Inefficiency of management of health care resources

For these and other reasons, MCOs use a variety of direct and indirect techniques to control their costs. Indirect methods include controls such as preventive health care services and prospective payment along with any contractual incentives. Direct controls often include the use of PCPs as gatekeepers, the various components of utilization review, case management, claims, and pharmacy reviews. Through these methods and others, controls can be set. Thus managed care is set apart from traditional indemnity health care insurance.

UTILIZATION CONTROLS

In many utilization review (UR) programs, the focus is on medical necessity, where the treatment is rendered, and the cost of such. However, they are not the key to quality or short- or long-term cost management. Effective UR programs must use solid processes and procedures as the basis for managing resource use, with the primary focus on identifying bad habits and correcting them.

When UR controls are used, they should not be treated as an end in themselves. They should be used as a stepping stone to effective utilization management. When an approach such as the latter is used, it can only occur through the use of individual and effective case management

services. Thus when the two elements are combined—utilization management and case management—one has managed care and not managed cost. Basic UR process include the identification of three major issues:

1. Is care medically necessary and appropriate? Medically necessary care is care that is required and consistent with the symptoms, diagnosis, and treatment of the patient's illness or injury; is considered safe and effective according to accepted clinical evidence; and is provided in the most appropriate setting.
2. Are there lower-cost forms of care that are available and as efficacious?
3. Is the patient improving at the rate anticipated as a result of the current treatment regimen?

Most UR programs divide review into categories such as the following:

- **Prospective review**—Review of the services before they are rendered.
- **Concurrent review**—Review conducted during the course of treatment. At this level the nurse may also be responsible for assisting the discharge planner when issues arise.
- **Retrospective review**—Review after services have been rendered.
- **Claims review**—Review, again after services have been rendered.
- **Case management**—The involvement of nurses in the more complex, intense, or severe or cases with multiple diagnoses or those that require very costly care.
- **Physician review**—This can be rendered at any time for one of the foregoing levels or at the frequency required by case events.

PROSPECTIVE REVIEW OR PRIOR AUTHORIZATION

Prior authorization is the process of reviewing medical services to ensure medical necessity and appropriateness of the level of care before delivery. Depending on the MCO's rules, many specialty visits and procedures require prior authorization. If specialty care or a procedure is required, most organizations require the PCP to submit his or her request for approval to the utilization department. Clerical staff members review the request first. Staff at this level will verify eligibility of both the patient and provider and ensure that all medical information is present to justify the request. The request is then submitted to a reviewer and reviewed against established criteria (e.g., InterQual, Milliman and Robertson criteria, or the MCO's internally developed criteria). If the request does not meet the criteria or is one that must be reviewed by a physician (e.g., cosmetic procedure, out-of-area care), it is forwarded to the medical director or a physician advisor for the final coverage determination.

A physician reviewer may believe that he or she cannot make the coverage determination without peer consultation, or possibly, review by the utilization management committee or special procedures committee. If this occurs, the request is then forwarded to the applicable review entity. In some cases (especially those considered experimental), the request might be sent for what is called *independent review* or *third-party review*. This level of review is outside the organization and is done by board-certified specialists in the field, who make the final recommendation.

Although review authority varies with the MCO, many use a tiered process for the prior review function. This can be divided into three categories such as the following:

- **Level I review**—Written justification is often not required or is a procedure that would be considered one that will fall into an automatic authorization category because it is rarely denied. This level can be performed by nonnursing personnel

who function under the direction of nursing personnel.
- **Level II review**—Written justification or specialty review is performed by professional nurses.
- **Level III review**—The medical director, physician advisor, utilization management committee, or a special procedures committee conducts the review.

Level I—Nonnurse Review

If Level I review is allowed, the utilization management or case management *clerical authorization representative*, using specific criteria developed for their level of review, may be allowed to authorize such services as the following:

- Breast biopsy
- Colonoscopy
- Contraction stress test/nonstress test (CST/NST)
- Doppler study
- Echocardiogram
- Endoscopy
- Electrocardiogram (ECG)
- Electroencephalogram (EEG)
- Fine-needle biopsy
- Gated cardiac scan
- Holter monitor
- Specific laboratory services
- Mammography
- Specific listing of nuclear medicine procedures
- Pulmonary function test–arterial blood gas
- Sigmoidoscopy
- Treadmill (including thallium treadmill)
- Medical supplies and dressings (expendable) less than $100
- Continued rental of DME items if the monthly rental rate does not exceed the purchase price and rental of the item is less than $100
- Other tests and procedures as outlined by the HMO's medical director

Level II—Nurse Review

Level II review is conducted by utilization management or case management professional nursing staff. The nurse may be given the authority to prior authorize such services and dollar amounts as follows:

A. Radiologic procedures without contrast and other procedures such as:
   1. Magnetic resonance imaging
   2. Digital subtraction angiography
   3. Myelogram
   4. Cardiac catheterization
   5. Electrophysiology study
B. Outpatient diagnostic procedures
C. Renal dialysis
D. Autologous blood transfusion
E. Outpatient surgery
F. DME if less than $1000 per item
G. Prostheses if less than $1000 per item
H. Rehabilitation therapy which often includes:
   1. Physical therapy: maximum of two times per week for four weeks
   2. Occupational therapy: maximum of two times per week for four weeks
   3. Speech therapy: maximum two times per week for four weeks
I. Home health agency and infusion therapy services within a specific limit of visits
J. Ambulance service, excluding air ambulance
K. Precertification of inpatient admission
L. Second opinion requests
M. Concurrent review authorizations
N. Skilled nursing facility admissions and concurrent review

If the review nurse specializes in mental health, he or she might be allowed to authorize services such as:

A. Day treatment service/partial hospitalization (alcoholism only)
B. Psychologic testing
C. Residential treatment center placement
D. Alcohol treatment program
E. Outpatient mental health visits
F. Precertification of admissions for mental health care

Level III—Physician Review

If level III review is required, the utilization management or case management staff members may refer the following cases to the medical director or physician advisor; or at times the medical director may refer the case to the utilization management committee, special procedures committee, a peer reviewer, or an outside reviewer:

A. All cases requiring a denial
B. All nonnetwork referrals
C. All transplants
D. DME requests greater than $1000
E. Requests for prostheses greater than $1000
F. Rehabilitation therapy when the specific therapy request goes beyond an eight-visit limit in four weeks
G. Air ambulance
H. Any case that fails criteria review or when benefits are in question
I. All experimental/investigational requests
J. All requests that exceed usual and customary costs and services for the condition
K. All plastic surgery procedures requests
L. Magnetic resonance imaging with contrast
M. All requests that exceed the maximum allowed by the level II reviewers
N. Any procedure for patient or physician convenience
O. When potential quality issues are identified

P. Refusal by patient or physician to use alternative level of care

Q. Refusal by patient or physician to use available network providers

R. Physician refusal to respond to a request for additional information

S. When overutilization or underutilization of health care services is an issue

Concurrent Review

Concurrent review is most often used for inpatient acute care, rehabilitation, skilled nursing care, and at times home care. The objective of concurrent review is to ensure that review is performed on an ongoing basis during the actual provision of services. This level of review is most often performed on inpatient stays and is used to ensure that the level of care is medically necessary, and if not, that an alternative level of care that can provide the same quality outcome is available. Once a case is known, the review nurse, using information and MCO protocols, establishes an estimated length of stay. This estimated length of stay will serve as a target date for possible discharge. Although the actual review is conducted by nurses, if the case does not meet review criteria or goes beyond the estimated length of stay, the case must be reviewed by a physician reviewer.

Most MCOs review inpatient stays by using established criteria (e.g., InterQual, Milliman, and Robertson criteria or the plan's approved criteria). All cases that do not meet the criteria should be reviewed by the attending physician before submission to the medical director. A process such as this allows the attending physician an opportunity to ensure that all pertinent information is present before the issuance of a coverage determination.

Most MCOs conduct concurrent review on a daily basis for inpatient stays. Others may allow the review to go to at least every third day, depending on the diagnosis and response to treatment. However, many MCOs do recognize that patients at specialty levels of care do not require daily review. This is true when the patient is receiving appropriate care, responding to the treatments, and progressing within the anticipated time frame for the treatments. Examples of such review are presented in Box 5-5.

When the concurrent review process is started, an admission review is always conducted first with the focus of review on the following areas:

- Severity of illness—duration of signs and symptoms and severity of symptoms and test results at the time of admission
- Intensity of service and initial treatments and frequency
- Appropriateness of admission level of care
- Anticipated length of stay

If review continues, the focus will be on the following:

- Intensity of service—ongoing plan of treatments and actual treatments, frequency, type, and patient responses

---

BOX 5-5
Examples of Concurrent Reviews

Type/Indication	Frequency of Review
Overestimated length of stay	Daily or as indicated
Acute-care rehabilitation	Minimum, once weekly
Skilled nursing facility or subacute-care facility	Minimum, once weekly
Neonates	Minimum, once weekly

- Appropriateness of the level of care
- Length of stay
- Identification of quality-of-care issues
- Discharge readiness and barriers to discharge

Effective concurrent review is used to facilitate referrals to or identify patients for the following:

- Discharge planning
- Case management
- Potential quality indicator reporting
- Potential reinsurance reporting

If the MCO desires NCQA or JCAHO accreditation, the organization must use standardized criteria for its reviews. The review criteria used will be those that are considered to be nationally recognized criteria sets. This includes InterQual, Milliman, and Robertson criteria and excludes internally developed criteria. In addition to the use of national criteria, organizations must require that the following to be taken into consideration when the review is performed and a coverage determination is rendered:

- Age
- Comorbidities
- Complications
- Progress in treatment
- Psychosocial situation
- Home environment when applicable
- Availability of skilled nursing facility, subacute-care facilities, or home health agency services to support the patient's medical care needs on discharge
- Coverage of benefits for skilled nursing facilities, subacute-care facilities, or home health agency care
- Ability of local hospitals to provide all recommended services within the estimated length of stay

Many large purchasers and some states also require UR programs to be certified by the American Accreditation HealthCare Commission (URAC). URAC's address is 1275 K Street NW, Suite 1100, Washington,

DC 20005. The phone number is 202-216-9010, and the website is www.urac.org. URAC's accreditation process closely follows that of NCQA but is a totally separate accreditation process. If an organization undergoes accreditation review by URAC, URAC evaluates the following areas:

- Written policy and procedure manuals
- Training course outlines and evaluation tools
- Job descriptions
- Flow charts, depicting work processes
- Correspondence or other evidence of communications with members and providers (e.g., newsletters, member handbooks, provider manuals, website pages)
- Meeting minutes that list attendees by name and affiliation
- Sections of contracts for contractual language
- Relevant sections of state or federal statutes (including attestation of compliance with the application)
- Quality measurements and improvement tools, analysis reports, and data from quality assessments
- Other materials as appropriate

During review of an organization, URAC uses the following standards:

- Standards UM 1 to 3 cover confidentiality of utilization management information
- Standards UM 4 to 10 cover utilization management staff qualifications
- Standards UM 11 to 13 cover utilization management program qualifications
- Standard UM 14 covers the scope of utilization management program
- Standards UM 15 to 19 cover utilization management program qualifications
- Standard UM 20 covers the organization's utilization management program

- Standard UM 21 again covers utilization program qualifications
- Standards UM 22 and 23 cover accessibility and on-site review procedures
- Standards UM 24 to 26 cover information on which utilization management is conducted
- Standards UM 27 to 30 cover standards for procedures for review determinations
- Standards UM 31 to 33 cover appeals of determination not to certify
- Standard UM 34 covers expedited appeals
- Standard UM 35 covers standard appeals

RETROSPECTIVE REVIEW CONTROLS

Retrospective review is the review of the services after they are rendered. Although some retrospective review is conducted before claims submission (e.g., it was found that a prior authorization was not obtained), most retrospective review occurs after claims submission and is used for review of such issues as the following:

- Elective admissions or services rendered without prior authorization
- Retrospective admission review showing the case did not meet medical necessity guidelines
- Use of nonparticipating provider or out-of-area services without prior authorization
- Services not provided in the appropriate setting

As with prospective and concurrent review, retrospective review is performed to ensure that services were medically necessary and provided at the appropriate level of care. It is also another way to assist with the reduction of unnecessary costs, to identify quality-of-care issues and risk or utilization problems, and to trend for quality management activities.

Although emergency services can be retrospectively reviewed, in many states or for plans that follow President Clinton's Consumer Bill of Rights, retrospective denials may not be issued for the medical screening portion of the care because the "prudent layperson" language and interpretation must be used. A denial can be issued to the provider when care continued despite the fact that services were performed for a condition that was nonemergent in nature. In cases such as these, the member, if part of a managed care plan, cannot be billed for the balance, and the provider is required to assume responsibility for all unpaid charges.

INCOMPLETE REQUESTS

Most MCOs have processes in place to handle requests that are incomplete (i.e., lack necessary information). Generally, the utilization management clerical staff will review the prior authorization request initially, and if it is noted to be incomplete, it will be forwarded to a nurse for review. Depending on the organization's policies, the request may remain suspended until a response is generated from the physician who submitted the original request.

Prudent MCOs or HMOs will make every attempt to obtain the information as quickly as possible, since most organizations follow NCQA's timeliness standards for the various authorization types (e.g., routine-nonurgent, urgent, concurrent review, and retrospective). If an incomplete request is submitted, the organization has a very limited time frame in which to obtain the information and make a coverage determination. Unfortunately, the clock starts at the time the original request is received.

PHYSICIAN REVIEW

Any case that does not meet review criteria at any stage of the prospective, concurrent, retrospective review processes, or any case that requires physician review as established by the MCO must be referred to a physician reviewer. This might be the organization's medical director, assistant medical director, physician advisor, or a peer reviewer. Cases are frequently referred for physician review when the following occur:

- The medical necessity or appropriateness of care cannot be determined by the utilization management staff.
- The proposed treatment is experimental or is not approved by the Food and Drug Administration (FDA).
- There is a potential denial of coverage for the care and/or services.
- The attending physician is refusing to cooperate with the review request.
- The utilization management staff identify an alternate place of service, the member is stable for transfer, and care needs can be met at the alternate level of care, but the attending physician or patient and family are not in agreement with the plan.

Although nurses can make a denial when the requested service is not a benefit or the member is not eligible, only physicians can make a "denial" recommendation or coverage determination when the denial involves medical necessity.

In most plans either the medical director or assistant medical director will issue the actual denial. This is true even when physician advisors are employed. The physician advisor will make his or her recommendations, but the actual denial will be made under the medical director's name. Most organizations allow the medical director to retain the right to submit any request to an outside specialist for a recommendation or to the organization's utilization management committee. This process is most often used for the review when the medical director believes another

level of review is warranted before the final coverage determination can be rendered. In some organizations the utilization management committee is used for all case reviews.

Although not all organizations require physician reviewers to use a physician review form, it is an excellent practice. Physician reviewers can use this form to document their recommendations or findings. To be valid, the form must be dated and signed by the physician. Use of a formal process such as this allows formal documentation of the coverage determination and recommendations, should questions arise at a later date.

PEER REVIEW

Peer review, or like-specialty review, is required when services are determined to be not medically necessary or when the medical director requires assistance with a determination for the issue at hand. If the medical director and attending physician do not concur on the coverage determination, the request is most often forwarded to a peer reviewer in the same medical specialty as the service being requested. Thus in addition to the medical director and physician advisors, many organizations also employ peer reviewers. Requirements for peer review are as follows:

- Only licensed physicians of medicine or osteopathy or doctors of dentistry can be used.
- They must be engaged in active practice.
- They must be in the same specialty as the requested service.
- They must have active admitting privileges in one or more hospitals in the contract area used for the peer review process

In most plans peer review physicians must be board-certified or board-eligible. If other types of reviews are needed (e.g., anesthesiology, pathology, radiology, some mental health services), these reviews can only be conducted by a peer reviewer who has the appropriate education and licensure.

THIRD-PARTY REVIEWS

The use of third-party review is due to recent laws and regulations geared toward MCOs and the backlash from lawsuits. Third-party reviews are frequently used when a denial is being appealed or when the requested services are experimental. In some cases it is used when a consensus cannot be reached or the expertise is not available locally or within the MCO. When third-party review is requested, it generally requires that at least three board-certified physicians review the case and issue their recommendations. To protect themselves from litigation, many MCOs now use this peer review process and the recommendations of the reviewers for the final determination. Many go as far as to say that if one reviewer out of three indicates the process is efficacious, the request will be allowed.

PHYSICIAN RESPONSIBILITIES

A physician reviewer's (e.g., medical director, physician advisor) responsibilities include the following:
- Review of the presented documentation
- Identification of additional data needs
- Application of medical expertise to define medical necessity/appropriateness of recommended care and setting
- Identification of health care alternatives

The final determination is based on communications and/or discussion of the case with the attending physician, the health plan's statements or policies on benefit coverage, and any information contained in the scientific literature. The nurse's role in the physician review process is described in Box 5-6.

In many MCOs a daily routine is established whereby a physician reviewer is present to ensure maximum effectiveness of the daily review processes. Thus physician review and case determinations can be completed within the strict time frames required by NCQA or contractually required by the health plans.

Most organizations follow NCQA's recommended time frames for their reviews and issuances of a coverage determination (Table 5-1).

Once the coverage determination is made, it is imperative that the nurse document all actions and retain copies of all documents. This is especially important when the request is one that is denied. Retrieval of documents will be vital if the denial is appealed or if an audit on the denial process is conducted.

PHARMACY REVIEW CONTROLS

Many MCOs use a pharmacy denial process. In cases such as these, if the request fails the pharmacy auto-adjudication process or if it is for an injectable drug, an off-label drug, or one that is investigational or experimental, the request will be forwarded first to the MCO's pharmacy

---

BOX 5-6
The Nurse's Role in Physician Review

To assist the physician reviewer with the case review and coverage determination, the nurse must ensure data are well prepared, concise, and presented in a comprehensive manner. Before any review with a physician advisor, the nurse may contact the attending physician to ensure all clinical information is presented and prepare any documents he or she believes the physician may need for review of the case. Ultimately, each case presentation includes clinical status that is based on data available, defined areas of concern, expected outcomes, and time parameters for determination and communication.

TABLE 5-1
Time Frames for Reviews and Issuances of a Coverage Determination

File Type	Decision-Making Time Frame	Initial Notification (Practitioners Only)	Follow-Up Notification to Members and Practitioners (Electronic or Written)
Precertification—nonurgent	Two working days (after receipt of all information)	One working day (after decision is made)	Two working days (denials only—after initial notification)
Precertification—urgent	One calendar day	Zero calendar days (same day as decision is made)	Two working days (after decision) Note: Must include expedited appeal information
Concurrent	One working day (after receipt of all information)	One working day (after decision is made)	One working day (after initial decision) Note: Must include expedited appeal information
Retrospective	30 working days (after receipt of all information)	NA	Five working days (after decision)

Data from NCQA: *Surveyor guidelines for accreditation for MCOs*, Washington, DC, July 1, 2000, to June 30, 2001, p 170-171.

manager. Depending on this person's level of review authority, he or she may be able to approve the drug. If not, the request will be forwarded to the HMO for the final coverage determination. As with the other review processes, if the drug in question does not meet the criteria and cannot be reviewed at the pharmacy manager's level, the request must be prepared and submitted to the medical director for the coverage determination.

TRACKING AND REPORTING OF DENIALS

Most MCOs use a method to track and report their denials, especially if the MCO is NCQA-accredited or is a Medicare + Choice or a Medicaid contractor. If tracking and reporting of denials is required, all denials will be entered into a database or hard copy log and will eventually be reported to the appropriate entity. Maintaining a denial log is important not only for reporting purposes but also for val-

idating that denial letters were issued correctly and within the allocated time frame.

Oversight of Denials

If utilization review is delegated, oversight of the denial process is only one of the utilization processes for which the MCO must conduct oversight activity. If oversight activity is required, the auditor will review the denial log and then select random denial files. This ensures that all processes were followed (e.g., physician opportunities were allowed for submission of the data, denial was made at the appropriate level, correct letter was used and was accurately completed and submitted within the appropriate time frame).

CLAIMS REVIEW CONTROLS

The claims processing department uses a process similar to the prior authorization process when claims must be reviewed. Most claims are processed without a hitch and by means of the auto-adjudication process (e.g., the claims processing database is set up with codes and linkages to other databases to ensure all the coded fields on the claims match the precoded database). If the claim fails review, it will require additional review before payment. If review is required, most MCOs assign specific reviewers for specific reasons for claims failure. Thus if a claim fails, it is then suspended to this specific area for review.

Claims processing is very similar to the front-end prior authorization system: some claims can be reviewed by nonprofessional nurses; others will require review by a nurse or at times a physician before any payment can be made. A physician's expertise is generally required when there are questions related to usual and customary issues or the medical necessity of the services or when the claim codes do not match those anticipated for the diagnosis and treatment of illness.

Goals of Claims Control

Claims review endeavors to promote good medical care, keep costs at a reasonable and predictable level, and ensure fairness and equity to both the patient and physician. Any claim found to be in excess of what is considered usual and customary for the final payment can be subject to review by a professional nurse, the medical director, and at times a peer reviewer. Peer review of claims is used to make recommendations for any service that is not indicated by the standards of medical care in the area. The claims review process strives to identify and then eliminate factors that are impediments to its goals and objectives:

- Overutilization of health care facilities or services by enrollees or providers
- Practice patterns, on the part of either the individual provider or group practice, that do not meet the community standards for quality care

- Unreasonable fees charged by practitioners
- Unfounded accusations against practitioners
- Underutilization of health care facilities or professional services

If issues are identified, the claim will be subject to a referral to the quality department for further investigation and reporting.

QUALITY STUDIES

Most MCOs have processes in place through their quality review departments to conduct studies that validate their actions toward quality of care and reduction of costs. For example, the study might be done to establish whether trends exist or to identify opportunities for improvement. If during the review processes, aberrations in physician practices are discovered, a physician might be placed under review. If it is found that his or her services are performed in excess of acceptable practice patterns, sanctions might be imposed on the physician under review. The same is true if it is discovered that the physician's practice patterns are below the standards desired for quality. In cases such as this, the ultimate consequence might be that the physician is sanctioned or terminated.

EMERGENCY SERVICES

As a result of the enactment of Emergency Medical Treatment and Active Labor Act (EMTALA) and its requirements to ensure antidumping, many states follow "prudent layperson language." Because the "prudent layperson" now has the ability to use emergency services without question, many organizations are struggling with how to handle the volume of claims related to emergency care.

A prudent layperson is considered to be a person who has no medical training and draws on his or her practical experience when making a decision regarding whether emergency medical treatment is needed. A prudent layperson is considered to have acted "reasonably" if other similarly situated laypersons would have believed, on the basis of observation of the medical symptoms at hand, that emergency medical treatment was necessary. Basically according to the prudent layperson definition, a person can seek medical care from any provider without prior authorization if he or she believes that life or limb is in danger.

According to the prudent layperson requirements, the MCO must pay for all costs necessary to perform the initial medical evaluation, including all tests and services ordered. Reimbursement must continue up to and including the decision-making processes (e.g., if an ECG or x-ray film is ordered but the interpretation is not immediately ready) until the patient is medically stable and requires admission or discharge. If treatment that could have been performed in an alternate setting is continued in the ED, this portion of the claim can be denied as not medically necessary. However, if the patient is an MCO member, he or she cannot be balance-billed, and the provider is the one who must assume the costs when such denials are issued.

With this in mind, most ED claims are processed according to CMS's guidelines or codes for what constitutes an emergent medical event. The system is also set up to allow for the smooth processing of at least the medical screening examination portion of the claim. A claim will be suspended for manual review when it contains codes for continued medical treatments that may not be medically necessary in the ED but could be performed at an alternate care site.

The biggest issue found with ED claims is upcoding. This is a process used by the ED physicians and claims billers to maximize reimbursement. The provider uses higher codes for the services rendered.

Consequently, many claims then require manual review to ensure all codes match the documented record of events as listed in the patient's ED medical record. The explosion of ED use is causing many organizations to review their processes and seek legal assistance as they develop policies, procedures, strategies, and processes to educate members of what constitutes emergency care versus urgent and routine care.

Historically, many organizations have used techniques such as frequent flyer mailers and frequent flyer call-back programs in their attempts to control ED use. What worked then may not work now; therefore the case manager should be aware of his or her organization's processes for dealing with frequent flyers or persons who use the ED frequently and inappropriately. This is important so as not to place the organization in a legal situation, or possibly worse yet, cause withdrawal of a large employer group's members because of complaints and issues raised by members as they relate to ED use.

CLAIMS INFORMATION

Claims are the bills submitted by providers to obtain payment. A claim form will identify at a minimum the following:

- Provider (name, address, license number)
- Member (name, address, date of birth, policyholder)
- Date, and at times, the actual time the services were rendered
- Diagnosis (coded)
- Services or procedures rendered (coded)

Claims are submitted in three common formats:

- **UB 92**—Hospitals and other institutional providers of inpatient services primarily use this form.
- **HCFA 1500**—This form is used by physicians and ancillary providers and for outpatient billing.

- **Super Bill**—Although less common because it does not capture the data often required by employers or for quality tracking and reporting, a super bill might be used by office-based physicians. This form is designed for ease of use, since it is preprinted and contains check-off boxes for the procedures and diagnosis. Each box is precoded for both the diagnosis and procedures (e.g., *ICD-9* for the diagnosis, *CPT* and *RBRVS* for procedures), and each box for a procedure performed lists a charge.

To assist with processing claims, a coding system is used to convey clinical and billing information. The standardized and universal codes used by providers are as follows:

- **UB-92 codes**—These identify the specific hospital department that provided the service.
- **ICD-9 codes** (*International Classification of Disease, Ninth Revision*)—These identify the diagnosis, and although not as common, can identify procedures.
- **DRGs**—This is a set of 468 codes used by Medicare to bill for hospital services by categorizing the patient by diagnosis and resources consumed.
- **RBRVS (resource-based relative value scale)**—This is another set of codes used by the Medicare program to bill for physician services.
- **CPT-4** (*Current Procedural Terminology, 4th Edition*)—This is the most recognized system for coding professional services and procedures.

AUTO-ADJUDICATION

Since many referrals and procedures require prior authorization, the organization's claims system will be linked to the prior authorization system, membership, and provider databases. To expedite claims processing an "auto-adjudication" process is used. Basically, as claims are processed, the information submitted will be data-entered (keyed), and then an automated search of the organization's databases will be conducted. In most cases this includes a search of the following:

- Membership database to validate that the member was eligible on the date the services were performed. If the member is not eligible, the claims processing stops here and the claim will be denied.
- Prior authorization system to ensure the service billed was authorized, or if not, whether it is one that does not require prior authorization or further review. It is also used to ensure that what was prior-authorized is what is billed.
- Provider database to validate provider eligibility or that the provider is not one whose claims require additional review.
- Claims database to ensure the present claim is not a duplicate claim that has previously been processed and paid.
- Claims database to ensure the diagnosis and procedure codes and sex of member are not mismatched (e.g., cardiac diagnosis, but the procedure billed was for a laminectomy; or, a sex-specific procedure is listed but the patient is of the opposite sex).

If no errors are found and no additional review of the claim is required, the claim will be processed smoothly and paid.

RETROACTIVE PROCESSING

An issue that stalls service, claims processing, or assignment to a provider is retroactivity. Retroactivity is the by-product of the lack of timely submission of data by the employer (e.g., enrollment applications,

COBRA, or terminations). In some cases this process will cause all services to be suspended for up to 90 days; thus, the person will be listed as not eligible for services that might have been otherwise prior-approved and rendered, and any care or services needed will cease until eligibility is proven.

Consequently, as MCOs train their prior authorization staff, it is important to have them say, "Prior authorization is contingent upon eligibility at the time of service." If the patient is eligible but not showing as such, tremendous collaboration is required until the issue of eligibility is resolved. Therefore one may need to work not only with the MCO's enrollment unit but also with member services staff, the sales staff, and the employer's personnel department. In the case of COBRA, patients often do not understand the importance of this benefit or of enrollment within any deadlines and paying the premiums on time. Thus they can be caught in a nightmare of needing services but having no health care coverage.

PREDICTING CLAIMS COSTS

Incurred but not reported (IBNR) claims tracking is a process used to forecast future claims expenses. IBNR tacking is necessary when a person has already received the care but the claim has not been received by the insurer. The period between the two is referred to as *claims lag*. Most providers want to be paid as soon as possible. However, with some providers' billing practices, it takes several months before the claim is submitted and processed. In these scenarios if the member is indeed eligible for services at the time the services were rendered, the insurer remains responsible for paying the claim.

Why are IBNRs tracked? The basic reason is simple—so the MCO can anticipate future expenses and have enough money to pay for the claims as they come due. One method of tracking IBNRs is using esti-

mates based on previous claims cost per member per month for the various services typically reimbursed by the MCO. The second method is using the prior authorization system and the number of authorizations issued for specific services and putting a value on the services. Most organizations use both methods in tracking and forecasting future claims expenses.

OTHER TECHNIQUES USED TO REDUCE AN MCO's EXPENSES

Coordination of Benefits

COB is by far the most important means to ensure the organization's claims expenses are kept to a minimum. The purpose of the COB program is to identify the health benefits available to a member, determine whether there is other insurance, and then coordinate the payment processing between the two insurers. The COB program involves the collection, management, and reporting of other insurance coverage. Information on eligibility and benefits entitlement is obtained from the COB central file and is used to facilitate accurate payment from each insurer.

COB applies to those cases in which a person has more than one insurer or another insurer is responsible for payment of the claims. Under COB rules, if the person has more than one insurance, the COB process prevents providers from being paid twice or patients from collecting the difference. When a person has two or more insurance policies, MCOs and insurers follow what are called *COB rules* for claims payment. The primary insurer pays according to the extent of benefits offered or the order in which the insured has coverage and then the secondary insurer picks up any differences.

THIRD-PARTY LIABILITY

Many cases in case management will fall under what is termed *third-party liability*

(TPL) for payment of the claims. In other cases the cost of care should be covered by workers' compensation (WC) because the injury occurred while the person was employed. The reason is the catastrophic event and resultant care was the result of a third-party injury or event. Therefore the charges related to care would be the responsibility of the other insurer and not the patient's primary health insurer.

TPL issues arise when the injury is caused by an automobile or other motor vehicular accident, when an injury occurs on another person's or place of business's property, or when work-related injuries occur during work hours for the employee.

Insurers and claims processing units have processes in place to monitor TPL cases. This is necessary, because it is a way to recoup expenses of providing care to the member when it is not the insurer's responsibility to assume such costs. If a person is covered by TPL, the insurer will have processes in place to identify such cases, place a lien on any further settlements, and recoup any claims costs once the settlement is reached. Unfortunately, the down side of TPL is the fact that many patients may have settled their claims long before the event is known to the primary health insurer; in some cases the settlement money has already been spent by the patient, and any ongoing medical care required becomes the responsibility of the health insurer.

In the event a case is the result of a TPL incident or WC event, the patient's primary health insurer remains responsible for all costs of care and services until the TPL or WC carrier acknowledges the event as its responsibility. Unfortunately, with TPL, the MCO can only recoup its losses after the TPL carrier settles the issue with the patient. In the case of WC, although the MCO may not have to wait until the claim is settled, the MCO remains responsible for all care until the employee files a first report of injury and the WC carrier deter-

mines the case is its responsibility. These two points are very critical when case managing a catastrophic case, and it is imperative that the case manager work closely with the claims processing unit to identify such cases as early as possible. For WC cases, the case manager may have to assume responsibility for educating the patient about the benefits of filing for WC.

BIRTHDAY RULE

The birthday rule is an important rule used by insurers to determine which plan pays first when a person has dual insurance (e.g., covered by both the mother and father). Under the birthday rule, the birthdays of both parents are considered, and the person with the first birthday in the *calendar* is designated as the primary insurer. Note, it does not matter which parent is older, since the *year* of birth is not a factor. Thus if one person's birthday is July 15, 1955, and the other's is September 17, 1953, the person with the birthday on July 15 would be considered the primary insurer because this birthday comes first in the calendar year.

OTHER COVERAGE RULES (NON-MEDICARE)

- **Same birthdays**—If both parents or spouses happen to have the same birthday, the plan that has covered one of the parents or spouses longer pays first.
- **Divorce or separation**—When two or more plans cover children as dependents when the parents are divorced or separated, if the divorce decree does not specify whose insurance is to pay first, the plan of the parent who has custody pays first. If a court has issued a divorce decree stipulating that one of the parents is more responsible for the health care expenses of the children than the

other parent, regardless of custody, the responsible parent's plan pays first. A divorce decree of this type supercedes the birthday rule. Therefore that parent's insurance is the primary insurer until the child reaches the age of 18 years or the maximum age stipulated by the insurer for cessation of insurance benefits (e.g., the child needs insurance because he or she is a full-time student and is covered under the other parent's insurance until age 23; if the child remains a full-time student, this parent's insurance would assume responsibility for coverage).

- **Active employees**—If the person is currently employed and has health insurance through his or her employer and the spouse also has coverage through a former employer (e.g., COBRA) and the children are listed as dependents on both plans, the employed person's plan would be considered primary.
- **Different plan types**—If the parents have two different types of health plans, the rules are also different. For example, if one person has a group health plan and the other has an individual plan, the group health plan pays first regardless of the birthday rule.
- **Coverage by more than one health plan**—It is common to find persons covered by more than one health plan. In most cases the person insured through their employer will be the subscriber, and this plan will be primary for this person. If this same subscriber is also covered as a dependent under another insurance, the second insurance will be the secondary insurer. Coverage by more than one health plan is a common practice, particularly for children of divorced parents. In these cases coverage is taken out by both parties to

maximize benefits. In the case of divorce, dual coverage might be in place to ensure the children are covered when visiting the noncustodial parent, especially when the custodial parent lives in another state. This is important because if one insurance is linked to an HMO in one state, the children will covered for only emergency care and will not be covered for any routine care while visiting the noncustodial parent.

- **None of the above**—When none of these rules determines the issue, the plan of the parent who has been covered longer is designated as primary.

MEDICARE COVERAGE RULES

For full specifics and details about Medicare coverage rules, please see CMS's website, www.cms.hhs.gov. Basically the rules are as follows:

- Employers must offer employees and their spouses who are 65 years of age or older Medicare coverage. The coverage must be the same as that offered to all employees and their spouses and dependents. The employer cannot deny a person coverage, nor can the employer offer a different set of or reduced benefits.
- If the person has Medicare (for a person older than 65 years as well as the disabled younger than 65 years) and either that person or his or her spouse continues to work, the employer provides group health insurance, and the employer has 20 or more employees, the employer group coverage will be primary. However, if the spouse or person covered by Medicare rejects the group health plan, Medicare is the primary insurer and there is no secondary insurer to serve as a Medicare supplement.

- If the employer has fewer than 20 employees, Medicare will pay as primary insurer.
- If the person is covered by Medicare and a group health plan as well but is working and is injured on the job, WC will always be primary.
- If the person has Medicare through the End-Stage Renal Disease (ESRD) Program, this is a separate program with specific criteria for eligibility. For specific details, see CMS's website at www.cms.hhs.gov. However, under the ESRD program, Medicare will begin in the third month of dialysis or within the same month that a person is admitted to a hospital for a kidney transplant. Basically, the ESRD program follows the same Medicare rules as listed above for determining the primary versus the secondary insurer.

NONCLAIMS TECHNIQUES TO CONTROL COSTS

In addition to utilization controls, MCOs use a variety of processes to contain costs. These efforts include activities such as the following:

- Preventive health services
- Use of PCPs as gatekeepers
- Case management
- Drug formulary
- Telephone advice lines health education
- Health education

Preventive Care Services

Since many MCOs target young healthy working people and many federal and large employers or purchasers require preventive services as part of the contractual negotiations, many organizations offer a variety of preventive care services to enrollees of the MCO. To ensure they are following guidelines, most MCOs follow the recommendations as outlined by the

U.S. Preventive Services Task Force. For guidelines see either of the following websites: www.ahrq.gov/c or www.odphp.osophs.dhhs.gov/pubs/guidecps/.

Health Education

As indicated earlier, health education is a technique used by many MCOs to encourage members to adopt a healthier lifestyle, take an active role in disease prevention, or in the case of an already diagnosed disease, a more active role in self-management and compliance. The scope of the health education programs offered depends on the organization's size, large purchaser demands, contractual requirements, and any state statutes on the issue.

Case Management

Case management can be thought of as an intensive, long-term, and concurrent review process for patients with complex medical diagnoses or those with long-term high-cost or high-risk needs. Case management as a tool for cost containment focuses on the following[4]:

- Prevention of readmissions
- Identification of new problems before they become serious
- Optimization of care while controlling costs
- Restoration of a patient's preillness level of functioning

Primary Care Physician as Gatekeeper

This has already been discussed in this section. Using the PCP as gatekeeper is an old technique that has been used by MCOs for years. In the role of gatekeeper, the PCP must make recommendations for all referrals to specialty services, for inpatient care, and some ancillary services.

Use of the PCP as a gatekeeper is one of the primary reasons cited by consumers for managed care backlash. For example, consumers believe they do not always receive the care that is necessary or they believe the PCP delays their care when a specialist might handle it more efficiently. Unfortunately, although the PCP should only manage those cases for which he or she is trained, if compensation is linked to incentive withholds or other bonus-type incentives, the PCP might keep the patient under his or her care too long before a referral is granted. A good reference on the tasks traditionally assigned to a PCP is Milliman and Robertson's physician guidelines, which can be found on their website at www.milliman.com or obtained by calling any of their main offices located throughout the United States.

Drug Formulary

A method used by MCOs to help in their control of pharmacy costs is the use of what is called a *drug formulary*. Although an MCO may offer this function, in most instances, it will be the HMO that retains this task, dictating what drugs will or will not be covered, as well as the patient's copayments. A drug formulary is a list of drugs that the MCO or HMO has determined it will allow to be prescribed for its members. The formulary is developed through use of a committee that comprises members of the MCO's or HMO's contracted pharmaceutical network, the medical director, and a mix of contracted network primary care and specialty physicians.

The task of the committee is to review the literature on new drugs and make a determination of the advantages and disadvantages of the new drugs' use versus those on the current formulary. Drugs are chosen for the formulary based on drug standards, Food and Drug Administration approval, efficacy, effectiveness, safety, and cost. In most cases the formulary will contain a number of drugs that can be used to treat a given condition, but those drugs may not be equally effective and they may have different side effects and costs as well. The formulary is also used when the MCO

or HMO requires certain generic drugs be substituted for their respective brand-name equivalents. With the cost of drugs skyrocketing, many MCOs and HMOs are leaning toward a policy of all generic drugs, or they have gone to a tiered system for copayments for various drugs. In essence, the higher the tier or cost, the higher is the copayment.

In addition to a drug formulary, some organizations have what is called an *open formulary*. If the drug is not on the formulary, a physician may request prior authorization of the drug. The drug can only be approved if the physician submits the required medical justification that validates the reasons that the current formulary drug is not effective. If the MCO or HMO maintains a closed formulary (or in some cases, an employer group may request it), this generally means no exceptions are permitted.

Another way to contain pharmacy costs is through the development of a mail-order pharmacy program. Although is set up to serve the member because it allows a 90-day supply of medications with a reduced copayment and direct mailing to a member's home, it also serves the MCO or HMO, since pharmacy operating costs can be lowered. Costs are lowered because the costs for staffing to refill prescriptions are lowered (rather than the prescription being filled three times in three months, there is one fill for the full 90 days).

Telephone Advice Lines

Some larger MCOs offer telephone advice line services. If an advice line is used, many MCOs require all callers to be screened by advice nurses before any appointments are made or any services are activated. Others use their advice lines for after-hours triage or for appropriate direction of members to services. The advice lines are offered directly through the MCO and its nurses or through contracts with companies specializing in telephone medical advice. In most cases advice lines are used to help members decide whether their symptoms require immediate medical attention. In many organizations, they are used as an attempt to keep ED use to a minimum.

When an advice line is used, it is staffed by registered nurses who practice under the direction of physicians, using very strict policies, procedures, and other criteria. The main task of the nurse is to help the caller separate routine issues from urgent or emergent ones. To do this, most advice lines require the use of criteria scripts for specific symptoms. From a script, the nurse can query the caller about symptoms, treatments rendered, and the responses to the treatments. From the caller's answers to the questions and description of the symptoms and events, the nurse is able to recommend the appropriate course of action (i.e., the nurse may call the on-call PCP, send the patient directly to the ED, give specific directions for at-home care, or advise the caller to seek medical care the next business day). Advice lines have two key advantages: (1) control of costs through the reduction of unnecessary emergency and urgent care use and (2) benefits to the caller. The benefits to the caller are personal attention, reassurance, and appropriate referral or directions for care for the issue at hand.

The inherent danger found with managed care and the variants used to control costs and reduce unnecessary utilization and costs—discounts, utilization management, restricted provider, autonomy risk contracts, capitation, and restricted access—is that many methods are designed to promote undertreatment and may at times limit access to necessary care. As a result of consumer backlash to managed care, purchasers, insurers, and regulators are increasingly demanding that providers develop policies and procedures for ensuring adequate quality: providers are expected to explain their quality processes,

how they are monitored, what they do when issues are discovered, and how they justify expenditures.

SUMMARY

Understanding the basics of health insurance and how services are paid is of key importance to case management. This is necessary because cases under case management could have more than one payer, and many payers use a managed care process in their attempts to control costs. It is also important because some patients will have insurance that is quickly exhausted or has limited or excluded benefits.

The HMO Act of 1973 changed health care by introducing managed care and a totally different way of paying for services and care. As managed care has evolved through the years, so have the processes and the ways care can be managed. Care is now offered from a variety of approaches —all with the intent of controlling soaring health care costs.

The initial focus of cost containment, in earlier models of managed care, was on cost-sharing and price negotiation. However, neither appreciably slowed the demand for services. This is in part due to increased consumer demand for more expensive care and a lack of knowledge or willingness, on the part of both the provider and the patient, to seek alternatives.

For containment of costs in the future, the focus of managed care will be on appropriate utilization and the effectiveness and efficiency of providers. This means the major players in the field—the government, all insurers and health plans, hospitals, physicians, suppliers, employers, and health and welfare trust funds—must reassess their willingness to compromise and make different trade-offs to frame a unified approach to dampening cost escalation while preserving "controlled access" and quality of care. This will require participating in rigorous programs, evaluations, audits, and quality assurance reviews and then acting on the findings in a meaningful way.[2]

The power of large employer groups cannot be underestimated. Because large employers control large numbers of an MCO's membership, they often demand that the MCO be held accountable for the health care services provided. More important, they are demanding that MCOs demonstrate and prove the value they bring to the marketplace. This must be done by providing the purchaser with more data in areas such as employee utilization, member satisfaction, and quality measures such as HEDIS reporting. Many large employers have their own formats for monitoring and reporting data and results. If not, they may use those developed by NCQA or consulting firms.

These same employer purchasers use these data to evaluate an MCO's ability to provide care, control costs, and prove the value of the premium dollars spent. In addition to this, many large employer groups use large auditing firms to annually audit an MCO's performance, policies, procedures, processes, and compliance with the contractual agreement. Plans that cannot meet these demands are at a competitive disadvantage.

Although their actions are not as strong as their philosophy, large employer purchasers are gradually moving away from buying health care based strictly on price. In addition to incorporating different factors in the decision-making process about what to buy and on what terms, purchasers are also starting to reduce the number of health care plans to cut administrative costs, gain efficiency in procurement, and increase control over health plan or vendor performance. By reducing the number of health plans, large purchasers can leverage their purchasing power and increase their market share. Some of the factors used by large pur-

chasers as they evaluate a health plan for inclusion in their employee benefits package are as follows[2]:

- Management experience
- Financial solvency
- Administrative flexibility
- Controls used to detect unnecessary utilization while ensuring quality
- Ability to provide meaningful utilization data, client reports, and quality data
- Capacity to meet the service needs of local company managers
- Ease of implementation and claims administration
- Willingness to stand behind their product with rate and performance guarantees

Chapter Exercises

1. Review the HMO Act of 1973 and list the requirements of a federally qualified HMO.
2. List the differences between a PPO, an indemnity insurance company, an EPO, and an MCO.
3. List at least three mechanisms used by MCOs to control costs.

Suggested Websites and Resources

www.insure.com/about.html—A website dedicated to information about health insurance

www.cms.hhs.gov—Centers for Medicare & Medicaid Services

www.census.gov/Press-Release/ inpovtab3a.html—U.S. Census Bureau

www.milliman.com—Milliman and Robertson website

www.ahrq.gov—Agency For Healthcare Research and Quality

www.odphp.osophs.dhhs.gov/pubs/guidecps/— Department of Health and Human

Services website for Preventive Health Services

www.urac.org—American Accreditation Healthcare Commission for Utilization Review

www.NCQA.org—National Committee for Quality Assurance

www.aahp.org—American Association of Health Plans (AAHP)

www.interqual.com—InterQual website

www.jcaho.org—JCAHO website

REFERENCES

1. Kirk R: *Managing outcomes process and cost in a managed care environment,* Gaithersburg, Md, 1997, Aspen.
2. Boland P: *Making managed care work: a practical guide to strategies and solutions,* Gaithersburg, Md, 1993, Aspen.
3. Kongstvedt PR: *The managed care handbook,* ed 2, Gaithersburg, Md, 1993, Aspen.
4. Jones RW: *HMO 101: introduction to HMOs,* ed 2, Colorado Springs, Colo, 1997, TTM Health Publishing.

Medicare and Medicaid

Peggy A. Rossi, BSN, MPA, CCM, CPUR

OBJECTIVES

■ To be able to differentiate between the benefits allowed by Medicare Part A and Part B and benefits allowed by Medicare + Choice

■ To be able to identify the primary law of 1997 that changed Medicare and now allows a structured managed care approach

■ To be able to identify the key organization responsible for the running and oversight of the Medicare program

■ To be able to list the basic eligibility categories of Medicaid and the criteria for eligibility for each

■ To be able to list the core benefits of Medicaid and optional benefits offered by most states

■ To be able to describe the Medicaid managed care requirements

■ To be able to describe the mechanism to measure quality of Medicaid managed care plans

MEDICARE

Title XVIII of the Social Security Act of 1965 created Medicare. The original intent of Medicare was to provide health care coverage for persons older than 65 years. Since its inception, Medicare has undergone multiple changes. Over the years, eligibility requirements have changed, and Medicare now covers persons younger than 65 years, if they meet the Social Security Administration's (SSA's) eligibility requirements. In recent years the most drastic changes to Medicare occurred under the Balanced Budget Act (BBA) of 1997. Under the BBA, the law now allows what is called *Medicare + Choice (M+C)*, a health maintenance organization (HMO) option for some Medicare beneficiaries who reside in specific areas of the United States. Another result of the act was that the payment methods used by Medicare were changed.

Medicare provides coverage for approximately 40 million people older than 65 years, as well as for persons younger than 65 years who meet the SSA's definition of disability. Medicare pays for most of the costs associated with acute-care hospitals and about one half of all other health care expenses.[1] Because it is a federal program, the basic benefits and eligibility are consistent nationwide. Medicare is divided into two parts, Medicare Part A and Medicare Part B. Part A is the hospital portion and pays for acute care and skilled nursing facility (SNF) care. Part B is the supplemental portion and pays for physician charges and outpatient and other ancillary charges.

Medicare is operated in cooperation with the SSA and by a division of the Department of Health and Human Services and the Centers for Medicare & Medicaid Services (CMS). Although the CMS (formerly the Health Care Financing Administration [HCFA]) allows HMOs to administer Medicare benefits under the M+C program, it is important for a case manager to understand the basics of the Medicare program as a whole. This is necessary for two primary reasons: (1) Medicare coverage guidelines are used as the basis for most insurance coverage guidelines and decisions (i.e., if coverage is allowed by Medicare, other private health insurers follow suit); and (2) although some persons will be eligible for the M+C program, the HMO can enhance benefits but cannot eliminate the core or basic benefits allowed by the basic Medicare program.

As indicated, with the enactment of the BBA, Medicare changed its HMO options title to M+C. As a result, organizations that want to offer this program are referred to as *Medicare + Choice organizations (M+COs)*. The new name is simply an umbrella title for the options now available to Medicare beneficiaries. In addition to the new + Choice option, several changes also occurred in the payment mechanism used by Medicare. As the new payment structure is implemented over the next few years, it will basically impose a prospective payment system for reimbursement to almost all levels and types of providers.

The original form of Medicare, which is still around, is known as *fee-for-service* (FFS). This means Medicare pays a set fee for each service, if the provider is a participating provider with the Medicare program. If the participating provider does not accept what Medicare allows, the patient must pay the difference between what was billed and what was paid, as well as any copayments or deductibles. For example, if the provider does not accept Medicare assignment (the amount that Medicare recognizes as what it will pay) and the provider bills $125 but Medicare only pays $57 of the claim, the patient is responsible for the difference, or $68. Most people with FFS Medicare have three choices:

1. Remain responsible for the out-of-pocket differences and find a way to pay the costs
2. Purchase a supplemental health insurance policy (called *medigap insurance*) that pays most or all of the difference
3. If eligible, qualify for their state's Medicaid program (in most cases, this means the patient must have low income and few liquid assets)

Because Medicare is such an important program, it is wise to keep the phone numbers in Box 6-1 handy should questions arise.

OVERVIEW OF THE BASIC MEDICARE PROGRAM

Eligibility

Most persons older than 65 years are automatically covered by Medicare Part A, which is the premium-free portion of Medicare. This occurs when they are entitled to retirement benefits from Social Security, the Railroad Retirement Fund, or a federal civil service retirement program. The two largest categories of persons eligible for benefits are as follows:

BOX 6-1
Key Phone Numbers

Medicare—800-633-4227 or TTY/TTD:
    877-486-2048
Railroad Retirement Board—800-808-0772
Social Security Administration—800-772-1213
Office of Personnel Management—
    888-767-6738
Veterans Affairs—800-827-1000
Department of Defense—800-538-9552

■ Persons who are eligible for Social Security retirement benefits or who have civil service or railroad retirement credits equal to an amount that would have made them eligible for Social Security retirement. Although a person can use retirement benefits before the age of 65 years, Medicare insurance does not start until he or she reaches the age of 65 years.

■ Persons who are eligible to collect Social Security benefits as a dependent or survivor. This means the dependent is older than 65 years but the actual worker or subscriber, who paid into Social Security or the Railroad Retirement Fund, might only be 62 years old and might not have actually filed a claim for retirement benefits.

Other categories include the following:

■ Persons who reached age 65 years before January 1, 1968, even if they are not eligible for Social Security benefits, but who are United States citizens or have lawfully resided in the United States or its territories for 5 consecutive years immediately before applying for Medicare (this means they cannot have a break in residence before their application).

■ Persons, regardless of age, who have been entitled to Social Security disability benefits for the required time (generally 24 months, but this period varies for some diagnoses such as quadriplegia and amyotrophic lateral sclerosis).

■ Persons who have permanent kidney failure, requiring either a kidney transplant or maintenance dialysis, and either they or their spouse has worked at a job covered by Social Security or Railroad Retirement

■ Persons who participated in a state, county, or nonprofit retirement plan but who did not pay into Social Security might also be eligible (if a person falls into this category, the case manager must direct the person to the nearest Social Security office for help).

■ Dependents and spouses. A person's eligibility could be based on the work history of a spouse or parent (again, if a person falls into this category, the case manager must direct the person to the nearest Social Security office for help).

Applications

Application for Medicare is made at the same time as application for retirement benefits. For benefits to start on time, this must be done approximately 3 months before the person's 65th birthday. Even though some people continue working after their 65th birthdays, they are still eligible to receive the free Medicare Part A benefits if they have an application on file with the SSA. Although a person can apply for retirement benefits earlier than age 65 years, Medicare eligibility will not start until he or she reaches the age of 65 years.

If the person is disabled and younger than 65 years, he or she must prove disability and remain disabled for 24 months before he or she will qualify for Medicare. The disability process takes at least 5 months from application to an initial determination that a person qualifies for Social Security Disability Income (SSDI). If eligible for SSDI, the person will not be eligible for Medicare for 24 months. Consequently, the person must pay privately, rely on private health care insurance, or qualify for Medicaid. As indicated previously, the only three exceptions to the 24-month waiting period are for quadriplegia, amyotrophic lateral sclerosis, and end-stage renal disease (ESRD). For persons with ESRD, eligibility for Medicare starts after the third month of dialysis or during hospitalization for kidney transplantation.

Enrolling in Part B

Medicare Part B, also known as *supplementary medical insurance*, provides optional additional coverage for doctors' visits and other outpatient services such as those provided by physician assistants, nurse practitioners, and clinical laboratories. Most people can be eligible for at least Part B; however, they must enroll and pay a monthly premium.

Many patients with Medicare Part B will also have Medicaid or other insurance. This is necessary because Part B does not cover hospitalizations. If the patient is hospitalized, Medicaid will be the insurer for any inpatient hospital services and any deductibles or copayments. Once the patient is discharged, Part B will pay for physicians' visits and other services the patient may require.

Enrolling When Not Eligible for Social Security

If a person is not eligible for Social Security benefits, he or she can purchase both parts of Medicare insurance through the local Social Security office. The person must pay a steep monthly premium for Medicare Part A and the monthly premiums for Part B. The amount of the premiums depends on the person's or his or her spouse's work credits with Social Security. If the person elects to purchase Medicare, he or she has the option of purchasing only Medicare Part B. However, if the person elects to purchase Medicare Part A, he or she must also purchase Part B, which has an additional premium.

Enrollment is limited to a period that extends for 7 months. The enrollment period begins 3 months before the person turns 65 years and ends 3 months after the month in which he or she turns 65 years. Therefore if the person enrolls during the first 3-month period, Medicare will start on his or her 65th birthday. If the person waits and enrolls toward the end of the 7-month period, Medicare will be delayed by 2 to 3 months.

If the person does not sign up for Medicare by age 65 years or during the

7-month period allowed, he or she must wait until the next general enrollment period, which is January 1 to March 31 of each year. If the person signs up during this enrollment period, Medicare will not start until July 1 of that year. In addition to waiting, the person is penalized by the fact that Part B premiums will be 10% higher.

Deductibles and Coinsurance

As indicated earlier, once enrolled in Medicare, the Medicare beneficiary will be faced with not only monthly and annual premiums or deductibles but other copayments and out-of-pocket expenses. Basic Medicare deductibles and coinsurance rates are as follows:

- **Deductible**—Medicare Part A is deductible-free. However, there is a $100 annual deductible for Medicare Part B.
- **Coinsurance**—Medicare Part A has a hefty coinsurance rate that is paid as a one-time fee at the time of admission to an acute-care hospital and the start of each benefit period (see Benefit Periods). If the patient requires a continued stay beyond 60 days, there is a daily coinsurance rate that is due for each day the patient stays up to and including the 150th day. Patients obtaining services under Medicare Part B have a 20% coinsurance payment due for almost all services.

Financial Help with Premiums and Other Medicare Charges

Under programs known as *Qualified Medicare Beneficiary (QMB)*, *Specified Low-Income Medicare Beneficiary (SLMB)*, and *Qualifying Individual (QI) Medicare*, beneficiaries who have low income and few assets may receive help with their basic Medicare expenses. For example, if a person qualifies for QMB Medicare, the state pays all Medicare premiums, coinsurance, and deductibles. If a person qualifies for

SLMB Medicare, the state pays the monthly Medicare Part B premiums but not any coinsurance or deductibles. Finally, if a person qualifies for QI Medicare, the state pays a portion of the Medicare Part B premium but no coinsurance or deductibles. Table 6-1 presents examples of income qualifications and the programs and amounts paid. For more information on these programs see the SSA's website at www.ssa.gov/notices/supplemental-secur. Note that these programs are not available outside the United States.

Medicare Card

When a person is enrolled in Medicare, he or she will receive a red, white, and blue card. This card lists several pieces of valuable information such as the following:

- Name

- Whether person has Medicare Part A and Part B, just Part A, or just Part B
- The effective date of Medicare coverage
- The claim number, which is the person's Social Security number followed by one or two letters of the alphabet

Unfortunately, many Californians are confused when they read their cards because they believe the part that says "Medical" Insurance means they have Medi-Cal coverage as well.

When Do Benefits Begin?

Once the application is processed, Medicare Part A benefits will start within 6 months after the person turns 65 years. However, if the person applies after his or her 65th birthday, coverage only dates back

---

TABLE 6-1
Examples of Programs for Which a Low-Income Beneficiary Might Qualify

Monthly Income (2000)	Program Name	Program Pays
$716 individual or $958 couple	Qualified Medicare Beneficiary (QMB)	Premiums, deductibles, and coinsurance. States have the option to pay HMO premiums, if the beneficiary is enrolled in an M+CO.
$855 individual or $1145 couple	Specified Low-Income Medicare Beneficiary (SLMB)	Medicare Part B premiums, any extra M+C premiums, deductibles, or copayments if the beneficiary has elected an M+CO.
$960 individual or $1286 couple	Qualifying Individual (QI-1)	Medicare Part B premiums and any extra M+C premiums, deductibles, or copayments if the beneficiary has elected an M+CO.
$1238 individual or $1661 couple	Qualifying Individual (QI-2)	A small part of the Medicare Part B premiums but only the portion of the Part B premium that finances home health costs; does not pay Part A premiums or any extra M+C premiums, deductibles, or copayments.
$1392 individual or $1809 couple	QDWI-Qualified Disabled Working Individual	Pays Part A premium, once it starts being charged to those who've completed their trial work periods and extended periods of eligibility (after 99 months back-to-work); does not pay Part B premium, any extra M+C premiums, or any deductibles, or copayments.

HMO, Health maintenance organization; *M+C,* Medicare + Choice; *M+CO,* Medicare + Choice organization.

to 6 months from the date of application. If a person continues to work after age 65 years but defers Social Security retirement benefits, he or she is still entitled to Medicare Part A benefits, if an application is on file with the local Social Security office. As indicated previously, for persons younger than 65 years, Medicare is based on disability, and Medicare coverage starts after they have received SSDI for 24 months.

If a person is covered by a group health plan, based either on his or her own or a spouse's current employment, he or she can enroll in Part B after his or her 65th birthday, and this can be done without penalty or having to wait for the next open enrollment period. A person can delay signing up for Medicare Part B if he or she is already covered by a health plan. Thus a person can sign up for Medicare Part B at any time while covered by the health plan or within 7 months of the date he or she or a spouse ends employment or the health plan coverage is terminated, whichever comes first. Benefits of signing up early are listed in Box 6-2.

Benefit Periods

A key feature of FFS Medicare Part A is its benefit periods. This may be the most difficult part of the Medicare program to explain to patients and families.

Under FFS Medicare Part A, a patient's inpatient hospital days are divided into benefit periods. If a patient continues to

---

BOX 6-2
Benefits of Signing Up Early for Medicare Part B

1. It ensures the coverage will start as soon as the person is 65 years old.
2. If the person waits more than 3 months after his or her 65th birthday to enroll in Part B, he or she must wait until the following open enrollment period (January 1 through March 31), but eligibility will not start until July 1.

---

require skilled nursing care and requires hospitalization, he or she can be covered for a period of 150 days. The benefit periods are divided into three categories:

1. The first 60 days—one coinsurance rate
2. The 61st to 90th day—daily coinsurance rate
3. The 90th to 150th day—daily coinsurance rate

Each benefit period has a specific coinsurance rate, and amounts are adjusted annually. For full details on the coinsurance rates, please refer to a current Medicare handbook (updated annually). Medicare handbooks can be downloaded from Medicare's website at: www.Medicare.gov.

For the first 60 days, the coinsurance is a one-time payment, and after the coinsurance is paid, Medicare pays 100% of a patient's bill for the 60 days if the patient continues to require skilled nursing care or remains an inpatient in an acute-care facility. If the patient requires skilled care beyond the 60th day, the patient is responsible for a daily coinsurance rate until the 90th day, should he or she require inpatient care for this duration. If the patient requires skilled care that extends beyond the 90th day, he or she is given a one-time option to use his or her last set of 60 days, called *reserve days*. Although the first 90 days are renewable if the patient can remain out of a hospital or SNF for 60 consecutive days, the reserve days, or last set of 60 days, are not. Reserve days carry with them a steep daily coinsurance rate, and only 60 reserve days are granted to a Medicare beneficiary in his or her lifetime. An example of benefit days and the coinsurance rates follows.

Mary Jones falls and breaks her hip and is in an acute-care hospital for 5 days, paying her annual coinsurance rate (i.e., $768). On discharge, she is sent to an SNF for her continued rehabilitation therapy where she stays for 10 days (this is 10 days of her SNF benefit period—so is paid at

100% for her stay with no additional coinsurance payment). On the 10th day, she is sent to a board-and-care home but falls that very day and dislocates her newly repaired hip. Mary is sent back to the acute-care hospital, and instead of entering a new benefit period, she continues with the previous benefit period and her day count starts at day 6. Consequently, there is not another coinsurance amount due. During this hospitalization Mary has a stroke and multiple complications, resulting in an 8-week stay in the intensive care unit and the need for ventilatory assistance. By the start of her seventh week in the intensive care unit, Mary has exhausted her initial 60-day benefit period and has entered her next benefit period (30 days), which carries with it a daily coinsurance rate (i.e., $192). Mary's condition is finally stabilized medically, and she is weaned from the ventilator and sent to a nursing unit. Because her sputum is now testing positive for methicillin-resistant *Staphylococcus aureus* and she has multiple deficits, it is determined that she will require SNF care on discharge. Because the discharge planner is not able to locate an SNF that can manage her level of care, Mary remains an inpatient, continuing to pay her daily coinsurance rate (i.e., $384) until her 90th day. At this time, Mary's family is given the option of continued use of her benefit days, and they agree to use these days. So, Mary begins using her lifetime reserve days, paying a hefty daily coinsurance rate, until she dies on day 125.

Following the Rules

Medicare does not pay for services considered not medically necessary or not skilled. This includes many elective and cosmetic surgical procedures and alternative medicine options. It also does not cover providers who are not certified by Medicare.

Thus all care, whether rendered in an inpatient or outpatient setting, must be reasonable and necessary for the condition. This requirement automatically eliminates reconstructive or cosmetic surgery, if it is not related to an accident or disfiguring illness or injury. There is absolutely no coverage for custodial conditions, and this is probably the biggest area of confusion for patients and their families. The patient and family should have an understanding of custodial care and how it applies to the patient's situation. The case manager must educate the patient and family about the differences between skilled and custodial care, giving simple examples of each.

Reimbursement from Medicare can only occur if Medicare certifies and approves the agency or facility. To be approved, the provider must meet Medicare's standards for quality of care and staffing. It is rare to find a facility that is not certified by Medicare. If in doubt, the best place to look is the provider's admissions office.

Fortunately, most providers have their certifications and licensing information displayed in an open public place within their offices or facility. If there are further questions or concerns about the provider, the best place to turn will be the state agency responsible for licensing and certification. To locate providers who participate in the Medicare program see CMS's website at www.medicare.gov/Physician/.

In the case of transplants, Medicare only allows reimbursement if the transplant is done at one of the Medicare-approved centers. For more information on the centers that are approved, please see the following websites:

- Heart transplants—www.cms.hhs.gov/providers/transplant/hartlist.asp
- Heart and heart-lung transplants—www.cms.hhs.gov/providers/transplant/lunglist.asp
- Liver transplants—www.cms.hhs.gov/providers/transplant/livrlist.asp

■ Intestine transplants—www.cms. hhs.gov/providers/transplant/ intstnlist.asp

Medicare allows all patients to have access to emergency care nationwide. However, emergency care outside the United States and its territories is not a covered benefit. If the Medicare beneficiary is linked to an M+C plan, the law prohibits restrictions on the use of hospitals or physicians and allows the patient treatment in any emergency facility, regardless of whether the facility is a network provider for the M+CO. The law also prohibits the requirement of prior authorization from an M+CO's utilization department or the patient's primary care physician.

By law (laws vary by state), nonparticipating providers cannot bill a Medicare beneficiary any more than what is called *the limiting charge.* The limiting charge is set at 15% more than Medicare's approved charges. What does this mean? Although a patient can be charged the 20% difference between Medicare's approved amount and the provider's charge, he or she cannot be balance-billed any more than 15% of the amount the physician charges.

Table 6-2 illustrates the difference between a provider who accepts the Medicare assignment and one who does not. When working with Medicare patients, the case manager must educate them about the advantages of using providers that accept assignment. If a provider accepts assignment, although the patient will still remain responsible for the 20% coinsurance payment, he or she will not have any additional balances due. The primary disadvantage of case-managed cases is that many patients require specialty care, the one category in which providers are least likely to accept assignment. To assist his or her patients, a prudent case manager will have knowledge of the providers in his or her area that do accept assignment.

Medicare Summary Notice

A Medicare summary notice is Medicare's statement of what was paid to the provider. Because these notices are often confusing for patients and families to read, case managers serving persons with Medicare must know how to read the notices so that they can help their clients interpret them and take action as needed. The Medicare summary notice contains the following elements:

■ Date of the notice (patients have 6 months from the date of the notice to appeal any decision they dispute)

■ Medicare intermediary's name, address, and phone number (listed in the upper right corner of the notice)

■ The type of claim (this will be in the middle of the page and will list the provider type)

TABLE 6-2					
Participating Versus Nonparticipating Providers					
Service	Amount Billed	Amount Approved	Amount Paid (80% of the Approved Amount)		Amount Patient Pays
Participating Provider—Assignment Accepted					
Office visit	$100	$75	$60		20%: $15
Nonparticipating Provider—Assignment Not Accepted					
Office visit	$100	$75	$60		35%: $26.25

- Services provided (this will list the provider's name and address and the date services were rendered, as well as a description of the services)
- How costs were paid (this includes amount charged, Medicare-approved amount for the services, and then the amount paid)

Comparison of Medicare and Medicaid

Many people confuse Medicare and Medicaid. As stated earlier, Medicare was created as an attempt to offer health coverage to older Americans. It also addresses the fact that older citizens and the disabled often have medical bills significantly higher than the rest of the population, and because of their age or disability, they may no longer be able to work to cover the costs of medical care.

Unlike Medicaid, Medicare is solely a federal program in which eligibility does not rest on individual need. Entitlement is based on work history and entitlement to Social Security or retirement benefits. On the other hand, Medicaid, although it is a federal program, is basically run by individual states and is designed for the low-income and financially needy population.

Depending on disability, age, or financial status, a person may qualify for both Medicare and Medicaid. However, there are separate eligibility requirements for the two programs, and a person may be eligible for one but not for the other. Unlike Medicare, in which eligibility and benefits are consistent nationwide, Medicaid has eligibility requirements and program benefits that vary drastically by state.

Box 6-3 offers a comparison of Medicare and Medicaid.

PART A COVERED CARE

If the patient has both Part A and Part B, Part A, which is known as *the hospital insurance*, is key for coverage of inpatient care. Inpatient care can be provided in either an acute-care hospital or an SNF. Part A also covers some home health care.

Basically, Part A, or inpatient acute-care hospital coverage, includes the following:

- Semiprivate room—two to four beds per room (a private room if medically necessity is so documented in the chart)
- All meals, including special or medically required diets
- All regular nursing services
- Special care units such as intensive care or coronary care
- Drugs, medical supplies, and appliances required during the inpatient stay

---

BOX 6-3
Medicare Versus Medicaid

Medicare	Medicaid
Eligibility	
Medicare is for persons older than 65 years (rich or poor) and for some disabled persons younger than 65 years or persons with kidney failure.	Medicaid is for low-income and financially needy persons, regardless of age.
Medicare is an entitlement program that is based on a person's (or spouse's) entitlement to Social Security because he or she paid into Social Security or the Railroad Retirement Fund.	Medicaid is a public assistance program for the financially needy and persons with low income.

Continued

BOX 6-3
Medicare Versus Medicaid—cont'd

Program Administration

Medicare is a federal program, and Medicare rules are the same across the United States and its territories.

Medicare information is available at the nearest local Social Security office or via a national toll-free number. The number is 800-772-1213.

The Medicaid program is administered by each state. Thus there are differences in eligibility and benefits from state to state.

Medicaid information is available from the local county welfare department, the county social services department, or a state's Department of Health and Human Services (DHHS).

Coverage

Medicare Part A, the hospital portion, provides basic coverage for acute-care hospitalizations and postacute-care services when a skilled nursing facility or home health care is required.

Medicare Part B, the medical portion, provides coverage for physicians' visits and many outpatient and medical services.

Federal guidelines require Medicaid programs to provide the following, at a minimum:
- Inpatient hospital services
- Outpatient hospital services
- Physician services
- Pediatric and family nurse practitioner services
- Medical and surgical dental services
- Nursing facility services for individuals 21 years of age or older
- Home health care for persons eligible for nursing facility services
- Family planning services and supplies
- Rural health clinic services and any other ambulatory services offered by a rural health clinic that are not otherwise covered under the state plan
- Laboratory and radiology services
- Federally qualified health center services and any other ambulatory services offered by a federally qualified health center that are not otherwise covered under the state plan
- Nurse-midwife services (to the extent authorized by state law)
- Early and periodic screening, diagnosis, and treatment (EPSDT) services for individuals younger than 21 years

States can provide additional benefits such as prescription drug coverage, coverage for preventive care services, dental care, and eyeglasses.

Costs

Both Medicare Parts A and B have deductibles. Part A has hefty copayments that must be paid for inpatient care if care goes beyond a specific number of days or if skilled nursing facility care is required beyond 20 days.

Under Part B, there is a monthly premium, and the person is responsible for 20% of the charges. If a provider selected does not accept Medicare assignment, the patient is responsible for the balance of the bill (between what Medicare paid and what was billed).

The cost share level paid by the patient is dependent on his or her income and the state's requirements for cost sharing.

Medicaid will pay the deductibles and copayments, and at times the premiums, when a person is also covered by Medicare.

BOX 6-3
Medicare Versus Medicaid—cont'd

Paperwork
If a patient has fee-for-service Medicare, although many providers will bill Medicare and be reimbursed directly, the patient has some responsibility for keeping paid claims organized. This is necessary to ensure any copayments required are paid, and if the person has a medigap policy, that the policy can be used for any remaining payments. In this scenario, Medicare sends the paid statement (called *Medicare summary notice*) to the patient once Medicare has paid its portion. The patient must then submit a copy of this notice along with a claim form to the medigap insurer.

The other paperwork sent to patients includes statements that describe any unpaid portion of the deductible, any coinsurance payments not paid, and the charges not covered by Medicare.

Remind patients to always review any statements they receive to ensure they are only charged for the services received. This also validates that any insurance they have has paid their amounts correctly. How can patients do this? They need to place all documents side by side for comparison (e.g., Medicare summary notice, any paid statement from a medigap policy, and the provider's itemized bill). In this case the patient is comparing all to ensure all charges were paid correctly while validating that the provider did not bill for services not rendered.

Generally, there is no paperwork if the patient has no cost share and the provider bills for services and is reimbursed directly. If there is a cost share, the patient may need to keep receipts to prove the monthly cost share was met.

- Laboratory testing, x-ray films, or other imaging services and radiation treatments
- Operating and recovery room charges
- Blood transfusion administration costs, as well as all blood charges after the first three pints
- Rehabilitation services
- Transplants—all Medicare-approved transplants

Part A does not cover the following:

- Personal convenience items (e.g., television or phone)
- Private duty nursing
- Private room, unless medical necessity is documented
- Care outside the United States

Payments by Medicare

Under Part A Medicare, Medicare pays all charges related to the hospital with the exception of the coinsurance rates. The patient is responsible for the deductibles and copayments (i.e., the one-time deductible for each benefit period and then the daily coinsurance rates for days 61 through 150 for short-term hospitalizations and from day 21 to day 100 for SNF care).

Psychiatric Hospitalizations

Medicare Part A covers a total of 190 days per lifetime for a patient needing inpatient care in a psychiatric hospital. One limitation to Medicare's psychiatric benefits is that if a patient is already hospitalized at the time his or her Medicare benefits go into effect, Medicare counts back to the date of admission and subtracts these days from the 190-day lifetime benefits. All other inpatient coverage rules listed previously apply to psychiatric hospitalizations.

Skilled Nursing Facility Care

To be eligible for SNF coverage under Part A, the person must meet two basic requirements:

1. There must be a prior acute-care hospital stay of 3 consecutive days for the same condition within the last 30 days (not counting the day of discharge).
2. The attending physician must certify that skilled nursing care or rehabilitation services are required on a daily basis. (Medicare defines daily as 5 days per week.)

If eligible for SNF care, a patient can have up to 100 skilled days. If a patient requires SNF care, Medicare pays up to the first 20 days at 100% (if the patient requires skilled care this entire time. Unfortunately, this is not the case because many patients have reached the goals of therapy and are ready for discharge within approximately 7 to 14 days after admission). However, if the patient continues to require skilled nursing or rehabilitation services, coverage can continue until the 100th day. From the 21st day to the 100th day, the patient is responsible for a daily copayment (i.e., $96 or the copayment amount for the year, since the copayment rate is adjusted annually). If the patient requires skilled nursing care beyond the 100 days, the cost of the continued stay is either paid privately or by Medicaid.

SNF care does not have reserve days as allowed for acute-care hospitalizations. However, if the patient can stay out of an acute-care facility and SNF and renew his or her 60-day benefit period, the patient qualifies for a new benefit period of 100 days for SNF care as well.

Part A coverage for SNF care includes the following:

- Basically the same coverage as outlined for inpatient acute care
- Hospitalizations outside the United States

Levels of Skilled Nursing Facility Care

Most SNFs divide their levels of care into two areas—skilled and custodial. This division can be confusing for families who are already struggling to understand custodial care and now are being advised by a case manager to place their loved one in a "skilled nursing facility." Depending on the patient's medical condition, care needs may shift from skilled to custodial and vice versa.

Custodial care is primarily personal in nature and is nonmedical; it is the care that is required when a person can no longer fully care for himself or herself. For the most part, custodial care is the assistance the person needs to perform what are called *activities of daily living*. These activities include bathing, dressing, grooming, moving about, getting up and down, eating, and toileting. Custodial care could involve help with medical care as well, and this might be help with medications (e.g., administration or monitoring as the person takes the medications), or it could involve some help with exercises (e.g., range-of-motion exercises or moving the person about). As a rule, custodial care is provided by health care professionals who are often not highly trained.

Unfortunately, the custodial care level can last for months or years. For this reason, it is a level of care that is not paid for by Medicare or most insurers (i.e., Medicaid, long-term care insurance, and workers' compensation are the only exceptions).

Medicare Hospice Benefit

Hospice care is generally the care a person receives at home (it can be provided in an SNF or board-and-care facility if the facility has a waiver) when the patient has a terminal illness and death is anticipated within 6 months. Hospice care, unlike care that is provided when a cure or recovery is anticipated, is not focused on treating the illness or fostering recovery. Its focus is on palliative care and keeping the patient as comfortable and pain-free as possible during the last stages of life. If the patient elects to participate in Medicare's hospice program, Medicare pays 100% of the claims with the exception of two charges. The two exceptions are prescriptions and inpatient care. If the patient receives prescriptions for pain control or symptomatic relief, the cost per prescription is $5. Similarly, if the patient requires an inpatient stay in either an acute-care hospital or SNF for respite care, the patient is responsible for $5 per day.

Hospice care centers on the patient and family and is a team approach that combines the efforts of the physician, nurse, social worker, dietitian, clergy, therapists, and trained caregivers. Generally, a hospice plan can only be established if support and care provided by the family, a friend, or other caregiver are available on a 24-hour basis. Twenty-four–hour coverage is necessary, because although the hospice team will make regular visits, they do not provide care for more than an hour or so at a time.

When care is provided under the hospice benefit, if the family or caregiver needs a break, respite coverage is available. Respite care is allowed for up to 5 days, and it is offered in either an acute-care or skilled nursing inpatient setting. For additional information on the Medicare hospice program or to download the Medicare Hospice Manual, see the CMS's website at: www.cms.hhs.gov/manuals/21_hospice/hs0-fw.asp.

Hospice Coverage Under Medicare

If a patient is accepted into a hospice program, Medicare covers nearly all the costs associated with hospice care, including the following:

- Physician services
- Nursing care
- Medical supplies and appliances
- Medications necessary for the management of pain and other symptoms
- Health aide and homemaker services
- Rehabilitation therapy (e.g., physical therapy or speech therapy)
- Medical social services and counseling
- Dietary counseling
- Clergy
- Respite care—up to 5 days in an inpatient setting for the caregiver to have a break (note: if the patient is not covered by Medicare, respite coverage may not be a benefit)

Hospice Restrictions

Because hospice does have restrictions, the case manager should prepare the patient for what entering a hospice program means. The patient and family should be informed that hospice treatments will focus on comfort care and not on curative care. It is wise for the patient to have an advanced directive prepared, indicating his or her wishes to the family. The advanced directive will be used in the event that the person's condition deteriorates and he or she is unable to make his or her wishes known.

Hospice restrictions on coverage include the following:

- Care must be provided by a Medicare-approved hospice agency.
- The hospice team and the patient's attending physician must develop a plan of care.
- The patient's physician and the hospice medical director must certify that the patient is terminally ill and life expectancy is less than 6 months.

■ The patient must sign a statement indicating choice of the Medicare hospice benefits rather than regular Medicare benefits.

Although a patient might sign the hospice statement on entry into the program, he or she has the right to cancel hospice care and return to regular Medicare coverage at any time.

Periods of Coverage

In the hospice program, a patient is allowed two 90-day benefit periods of hospice care, followed by a 30-day period if deemed necessary. In some circumstances these periods can be extended indefinitely. Thus if a patient elects hospice, he or she could receive care for a total of 210 days. The benefit periods can be used together or separately. Although rare, if a patient cancels the hospice program during a benefit period, he or she will lose any remaining days in the benefit period. However, if the patient later elects to reenter a hospice program, the previous cancellation does not affect future benefit periods.

Home Health Care

Benefits for home care are available under both Medicare Part A and Part B. However, unlike coverage under Part B where a qualifying acute-care inpatient stay is not required, to qualify for coverage under Part A, the patient must have a 3-day inpatient hospital stay.

Under each part, if the patient meets Medicare's criteria for skilled home care, Medicare pays 100% of the cost. As with all other services, if Medicare is to reimburse for costs, the agency must be Medicare-certified. If a patient continues to require skilled nursing care, there are no limits on the number of visits he or she might receive. Further information on home health services can be found on CMS's website at www.cms.hhs.gov/manuals/11_hha/HH00.asp.

Home health services (paid by either Part A or Part B) include the following:

■ Part-time skilled nursing care—usually two to three visits per week at about 1 to 2 hours per visit. Patients may require more visits, and this can include up to two visits per day in some cases, if medically necessary and the physician's orders support this intensity of need Physical therapy or speech therapy.

If a patient is receiving skilled nursing or rehabilitation services or both, he or she will also qualify for the following:

■ Occupational therapy
■ Part-time home health aide services (bathing and personal care)
■ Medical social worker services
■ Medical equipment and supplies provided by the agency (e.g., bed, walker, or medical supplies for dressing changes)

Services not covered for home care include the following:

■ Full-time nursing care
■ Medications for home use
■ Meals or meal preparation
■ Housekeeping services
■ Transportation

Restrictions on Home Health Care

Despite the obvious benefits of home care for most patients, coverage for home health services is severely restricted, and the restrictions include the following:

■ The physician must certify that the patient requires intermittent nursing care and is homebound.
■ The care plan must be set up in collaboration with the attending physician.

The two biggest restrictions are that the person must be classified as homebound and that the person must require only intermittent skilled nursing care. If the person is not homebound and is able to safely leave the house for his or her medical care (e.g., dressing changes or rehabilitation therapy), the person may not be eligible for home health care services.

If the person requires more care than the agency is allowed to provide under the home health care benefit, the case manager must explore the options of SNF care versus hiring private help in the home. The other option the family has is to learn how to do the care themselves. This option involves the agency supervising and teaching the care at a schedule determined by the type of care required, the frequency of care, and the abilities of the caregivers.

Home care, when properly administered, can afford enormous benefits: the patient is in his or her own familiar surroundings among family and friends and has privacy and freedom from routines—all of which are conducive to a speedy recovery. However, home care is not always the right solution for everybody. Case managers must therefore constantly evaluate their patients for the appropriate level of care. Of equal importance, they must be honest with patients and families if a home plan is not in the patient's (or caregiver's) best interest. Certainly, the patient has the right to make choices, but a wise case manager will educate patients and families about the pros and cons and alternative options.

However, some patients and their families will make unwise choices and not accept alternatives or options, and this scenario is not limited to home care issues. If this occurs, the case manager must not intimidate the clients or impose his or her own beliefs on them. If unwise choices are made, the case manager must keep the team apprised, document all events, and summarize reasons. If the decisions made place the patient or others at risk, a report to Adult Protective Services or Child Protective Services may be required. In some cases the police might need to be involved as well.

PART B MEDICARE COVERAGE

Medicare Part B, referred to as *supplemental medical insurance*, covers doctors' bills, outpatient services such as laboratory testing, therapy, and home health care. For a full list of medical benefits, supplies, and diagnostic and other services covered by Medicare Part B, see CMS's website at www.medicare.gov.

Before Medicare pays any portion of the Part B services, the patient is responsible for an annual deductible of $100 at this writing. However, in all likelihood this amount will increase over the next few years.

Part B Medicare covers the following:

- Physician services
- Services of practitioners such as clinical psychologists, social workers, and nurse practitioners
- Outpatient services, laboratory tests, radiologic and imaging services
- Ambulances
- Medical equipment, braces, and medical supplies
- Prosthetic devices including breast prostheses after mastectomy
- Oral surgery
- Outpatient rehabilitation therapy
- Drugs administered in a physician's office or outpatient hospital setting
- Immunosuppressive therapy (limited) for transplant recipients and some patients with ESRD
- Kidney dialysis
- Home health care
- Chiropractor care (limited)
- Preventive screening examinations, including the following:
  - Bone mass measurements (e.g., for persons at risk of losing bone mass)
  - Colorectal screening (e.g., fecal occult blood test, flexible sigmoidoscopy, colonoscopy, or barium enemas)
  - Diabetic services (monitors, test strips, and lancets and self-management training programs)

- Mammography screening
- Papanicolaou smears and pelvic examinations (includes clinical breast examinations)
- Prostate cancer screening
- Influenza, pneumonia, and hepatitis B vaccinations
- Podiatry services
- Optometrists
- Clinical psychologists or social workers
- Outpatient mental health treatment

Services not covered by Part B Medicare include the following:

- Drugs and medications for home use
- Acupuncture
- Treatment that is not medically necessary or that is custodial in nature
- Routine physical examinations
- Vaccinations and immunizations
- Eyesight and hearing examinations
- Hearing aids
- Orthopedic shoes
- General dental care and dentures
- Cosmetic surgery
- Any services obtained outside the United States

Finding a Medicare-Participating Provider

To assist in locating a provider that participates in the Medicare program, Medicare maintains a national participating physician directory. The directory contains names, addresses, and specialties of Medicare-participating physicians who have agreed to accept assignment on all Medicare claims and covered services. Assignment only works with the original Medicare plan. It does not apply if a patient has selected an M+C plan or a private FFS plan.

Home Medical Equipment

Medicare Part B pays for home medical equipment (e.g., walkers, wheelchairs, and beds), splints, prosthetic devices, body braces, therapeutic shoes for patients with diabetes and certain other conditions, glucose monitoring equipment, corrective lenses after cataract surgery, and other recognized and Food and Drug Administration–approved items or devices. The key to coverage is that the item must be medically required for the condition at hand and cannot be used for convenience. Additionally, a physician must prescribe the requested item.

Because of the increase in fraud and abuse of the program, Medicare has cracked down on its requirement for the physician's signature. Now most durable medical equipment companies will not honor orders for equipment unless it is accompanied by an original and signed prescription from the attending physician. Additionally, the prescription must indicate: the name of the item, medical diagnosis, and reason for and duration of need, at a minimum. If the equipment meets Medicare's guidelines for coverage, Medicare reimburses 80% of the equipment costs, with the patient responsible for the remainder of the charges. For a full listing of Medicare-approved items, see Medicare publications at the Medicare website: www.medicare.gov/Publications/Search/View/ViewPubList.asp?Language=English.

Ambulances

Medicare Part B covers the cost of ambulances as long as they are medically necessary and the patient meets specific conditions. Coverage for ambulance fees is generally limited to a trip to the hospital. It might be covered on discharge to home or an SNF if the patient meets specific requirements related to bed confinement.

Medicare does not cover routine transportation to and from doctors' appointments or dialysis, despite the fact that patient may not be able to get in and out of a car. Case managers must work closely with the patient and family in these situations because if community resources are not available, the patient or family must assume responsibility for such costs or arrangements for a ride.

Dental Care

Medicare does not pay for routine dental care. However, like all health care insurers, it does pay for dental care if the care required is related to an underlying medical condition or conditions that resulted from radiation therapy or an injury. Keep in mind that if dental care is covered, the care must not be related to normal tooth decay or gum disease.

Eyesight and Hearing Examinations

Medicare Part B does not cover routine eye or hearing examinations, nor is coverage allowed for hearing aids, eyeglasses, or contact lenses. The only exceptions are for lenses after cataract surgery and for vision or hearing conditions that are the result of an injury or illness. Medicare does cover some aids for the blind.

Medications

Possibly the biggest void in the Medicare program is the lack of drug coverage. Because of this void persons often choose a medigap policy, join a local M+CO, or file for Medicaid, if they are financially eligible. If an M+CO is in the local area, many patients elect this option, since these plans offer an enhanced benefit of some drug coverage without an additional premium.

Medications are possibly the most costly area of medical care that is not covered. This is often the area that disturbs case managers working with the elderly the most. The case manager may find that the patient is noncompliant with treatment merely because he or she cannot afford the costs; the patient may have to choose between paying for medications and buying food.

Medicare Part A will cover medications administered in a hospital or an SNF. Part B does cover drugs that cannot be self-administered but must be given in an outpatient setting, clinic, or physician's office. Medicare Part B does allow coverage for some cancer drugs and some drugs required after organ transplantation. It also allows coverage for influenza and pneumonia vaccinations. If such vaccinations are administered, Medicare pays 100% of the approved charges for such, if the provider accepts assignment. In cases such as this, the person's annual $100 deductible does not apply.

Although many Medicare beneficiaries travel and could be exposed to communicable diseases, Medicare does not cover any immunizations required for travel. If the person's private physician's office cannot supply these immunizations, local public health clinics can administer them at a cost to the patient.

Although insulin for patients with diabetes is medically necessary, Medicare does not pay for this drug, because it is classified as self-administered. It is not covered even when administered by a family member or friend. Insulin administered in an SNF is not covered if it is for routine use. However, if the dosage of insulin is being regulated and the patient is being monitored for responses to the dosage, insulin and facility charges will be covered until the appropriate dosage is established because the care is considered skilled. Once the patient's glucose level is stabilized, coverage ceases because the patient is then reclassified at a maintenance or custodial level.

How can case managers help patients find some coverage for their medications? The first question to ask patients is, "What is your income?" This simple little question can help in guiding patients to the state's Medicaid program if necessary. Other options include the use of samples if the organization or physician's office is allowed to maintain sample stock. If the physician prescribing the medication does have samples, one solution is to ask the physician for them. Another way is to contact the pharmaceutical company directly and ascertain whether it has a program that allows patients to purchase medications at a discount. Another alternative is to assist the patient in exploring the possibility of home delivery of drugs from mail-order pharmacies. Drugs are often mailed in bulk, and the patient is given a price break, since the costs are lower because dispensing fees are lowered.

Clinical Laboratory Services

Medicare pays 100% of the approved amount for laboratory testing without payment of the annual $100 deductible. All laboratories accept assignment except those in Maryland, where a hospital can bill a 20% coinsurance rate for outpatient laboratory services.

Outpatient Hospital Services

For most outpatient services, Medicare pays 80% of the Medicare-approved amount. However, if the patient receives care from a hospital as an outpatient, the patient is responsible for not only the 20% coinsurance payment but also 20% of whatever the hospital charges. This difference is not limited in any way by the Medicare-approved charges as are physician fees. This means that if a patient has surgery, radiology testing, other diagnostic testing, or radiation therapy as an outpatient in a hospital, charges and then differences between what is approved and paid will be higher than if the same services were provided by a independent community-based outpatient provider. Therefore case managers should continually attempt to assist patients in obtaining services from non–hospital-based providers whenever possible.

Outpatient Mental Health Services

Medicare Part B covers outpatient mental health services at 50% of the approved charges. This is true regardless of whether a psychiatrist, psychologist, or clinical social worker in a hospital, SNF, clinic, or rehabilitation unit provides the services. The patient is not only responsible for the balance of the 50% but also the yearly Part B deductible, as well as any charges above the Medicare-approved amount when the provider does not accept assignment.

Appealing Denial of Coverage

Unfortunately not every Medicare service coverage determination is made as the patient thinks it should be. Therefore Medicare allows beneficiaries to appeal a denied service. Although this could happen with a claim for outpatient care or services, one area that dominates the appeal process is inpatient care, whether provided at an acute-care hospital or an SNF.

ROLE OF THE CMS

The CMS is responsible for the Medicare program and its policy formulation. Their offices are further broken down into a central office and regional offices. Each office has different accountabilities for general management and operations. The overall responsibilities of the CMS central office include the following:

- Determining, in consultation with the SSA, an individual's entitlement to benefits
- Determining the nature and duration of services for which benefits may be paid
- Establishing, maintaining, and administering agreements with state agencies, providers of services, and contractors
- Formulating major policies regarding conditions of participation for providers
- Developing and maintaining statistical research and actuarial programs
- Managing general finances of the program

- Determining costs and amounts to be paid to providers, physicians, and suppliers

Regional office responsibilities include the following:

- Exercising the authority to implement the Medicare program in various geographic areas
- Serving as the focal point for control and liaison for intermediary carrier and SSA activities
- Providing the following administrative functions:
  - Emphasizing and reiterating program instructions from the central office to intermediaries and carriers (the organizations that pay Medicare Part A and Part B claims)
  - Appraising current specific program or operational issues that may require compiling and reporting selective data within designated periods to CMS
  - Communicating directly with carriers and intermediaries concerning operational activities and program effectiveness
  - Working with other agencies and organizations that are directly or indirectly involved in the Medicare program

Role of Part A Intermediaries

Part A intermediaries are national, state, public, and private agencies or organizations that have entered into an agreement with CMS to process Medicare Part A claims for providers who provide services under Part A. These agencies or organizations perform such administrative duties as the following:

- Determining covered services furnished by providers under both Part A and Part B
- Providing consultative services to assist providers in maintaining necessary fiscal records and participation qualifications

- Conducting provider records audits
- Helping providers with utilization review procedures
- Providing the Office of Inspector General (OIG) with needed information and assistance in fraud and abuse investigations
- Establishing controls, developed in conjunction with the OIG, to minimize the possibility of incorrect Medicare payment
- Applying safeguards against unnecessary use of covered services
- Serving as a center for communication with providers
- Assisting the beneficiary in the appeal process

Role of Part B Carriers

Like Part A intermediaries, the Part B carriers can be national, state, public, or private agencies that contract with CMS to process the Part B claims. Carrier responsibilities include the following:

- Determining the amount of Medicare payment for covered Part B services
- Making payments
- Maintaining payment and related program records that demonstrate the quality of carrier performance
- Relaying to the physician and supplier community information pertinent to the administration of the program
- Providing the OIG with needed information and assistance in fraud and abuse investigations
- Establishing controls developed in conjunction with OIG to minimize the possibility of incorrect Medicare payments

MEDICARE MANUALS AND PUBLICATIONS

Information on Medicare and its deductibles and copayments can be found in any Medicare handbooks that can be downloaded from Medicare's website at www.medicare.gov/publications/. Medicare's SNF manuals also can be found at www.medicare.gov/Publications/Pubs/pdf/snf.pdf or www.cms.hhs.gov/manuals/12_snf/SN00.asp. To keep the Medicare and Medicaid program manuals current, CMS uses transmittals. To introduce changes to Medicare, CMS uses documents that are called *operation policy letters*. Copies of such documents can be located at the following CMS websites:

- Operation policy letters—www.mcol.com/armenu3.htm and www.cms.hhs.gov/healthplans/opl/index.pdf
- Transmittals—www.cms.hhs.gov/manuals/transmittals/comm_date_dsc.asp

MEDICARE MANAGED CARE ORGANIZATIONS

Managed Medicare since the BBA of 1997 is now referred to as *Medicare + Choice*. If a patient joins an M+CO, he or she must sign over his or her Medicare fee for service to the managed care organization (MCO). This means that although the patient will still have the basic Medicare benefits as outlined previously, the organization selected is paid to administer the Medicare benefits, as well as to provide the care and services the patient requires. To join an M+CO, the patient must have both Medicare Part A and Part B.

The BBA also created a program known as the *private fee for-service plan*. A private FFS plan is Medicare, but the benefits are administered by a private health insurance company. Under this plan the federal government pays the health plan a set amount of money each month to provide health coverage. Because the health plan is in control, it determines the areas in which coverage is offered. It also has the ability to offer different plans with different benefits and costs.

Under a private FFS plan, the beneficiary has the same benefits as allowed by Medicare Part A and Part B. The big difference with the private FFS plans is that the person has the right to use any physician or hospital and can obtain services outside the plan's service area. However, there are several down sides. One is the fact that M+C and private FFS plans are not available in all areas of the United States. Another is the amount that private FFS plans can charge the beneficiary—because this can be more than the traditional costs related to Medicare FFS. Still another is related to persons with ESRD requiring dialysis or a kidney transplant. If a patient has a diagnosis of ESRD at the time of enrollment, he or she is excluded from enrollment in either plan.

When a patient signs up with an M+CO or a private FFS plan, he or she can do so regardless of any preexisting conditions except as stated earlier, those persons previously diagnosed with ESRD before enrollment. Fortunately, if the patient is diagnosed with ESRD *after* enrollment, he or she is not required to disenroll. Thus patients with a preexisting diagnosis can enroll in a plan at any time if there are openings for new members. Every plan must offer its Medicare plan during an open enrollment period starting November 1 of each year. Coverage then begins the following January 1.

CHANGING PLANS

If the patient is hospitalized and changes from one plan to a similar plan, the first M+CO or private FFS plan remains responsible for care until discharge. The same is true if the patient is an FFS Medicare patient and joins an M+CO or private FFS plan: FFS Medicare remains responsible for the charges until discharge. This rule does not apply to SNFs, psychiatric hospitals, cancer hospitals, children's hospitals, or rehabilitation facilities. If the person moves out of the health plan's service area, he or she must disenroll. Once disenrolled, the patient's coverage reverts to the original FFS Medicare.

Until the end of 2001, Medicare beneficiaries could enroll in and disenroll from M+CO or a private FFS plan at any time. Beginning in January 2002, the BBA required that elections be limited. This change in election period limitations is termed a *lock-in*.

Beginning January 1, 2002, beneficiaries will be limited to the following periods for enrollment:

- The annual election period in November
- An open enrollment period from January through June
- Any time during a special election period

In 2003 the open enrollment period will be reduced in length and will last from January through March. This new requirement will limit a Medicare beneficiary's enrollment, and the beneficiary cannot enroll in a new plan or disenroll into the FFS Medicare plan except during set periods. However, in the event a beneficiary

---

TABLE 6-3
Comparing Medicare + Choice and Medicare Fee-for-Service Plans

Service	Medicare Fee-for-Service	Medicare + Choice
Choice of providers	Can use any physician as long as the provider is a Medicare-approved provider.	Must use the Medicare + Choice plan's network of providers.
Access to specialists	As long as the provider accepts Medicare and the patient has a medigap policy or can pay the balances of any bills. If the patient has Medicaid, the provider must be willing to accept Medicaid's allowed amount.	In most plans the patient can only be seen on referral from the PCP. If the specialist is not available within the network, the plan must authorize an out-of-plan provider.
Premiums	Medicare Part A is premium-free if the person obtains it through retirement or by meeting SSDI requirements. Part B has a monthly premium.	No premium for basic benefits but patient has broader coverage.
Deductibles and copayments	Deductibles and copayments are as described above in the Medicare Part A and Part B section.	Most services require a copayment.
Prescription coverage	Limited to drugs as described above under Medicare Part B.	Most plans offer some prescription coverage, but it is often limited to a specific amount per year. Drugs covered will be listed in the plan's drug formulary. Depending on the drug used, copayments can vary (e.g., $5-$25) per prescription.
Treatment approval	None if the service is one allowed by Medicare.	Many services will require prior authorization.
Geographic mobility	Anywhere in the United States and its territories. Care outside these areas is not covered.	Except for emergency medical care, most care is restricted to the plan's service area. Medicare beneficiaries are allowed to remain "temporarily" out of a service area, and the plan must cover such services when notified.

Continued

TABLE 6-3
Comparing Medicare + Choice and Medicare Fee-for-Service Plans—cont'd

Service	Medicare Fee-for-Service	Medicare + Choice
Emergency care	Covered anywhere in United States and its territories. No coverage for care outside the United States and its territories.	Covered anywhere in United States and its territories. No coverage for care outside the United States and its territories. Emergency care and urgent care both have copayments (e.g., $50 for ED care and $25 for urgent care). Copayments are waived if the person is admitted.
Home care	Covered under both Part A and Part B. Covered at 100% if the patient meets criteria and is homebound.	Covered at 100%.
Preventive care services	Only those as listed above under Part B	Most plans offer preventive services that are free or low-cost.
Eye examinations and glasses	Not covered unless related to an accident or injury. If contact lenses are required after cataract surgery, Medicare Part B covers.	Many plans offer limited discounts on both exams and eyewear, whether related to an eye injury or accident or not. Contact lenses are covered after cataract surgery.
Hearing aids and examinations	Not covered unless related to an accident or injury.	Many plans offer limited discounts on both exams and hearing aids.
Dental care	Routine dental care is not covered. If dental care is related to an accident, injury, disease, or treatments for a disease, coverage is allowed.	Some companies offer some limited discounts or services. If dental care is related to an accident, injury, disease, or treatments for a disease, coverage is allowed.
Wellness programs	Not covered	Many plans offer low cost or free wellness programs designed for specific diseases.
Chiropractic care	Covered but a limited benefit.	Broader coverage than allowed by Medicare FFS.
Alternative medicine	Not covered	Some plans offer a limited number of alternative medicine benefits.

ED, Emergency department; *FFS,* fee for service; *PCP,* primary care provider; *SSDI,* Social Security disability income.

moves or the plan terminates its contract, disenrollment can occur.

Requirements of Organizations Under M+C

CMS requires that each M+CO be licensed under any state law in every state in which it operates. CMS also requires the organization to be a risk-bearing entity that offers health insurance or health benefits coverage in each state in which it offers one or more managed care plans. The intent of this requirement is to ensure that each organization offering M+C has the state authority to do so and that each organization will meet state solvency standards.

Under M+C, federal law preempts state law in three specific areas: (1) benefits, (2) inclusion and treatment of providers, and (3) coverage determinations (including related appeals and grievances). Other than these three areas, M+COs must comply with *all* state laws and standards applicable to all insurers or health plans. Additionally, M+COs that elect to offer Medicare must comply with *all* federal laws and standards. If state laws are inconsistent with the standards required for Medicare operations, insurers and health plans are not required to adhere to the state's laws and standards. However, if the state laws or standards are more stringent than the federal standards, CMS does not consider this an aberration to its rule on inconsistency. Therefore federal law will rarely preempt these standards.

M+C APPEALS PROCESS

The definitions of an appeal and a grievance are often confusing for beneficiaries. However, CMS classifies an appeal and grievance as follows:

- An appeal involves a request for a re-review of a coverage determination. An appeal can be invoked when payment is denied or the services for which the enrollee believes to be covered are denied.
- A grievance is basically a complaint relating to issues such as those in the following examples. The beneficiary had difficulty in accessing services or scheduling an appointment; the demeanor of the person providing the service was insulting or otherwise inappropriate; or the beneficiary did not like the amount of time he or she had to spend in a waiting room.

Although re-review of coverage determinations must go through CMS's mandated appeals process, the beneficiary has the right to obtain an attorney and file a valid claim under state tort or contract law. Thus states are allowed to investigate consumer complaints to determine whether the complaint falls outside of the specific preemption area and is therefore subject to state jurisdiction.

Medicare beneficiaries enrolled in any health plan that offers an M+C plan have the right to request timely coverage determinations, and if they are dissatisfied with the determination, to file an appeal. An appeal includes any of the procedures that pertain to the re-review of a case when an adverse determination was made or the request for payment for the service was denied either in whole or in part. Only complaints concerning denials or organization determinations are subject to the M+C appeal process.

Although it appears that the appeals process stops once a determination is made to uphold the denial or overturn it, this is not the case. The beneficiary is given other options for appeal if he or she continues to be unsatisfied with the determination. Thus the appeal process includes the following:

- Reconsiderations by the M+CO as a second-level appeal
- If necessary an independent medical review entity
- A hearing before an administrative law judge
- Review by the departmental appeals board (DAB)
- Judicial review

All other complaints are subject to the M+CO's grievance requirements. As indicated earlier, a grievance is any complaint or dispute other than one involving a denial or organization determination. Grievance procedures also apply when a beneficiary disagrees with the M+CO's decision not to provide an expedited determination.

CMS requires M+COs to make the decision as quickly as the beneficiary's health requires. Thus the organization must make its determination according to the beneficiary's health needs, but in no case later than 14 calendar days after the M+CO receives the request.

Standard Appeal

A beneficiary has the right to file a standard appeal if the M+CO denies a service, terminates coverage, or refuses to pay for services that the beneficiary believes should be covered. For a standard appeal, the M+CO has 30 calendar days to render its decision on the issue. If the beneficiary's appeal is related to a request for payment, the M+CO has 60 calendar days to render its decision.

Expedited Appeal

A beneficiary or a physician has the right to file an expedited appeal if he or she believes that the waiting time for a standard appeal would seriously jeopardize life, health, or the ability to regain maximum function. For an expedited appeal, the M+CO has 72 hours to reconsider the original determination. A physician, regardless of his or her network status with the M+CO, has the right to support the beneficiary's request for the expedited review.

In the case of either an expedited or a standard appeal, an extension of up to 10 days can be allowed if either the beneficiary or the M+CO can justify that the additional time will be in the best interest of the beneficiary. For example, this additional time might justify the use of an extension if it is used to obtain additional medical records that can support the reconsideration determination (Box 6-4).

Additional Appeal Facts

In recent years the time frames during which appeals are considered and a new determination is made have decreased, and other requirements for appeals processing have surfaced. For example, with

---

BOX 6-4
Comparison of Standard and Expedited Appeals Under Medicare + Choice

Standard Appeals 60-Day Process	Expedited Appeals 72-Hour Process
Standard appeals may be filed for the following disputed reasons: 1. Payment for emergency or urgently needed services received 2. Any other health services furnished by a provider or supplier other than the health plan that the beneficiary believes are covered under Medicare or should have been furnished, arranged for, or reimbursed by the health plan 3. The health plan's refusal to provide services that the beneficiary believes should be furnished or arranged for by the health plan and the beneficiary has not received the services outside the health plan. 4. Decisions to discontinue services when the enrollee believes there is a continuing need for the service. Health plans must notify the beneficiary within 60 calendar days of receiving the beneficiary's request for payment or services. The letter must contain the reasons for the determination and inform the beneficiary of his or her appeal rights.	Expedited appeals may be filed for the following reasons: 1. The health plan's refusal to provide services that the beneficiary believes should be furnished or arranged for by the health plan and the beneficiary has not received the services outside the health plan. 2. Decisions to discontinue services when the beneficiary believes there is a continuing need for the service. Health plans have 72 hours in which to re-review a request. In most cases the provider and beneficiary will be notified by phone of the determination. This is followed by notification in writing, and the letter must include the reasons for the determination and further appeal rights. Under the expedited rule, a health plan must grant all physician requests (network or nonnetwork) and the beneficiary's request for physician support for an expedited appeal. If the provider assisting the beneficiary is a nonnetwork provider, the health plan begins the appeal process with the receipt of the information.

BOX 6-4
Comparison of Standard and Expedited Appeals Under Medicare + Choice—cont'd

Standard Appeals 60-Day Process	Expedited Appeals 72-Hour Process
Requests for reconsideration must be made in writing and filed with the health plan, the Social Security Administration, or the Railroad Retirement Board. Requests must be filed within 60 calendar days of the denial.	Requests for an expedited reconsideration may be made either orally or in writing to the health plan. If for some reason the beneficiary calls the health plan and requests an expedited appeal, the health plan is to assist the beneficiary by documenting such oral requests in writing.
	If the health plan determines the standard 60-day appeal process could seriously jeopardize the life or health of the beneficiary or the beneficiary's ability to regain maximum function, the beneficiary the must be notified of such and that the request for the appeal will be handled as expedited.
	If the health plan determines the expedited request for an appeal does not qualify for expedited review, the beneficiary must be notified orally that the appeal will be processed according to the standard appeal process and time frames. This oral report will be followed by notification in writing within 2 working days.
If additional information is needed, the health plan must provide the beneficiary the opportunity to present additional evidence related to the issue in dispute. Beneficiaries can do this either in person or in writing.	Despite the fact that time frames are so short with an expedited review, the health plan must still allow the beneficiary an opportunity to present additional evidence to support his or her request. The beneficiary may do so either in person or in writing, and written information can be received via fax or e-mail.
The health plan has 60 calendar days (CMS does allow extensions to the time limit for good cause) in which to make its reconsideration determination and if it does the following:	If the health plan makes a favorable decision, it must do so within the 72 hours from the date of receipt of the request. If the beneficiary requests additional time or if the health plan finds that additional information is necessary and the delay is in the interest of the beneficiary, an extension of no more than 10 working days can be allowed. This request can be made orally, but written confirmation must be mailed within 2 working days. If the health plan, on review, determines:
1. Make a decision to rule fully in the beneficiary's behalf, the health plan must issue its decision within the 60 calendar days.	
2. Make a recommendation to partially or completely uphold the original denial, the health plan must prepare a written explanation and send the entire case to CHDR within the 60 calendar days for CHDR to issue the final reconsideration determination.	If the denial is overturned in the beneficiary's favor, the beneficiary must be notified orally and the written notice mailed within 2 working days.
3. Should the health plan fail to issue a reconsideration determination within the 60-day time frame, this constitutes a denial, and the case must be filed with CHDR for the decision.	If the denial is to be partially or wholly upheld, the health plan must prepare a written explanation and send the entire case to CHDR within 24 hours of its determination.
4. If the case is forwarded to CHDR, the health plan is required to keep the beneficiary informed concurrently of this fact.	If the health plan fails to issue a reconsideration determination within the 72-hour limit or before expiration of an extension, this constitutes an adverse determination, and the file must be submitted to CHDR. If the case is forwarded to CHDR, the health plan must concurrently keep the beneficiary informed of the facts.
CHDR has 30 working days to issue its determination.	CHDR has 3 working days to issue its determination.

CHDR, Center for Health Dispute Resolution; *CMS,* Centers for Medicare & Medicaid Services.

regard to the M+C program, any supplemental benefits allowed by the M+CO are also subject to the new time frames for the appeals process. Additionally, any denial that is based on lack of medical necessity must now be reconsidered by a physician who has expertise in the field of medicine appropriate to the issue at hand. This physician must be one who did not participate in the initial coverage determination. For this reason, many organizations use third party reviewers who are not part of their organization for this level of review. M+COs are prohibited from taking any punitive actions against providers who support or request an appeal on the beneficiary's behalf.

Another requirement is that if the M+CO reverses its determination and rules in favor of the beneficiary, the organization is required to authorize or provide services as quickly as the beneficiary requires, but no later than 30 days from the date of its decision. If an independent reviewer or higher entity issued the favorable determination, the plan must pay for the service within 60 days.

Appeal Levels Beyond the Health Plan

If, on reconsideration, the M+CO upholds its original denial (wholly or partially), the organization must forward the beneficiary's case to an independent medical review entity that contracts with Medicare (currently the Center for Health Dispute Resolution [CHDR]).

For its review determinations CHDR is under the following time constraints:

- **Expedited appeals**—Within 3 days from the date of request
- **Preservice cases not expedited**—Within 10 days from the date of request
- **Retrospective cases**—Within 15 days from the date of request

In the event CHDR requests additional information and the health plan does not comply, CHDR will issue its determination based on the information originally submitted. If CHDR denies any part of the beneficiary's request (the dispute must be over a request that is greater than $100), CHDR advises the beneficiary of his or her right to appeal to an administrative law judge from the SSA. The beneficiary has 60 days to file an appeal with an administrative law judge. Although the M+CO does not have a right to request an administrative law judge hearing, the organization is allowed to be a party to the administrative law judge hearing. If the administrative law judge agrees and upholds the denial, the beneficiary has another level of appeal he or she may pursue. This level is called the *DAB*. When a beneficiary files with the DAB, he or she has 60 days to request a review. At the DAB level there is no dollar limit for the amount in dispute. If the beneficiary remains unsatisfied with the outcome at the DAB level, he or she has 60 days to file a suit in federal court. However, for the appeal to reach the judicial review level, the amount in dispute must be at least $1000.

Discharge Appeal Rights

Possibly the biggest upheaval with hospital discharges for M+CO beneficiaries occurs with the newest requirements of CMS for advising Medicare beneficiaries of their appeal rights on discharge. As a result, hospitals over the past few years have scrambled to ensure they are in compliance with CMS's requirements with the letters. The letters are currently called *Notice Of Discharge and Medicare Appeal Rights (NODMAR)*.

According to guidelines for the NODMAR, if the beneficiary believes he or she is being discharged too soon from a hospital, he or she has the right to immediate review by the state's peer review organization. During this review the beneficiary has the right to remain hospitalized at no charge, and the hospital cannot discharge the beneficiary before the peer review organization reaches a decision. CMS appeal information can be found at www.cms.hhs.gov/healthplans/appeals/sanqna.asp, and Medicare appeal information can be found in the current Medicare handbook on the website at www.medicare.gov/Publications/Pubs/pdf/10050.pdf.

Clinical Trials—Medicare FFS and M+C

Because many patients who are followed up by case management might be candidates for clinical trials, case managers must be familiar with Medicare's stance on the issue. Medicare describes clinical trials in more detail in its *National Coverage Determination* manual. A quick reference guide to clinical trials can be found on the CMS website at www.medicaid.com/medlearn/refctmed.asp or at www.cms.hhs.gov/coverage/8d.asp or by calling 800-MEDICARE.

Because the costs of clinical trials are outside the national coverage determination, the M+CO is not required to cover the cost of a trial, and costs are passed on to Medicare FFS for payment. Medicare FFS continues to pay these costs until it is determined that ongoing costs can be included in future capitation rates negotiated with the M+CO. If costs for the trials are passed on to Medicare FFS, Medicare FFS assumes responsibility for payment to the providers. Thus Medicare pays providers directly for their services regardless of whether they are network providers for the M+CO. The reason for this arrangement is that clinical trials will rarely be available within an M+CO's network. Although Medicare FFS assumes responsibility for the costs of the clinical trial, M+COs cannot limit clinical trials to those provided within their network.

If a beneficiary is enrolled in a clinical trial and also in an M+CO, although payments for the clinical trial will be assumed by Medicare FFS, the patient will not be responsible for any Part A or Part B deductibles. However, the patient is required to pay the coinsurance amounts applicable to any of the services paid for under the Medicare FFS rules. Because these amounts could be substantial, case managers must inform their patients of any funding programs (e.g., Medicaid) for which the patients might be eligible. If the patient is enrolled in a clinical trial, his or her M+CO remains responsible for all care and services *not related to the condition covered by the clinical trail*. Additionally, the organization is not required to pay any additional or supplemental costs of the clinical trial.

THE BBRA AND OTHER MEDICARE RULES

The following were results of the passage of the Balanced Budget Refinement Act (BBRA) of 1999:

- Extension of Medicare benefits for coverage of immunosuppressive drugs after organ transplantation
- Placement of a 2-year moratorium on the cap of $1500 for outpatient therapy visits that was to have been implemented under the BBA of 1997; as a result of the BBRA change, therapy will now be covered that would not otherwise have been covered
- Coverage of adult liver transplantation to persons given a diagnosis of hepatitis B

The BBRA extends Medicare benefits for immunosuppressive drugs after organ transplantation. Before this act, coverage was limited to 36 months after transplantation. Starting on January 1, 2000, coverage was extended an additional 8 months for a total of 44 months. Although this affects FFS Medicare, it has a greater impact on M+COs when such beneficiaries are enrolled, because the organizations must now assume the costs of these drugs from their capitation payment.

Unfortunately, any extended Medicare coverage does not affect beneficiaries with ESRD who have undergone successful kidney transplantation. They continue to lose Medicare eligibility after 36 months, unless they are eligible for Medicare because of age or disability.

Additional benefits allowed by CMS under the act for M+COs include the ability to offer in-home accessibility aids, provided certain conditions are met. If an M+CO offers this as a benefit the following conditions must be met:

- The health care items or services must be intended to maintain or improve the health status of enrollees.
- The plan must incur a cost or liability directly related to the item or service and not just an administrative processing cost.
- The item or service must be submitted and approved through the benefit rating process.
- The benefit must be classified as an additional benefit, mandatory supplemental benefit, or optional supplemental benefit.
- The benefit must be established by the plan as "reasonable and appropriate" according to standards for the provision of in-home accessibility aids. Additionally, the plan must apply those standards equitably to all members within their managed care plans. If the benefit is offered as an optional supplemental benefit, the organization must apply the standards equitably to all members within the organization. If the organization wants to offer the item or service to some but not all members, the item or service cannot be offered as part of an M+CO's benefits. The "uniformity of benefits" requirement of the Social Security Act stipulates that all benefits must be available to all enrollees in the MCO.

OTHER RULES FOR M+C BENEFICIARIES

Because many patients followed up by case management will be undergoing dialysis or will have ESRD, it is imperative that case managers understand the rules of the M+C program on this issue. Under the M+C option, all beneficiaries, regardless of diagnosis, have the right to be out of a service area on a temporary basis. A temporary status can be allowed when the beneficiary (1) is absent from the service area for 12 months or less and (2) continues to maintain a permanent address/residence within the service area. When they are out of a service area, beneficiaries are entitled to emergency or urgent services without direction from their primary care provider or prior authorization; and for beneficiaries with ESRD, this means having their dialysis treatments.

If the beneficiary is outside the service area on a temporary basis, the M+CO remains responsible for payment of all medically necessary dialysis treatments and related care. The only restriction is that the dialysis must be obtained from a participating Medicare dialysis provider, but it can be provided by anyone selected by the beneficiary. Although it is advisable for such patients to inform the M+CO of their intent to be absent from the service area, they are not obligated to do so. Nor are they required to obtain prior authorization. Similarly, the beneficiary is not required to give advance notice that he or she will be using dialysis services while temporarily absent from the organization's service area.

To ensure timely payments and prevent unnecessary hassle, case managers assisting patients with ESRD must educate them about their rights to services. Patients must also be informed that they have the right to independently select a dialysis provider and that the M+CO remains responsible for payment of the claims.

Also, as case managers work with beneficiaries, it is important to build their confidence so that once beneficiaries are away from the service area, they will call as medical needs or issues arise.

M+COs are allowed to consider a beneficiary's move permanent when they are notified from the beneficiary of such a move or documents reveal a permanent residence (e.g., voter registration or driver's license) that indicates that the beneficiary is outside the organization's services area. Any change in residence that lasts longer than 12 months is considered a permanent move. If the beneficiary moves out of the service area permanently, he or she must disenroll from the M+CO. When he or she disenrolls, the effective date is the first day of the month after receipt of the disenrollment request.

Quality and Medicare

For quality monitoring, M+COs are required to achieve compliance through what is termed by CMS its *quality improvement system for managed care*, more commonly known as QISMC. Although QISMC remains under development, its interim standards and guidelines are being used as a tool for states as they measure performances of their Medicare and Medicaid managed care plans. The final QISMC standards will eventually be the document used for Medicare's quality assurance and will be outlined in the Medicare program manuals. For more information on QISMC see CMS's website at www.cms.hhs.gov/cop.2d.asp.

QISMC represents CMS's attempts to implement quality requirements for organizations that participate in the M+C program. The standards are designed to measure an organization's operations and performances in the areas of quality measurement and improvement. The primary intent of QISMC is to assist organizations in the development of mechanisms to measure and improve outcomes, with the ultimate goal being high-quality and cost-effective care. QISMC's interim standards and guidelines apply to all services provided by the organization not only for Medicare enrollees older than 65 years but also for Medicare enrollees younger than 65 years with special needs.

The BBA gives CMS the authority to deem that an M+CO meets certain quality assurance requirements if the M+CO is accredited and periodically reaccredited by a private organization (e.g., National Committee for Quality Assurance). Thus the national accrediting organization may "deem" the organization is compliant in its quality program. If deeming is used, it is based on rigorous standards established to ensure quality for both the Medicare and Medicaid programs. Therefore the following six specific areas are reviewed:

1. Quality assurance
2. Antidiscrimination
3. Access to services
4. Confidentiality and accuracy of enrollee records
5. Information on advance directives
6. Provider participation rules

MEDICAID

Title XIX of the Social Security Act created Medicaid, a program that provides medical assistance for certain individuals and families with low incomes and few resources. The program became law in 1965 and is a jointly funded cooperative venture between the federal and state governments. Medicaid is the largest insurance program that provides medical and health-related services to the poorest people in the United States.

The basic differences between Medicare FFS and Medicaid are simple. Medicare FFS is primarily available to persons older than 65 years, regardless of income and benefits, and the criteria for eligibility are the same, no matter where in the United States the beneficiary resides or what benefits are used. Medicaid, on the other hand, is available to persons of any age, and eligibility is based strictly on financial need. However, eligibility criteria and benefits vary from state to state. Another big difference between Medicare and Medicaid is that although both cover short-term care, Medicaid is the primary funding source for long-term care, covering more than half of all long-term custodial care costs.

Intent of Medicaid

The intent of the Medicaid program is to assist states in the provision of adequate medical care to eligible financially needy persons. Although the states administer their own programs, they do so under broad federal guidelines that allow them to do the following:

- Establish their own eligibility and financial criteria standards
- Determine the type, amount, duration, and scope of services
- Set the rate of payment for services
- Administer its program

Initially, Medicaid provided medical care to federally funded income maintenance programs for the poor. The emphasis of the initial program was on the aged, the disabled, and dependent children and their mothers. However, recent legislation has allowed the following:

- Expansion of the Medicaid program to cover low-income pregnant women, poor children, and some Medicare beneficiaries who are not eligible for any cash assistance program and would not have been eligible for Medicaid under earlier Medicaid rules
- Continued specific benefits beyond the normal run of Medicaid eligibility
- Continued sharp increase in expenditures for short-term intensive care, for home health care, and for skilled nursing services for the elderly and disabled

Eligibility
Categorically Needy

There are wide variations found in Medicaid eligibility. To qualify for Medicaid as categorically needy, a person must have income and assets at or below the state's predetermined dollar amounts. Most states use the same formula that is used for the federal Supplemental Security Income (SSI) program to determine eligibility for Medicaid. Unfortunately, other states establish their own Medicaid eligibility formulas and standards, which are more difficult to meet than those set for SSI.

To be eligible for federal funds, states are required to provide Medicaid coverage for most individuals who receive federally assisted income maintenance payments. In addition, each state is allowed to cover some related groups not receiving cash payments. Some examples of the mandatory Medicaid eligibility groups are as follows:

- Low-income families with children who meet the state's Aid to Families with Dependent Children (AFDC) plan
- SSI recipients
- Infants born to Medicaid-eligible pregnant women; in these cases Medicaid eligibility continues throughout the first year of life or as long as the infant remains in the mother's household and the mother remains eligible or would be eligible if she were still pregnant
- Children younger than 6 years and pregnant women whose family income is at or below 133% of the federal poverty level
- Recipients of adoption assistance and foster care under Title IV-E of the Social Security Act
- Certain Medicare beneficiaries
- Some special protected groups who may continue to receive Medicaid

for a limited amount of time (e.g., persons who lose SSI payments because of earnings from work or increased Social Security benefits and families who are provided 6 to 12 months of Medicaid coverage after loss of eligibility because of earnings or 4 months of Medicaid coverage after loss of eligibility because of an increase in child or spousal support)

States have the option (for which they will receive federal matching funds) of providing Medicaid coverage for other "categorically needy" groups. Although these groups share some characteristics of the mandatory groups, the eligibility criteria are more liberal. In most cases the categorically needy persons will be eligible for Medicaid but may or may not receive cash assistance from a state's SSI program. Examples of the optional groups states may cover are as follows:

- Infants until the age of 1 year and pregnant women who are not covered under the mandatory rules when the family income falls below 185% of the federal poverty level
- Low-income children
- Certain elderly, blind, or disabled adults with incomes below the federal poverty level but above incomes requiring mandatory coverage
- Children younger than 21 years who meet income and resources requirements for AFDC but who otherwise are not eligible for AFDC
- Institutionalized individuals with income and resources below specified limits
- Persons who, if institutionalized, would be eligible but are receiving care at home under a Medicaid home- or community-based services waiver
- Recipients of a state's supplementary payments

- Persons with tuberculosis who would be financially eligible for Medicaid at the SSI level but cannot afford the tuberculosis-related ambulatory services or tuberculosis drugs
- Low-income or uninsured women who have been screened, given a diagnosis of, and determined to be in need of treatment for breast or cervical cancer

Even under the broadest provisions of the federal statute, not all poor people are eligible for Medicaid. Unless they are in one of the groups designated previously, patients will be excluded from eligibility and any Medicaid benefits. In most states a person can qualify for Medicaid if he or she is eligible for SSI assistance. This means the person can own a home, regardless of value, and a car worth a certain value. To qualify for Medicaid, a person must have a monthly income that is no more than a specific amount (i.e., $450 for an individual or $600 for a couple). The person can also have assets worth up to a specific dollar amount (i.e., savings of $2000 per individual or $3000 per couple plus some household goods and a burial plot).

States and Eligibility for the Categorically Needy

States that follow SSI standards to determine Medicaid eligibility for the categorically needy are as follows:

- Alabama
- Alaska
- Colorado
- Idaho
- Mississippi
- Nevada
- New Mexico
- Oregon
- Rhode Island
- South Carolina
- South Dakota
- Tennessee
- Wyoming

If the state uses the more stringent standards to determine Medicaid eligibility, the person must have assets and income even lower than SSI standards including lower values on the home, automobile, or personal property. These states include the following:

- Connecticut
- Hawaii
- Illinois
- Indiana
- Minnesota
- Missouri
- New Hampshire
- North Carolina
- North Dakota
- Ohio
- Oklahoma
- Virginia

Medically Needy

The ability to offer a "medically needy" program allows states to extend Medicaid eligibility to persons who may have too much income to qualify under the mandatory or optional categorically needy groups but too little to pay for needed services. Basically, this program examines only income and assets. However, some states do take into consideration a person's medical bills, whether current or anticipated. Therefore medically needy persons who would be categorically eligible except for income or assets may become eligible for Medicaid solely because of excessive medical expenses.

The following states offer Medicaid coverage for the medically needy based on income and assets plus their current or anticipated medical expenses[1]:

- Arizona
- Arkansas
- California
- Connecticut
- District of Columbia
- Florida
- Georgia
- Illinois

- Iowa
- Kansas
- Kentucky
- Louisiana
- Maine
- Maryland
- Massachusetts
- Michigan
- Minnesota
- Montana
- Nebraska
- New Hampshire
- New Jersey
- New York
- North Carolina
- North Dakota
- Oklahoma
- Pennsylvania
- Texas
- Utah
- Vermont
- Virginia
- Washington
- West Virginia
- Wisconsin

Persons in this category are allowed to "spend down" to Medicaid eligibility by incurring medical care expenses to offset their excess income. Thus they are allowed to reduce their assets to a level below the maximum allowed by the state's Medicaid plan. A family may establish medically needy eligibility by paying monthly premiums to the state in an amount equal to the difference between family income (reduced by unpaid expenses if there are any incurred expenses for medical care in previous months) and the income eligibility standard.

Many Medicaid beneficiaries are not required to pay premiums, deductibles, copayments, or other out-of-pocket fees (also referred to as *cost-sharing* or *SOC [share of cost] fees*).

Many states have elected to provide Medicaid to people who qualify as "medically needy." Even though these people may not qualify based on their incomes or assets, they are accepted because they face huge medical bills.

The Dual Eligible—Medicare and Medicaid

Some low-income Medicare beneficiaries may receive help paying for their out-of-pocket medical expenses or the cost of premiums from their state's Medicaid program. There are various benefits available to "dual eligible" beneficiaries, those eligible for both Medicare and Medicaid.

When a person is eligible for full Medicaid coverage, his or her Medicaid program supplements Medicare coverage by providing coverage for deductibles and copayments for any services or supplies. When a person has dual coverage, Medicare is considered the primary insurer with the difference paid by Medicaid, up to the state's payment limit (i.e., if Medicare pays what the state would have paid, Medicaid will pay no more). As indicated previously, Medicaid is the major insurer for long-term care and it covers additional services not covered by Medicare (e.g., nursing facility care beyond the 100-day limit, prescription drugs, eyeglasses, and hearing aids).

Medicaid can help some other low-income Medicare beneficiaries pay for out-of-pocket Medicare cost-sharing expenses. If a person is receiving SSDI and loses entitlement to Medicare benefits because of a return to work, he or she is given an option to purchase Part A of Medicare. However, if this person's income meets Medicaid eligibility requirements, he or she may qualify to have Medicaid pay their monthly Medicare Part A premiums through a program known as *Qualified Disabled and Working Individuals*. For more information on this topic, please see the CMS website at cms.hhs.gov/manuals/45_smm/sm_03_3_toc.asp.

Retroactive Coverage

If an individual is deemed eligible for benefits, retroactive coverage can occur. When this happens, eligibility actually starts 90 days before the actual date of application. Retroactive eligibility is allowed when it is deemed that the individual would have been eligible but for some reason did not enroll.

Termination

If an individual is deemed ineligible, coverage stops only at the end of the month in which a person's financial circumstances change.

MEDICARE CATASTROPHIC COVERAGE ACT OF 1988

Although significant changes were anticipated for Medicare under the Medicare Catastrophic Coverage Act (MCCA) of 1988, the act was repealed. However, the portions intended for Medicaid remain in effect. Beginning in 1989, Medicaid eligibility rules for persons needing nursing facility (NF) care were changed. As a result of this change, Medicaid eligibility for persons needing nursing home care was accelerated. This is allowed under a rule called *spousal impoverishment*. The MCCA requires states to permit the at-home spouse to retain a "maintenance needs allowance." Thus the spouses of NF residents are protected from impoverishment.

Basically, the law allows the couple to split and protect assets. It also allows an amount to be deducted from the institutionalized spouse's income that is added to the at-home spouse's income. Consequently, most states look only at the income of the SNF resident, but some states do take into consideration the joint income of both parties. For example, before an institutionalized person's monthly income is used to pay for the cost of institutional care, a minimum monthly maintenance needs allowance is deducted from the spouse's income. This brings the income of the at-home or community spouse up to a moderate level. Depending on the state, the at-home spouse is allowed a monthly income while he or she retains the home, as well as a specific amount of cash assets (i.e., $84,000).

However, if the state allows these new rules, the state also has the ability to place a lien on the assets and property equal to the amount spent on care for the spouse in the SNF. When the at-home spouse dies or sells the house, the state will enforce the lien, taking money the at-home spouse would leave to survivors.

CORE BENEFITS

According to Title XIX of the Social Security Act, for a state to receive federal matching funds, certain basic services called *core benefits* must be offered. Medicaid core benefits include the following:

- Inpatient hospital services
- Outpatient hospital services
- Physician services
- Pediatric and family nurse practitioner services
- Medical and surgical dental services
- NF services for individuals 21 years of age or older
- Home health care for persons eligible for nursing facility services
- Family planning services and supplies
- Rural health clinic services and any other ambulatory services offered by a rural health clinic otherwise covered under the state plan
- Laboratory and radiology services
- Federally qualified health center services and any ambulatory services offered by a federally qualified health center otherwise covered under the state plan
- Nurse-midwife services (to the extent authorized under state law)
- Early and periodic screening, diagnosis, and treatment (EPSDT) services for individuals younger than 21 years

In addition to federally mandated coverage of physician, hospital, and nursing facility services, most states have chosen to cover what are termed *optional services* and these include the following:

- Eye care (includes eye examinations and eyewear)
- Dental care (dental examination and dentures)
- Prescription drugs

Almost all states also include the following:

- Physical therapy
- Hospice care
- A variety of rehabilitative services
- Nonemergent transportation
- Various preventive screening and services
- Inpatient psychiatric care for those 65 years old and older
- Prosthetic devices
- Podiatry
- Chiropractic care

The types and amounts of optional services vary from state to state. States may also receive federal funding if they elect to provide other optional services. The most commonly covered optional services under the Medicaid program include the following:

- Clinic services
- Nursing facility services for persons younger than 21 years
- Intermediate care facility/mentally retarded services
- Tuberculosis-related services for persons with tuberculosis

Additional optional services might also include the following:

- Durable medical equipment and medical supplies
- Artificial limbs, braces, and eyes
- Acupuncture
- Blood and blood derivatives and their administration

If a state chooses to include the medically needy population, the state's Medicaid plan must provide the following services, at a minimum:

- Prenatal care and delivery services for pregnant women
- Ambulatory services to individuals younger than 18 years and individuals entitled to institutional services
- Home health services to individuals entitled to nursing facility services

Excluded Services

The following is a list of services most often excluded from Medicaid coverage:

- Administration of routine oral medications
- Any service or supplies covered under workers' compensation benefit plans, conditions resulting from acts of war (declared or not), court- or employer-ordered care, and school recreation or work physical examinations
- If the person is enrolled in a Medicaid managed care plan, any service received before the beneficiary's effective date of coverage or after the effective date of termination
- Circumcision, unless medically indicated
- Cosmetic surgery, unless medically indicated
- Eating disorders
- Experimental drugs, services, items, or procedures or devices that have not been tested in humans
- Eye surgery for the sole purpose of correcting refractive error (i.e., radial keratotomy), orthoptic services (a technique of eye exercises designed to correct the visual axes of eyes not properly coordinated for binocular vision eyeglasses), contact lenses or low vision aids more than once every 24 months; also excluded are routine vision examinations and eye refractions for the fitting of glasses, more than once every 12 months
- Hair transplantation

- Hysterectomy for the sole purpose of sterilization
- In vitro fertilization, artificial insemination, gamete intrafallopian transfer, zygote intrafallopian tube transfer, or any other procedure involving combining of ovum and sperm outside the body, costs of donor sperm storage, and so forth
- Liposuction
- Loaner hearing aids during repair periods covered under guarantee and replacement batteries
- Morbid obesity surgery
- Nonmedically necessary services or procedures
- Physical examinations related to school, employment, marriage licenses
- School supplies (e.g., computers)
- Services related to learning disorders
- Sex transformation
- Some outpatient prescription and nonprescription drugs such as the following:
  - Drugs or supplies provided for cosmetic purposes including drugs for hair regeneration
  - Nutritional supplements
  - Experimental drugs or supplies
  - Investigational drugs or supplies except for those that meet the state's Medicaid criteria
  - Anabolic steroids
  - Vitamins (other than pediatric and prenatal)
  - Topical fluoride preparations
  - Anorexiants (subclassification of antiobesity drugs)
  - Noninjectable and injectable drugs or supplies customarily dispensed from physician's offices

Amount and Duration of Services

Although federal guidelines define core benefits, each state is allowed to determine the amount and duration of services offered under its Medicaid programs. However, states are required to set the amount, duration, and scope of each service to be sufficient to reasonably achieve its purpose. States are also allowed to place appropriate limits on Medicaid services based on criteria such as medical necessity or any utilization controls it requires (e.g., states may place a reasonable limit on the number of covered visits to a provider or may require prior authorization from a local field office before the service is rendered).

Each state can determine the amount and duration of services, but the scope and duration of each service must be sufficient to reasonably achieve its purpose and care must be medically necessary.

ADDITIONAL MEDICAID MANDATORY BENEFITS

In addition to core benefits, state Medicaid programs must include the following as mandatory benefits:
- Nursing facility services for individuals 21 years of age and older
- Home health services
- EPSDT

Nursing Facility Services for Individuals Aged 21 Years and Older

Nursing facility services for individuals aged 21 years and older are a mandatory Medicaid benefit and are performed in facilities that primarily provide the following:
- Skilled nursing care and related services for residents who require medical or nursing care
- Rehabilitation services for injured, disabled, or sick persons
- Health-related care and services to individuals who, because of their mental or physical condition, require care and services above the level of room and board, which can only be made available to them through institutional care

A nursing facility that is a participating provider in a state's Medicaid program must provide or arrange for the full range of services for residents who need them. Nursing facilities are required to meet a number of requirements relating to provision of services, residents' rights, and administration. To fulfill all plans of care, a nursing facility must provide or arrange for the provision of the following:
- Nursing and related services and specialized rehabilitative services to attain or maintain the highest practicable physical, mental, and psychosocial well-being of each resident
- Medically related social services to attain or maintain the highest practicable physical, mental, and psychosocial well-being of each resident
- Pharmaceutical services to meet the needs of each resident (including procedures that ensure the accurate acquisition, receipt, dispensing, and administration of all drugs and biologic agents)
- Dietary services that ensure that meals meet the daily nutritional and special dietary needs of each resident
- An ongoing activity program, directed by a qualified professional designed to meet the interests of and enhance the physical, mental, and psychosocial well-being of each resident
- Routine dental services (to the extent covered under a state's plan) and emergency dental services to meet the needs of each resident
- Treatment and services required by mentally ill and mentally retarded residents not otherwise provided or arranged for (or required to be provided or arranged for) by the state

Home Health Services

Home health services are a mandatory benefit for individuals who are entitled to nursing facility services under the state's

Medicaid plan. Services must be provided at a recipient's place of residence and must be ordered by a physician as part of a plan of care that is reviewed every 60 days. Home health services must include nursing services as defined in a state's Nurse Practice Act and must be provided on an intermittent basis. Also covered are home health aide services provided by a home health agency, medical supplies, equipment, and appliances deemed suitable for use in the home. Physical therapy, occupational therapy, speech therapy, and audiology services are optional services states may choose to provide. To participate in the Medicaid program, a home health agency must meet the conditions of participation for Medicare.

EPSDT Services

Under the Omnibus Budget Reconciliation Act of 1989 states are mandated to provide EPSDT. The act mandates that preventive screenings be made available to children, as well as any federally allowable diagnostic and treatment service determined to be medically necessary. EPSDT services are very specific and detailed and are to include periodic health assessments, beginning at birth and continuing through age 20 years; all age-specific immunizations; and age-appropriate assessments. All of these services must be provided at intervals, according to defined periodicity schedules.

EPSDT is a program that offers Medicaid-eligible individuals access to Medicaid services that are medically reasonable and necessary. The program goals are to periodically screen Medicaid enrolled children for correctable health problems throughout their development and to provide appropriate treatment for identified problems.

The EPSDT program requires every child to have a complete examination at regular intervals. Services identified as medically necessary must be provided by a state's Medicaid plan, even if those services are not included as part of the covered services in that state's plan. The physical examinations provide important information for other services and also the following:

- Evaluate the form, structure, and function of particular body regions and systems
- Determine whether these regions and systems are normal for the child's age and background
- Discover those diseases and health problems for which no standard screening test has been developed, including evidence of child abuse and neglect

Since many children served by case management will be eligible for Medicaid, case managers assisting pediatric patients must be very familiar with the state's and program's requirements.

OPTIONAL SERVICES

State Medicaid programs are allowed flexibility as they create their programs. Therefore they may or may not offer the following optional benefits:

- Hospice services
- Rehabilitation services
- Personal care services
- Targeted case management
- Home- and community-based service (HCBS) waivers
- Programs aimed at institutionalization of persons with mental disorders older than 65 years
- Programs designed for women with cancer
- Programs designed for persons with HIV infection
- The Program of All-Inclusive Care for the Elderly (PACE)
- Work incentive programs

Hospice Services

Hospice services are an optional benefit states may choose to make available under their Medicaid program. As with all hospice programs, the intent of the program is to provide for the palliation or management of the terminal illness and related conditions. Under federal qualifications for hospice, a physician must certify the individual to be terminally ill. An individual is considered to be terminally ill if the medical prognosis is life expectancy of 6 months or less. Individuals who meet these requirements can elect to use the state's Medicaid hospice benefit.

To receive Medicaid payment, the provider must meet Medicare's conditions of participation and have a valid provider agreement with the state agency overseeing the Medicaid program. As with any hospice program, the overall intent is to provide care in the home and avoid an institutional setting, as well as to improve the individual's quality of life until he or she dies. Although the programs are generally geared to care within a home setting, some patients receiving hospice will reside in an SNF or board-and-care home as they receive their hospice care (this allowance will be facility-specific because not all facilities are licensed to provide or participate in a hospice program).

As a rule, the services provided by hospice must be related to the palliation or management of the patient's terminal illness, offering pain and symptom control while enabling the individual to perform activities of daily living and basic functional skills as normally as possible. To ensure coverage, a plan of care must be established before the actual rendering of any services. To meet the plan of care goals, the following disciplines are used and covered by hospice:

- Nursing care
- Medical social services
- Physicians' services
- Counseling services
- Home health aide
- Medical appliances and supplies, including drugs and biologic agents

- Physical and occupational therapy

Depending on case needs, continuous home care can be provided in periods of crisis. If continuous home care is required, it consists primarily of nursing care for a short period—usually only a day or so. If care is needed for a longer period, the patient may require placement in an SNF or a short-term hospital stay. If short-term inpatient care is required, it can be covered as long as it is provided in a participating hospice hospital or SNF. Generally, if inpatient care is needed, it is for procedures necessary for pain control or for the immediate management of symptoms that cannot be accomplished in an alternate setting. At times it may be needed for respite for the caregiver.

If respite care is required, it will be short-term. In most cases it will be provided in an inpatient setting, since it is used to give the family members or caregiver a period of rest from the responsibilities of continuous care of the patient. Respite care is provided on an occasional basis and is reimbursed for no more than 5 days at a time. The respite care benefit does not extend to patients residing in an SNF.

Rehabilitation Services

Another optional Medicaid benefit is rehabilitation services. Rehabilitation, according to this definition, is broad, since it not only covers traditional physical medicine and rehabilitation but also care that might be related to mental health services.

Physicians or other licensed health care providers practicing within their scope of expertise can prescribe mental health rehabilitation services. The services may be provided in any setting and are generally supplied in a variety forms such as those used in mental health services (e.g., individual and group therapy and psychosocial services).

States may also provide services aimed at improving physical functional abilities, including physical, occupational, and speech therapy. A licensed physician must prescribe the therapy, and the therapy must be provided under the direction of a licensed and qualified physical, occupational, or speech therapist. Included are any medically necessary supplies and equipment.

Personal Care Services

Personal care services are another optional Medicaid benefit. Personal care services are provided to individuals who are not inpatients or residents of a hospital, nursing facility, intermediate care facility for the mentally retarded, or institution for mental disease. The following requirements apply to reimbursement for personal care services:

- Must be prescribed by a physician in accordance with a plan of treatment and authorized for the individual in accordance with a service plan approved by the state
- Must be provided by a qualified individual who is not a member of the individual's family
- Must be furnished in a home or home-like setting

Personal care services include a wide range of human assistance provided to persons with disabilities and chronic conditions of all ages and can be provided on a continuous or episodic basis. The intent of the services is to enable the person to accomplish tasks he or she would normally perform if he or she did not have a disability. Personal care services are most often in the form of hands-on assistance or cueing so that the patient or client performs the task by himself or herself and include such assistance with the performance of activities of daily living and instrumental activities of daily living, which include eating, bathing, dressing, toileting, transferring, personal hygiene, light housework, and medication management. Although personal services can augment skilled services, they must not be confused with skilled services, which must be performed by a licensed health care professional.

Targeted Case Management

States are allowed to provide optional targeted case management services to recipients as part of their state Medicaid statutes. The specific statute defines targeted case management services as "services which assist an eligible individual in gaining access to needed medical, social, educational and other services." Targeted case management enables states to reach beyond the boundaries of the Medicaid program to coordinate a broad range of activities and services necessary to maximize the optimal functioning of select categories of Medicaid beneficiaries. States providing such case management services do so by amending their state plans with a separate plan approved for each targeted group. If targeted case management services are allowed, states frequently use case management vendors to supply the services required.

If the Medicaid beneficiary is enrolled in a Medicaid managed care plan, targeted case management is often a carve-out between the MCO and the state's department of health services. This means that if the patient requires intensive case management services, the department of health services may allow disenrollment of the beneficiary from the managed care plan, reverting the patient's coverage to FFS Medicaid and linking the patient to a department of health services case management vendor. As with traditional case management services, targeted case management is used to monitor high-risk Medicaid patients, a group that may include the following individuals:

- Certain women, infants, children, and young adults (until the age of 21 years) who have a high-risk diagnosis or medical condition
- Persons with human immunodeficiency virus or acquired immune deficiency syndrome

- Persons who are technology-dependent. Solely for the purposes of the targeted case management services program, *technology-dependent persons* are those persons who use a medical device that compensates for the loss of normal use of a vital body function and require any amount of skilled nursing care to avert death or further disability (can be 24-hour care)
- Persons with multiple diagnoses who require services from multiple health care or social service providers
- Persons who are medically fragile (often the elderly)

Solely for the purposes of the targeted case management services program, *medically fragile persons* are those persons who require ongoing or intermittent medical supervision without which their health would deteriorate to an acute episode.

Targeted case management services are designed to assess beneficiaries, develop a written plan, link the patient to specific services and resources designed to meet his or her needs, and conduct follow-up to ensure the required services are implemented. The case manager may assist the beneficiary in gaining access to services through such activities as actually making the appointment and coordinating the necessary transportation, arranging for translation services, or making arrangements for any nonmedical crisis assistance planning.

Home- and Community-Based Waivers—1915(c) Waivers

Section 1915(c) of the BBA created the Medicaid HCBS waivers. Under this section of the act, states are afforded the ability to be flexible as they develop and implement creative alternatives aimed at placing Medicaid-eligible individuals in hospitals, nursing facilities, or intermediate care facilities (e.g., facilities for persons with mental retardation). The act specifi-

cally lists seven services that must be provided in HCBS waiver programs:

1. Case management
2. Housekeeping
3. Home health aide services
4. Personal care services
5. Adult day health
6. Habilitation
7. Respite care

If patients are to avoid placement in a medical facility, states may request such services as the following (must be approved by CMS):

- Nonmedical transportation
- In-home support services
- Special communication services
- Minor home modifications
- Adult day care

The goal of the HCBS waiver program is to provide care to those individuals at risk of being placed in these facilities in their homes and communities. Thus their independence is preserved, as are the ties to family and friends. Therefore all states have federal waiver status allowing them to pay for home and community care for elderly beneficiaries who otherwise would end up in nursing homes. States are not limited in the scope of services they can provide for patients covered by a waiver. The key is the cost-effectiveness of the plan of care because care can cost no more than institutionalization.

For the purpose of developing Medicaid-financed community-based treatment alternatives, section 1915(c) allows states to request waivers of certain federal requirements. The three requirements that may be waived for the medically needy are "statewideness," comparability of services, and community income and resource rules. The law allows states the flexibility to design their waiver programs and select the mix of waiver services that best meets the needs of the population to be served. HCBS waiver service may be provided statewide or may be limited to specific geographic subdivisions.

Federal regulations allow HCBS waiver programs the ability to target specific illnesses or medical conditions, technology-dependent persons, or individuals with AIDS. HCBS waiver programs also have the ability to serve elderly persons with physical disabilities, developmental disabilities, mental retardation, or mental illness. For persons with chronic mental illness, the law permits day treatment or other partial hospitalization services, psychosocial rehabilitation services, and clinic services (whether or not furnished in a facility). Room and board are excluded from coverage except for certain limited circumstances.

To receive approval for an HCBS waiver program, the state Medicaid agency must assure CMS that the cost of providing HCBS will not exceed the average per capita cost of care for an identical population in an institution. Additionally, the state agency must document the safeguards it will have in place to protect the health and welfare of beneficiaries. Because waivers are so valuable and patients who are technology-dependent can quickly exhaust any health care benefits allowed, case managers must be very knowledgeable about their state's or the patient's state's waiver program. At a minimum, this includes knowledge of the application process and basic requirements of the program.

Institutions for Mental Disorders

Federal law allows states the ability to offer optional coverage for persons aged 65 years or older who are institutionalized because of a mental disorder. Additionally, states are allowed to provide similar optional coverage for individuals younger than 21 years if they are institutionalized. Medicaid programs are not required to cover medical services provided to any individual who is younger than 65 years and who is a patient in an institution for mental disorders unless the payment is for inpatient psychiatric services for individuals younger than 21 years.

Medicaid and Cancer

The Breast and Cervical Cancer Prevention and Treatment Act of 2000 gave states the option of providing medical services to certain women who have been found to have breast or cervical cancer or precancerous conditions. This law allows states to expend their Medicaid coverage to cover the cost of treating poor women who have been given a diagnosis of breast cancer. Under this act, the federal government is allowed to reimburse states for a portion of the treatment costs.

Medicaid and HIV

Many persons infected with HIV are eligible for Medicaid, especially if they are disabled, have low income and limited assets, or meet certain income and resource standards. Many states base eligibility on the person's medical expenses. Each state must provide the full range of Medicaid services covered in its plan to eligible persons with HIV infection. States may also provide optional services that are appropriate for people with HIV and AIDS, such as targeted case management, prevention services, and hospice care.

Medicaid and the Elderly—The PACE Program

Another program authorized by the BBA of 1997 is PACE. PACE is a permanent entity within the Medicare program and enables states to provide PACE services to Medicaid beneficiaries as a state option. This program is a new capitated benefit featuring a comprehensive service delivery system paid through integration of both Medicare and Medicaid payments. The PACE model uses a multidisciplinary team approach in an adult day health center. The model is further supplemented by in-home and referral services in accordance with the participants' needs. The goal of the program is to use a comprehensive service package, allowing most participants to remain at home rather than be institutionalized. To enter the program participants must be the following:

- At least 55 years old
- A resident of the PACE service area
- Certified as eligible for nursing home care by the appropriate state agency

Once an enrollee is certified as eligible, the PACE program serves as the sole source of services. The participant's care plan is developed by using assessment data through a team approach, with the team comprising both professional and paraprofessional staff. The plan and services provided include acute-care services and nursing facility services when necessary. The core program provides social and medical services primarily in an adult day health care center and this is supplemented by in-home and referral services as dictated by the participant's needs.

Financing for the program is through a capitated model that places full risk on the providers. This model requires providers to deliver all the services participants require (i.e., there are no limits on amount, duration, or scope of services). Thus participants are not subjected to piecemeal or limited services as they might be in the traditional Medicare FFS and Medicaid FFS service systems. In the reimbursement model, providers receive monthly Medicare and Medicaid capitation payments for each eligible enrollee. Medicare-eligible participants who are not eligible for Medicaid pay monthly premiums equal to the Medicaid capitation amount. However, they do not have a deductible or coinsurance payment.

WORK INCENTIVES

A new set of rules, which also came from the BBA, allows states to provide Medicaid coverage to working individuals with disabilities, who were historically excluded from coverage because of their earnings, through the creation of an optional categorically needy eligibility group. Under this rule, an individual's disability and family income is used to determine whether the person meets the SSI program's standards, since this is the key factor used to determine eligibility.

Two additional categories for eligibility were created under an act termed the *Ticket to Work and Work Incentives Improvement Act of 1999 (TWWIIA)*. This act created two new optional categorically needy Medicaid eligibility groups: (1) the basic coverage group and (2) the medical improvement group. States can elect to cover only the basic coverage group; however, if they do cover the medical improvement group, they must also cover the basic coverage group. Under the basic coverage group, the following rules apply:

- There are no federal required income or resource standards.
- The individual must be at least 16 years old and not more than 64 years old.
- Individuals covered must be disabled, as defined by SSI.
- Earned income is not automatically disregarded.
- If states establish income and resource standards, SSI income and resource methods must be used to determine eligibility.

The medical improvement group is similar but requires the following:

- The individual must be at least 16 years old but not more than 64 years old.
- The individual covered must have a medically improved disability.
- The individual covered must have been eligible under the basic coverage group but lost that eligibility because his or her medical condition improved to the point that he

or she was no longer disabled as defined by SSI.

- Earned income cannot be automatically disregarded.
- Federal requirements for income and resource standards cannot be applied.
- If states establish income and resource standards, SSI income and resource methods must be used to determine eligibility.

The new BBA rule allows states the freedom to establish their own income and resource standards, to have no income and resource standards if they choose, and to use more liberal or more restrictive income and resource eligibility criteria than those used by SSI. In addition, states can require payment premiums or other cost-sharing charges on a sliding scale based on income.

The health care provisions of the TWWIIA are covered under Title II of the act, and health care provisions are administered by The Department of Health and Human Services through CMS. Title II establishes a grant program that allows states to provide benefits equivalent to or greater than those provided by Medicaid. The group served is the categorically needy workers who have physical or mental impairments that will result in disability if they do not receive medical assistance.

The TWWIIA requires the establishment of a demonstration project called *The Demonstration to Maintain Independence and Employment*. This project is authorized for 6 years, and the goal of the project is to address the needs of those people who have specific physical or mental impairments that have the potential to lead to disability. The demonstration project has two advantages: (1) states are allowed to assist working individuals by providing the necessary benefits and services required for covered persons to manage the progression of their conditions and remain employed; and (2) results will be used to evaluate the effects of the provision of Medicaid benefits and services as they relate to extended productivity and improved quality of life. CMS is the designated Department of Health and Human Services agency with administrative responsibility for this grant program.

Before TWWIIA, people with disabilities who met the SSA's criteria for disability but who returned to work were covered by Medicare for at least 39 months (3 years and 3 months) after they completed a 9-month return-to-work trial period. Workers were allowed Medicare hospital insurance (Part A) premium-free and were allowed to retain their Medicare medical insurance (Part B), if they paid their monthly premiums.

The TWWIIA extends Medicare coverage for this category of people for an additional 4½ years beyond the current limit. This means their Medicare coverage continues for at least 93 months (7 years and 9 months) after a 9-month return-to-work trial period. As described previously, they are entitled to Medicare Part A premium-free and Part B, if their monthly premiums are paid. The program is administered by the SSA and began in January 2001. The following individuals now qualify for the additional 4½ years of Medicare coverage:

- Those starting to work for the first time after disability benefits began
- Those in a trial work period
- Those in a 36-month extended period of eligibility that began after June 1997
- Those covered by Medicare before TWWIIA, which is not due to end until after September 30, 2000

MEDICAID AND CHILDREN'S MEDICAL SERVICES PROGRAMS

When a child is screened for eligibility for a state's children's medical services program, he or she is also screened for eligibility for

Medicaid. If the child is eligible for both programs, Medicaid will be the primary insurer.

TRANSPLANTS

A medically necessary transplant is covered by Medicaid if the following conditions are met: it is a Medicare-approved transplant for the diagnosis in question, the patient meets eligibility requirements for the transplant, and transplantation will be performed in a Medicare-approved transplant center. However, the final coverage determination, unlike a general request handled at the local county level, is often issued by a Medicaid division that handles only transplant requests.

Case managers working with transplant candidates or patients must be very familiar with their state's requirements for submission of information for the coverage determination and should know where requests are submitted and reviewed.

For patients enrolled in a Medicaid MCO, the actual pretransplantation and immediate posttransplantation costs are a carve-out from the MCO's contract. This means that although the MCO will be responsible for all requests for coverage until a decision is made that the patient is a candidate for transplantation, once this decision is made, the patient is disenrolled and his or her coverage reverts to Medicaid FFS. Depending on the state's requirements, the patient is often free to re-enroll in an MCO plan within a month or two of the transplantation. The burden of costs for antirejection drugs and follow-up testing and care is shifted back to the MCO chosen by the patient. Case managers working with Medicaid MCO patients must be keenly aware of the MCO's contractual requirements for disenrollment and potential re-enrollment and educate the patient about what the transition in coverage means and why it is necessary.

MEDICAID AND NURSING FACILITY CARE

The largest portion of public expenditures for SNFs, nursing homes, and long-term care is financed by a state's Medicaid program. Any patient who has exhausted his or her health care benefits but must remain hospitalized in an SNF or nursing home because of a need for maintenance care or custodial care must either pay privately or apply to Medicaid for this level of care. If the patient cannot pay, Medicaid will finance the care if the patient meets financial eligibility criteria. If for some reason the patient does not qualify, arrangements must be made for an alternate level of care at the patient's or family's expense.

For nursing home care, Medicaid is the most frequently encountered alternate funding source. However, only those with very limited assets and property qualify for this program. Unfortunately because not all patients qualify, they may "fall through the cracks" or be in the "gray area"—they have too much income to qualify but too little to pay the high cost of medical care themselves.

Medicaid FFS Payments

Medicaid covers the same kinds of services as most insurance plans including Medicare. However, in most states it covers a number of services not covered by insurance or Medicare. For example, Medicaid is almost always the insurer for long-term care both at home and in a nursing facility. It covers not only long-term SNF care but also, in some states, nonmedical care such as personal care. If the person is eligible for Medicaid, Medicaid covers the patient's inpatient deductibles and coinsurance payments.

To receive care from a Medicaid provider, the provider must participate in a state's Medicaid program, and if they do so, they must be willing to accept the amount Medicaid pays them as payment in full.

Each state has relatively broad discretion in determining (within federally imposed upper limits and specific restrictions) the reimbursement method and resulting rate for services, with the following three exceptions: (1) institutional services, for which payment may not exceed amounts that would be paid under Medicare payment rates; (2) disproportionate share hospitals, for which different limits apply; and (3) hospice care.

Federal law allows states to charge a nominal fee to persons who qualify for the Medicaid medically needy program. If a person qualifies for the categorically needy program, only those services considered optional can have any fees imposed. In addition, some states charge a one-time-only enrollment fee or premium that can be charged to the medically needy but not the categorically needy.

Emergency services and family planning services must be exempt from such copayments. Certain Medicaid recipients must be excluded from this cost sharing: pregnant women, children younger than 18 years, hospital or nursing home patients who are expected to contribute most of their income to institutional care, and categorically needy MCO enrollees.

The portion of the Medicaid program that is paid by the federal government is known as the *Federal Medical Assistance Percentage (FMAP)*. The FMAP is determined annually for each state by a formula that compares the state's average per capita income. The amount of federal money used in the Medicaid program has no set limit or cap, and thus the federal government must match whatever the individual state decides to provide within the law for its eligible recipients. The law requires that reimbursement rates be sufficient to enlist enough providers. This is necessary to ensure that Medicaid-reimbursable care and services are available to Medicaid recipients at least to the extent that such care and services are available to the general population in the geographic region. However, because of issues related to low reimbursement, finding providers who are willing to accept and treat a new Medicaid patient is often one of the biggest challenges for case managers.

Medicaid FFS Payments for Nursing Facility Services

Before 1980, Medicaid and Medicare reimbursed nursing facilities on what was called *a retrospective reasonable cost basis*. In 1980 the Boren Amendment was passed, changing the reimbursement method for SNF services.

Under the Boren Amendment, states were required to provide for payment of SNF services through the use of rates that were reasonable and adequate to meet the costs incurred by efficiently and economically operated providers to supply care and services in conformity with applicable state and federal laws, regulations, and quality and safety standards. In 1997 the BBA repealed the Boren requirements and replaced them with a requirement that states implement a public process when changes in payment rates or methods are proposed. As long as states conform to any requirement of federal laws and regulations, they may develop their own Medicaid reimbursement methods.

Therefore because there is no requirement that states develop and use a single payment method for all facilities providing SNF services, a wide variety of mechanisms may be used, and even within a state, mechanisms may vary among providers and provider types. Medicaid SNF payments are generally made by using one of three payment systems: cost-based, per diem, and case mix. As a rule, prospective payment systems (per diem or case mix) are used more frequently than cost-based reimbursement for SNF services. Although the payment systems can be categorized in general terms, specific methods vary from state to state.

MEDICAID AND MANAGED CARE

The BBA of 1997 enacted the first major revision of the statutes governing Medicaid managed care. Under the BBA, the law established new beneficiary protection that includes beneficiary information, quality assurance, and enrollee rights. A key feature is that it allows states greater flexibility in the design of their managed care initiatives. This was achieved by elimination of certain requirements such as those pertaining to the composition of enrollment in a Medicaid MCO and by allowing enrollees the freedom to disenroll from the MCO without cause at any time. Thus the most significant trend in service delivery for Medicaid is the rapid growth in Medicaid managed care enrollment. One vehicle for the expansion of managed care is the waiver process allowed by Section 1915(c) of the BBA. This waiver process allows states the flexibility to research and implement alternatives for health care delivery if the selected program can control program costs.

As a result of the new flexibility of Medicaid managed care, the federal government has given approval to 13 states to carry out ambitious Medicaid managed care demonstration programs. These programs are designed to expand Medicaid coverage and program benefits for low-income adults and their children rather than concentrating efforts only on the disabled and elderly. Most of those enrolled in Medicaid managed care plans are poor children or families receiving AFDC. States have the option to enroll beneficiaries either on a voluntary basis or on a mandatory basis. If a person has special needs, he or she can enroll in either of the foregoing or through section 1915(c) waivers or mandatory enrollment demonstration waivers.[2]

Once a person is enrolled in a Medicaid managed care plan, his or her care is managed by the health plan selected and in the same way that the organization provides managed care to its other enrollees. Each health plan participating in a state's Medicaid managed care plan does so under contract with the state agency responsible for managing the Medicaid program. The health plans are contractually required to follow very specific provisions for such processes as the following:

- Marketing and enrollment
- Disenrollment and terminations
- Determining beneficiary rights and responsibilities
- Ensuring services are culturally and linguistically appropriate for enrollees
- Providing health education services and opportunities
- Establishing rules to contractually provide routine services and care and rules applying to services considered direct access services and any services excluded or carved out
- Ensuring beneficiaries with special needs are identified and services to meet their needs are adequate and provided by qualified medical health care professionals
- Ensuring systems are in place for continuity of care when beneficiaries terminate or are moved to other programs (e.g., in the case of a carve-out service such as a transplant when the patient must be moved to Medicaid FFS); in such cases, the MCO's transition plan must allow the patient to continue to see the MCO provider(s) during the period of transition or up to 90 days, if necessary
- Ensuring that EPSDT services are performed as obligated by state statutes
- Ensuring providers used meet the Americans with Disabilities Act requirements for physical accessibility
- Financial reporting

- Handling of grievances, appeals, and state fair hearings
- Meeting the mandated requirements for quality assessment and improvement strategies, as well as the requirements for collecting and validating encounter data to assist in the management of Medicaid managed care initiatives

CARVE-OUT SERVICES

Carve out is a term often used in managed care when specific services are excluded from a contract and either retained by the entity generating the contract or contracted to another provider (e.g., often mental health or transplant services are carved out; mental health services may be provided by an entity other than the one providing medical surgical care, and because of their costs, transplants are often retained by the insurer or HMO). In most cases it pertains to the contract between the state agency and the MCO that agrees to offer managed care to Medicaid beneficiaries. Carve-outs basically mean those services for which the MCO is not held at financial risk. The state Medicaid agency will carve out specific services, and these are handled either by another vendor or the staff at a specific Medicaid field office will handle the processes related to the rendering of the coverage determination and claims payment. Services commonly carved out are targeted case management services, transplants, children's medical services, and mental health services.

QUALITY AND MEDICAID

The QISMC standards and guidelines are key tools used by CMS and states as they implement the quality assurance provisions required by the BBA and further amended by the BBRA of 1999. QISMC is a process used by CMS to monitor the quality of services provided by MCOs for either their enrolled Medicaid or Medicare beneficiaries. QISMC is a rigid and demanding quality monitoring system and because of the details involved with QISMC, this section only briefly covers the basics of the program.

Because the cases found within a case manager's caseload are often the ones that will be under scrutiny for quality, it is important to understand at least the basics of QISMC and its requirements. QISMC's standards and guidelines are intended to achieve four major goals:

1. To clarify the responsibilities of both CMS and states in promoting quality as value-based purchasers of services for vulnerable populations
2. To promote opportunities for partnership among all entities involved with quality improvement efforts (i.e., CMS, the states, and other public and private entities)
3. To develop a coordinated quality oversight system for Medicaid and Medicare with the intent of reducing duplicate or conflicting efforts while sending a uniform message on quality to organizations and consumers
4. To ensure effective use of available quality measurement and improvement tools and the flexibility to incorporate new techniques or processes

The QISMC standards and guidelines are equivalent to a Medicare program manual. However, for Medicaid, the standards and guidelines serve merely as guidelines for states to use as they implement and monitor quality initiatives. Thus states may use their discretion as standards are applied to achieve compliance with BBA requirements as they relate to quality measurement and improvement as well as for the delivery of health care and enrollee services. QISMC is a highly detailed and specialized process. For full details of QISMC, see CMS's website at www.cms.hhs.gov/cop/2d.asp. Basically, QISMC standards and guidelines direct an MCO serving Medicare or Medicaid beneficiaries to do the following:

- Operate an internal program of quality assessment and performance improvement. The program must achieve demonstrable improvements in enrollee health, functional status, and satisfaction across a broad spectrum of care and services.
- Collect and report data as required contractually with CMS or the state. The data must be reflective of the organization's performance on standardized measures of health care quality.
- Demonstrate compliance with basic requirements for administrative structures and operations. The administrative structure and operations must promote quality of care and ensure beneficiary protection.

The standards are applicable to all services provided by any MCO that provides services to Medicare or Medicaid beneficiaries, including medical care, mental health and substance abuse services, and any additional services (e.g., dental care) included in a Medicaid contract or furnished as a mandatory or optional benefit. Although the standards are not disease-specific, they do require organizations to evaluate and improve care for all enrollees, including persons with special needs. The standards are divided into four domains with detailed expectations and requirements for each.

Domain 1

Quality Assessment and Performance Improvement Program. The intent of the program is to focus on three distinct but related strategies for promoting high-quality health care in organizations serving Medicare or Medicaid beneficiaries. The three strategies are as follows:

1. MCOs must meet certain required levels of performance when providing specific health care and related services to enrollees. The performance level (e.g., a specific numerical rate for immunizations) will be determined by CMS for Medicare and by the state Medicaid agencies for Medicaid.
2. MCOs must carry out performance improvement projects that are outcome-oriented and achieve demonstrable and sustained improvement in care and services.
3. MCOs must take timely action to correct significant systemic problems brought to their attention through internal surveillance, complaints, or other mechanisms.

Domain 2

Enrollee Rights. The intent of the program focuses on articulation of the enrollees' rights, promotion of these rights, and ensuring that the MCO's staff and affiliated providers are familiar with enrollee rights and treat enrollees accordingly. This area closely follows the recommendations of the 1997 President's Advisory Commission on Consumer Protection and Quality in the Health Care Industry and its document, the Consumer Bill of Rights and Responsibilities.

Domain 3

Health Services Management. The focus of the program is on the ability of the MCO to ensure all services are available and it has employed or contracted with appropriately qualified institutional and individual providers and these providers have sufficient capacity to make services available to the organization's enrollees. Additionally, the MCO must ensure the following:

- Services and providers are accessible.
- Enrollees are educated about the existence and availability of the services offered.
- Procedures necessary for obtaining such services are clear.

- Services are geographically reachable and consistent with local community patterns of care.
- Enrollees do not experience undue waiting periods, either for obtaining an appointment or at the time of the appointment.
- Enrollees are offered care and services that are culturally and linguistically correct, and barriers for the mentally or physically challenged are eliminated.

The organization's initial assessment of availability must take into consideration:

- Expected use of services according to enrollee characteristics and health care needs
- The numbers and types of providers needed to furnish these services
- The geographic location of providers and enrollees

Domain 4

This domain requires that any MCO delegating functions (e.g., carve-out services or specific MCO areas of responsibility such as utilization management or case management) to another entity to remain wholly accountable to CMS or the state for performance of any delegated function. This domain does not pertain to those services considered carve-outs. If the state agency lists these as a contractual carve-out and enters into a separate contract with another MCO vendor or other service delivery system for a specific set of services (e.g., mental health and substance abuse, EPSDT, or dental services), the MCO offering primary medical care is not considered to have delegated these carved-out services. Therefore it is not expected to oversee or be accountable for such services.

SUMMARY

Multiple changes have occurred in the Medicare program, originally written as Title XVIII of the Social Security Act.

Despite its complexity, criteria for eligibility and benefits are consistent nationwide. Because many patients served by case managers will receive Medicare, it is imperative that case managers understand the basic Medicare FFS program. An understanding of this program is important for two reasons. First, it will help case managers educate patients as they traverse the health care system. Second, it will provide a better understanding of health benefits and utilization review, since Medicare is often considered the grandfather of utilization review and is the basis most insurers use for development of their programs and policies and procedures.

Medicaid was created in 1965 as Title XIX of the Social Security Act. Its primary intent, from its inception, has been to provide medical care and services to persons with low income or the needy. Because so many case management patients exhaust their health care coverage or their care becomes long-term and payment for such is not allowed, case managers must be very familiar with the state's Medicaid program. This also requires a general knowledge of the processes necessary to establish eligibility for benefits.

For case managers working with a Medicaid managed care plan, the requirements of QISMC are very rigid. An MCO that offers a Medicaid managed care plan will have stringent quality reporting requirements to capture the data required by CMS for reporting compliance for quality improvement activities.

Chapter Exercises

1. List the benefits allowed under Part A and Part B and compare them with those allowed under an M+C plan in your local area.
2. Research the BBA and identify four key components of the act that affect an M+C plan.

3. Describe the role of CMS in the oversight of Medicare and how local state agencies interface with CMS.
4. List the categories for eligibility and the criteria for each.
5. Describe the core benefits of Medicaid and those often offered by states as optional benefits and programs.
6. List the contractual requirements of a health plan if it is to offer a managed care product for Medicaid-eligible persons in the area.
7. Describe the primary processes used to measure quality in Medicaid managed care and list the domains and characteristics of each.

Suggested Websites and Resources

Medicare
www.cms.gov/—CMS's main website
www.medicare.gov/—Medicare's main website
www.medicare.gov/Publications/—Medicare publications (contains downloads in regular print, as well as a large-print edition)
www.governmentguide.com/govsite.adp?bread=*Main&url=http%3A//www.governmentguide.com/ams/clickThruRedirect.adp%3F55076483%2C16920155%2Chttp%3A//www.ssa.gov/—Social Security Act website
www.medicare.gov/Physician/Home.asp—Medicare's Participating Physician Directory
www.medicare.gov/Publications/Search View/View PubList.asp? Language=English—Medicare Manuals
www.cms.hhs.gov/healthplans/default.asp—Medicare managed care
www.medicare.gov/Contacts/Home.asp—Link to phone numbers of government health programs
www.mcol.com/armenu3.htm and *www.cms.hhs.gov/healthplans/opl.*

index.pdf—Medicare's operational policy letters
www.cms.hhs.gov/manuals/19_pro/pr07.asp—Sample NODMAR letter
www.cms.hhs.gov/manuals/transmittals/comm_date_dsc.asp—Medicare transmittals
www.cms.hhs.gov/cop/2d2.asp—QISMC standards
www.medicare.gov/Physician/—CMS website to locate physicians that participate in Medicare
www.cms.hhs.gov/providers/transplant/hartlist.asp—CMS website for heart transplant centers
www.cms.hhs.gov/providers/transplant/lunglist.asp—CMS website for lung transplant centers
www.cms.hhs.gov/providers/transplant/livrlist.asp—CMS website for liver transplant centers
www.cms.hhs.gov/providers/transplant/intstnlist.asp—CMS website for intestine transplant centers
www.cms.hhs.gov/coverage/8d.asp—CMS website for information on clinical trials
www.cms.hhs.gov/healthplans/appeals/sanqna.asp—CMS website for more information on Medicare appeal processes

U.S. Department of Health and Human Services

CMS or the Centers for Medicare & Medicaid Services—Formerly the Health Care Financing Administration or HCFA
7500 Security Boulevard
Baltimore, MD 21244-1850
Website: *www.dhhs.gov*

Medicaid
www.cms.hhs.gov/medicaid/eligibility/—CMS Medicaid eligibility website
www.cms.hhs.gov/hiv/hivfs.asp—CMS HIV website
www.ssa.gov/work—Social Security Administration

*www.aspe.hhs.gov/progsys/homeless/Programs.
htm*—Homeless information

*www.bphc.hrsa.dhhs.gov/*and
www.bphc.hrsa.dhhs.gov/databases/fqhc—
Primary care for the underserved

*www.cms.hhs.gov/medicaid/managedcare/def
ault.asp*—Medicaid managed care

*www.cms.hhs.gov/states/letters/bbapace.
asp*—CMS website on the elderly and
the PACE program

www.cms.hhs.gov/medicaid/waiver1.asp—
CMS website on Medicaid waivers and
demonstrations

*www.cms.hhs.gov/medicaid/meqc/mqcguide.
asp*—CMS and Medicaid quality control
projects

*www.cms.hhs.gov/manuals/45_smm/sm_
07_7_toc.asp*—CMS state Medicaid
manual on quality

www.cms.hhs.gov/medicaid/tollfree.asp—
CMS website for toll-free numbers for
state Medicaid programs

Medicaid Publications

For specifics on a state's Medicaid eligibility and the health services offered, contact
the local state Medicaid program office.

General information on the Medicaid program is given in the *Medicaid Fact Sheet*. For
a free copy write to the CMS at the address
given previously. For specifics on Medicaid
eligibility and the health services offered,
contact your State Medicaid Program
Office. The toll-free number for the Social
Security Administration is 800-772-1213.

REFERENCES

1. Mathews JL, Berman DM: Social security Medicare
   pensions, 7th ed, Berkeley, Calif, 1999, nolo.com.
2. Medicare website: www.hcfa.gov.

BIBLIOGRAPHY

Department of Veterans Affairs website: www.VA.gov.
Food and Drug Administration website: www.fda.gov/.
Health Affairs website for Information from the Office
   of CHAMPUS: www.ha.osd.mil.
Health Insurance Association of America website:
   www.hiaa.org/.
Indian Health Services website: www.ihs.gov/.
National Cancer Institute and National Institutes of
   Health website: www.nci.nih.gov/.
National Patient Travel Center website: www.patient-
   travel.org/afas/nptc.htm.
United States Code Service: Social security act. Title XVI:
   Supplemental security income for the aged blind and
   disabled, 1993, 42 USCS §1381–1385.

CHAPTER

7

Children's Health Coverage—Programs and Services

Peggy A. Rossi, BSN, MPA, CCM, CPUR

OBJECTIVES

- To identify four major federal laws that affect children with special needs
- To know which state agencies are responsible for assisting children with special needs and how to contact such agencies
- To know what services are mandated by federal law to be provided to children with special needs and what services are actually available in the local region

CHILDREN WITH SPECIAL HEALTH CARE NEEDS

The Social Security Act covers Children with Special Health Care Needs (CSHCN). The original act was passed as Title V of the Social Security Act of 1953. This program is known by a variety of names and is commonly referred to as *children's medical services, crippled children's services,* or *handicapped children's services.* Although CSHCN programs use a combination of federal, state, and county funds, each program is administered locally by state or county offices and is governed by the Civil Rights Act of 1964. Because CSHCN programs receive federal funds, they are available in every state, but benefits and eligibility vary from state to state and often even from county to county within a state. Each state's name for its CSHCN program also varies.

Eligibility for care and services is based on diagnosis, income, and state or county of residence. CSHCN is not an income-based program but one that provides payment for medical services to persons who qualify, and although some families may pay a portion of the medical care, in most cases, if families are eligible, services are free. Retroactive payments are not allowed, and as stated earlier, if the child has private insurance, this insurance will serve as the primary payer and must be used before any payment is made by CSHCN. Even if the child is eligible for the state's Medicaid program, the CSHCN program will always be the payer of last resort.

CHILDREN WITH SPECIAL NEEDS

Because of the large numbers of children with disabilities or serious medical problems and children with little or no insurance, it is imperative that case managers understand the various insurance and coverage options now available to children. Although a child may have private insurance, this does not mean he or she will be excluded from other funding programs. However, if a child does have private health care insurance, that insurance will always be the primary payer, with the public funding program used when the primary insurer limits or excludes specific services or when the child has exhausted his or her benefits. Unfortunately, all too often laypersons and professionals are not aware that a child may be eligible for additional funding. Under such circumstances, it is often believed that the only time the child will be eligible is when benefits are exhausted, and this is not true.

Although children may be covered by Medicaid, and some by Medicare, this section covers several public funding programs designed to specifically serve children if they meet eligibility requirements. The programs are as follows:

- CSHCN provisions of the Social Security Act (sometimes referred to as *Title V programs*)
- Special education
- The State Children's Health Insurance Program (SCHIP)
- The Department of Developmental Disabilities
- Special Supplemental Nutrition Program for Women, Infants, and Children (WIC)
- Supplemental Security Income (SSI)

The programs funded under CSHCN are designed to meet the medical needs of handicapped or disabled persons younger than 21 years when the families are unable to pay either part or all of the cost of recommended treatment. The intent of the program is to provide services to low-income children when a need is identified and the child meets certain eligibility criteria. Application is made in the county or state where the patient lives,

not the county or state in which care is supplied.

Purpose and Objectives

Because eligibility criteria vary from state to state, the purpose and objectives of each state's CSHCN program also vary. All programs must offer diagnostic capabilities and case management services. Despite the variations in scope, most programs have the following purposes and objectives:

- To locate eligible handicapped persons younger than 21 who need care
- To provide diagnostic and preventive services and early detection of handicapping conditions
- To enable eligible persons to obtain medical services to maximize their physical, mental, social, and educational development
- To provide funding for preventive and diagnostic services when funds are not available through private insurance or the family is unable to pay for the services
- To obtain the highest quality care for persons treated in the program
- To coordinate these services with those offered by other state and county agencies or departments to ensure that eligible persons receive the benefits to which they are entitled (e.g., visits by public health nurses, rehabilitation and vocational retraining, and mental health treatment)
- To serve as the cognizant public official or provide the public official statement necessary for receipt of benefits from TRICARE's Program for Persons with Disabilities. Although the public official may be any public official from the state's CSHCN program, Medicaid, or the Department of Developmental Disabilities or the superintendent of schools or director of special education, this official in many cases will

be the director or local official of a CSHCN program who attests to the fact that public agencies or services are not available or adequate to meet the needs of a particular child

- To work with local Planned Parenthood units to recommend therapeutic abortions when amniocentesis reveals that a fetus has an eligible condition (e.g., known life threatening birth anomaly) or to prevent AIDS in newborns

Typical Eligible Diagnoses

Although the following list of "eligible medical conditions" covered by a CSHCN program is fairly extensive, the actual diagnosis and level of services provided will vary from state to state. Thus a diagnosis that is eligible for services in one state may not be eligible in another (i.e., not all states allow coverage for acute care, since they may concentrate only on chronic conditions). Occasionally, a condition that is not listed below may be eligible. Therefore because of inconsistencies, it is wise for the case manager to make the referral even if in doubt. The key is to let the experts from the CSHCN office determine whether the child qualifies. Conditions frequently recognized as eligible include the following:

- Orthopedic conditions caused by infection, injury, or congenital malformations
- Conditions requiring plastic surgery or reconstruction such as cleft lip, facial anomalies, and burns
- Conditions requiring orthodontic reconstruction such as cleft palate, severe malocclusion, and orificial anomalies
- Eye conditions that lead to loss of vision
- Ear conditions that lead to loss of hearing
- Rheumatic fever
- Nephritis, nephrosis, or nephrotic syndrome

- Phenylketonuria
- Hemophilia
- Hyaline membrane disease (bronchopulmonary dysplasia)
- Endocrine or metabolic disorders that pose problems in medical management or problems with the establishment of a diagnosis
- Convulsive disorders that pose problems in medical management or problems with the establishment of a diagnosis
- Blood dyscrasias
- Neoplasms
- Severe skin disorders such as epidermolysis bullosa
- Chronic pulmonary conditions such as cystic fibrosis, bronchiectasis, and lung abscess
- Congenital anomalies that cause disabling or disfiguring handicaps
- Conditions of the nervous system such as inflammatory diseases that produce motor disability, paralysis, or ataxia or other neuromuscular diseases that may include cerebral palsy, muscular dystrophy, or stroke
- Conditions resulting from an accident or poisoning that are potentially handicapping such as complicated fractures, brain or spinal cord injuries, or stricture of the esophagus
- Severe adverse reactions to an immunization requiring extensive medical or related care
- Any disabling or disfiguring condition that may be long term and handicapping
- AIDS, AIDS-related complex, human immunodeficiency virus infection (this category of disease and the services provided vary drastically from state to state)

Referrals

Timeliness of referrals is of critical importance because it is the key to when coverage begins. This is especially true for the technology-dependent child for whom health care coverage is limited or benefits are excluded or exhausted. Although the actual medical diagnosis, family income, and place of residence are the three keys to referral, case managers should not hesitate to make a referral if they think the child may qualify for benefits (Box 7-1).

Eligibility Requirements

Once the child has been referred, the county or state agency must determine his or her family's financial eligibility before authorization for any services can be granted. Although this process can consume several weeks after the referral, actual coverage can be retroactive because all coverage starts with the day of the referral. There will be times when a child merely requires confirmation of eligibility to assist with the establishment of a diagnosis or referral to a school therapy program. If this is the case, financial screening for eligibility may not be necessary. With such time constraints in place, if it appears that the child may be eligible, the case manager should not hesitate to make the referral. Eligibility for a CSHCN program is based on three key components:

1. A medically eligible diagnosis
2. Family income or ability to pay for medical care
3. Place of residence

At the same time the child is screened for CSHCN eligibility, his or her family will also be screened for the state's Medicaid program. If eligibility for both Medicaid and CSHCN is established, Medicaid will become the primary payer, and the CSHCN program will be the secondary payer. When the formal eligibility screening process begins, the case manager may wish to inform the family that they must be prepared to provide the following information:

- Patient's name
- Patient's (and family's) addresses and phone numbers
- Patient's date of birth
- Proof of Medicaid eligibility, if applicable
- State tax records (In some states this is the basis for eligibility and determines the amount of the repayment obligation when appropriate; however, for states without a state tax this requirement is waived.)
- Amount of family income (including any Social Security benefits from a deceased parent or child support payments from an absent spouse)
- Names of family members earning income
- Number of persons dependent on family income
- Each employer's name and address
- Name and address of any company or agency providing health care insurance
- A signed release of information form allowing release of the patient's medical records, if medical records have not already been obtained

Once the eligibility screening process has been completed, the application and

---

BOX 7-1
Important Points to Remember About Referrals

- Can be accepted from anyone (e.g., health care professional or family member)
- Are made to the county or state in which the child lives, not the county or state in which he or she will receive care (the county or state of residence is determined by the residence of the father or legal guardian)
- Are encouraged, regardless of whether the patient has insurance or the family has income

any medical information or records supporting the diagnosis or condition are collected and forwarded to the unit responsible for determining the patient's medical eligibility. Medical eligibility is based on the following criteria:

- Evidence of need for care
- Prognosis
- Reasonable expectation of recovery
- Availability of treatment
- Priority of need for treatment

Case managers may want to inform the family of the following facts:

- All CSHCN funds are secondary to any health care insurer (including Medicaid), and if the child is linked to a managed care organization (MCO), benefits from a CSHCN program may not be available unless the child's health care benefits are limited, excluded, or exhausted.
- If income exceeds the basic standard amount needed by the family to live, the family is responsible for repayment of any portion in excess of this standard.
- If the family moves from one county or state to another during the course of the treatment, benefits cease and the family must file for a reevaluation and determination of financial eligibility in the new state or county.
- If the family is not eligible for the services of the CSHCN program, staff will assist the family in identifying community agencies that can provide assistance.
- All services require authorization before they are provided, and without authorization, the program is not obligated to pay for services.
- Most programs use only facilities, physicians, agencies, and other providers that have met the state CSHCN agency's standards for care.
- Families with health care insurance may be considered eligible for care if it is determined that their insurance coverage or income is insufficient to cover the needed care.
- When treatment reaches a plateau or when it becomes evident that treatment is not or will not significantly influence the eventual outcome, health care coverage ceases.
- These programs do not pay for custodial care, homemaker services, experimental treatments, education, or alterations to the home.

Services Provided

Although services vary, most CSHCN programs pay for services necessary to establish a diagnosis, provide basic treatment consistent with federal program objectives, and allow the establishment of a treatment plan. If the child has been enrolled in a Medicaid MCO, services related to the child's CSHCN diagnosis and treatments are often a "carve-out" for the MCO. If this is the case, the MCO is not financially responsible for the cost of any treatments or services related to the child's eligible CSHCN condition. In these cases the child must receive routine and preventive care or any medical care necessary not related to the CSHCN-eligible diagnosis from the MCO. If treatment is required for the CSHCN condition, the MCO's case manager must work closely with the CSHCN case manager to ensure that a transition is made and that the child obtains the care and services required for the CSHCN-eligible condition.

Case management services are a key element in most CSHCN programs. To ensure that the goals of treatment and case management plans are reached, case managers at all levels must work closely together. Case manager collaboration is especially necessary if dual coverage exists (e.g., CSHCN and private health care insurance) and services are carved out. The following services are commonly authorized for eligible persons:

- Hospitalization
- Outpatient treatment or services
- Physician, dental, optometrist, orthodontist, or other professional health care services
- Blood and blood products
- Medications
- Transportation
- Social worker services
- Nursing services for skilled care
- Braces and other prosthetic devices
- Laboratory or radiology services
- Radiation therapy
- Physical, occupational, or speech therapy
- Psychologic evaluation
- Durable medical equipment and accessory supplies
- Dressings and supplies

SPECIAL EDUCATION

The Individuals with Disabilities Education Act (IDEA) of 1991 declared that all individuals for whom special or exceptional needs have been identified have a right to a free and appropriate public education. Section 504 of the Rehabilitation Act of 1973 also protects children requiring special education. Both acts specify that a child is protected and must have reasonable accommodations to ensure that he or she receives a free and appropriate public education, including any special instruction, other services, or adaptive environment necessary to provide the education. The programs covered by this act are frequently referred to as *special education*.

Purpose

Special education is specially designed instruction or schooling and is provided at no cost to the parent to allow children with special or exceptional needs to obtain an education if their needs cannot be met by modifying the regular school program. Information about the program is available from the state or county department of education.

Because many case management caseloads include a significant number of children with special needs, case managers must be familiar with special education processes and understand what the program can and cannot provide for this category of children. Depending on the needs of the child and the problems the parents are experiencing in establishing services for the child, case managers may be invited by the parents to assist in any processes to establish need. One such process is an independent evaluation of the child during which needs for specific services are identified, and this is called *an individualized educational plan (IEP)*.

Because benefits vary from state to state, case managers should be aware of the federal benefits allowed, as well as those of the state in which the child resides. Also, because of the complex processes involved in obtaining special education services, many families are intimidated and therefore will need the help of a case manager who can act as their advocate. Serving as the advocate often means assisting the family when problems arise as they attempt to gain access to services or when the patient is denied benefits inappropriately (Box 7-2).

Criteria for Eligibility

Persons with exceptional needs are those who have a low-incidence disability or a chronic or severe handicapping condition (e.g., autism, blindness, deafness, severe orthopedic impairment, or severe emotional disturbance). A low-incidence disability is defined as a severe handicapping condition that has an expected incidence rate of less than 1% in the total statewide school population from kindergarten through grade 12.

Special education is not intended for persons whose educational needs are due primarily to unfamiliarity with the English

---

BOX 7-2
IDEA Rights

The Individuals with Disabilities Education Act (IDEA) protects all persons from birth to age 21 years who need special education and basically stipulates the following:
■ Education shall be offered at no cost in the most appropriate and least restrictive environment possible.
■ Once a person has been referred, an assessment and IEP must be developed within a specified period (ranging from 50 to 90 days, depending on the requirements in the individual state).
■ Noneducational public agencies cannot reduce eligibility for medical or other assistance due the person under the CSHCN program or Medicaid.
■ All state and federal resources must be used when necessary to provide the education, and all benefits must be coordinated to ensure there is no duplication.

IEP, Individual educational plan; *CSHCN,* Children with Special Health Care Needs.

---

language; a temporary physical handicap; or maturational, environmental, cultural, or economic factors. Special education is intended for individuals who have problems associated with the following:
■ Function below the normal level for chronological age
■ Impaired fine or gross motor control or a severe orthopedic impairment
■ Abnormal receptive or expressive language development
■ Abnormal social, emotional, or psychologic development
■ Impaired cognitive development
■ Deafness or impaired hearing development
■ Blindness or impaired visual development
■ Disabling medical or congenital syndrome

Services Provided

All services needed by children with the foregoing disorders are performed by qualified professionals and may be of many types:
■ Referrals and assessments
■ Any special instruction the pupil requires
■ Consultation
■ Coordination with other agencies or individuals

To enable the person to participate in any special education program, the school district must provide any related services at no cost if the services are not covered by insurance. However, if health care coverage is available, the school district has a right to seek reimbursement for the services to the extent permitted by federal law or regulation.

Special education services are developed and provided according to the following age categories:
■ **Birth to 3 years:** This is called *early intervention,* and the child's needs, developmental goals, and services required are documented in what is termed an *individualized family service plan.*
■ **3 to 5 years:** This is called *early childhood education,* and the child's needs, school readiness goals, and the services required are documented in what is termed an *IEP.*
■ **5 to 21 years:** This is called *special education,* and the child's special educational needs, annual goals and objectives for the school year, and the services required are documented in what is termed an *IEP.*

A confusing area of utilization review is that pertaining to speech therapy for a child. Case managers must keep in mind that health care insurers generally do not pay for speech therapy when such therapy is required because of a learning disorder rather than a medical disability. Consequently, once a diagnosis not related to a medical disability has been made, the parents must be informed of this fact and encouraged to apply for special education for the child. If the child is accepted as a client for special education, he or she may be entitled to "direct" or "related" services.

As with all services, the direct and related services that may be available in special education programs also vary from state to state.[1] This is very confusing to families, especially if they are in the military and move from state to state, because one state may allow a higher level of care and related services for the child than another. For instance, in one state, the care and related services may be provided by teachers who have been trained to perform the services; in another, services may be provided by qualified individuals or a home health agency under contract with the state; and in still another, services may be limited to personal care (e.g., helping the child use the toilet). Thus in these states the family or health care payer must provide the bulk of any skilled care needed (Box 7-3).

Sites for Schooling

In addition to providing special education within the confines of a specially designated classroom or public school, the local school district or county department of education is responsible for providing schooling in a full range of other locations. This continuum of responsibility covers all persons placed in a licensed children's institution, foster family home, special center or state hospital, psychiatric hospital, or other health facility located within or functioning under the district's jurisdiction.

A school district is also responsible for providing instruction to a pupil confined to a hospital or home with a medical condition related to surgery, an accident, a short-term illness, or medical treatment for a chronic illness. When home teaching is required, it is not classified as special education but is called *home tutoring*. Home tutoring can be obtained by calling the school district and making the necessary arrangements.

Referrals for Special Education

Referrals for special education should be made in writing to the local school district

---

BOX 7-3
Special Education Services

Direct Services	Related Services
Direct services are those specifically designed to address the educational component. Related services may be therapeutic, medical, or physically necessary "health care"–type services. If related services are required, they are generally provided by such health care professionals as the following: ■ Occupational, physical, or speech therapists ■ Nursing aides (who provide personal care or assistance) ■ Special nurses (who provide such services as gavage feedings, suctioning, catheterization, or other medically related services)	Related services are those services that might be provided if the child is deemed eligible for special education and may include the following: ■ Assistive technology or specialized equipment (e.g., computers) ■ Transcribers, readers, or interpreters ■ Transportation between home and school

or county office of education in which the pupil is enrolled. The school district must complete the needed assessments and tests and develop the IEP within a relatively short period (on average, 50 to 90 days) from the date of referral. When a referral is made, the information submitted should include the following:

- The type of illness or disability
- The possible medical side effects, complications, or treatments that could affect school function
- The educational and social implications of the disease and its treatment including the likelihood of fatigue, absences, changes in physical appearance, amputation, or problems with fine and gross motor control
- Any special considerations for a child with an infectious disease

Case Study Evaluation

The case study evaluation (CSE) is the initial step in determining eligibility for special education. A CSE may be requested or recommended when it is suspected that the child is having difficulty learning because of a disability. Before the CSE is done, a child's vision and hearing must be screened; this must be done within 6 months and is necessary to rule out any visual or hearing deficits. The CSE includes the following:

- Meeting with the child and parent/guardian or surrogate parent
- A social developmental examination
- Review of the child's medical history and the reports on the vision and hearing screening examinations
- If the child has been attending school, his or her school performance including observation of the child in the learning environment, achievement testing, and cognitive testing (e.g., IQ tests, memory assessments)

- If the child is younger than school age or is not attending school because of a suspected disability, observation and testing during a home visit
- Other specialized tests such as psychologic evaluations, speech-language assessment, learning disability assessment, and social work report

The CSE assessment report must include the following:

- A summary of the medical, physical, developmental, and/or psychologic findings
- A statement regarding whether the pupil needs special education or related services
- The basis for making the determination
- The relevant behavior noted during the observation of the pupil
- The relationship of the behavior to the pupil's academic and social function
- A determination about the effects of environmental, cultural, or economic disadvantages on the pupil
- Recommendations for specialized services, materials, and equipment necessary to provide the education

Assessment reports for pupils with learning disabilities should state whether there is a discrepancy between the child's achievement and his or her ability and should include information supporting the fact that the disability cannot be corrected or treated without special education or related services.

Assessments

After the referral has been made, assessments and testing must be completed within a specified time from receipt of the request for special education. These assessments and tests are performed at no charge to the parent. Parents should be aware that permission, or consent, for the tests or assessments must be provided in writing and that medical records, as well as a written report from the child's physician, might be needed. At no time is a single test procedure used as the sole criterion for determining the appropriate educational program. Testing, assessment materials, and procedures used must do the following:

- Cover all areas of function related to the suspected disability
- Be performed by competent credentialed persons
- Be selected and administered to avoid racial, cultural, and sexual discrimination
- Be provided in the person's primary language or mode of communication
- Be selected and administered to ensure that the test results accurately reflect the person's aptitude, achievement level, or other factor purported to be measured by the test
- Not measure the person's impairment, unless this is indicated

Regardless of who conducts the assessments, the written assessment report serves as the basis for the final IEP and the specific instruction and services eventually designed for the child.

Multidisciplinary Conference

Once a CSE is requested, the local school district has 60 school days from the date of the request to complete the CSE and convene the multidisciplinary conference (MDC). Written notice of the MDC must be sent to the parent or guardian at least 10 days before the day of the meeting. The MDC meeting must be held at a mutually agreed upon time and date. Persons who can attend the MDC include the following:

- Child's parent, guardian, surrogate parent
- Child's teacher, if child is attending school

- School district representative
- Director of special education
- Everyone involved in testing the child
- People who provide services to the child (e.g., therapist, social worker, caseworker, foster parents, doctors)
- Child, as appropriate
- Other school personnel familiar with child
- Other people who have information to share about the child
- Attorney or nonattorney advocates representing the child
- Other persons who can support the parents or offer additional information

The following happen at the MDC:

- Those who tested the child will present their test results.
- Child's problems and special needs are described.
- Recommendations are made as to whether the child needs special education services.
- School writes a multidisciplinary summary report listing the child's test results and the special education services for which the child is eligible.
- The parent, guardian, or surrogate parent receives a copy of the summary report at the end of the MDC.
- Dissenting opinions may be documented in the MDC summary report.

Individualized Education Plan

Any person who does not meet predetermined criteria for an area assessed in the CSE is further tested by another specialist who has credentials in the same area. If this is the case, case managers must be aware that parents have the right to request retesting at the department of education's expense. Parents also have the right to obtain at their expense, independent educational assessments, as long as qualified specialists perform the assessments. To ensure that the eventual IEP is tailored to the child's needs, the assessments must cover the following areas:

- Relevant health and development or medical condition
- Visual ability (including poor vision)
- Hearing ability
- Motor self-help and mobility abilities
- Interests (including social interests)
- Emotional and psychologic status
- Language functions
- General ability
- Academic performance
- Orientation
- Vocational abilities and interests

On completion of the tests and assessments, the findings are presented at an IEP meeting. This meeting must include qualified persons who can develop the pupil's IEP. The team members selected often include the following:

- A school representative who is knowledgeable about program options appropriate for the pupil and is qualified to provide or supervise the special education program
- The pupil's teacher or a special education teacher who is qualified to teach pupils of this child's age and level of impairment
- One or both parents or their representative
- When appropriate, the pupil
- If approved by the parents or school district, any other individual who possesses expertise or knowledge about the development of the pupil's IEP
- The person or persons who conducted the assessment
- A representative from the county mental health department, if the child has a severe emotional disturbance and the final recommendation will be residential placement
- A representative from the county welfare department, if the child will

be placed in an out-of-home setting (This person will help in identifying a facility suited to the child's needs.)

The team is responsible for reviewing the assessment results, determining eligibility, and reviewing the contents of the IEP plan. In making their recommendations, the team must consider any transportation needs, any related services, and when appropriate, placement alternatives.

The IEP is a written statement that serves as the basis for the designed instruction and any services the pupil requires. The plan must be maintained at each school site where the pupil is enrolled. Parents must be aware that they have a right to obtain a copy for their records, and this should be encouraged. When possible, case managers should request a copy for the child's file because it will be helpful in establishing the case management plan and identifying any gaps, fragmentation, or duplication of services.

At a minimum, the IEP must note or describe the following:

- The present level of the pupil's educational performance
- A list of annual goals, including short-term objectives
- The special education program and any related services required
- The extent to which the pupil is able to participate in regular educational programs
- The date for initiation of and anticipated duration of the special education program or services
- Appropriate objective criteria and evaluation procedures to be used and a schedule or time frame from which it can be determined whether goals are being achieved
- When appropriate, the plan should also include the following:
  - Recommendations for prevocational career education for pupils in kindergarten through grade 6

- Recommendations for vocational education or work experience or both for pupils in kindergarten through grade 12
- Linguistically appropriate goals, if the pupil's primary language or mode of communication is other than spoken English (e.g., other spoken language or sign language) and an outline of the programs and services necessary to reach these goals
- A description of the specialized services, material, or equipment necessary to reach the outlined goals when the pupil has a low-incidence disability

Depending on the child's age and needs, the IEP may also address such issues as the following:

- Whether the child will require regular class in a regular school with extra help or will require
- Special education class in a regular school for part of school day and transfer to a regular class for the rest of the day with extra help or will require
- Special education class in a regular school for the entire day
- Transition services and goals, intended for children 14½ years old or older who will need help preparing for life after school
- Transportation services for those children who, because of their special needs, are unable to walk or ride the bus with students without disabilities
- Parent counseling and training—for parents of disabled students (includes advice on how to help their children with schoolwork and more specific information about their children's special needs)
- A bilingual and English as a second language program, adjusted according to the child's abilities

- Adaptive physical education
- Behavior management plan
- Vocational education
- Graduation planning (begins at least 4 years before he child is scheduled to graduate)

If the school district and parent agree and if it is appropriate and required to implement the child's IEP, a child can be "tuitioned-out" to a private or public school out of the district or out of the state. When a child's IEP cannot be implemented at the local level, the following more restrictive environments may be considered:

- Special education at a public day school where all children have special educational needs
- Private day school where all children have special educational needs
- Residential program in a state facility
- Private residential school
- Special educational class in a hospital (medical or psychiatric)
- Special educational classes provided through special tutoring in a hospital or at home when the child has been homebound for more than 2 weeks

Once the initial plan has been developed, future planning meetings are held annually or:

1. When the pupil receives or requires any subsequent formal assessment or testing
2. When the pupil demonstrates lack of anticipated progress
3. When the teacher or parent requests a review or revision of the plan

Designed Instruction and Services

From the IEP, specifically designed instruction and services are developed with the intent of meeting the unique needs of the pupil. Before actual implementation of the pupil's special education program, the designed instruction and services must meet standards established by the local school board.

The designed instruction and services may include the following:

- Language and speech development and remediation
- Audiology services
- Orientation and mobility instruction
- Instruction in the home or hospital
- Adapted physical education
- Physical or occupational therapy
- Vision services
- Specialized driver education
- Counseling and guidance
- Psychologic services, other than those necessary for the assessment and development of the IEP
- Parent counseling and training
- Health and nursing services
- Social worker services
- Specially designed vocational education and career development
- Recreational services
- Specialized services for low-incidence disabilities (e.g., readers and transcribers)
- Transportation

In some circumstances, special education centers or state schools must be used when the nature and severity of the handicap are such that education cannot be achieved satisfactorily in the local school district. If the pupil is placed in such a center, nonacademic extracurricular services and activities must be provided to allow the handicapped pupil to participate with nonhandicapped pupils to the maximum extent possible considering the pupil's condition.

Schools for the Blind and Deaf

In the United States there are approximately 60 special schools for the blind and more than 60 public residential schools for the deaf. In addition to the full range of regular academic curricula, schools for the blind offer courses in braille, instruction in skills of daily living, and orientation and mobility training. Schools for the deaf accept children from infancy through grade 12. If accepted, the child receives, in addition to a standard education, speech therapy and training in lip reading, use of hearing aids, and sign language. Parents who need information about these schools should be encouraged to contact their local state department of education.

Placement

Parents should know that if their child cannot be placed in a regular classroom and there are no other provisions for special education in the local public school district, the child can be placed in a private school designed to assist persons with exceptional needs. In this case, pupils placed in a nonpublic, nonsectarian school are considered to be enrolled in the public school. The school district remains responsible for paying the full tuition. However, before state funds are used for this purpose, there must be documentation that attempts were made to place the pupil in an appropriate alternative public setting. This setting can either be within or outside the state, and before any payments are made, the state superintendent of schools must approve the use of funds.

Disabilities Covered Under the Individuals with Disabilities Education Act

The following disabilities are the ones most frequently covered by a school district for children who need special education:

- Autism
- Long- or short-term health impairment
- Cognitive impairment
- Emotional/behavioral disorder
- Hearing impairment
- Learning disability

- Orthopedic impairment
- Speech/language impairment
- Traumatic brain injury
- Visual impairment

Related Services Provided Under IDEA

The following is a partial list of related services that may be provided under IDEA:

- **Audiology**—Audiometric testing; recommendations for amplification systems, hearing aids, orientations, or habilitative activities (e.g., language habilitation, auditory training, speech reading, hearing conservation); counseling and guidance of children, pupils, teachers, and staff regarding hearing loss.
- **Braillist/reader**—Aide for students with visual disabilities who augments the educational program (e.g., by reading or taping materials, transcribing materials in braille, or thermoforming materials).
- **Counseling services**—School guidance counselors, social workers, or psychologists who provide guidance directly in small groups or individual sessions through consultation with teacher or through crisis intervention.
- **Adapted driver education**—Specially designed course to teach student with a disability to operate a car.
- **Adaptive technology**—Specially designed devices or processes that enable a student with a disability to perform tasks more independently.
- **Interpreter**—Specially trained individual who either interprets or translates.
- **Occupational therapy**—Services designed to improve, develop, or restore functions impaired or lost through illness, injury, or deprivation; to improve ability to perform tasks required for independent functioning; or to prevent, through early intervention, initial or further impairment or loss of function.
- **Orientation and mobility**—Services designed to increase a visually disabled child's ability to perceive and move about within his or her environment with a goal of independent movement and living.
- **Parent counseling and training**—Assistance to parents in understanding and managing the special needs of their child and provision of information about child development.
- **Physical therapy**—Services recommended and prescribed by a licensed physical therapist as necessary for student to benefit from an education.
- **Recreation**—Therapeutic activities that are designed to accomplish behavioral or cognitive goals and objectives or activities that develop the constructive use of leisure time.
- **Rehabilitative counseling**—Services focused specifically on career development, employment preparation, achievement of independence, and integration in the workplace and community
- **School health services**—Administration of medication necessary to help the student function during school hours.
- **Social work**—Services that address problems in a student's living situation that affect his or her adjustment in school and mobilization of school and community resources to enable him or her to receive maximum benefit from his or her educational program.
- **Speech and language**—Habilitation or prevention of communicative disorders.
- **Transportation**—Services different from those normally provided that are required because of student's disability.

STATE AGENCY FOR DEVELOPMENTAL DISABILITIES

Although developmental disability services are not limited to children, for a person to be entitled to the program beyond initial age requirements, the need for services must be identified before the age of 22 years. Thus it is important to add developmental disability services in this section because, if the individual is eligible, some funding and services may be available.

The rights of the developmentally disabled are protected under federal legislation and the Developmental Disabilities Act of 1984. In addition, they are protected by other federal acts such as the Americans with Disabilities Act, the Rehabilitation Act, and the Privacy Act. Under the Developmental Disabilities Act, states are required to provide specific services that will meet the needs of the developmentally disabled.

The major goal of developmental programs is to assist people with developmental disabilities (DD) to reach maximum potential through increased independence, productivity, and community integration. Programs are designed to address all elements of the life cycle: disease and injury prevention, diagnosis, early intervention, therapy, education, training, employment, and community living and leisure opportunities.

Because persons with DD constitute a large percentage of many caseloads, case managers must be familiar with the requirements for referral for this category of patients. If the state agency's name is not known, one of the best resources for locating it is the state capital's telephone directory service.

Definitions of Developmental Disability

The federal law defines a developmental disability as "a substantially handicapping disability which originated prior to an individual attaining the age of 22 years and continues or is expected to continue indefinitely. These handicaps include such conditions as: mental retardation, cerebral palsy, epilepsy, autism, stroke, traumatic brain injury, or any condition which is attributable to a mental or physical impairment and results in substantial functional limitations." It further states, "to be considered developmentally disabled, the functional limitations must be in three or more of the areas which affect major life activity. These are areas such as: self-care, receptive and expressive language disorders, learning, mobility, self-direction, capacity for independent living, and economic self-sufficiency."[2]

Another key definition is the one for mental retardation that was offered in 1992 by the American Association on Mental Retardation. According to the American Association on Mental Retardation, mental retardation is characterized by significantly subaverage intellectual functioning that exists concurrently with related limitations in two or more applicable adaptive skill areas—communication, self-care, home living, social skills, community use, self-direction, health and safety, functional academics, and leisure and work—and presents substantial limitations in functioning and manifests before the age of 18 years. Subaverage intellectual functioning means an IQ score of 70 to 75 or below on a standardized individual intelligence test. Related limitations refers to adaptive skill limitations that are related more to functional applications than to other circumstances such as cultural diversity or sensory impairment. For more information on mental retardation see the association's website at www.aamr.org/.

Services can be provided in any combination to meet the developmentally disabled person's needs and allow him or her to function as independently as possible and in the least restrictive environment.

These services may include diagnosis, evaluation, treatment, personal care, day care, domiciliary care, special living arrangements, training of the parents, education, sheltered employment, recreation and socialization, counseling for both the patient and the family, protective services, information and referral, transportation, and any other services that promote and coordinate the activities and services required by the person with a developmental disability.

Responsible State Agency

The actual name of the agency responsible for administering services to the developmentally disabled varies from state to state. However, in most states the point of entry is often the state department of mental health, the department of mental retardation, or whatever state department or private agency has been designated as responsible for the delivery of services to this category of clients. As with so many state programs, the processes required for application, services, and access to care from this agency vary greatly from state to state.

Unlike other states, California's point of entry into the state's continuum of care system for people with DD is a network of 21 private nonprofit units called *regional centers*. These centers are contracted by the state department of developmental services and are legislatively funded. Regardless of which agency is responsible for providing services, the intent is to provide services to any person regardless of current age (as long as the developmentally disabling condition occurred before age 22). Services are also intended to reach persons who are believed to have a developmental disorder or a high risk of parenting a developmentally disabled infant.

Referrals

Referrals must be made as soon as the developmentally disabling condition has been identified. Unfortunately, not all persons will be eligible for services. If a person is not eligible, the DD counselors are in a position to offer assistance consisting of, at a minimum, information and referral. The important thing for the case manager to do is to refer the patient and allow the DD staff to determine eligibility. Once a referral has been made, an initial data intake session is scheduled. At this time, the person or parents must provide the following information:

- Name
- Address
- Social Security numbers of both patient and parents
- Birth dates of patient and parents
- Disability status of parents, if applicable
- Whether parents are living or deceased
- Any insurance coverage
- Proof of receipt of SSI or other state or federal aid or other income
- Proof of residence
- Copies of any medical records, psychologic or intelligence evaluations, or an IEP

During this initial session, the counselor may provide the patient and family with information or advice on the following:

- The nature and availability of the services provided by the DD programs and other community agencies (e.g., Title V or Children's Medical Services program, Medicaid, or any services from mental health)
- The conservatorship process
- Exploration of income maintenance, money management, and financial programs or funding sources
- The extent of training for the parents, volunteers, or other professionals
- Supportive services to which the person is entitled

- Housing or placement services to which the person is entitled (e.g., board and care, residential care, intermediate facility care, domiciliary care, nursing facility care, or home care)
- Education entitlement
- Work opportunities and training
- Medical and dental services
- Recreational activities within the community
- Preventive services for high-risk parents and individuals
- Other services as determined by need

Many children referred to this program are also eligible for benefits from the Title V Children's Medical Services program and Medicaid. Consequently, children with special needs may have one or more payers for their care needs. However, in all cases if the person has health coverage from a health insurer, this will be the primary payer for services unless services are limited, excluded, or exhausted.

Because many persons with DD are receiving services or input from a number of different agencies, coordination of case management activities is imperative. This is needed when a variety of agencies are assisting the person and each offers a form of case management services for its clients. As stated in several sections of this manual, when multiple agencies are involved in the care of one patient, it is imperative for all case managers to confer, select one case manager to serve as the primary case manager for the case, and jointly develop the case management plan. A process such as this helps to eliminate confusion, frustration, gaps, fragmentation, and duplication of care.

Assessment

Once referred to the DD agency, a complete medical and psychologic assessment will be required. This assessment includes the following:

- Collection and review of historical medical and diagnostic data.
- Provision or procurement of necessary tests and evaluations from which a determination for coverage can be made. These tests often include intelligence or psychologic tests and occupational, physical, and speech therapy evaluations.
- Summary of the developmental disability levels and recommendations for services.

"Habilitation" Plan

If after the initial data intake and assessment procedures, the person is found to be eligible for DD services, a "habilitation" plan is developed. This plan must be completed within the state's specified time frame (e.g., in California, this habilitation plan is referred to as an *individual program plan* and must be completed within 60 days of the assessment). The individual program plan is prepared jointly by one or more representatives from the DD agency staff, the patient, and when appropriate, the parents or conservator.

The final habilitation plan must contain the following information:

- Summary of the person's specific capabilities and problems
- Time-limited goals and objectives
- The type and amount of services, and if known, the providers of services necessary to achieve program objectives
- Scheduled dates for review and reassessment to determine whether the planned services have been provided within the time frames established for the goals and objectives
- Identification of the person responsible for program coordination. This person may be a DD staff member, a qualified individual or employee of another agency contracted by the department to provide program

coordination, or the patient's parent or legally appointed conservator

Services Provided

To achieve the stated objectives of the habilitation plan, the DD agency can contract for services from local providers or vendors.

As with all state agencies, the ability to contract with vendors for services varies from state to state, but the following services are commonly provided:

- Training of parents, volunteers, or health care professionals as required
- Purchase of and referral for services
- Collection and dissemination of whatever information is necessary to coordinate and establish the programs
- Placement in a licensed community care home or other health care facility
- Monitoring of services for any person placed outside the home
- Advocacy and protection of the patient's civil and legal rights
- Termination of services if the provider is ineffective or noncompliant
- Identification, maintenance of listings, and use of every appropriate and economically feasible alternative for care available within the region, and if services are not available in the immediate area, provision and coordination of services outside the region
- Authorization of medical, dental, and surgical treatment if the patient's parent or conservator does not respond to the request, if the patient has no parent or conservator, or if the patient is mentally incapable of authorizing such treatment
- Initiation of conservatorship proceedings, when appropriate

- Referral for SSI and Medicaid or Social Security Disability Income and Medicare
- Identification and use of all governmental or other income or insurance sources available and necessary for payment of the person's care, including school district funds allotted for special education for handicapped pupils

All habilitation plans are reviewed and modified at least annually by the DD counselor, the program coordinator, the patient, and the parents or the conservator. In order to establish or maintain the appropriate level of care for a patient, the DD counselor has the ability to purchase services that allow the person to live outside of an institution. Priority is given at all times to supporting the patient at home if this is feasible and acceptable to the parents. Supportive services for the patient living at home may include the following:

- Advocacy
- Specialized medical or dental care
- Specialized training for parents or caregivers
- Infant stimulation programs
- Respite care for parents or caregivers
- Homemaker services
- Babysitters
- Camping or outings
- Day care
- Short-term out-of-home placement or care
- Psychologic counseling
- Behavior modification programs
- Special equipment and accessories or other self-help devices
- Adult vocational training programs
- Placement in a community day-care program

If the person cannot be assisted at home, services may include placement in a facility such as the following:

- Community care home (board and care)

- Residential care facility
- Intermediate care facility; in California these facilities are referred to as *intermediate care facilities for the developmental disabled*; in other states they might be referred to as *intermediate care facilities for the mentally retarded*
- State institution

In all cases the patient is placed in the least restrictive facility that can manage the level of care and provide the services required. Persons are placed in an intermediate care facility when they cannot be assisted at home or in a community care facility (i.e., a home providing board and care). Patients placed in an intermediate care facility frequently have problems with self-care skills and require a structured environment that permits behavior modification or training.

Patients placed in residential or intermediate care facilities often cannot participate in any day program activities because of the severity of their disabilities. Actual licensed nursing care in these facilities ranges from less than 1 hour per day to 8 hours per week. Although short-term placement is the goal of any DD facility, these facilities are designed to provide long-term care if it is needed.

If the patient is self-destructive or his or her behavior is unmanageable in a board and care or intermediate care facility, placement options are limited. Generally, this type of patient is placed in a state developmental center, a state-operated facility, or a state hospital. Entrance into a state facility requires a court order if the person is older than 18 years; if he or she is younger than 18 years, the parents or legal conservator must grant permission for entrance, or referral must be generated by the DD counselor responsible for the case.

Payment and Alternate Funding

Most of the care and services provided by the DD agency are free of charge. However, in some circumstances parents may be required to pay a fee for a child younger than 22 years who is placed outside the home. This fee is based on a sliding scale or the ability to pay and cannot exceed the cost of provisions of care for a healthy child living at home. Many patients with DD, especially those placed in a facility, will qualify for SSI and Medicaid.

As with most public funding or entitlement programs, all DD services require that any health care insurance benefits or other funds be used before DD funds can be released. Again, this stipulation must never negate a referral because there is always a possibility that insurance benefits may be limited, exhausted, or excluded.

AID TO FAMILIES WITH DEPENDENT CHILDREN

Aid to Families with Dependent Children (AFDC) is a program administered and funded by federal and state goverments. The intent is to provide financial assistance to needy families. Although the majority of a state's program is funded by the federal government, the state provides the balance of payments, manages the program, and detemines eligiblity for benefits and the scope of services to be included. To be deemed eligible and receive AFDC payments, a family must have a dependent child who meets the following criteria:

- Younger than 18 years and living at home with the parent(s)
- Deprived of financial support from one parent because of the parent's death, continued absence, or incapacity (this area also includes children in two-parent families in which the principal earner is unemployed)
- A resident of the state
- A U.S. citizen or an alien who is permanently and lawfully residing in the United States

AFDC provides cash grants to families and children whose incomes are not adequate to meet their basic needs. AFDC has three groups for which eligibility can be issued:

1. **AFDC-Family Group (AFDC-FG)**—Families are eligible if they have a child who is financially needy because of death, incapacity, or continued absence of one or both parents.

2. **AFDC-Unemployed Parent (AFDC-U)**—Families are eligible if they have a child who is financially needy because of the unemployment of one or both parents.

3. **AFDC-Foster Care (AFDC-FC)**—A child can be eligible if he or she is living with a foster care provider under a court order or through a voluntary agreement between the child's parent and a county welfare or probation department.

To assist clients in obtaining employment, AFDC uses a program called *The Greater Avenues for Independence.* The Greater Avenues for Independence program provides basic education and job search and training for adults receiving AFDC. The intent of the program is to give adult recipients, who have been receiving AFDC for 2 years, an opportunity to participate in a work preparation assignment during which adults can complete training and education. Participants who refuse a work preparation assignment can be subject to a reduction in the family's cash grant.

For more information on AFDC, see the Department of Health and Human Services' website at www.acf.dhhs.gov/programs/afdc/reports.

SPECIAL SUPPLEMENTAL NUTRITION PROGRAM FOR WOMEN, INFANTS, AND CHILDREN

WIC is a short-term low-cost preventative health care program. WIC is designed to assist young families, mothers, and children who are at risk for poor nutrition because of low income or poor nutrition–related health conditions. The intent of the program is to do the following:

- Enable parents to properly feed their children during critical periods of growth and development
- Ensure normal childhood growth and development
- Reduce early childhood anemia
- Increase immunization rates
- Improve access to pediatric health care

Benefits allowed by WIC include the following:

- Quality nutrition education and services
- Breast-feeding promotion and education
- A monthly food prescription package
- Access to maternal, prenatal, and pediatric health care services

The average period that a person receives WIC is 13 months, and eligibility is based on the following:

- Income level less than or equal to 185% of the poverty level
- Documented nutrition risk
- For full information on WIC, see its website at www.nwica.org/

THE STATE CHILDREN'S HEALTH INSURANCE PROGRAM

The SCHIP was created as a part of the Balanced Budget Act of 1997 as Title XXI of the Social Security Act. The program is designed to offer insurance coverage to children, many of whom come from working families in which incomes are too high for them to qualify for Medicaid but too low for them to afford private health insurance.

Eligibility

The federal statute clearly requires states to screen every child for Medicaid eligibility before determining eligibility for SCHIP.

By requiring such a process, Congress wants to ensure that every child is enrolled in the correct program and that SCHIP will help to increase the number of insured children across the nation.

Under this initiative, states are able to use part of their federal funds to expand outreach and ensure that all eligible children are enrolled in either Medicaid or SCHIP. Each state has different eligibility rules, but in most states, uninsured children 18 years old and younger whose families earn up to $34,100 a year (for a family of four) are eligible. Patient out-of-pocket cost sharing for this program is allowed, but limited. If cost sharing is applicable for the family, no cost sharing is required for preventive care services or well-baby and well-child care including age-appropriate immunizations. Under the program states have the flexibility to target eligible uninsured children and they can do this through the following:

- Expansion of their current Medicaid program (if this is done, financial limits and cost sharing can vary but can only be based on income in a manner that does not favor higher-income children over lower-income children)
- Designing a new child health insurance program
- A combination of the two

States are allowed, under their Medicaid programs, to make medical assistance available to children who are presumptively eligible, and this includes all persons younger than 19 years. The presumptive period begins with the date on which a qualified entity determines, using preliminary information, that the family's income does not exceed the income eligibility level. The period ends with the eligibility determination or if an application for eligibility has not been filed on the last day of the month following the month in which the entity makes the preliminary determination.

States are not allowed to tighten Medicaid eligibility standards for children to prevent them from shifting children from the traditional Medicaid program to SCHIP. In addition, states must screen all applicants for Medicaid eligibility, and if applicants are eligible, they must be enrolled in the Medicaid program instead of SCHIP. States are further required to continue Medicaid eligibility for disabled children who would have lost or did lose their SSI benefits because of the change in the definition of childhood disability. State programs may not impose preexisting condition exclusions for covered benefits. The only exception to this rule is for states that provide for benefits through a group health plan or group health insurance coverage. In these circumstances, preexisting condition exclusions may be allowed because they fall under the applicable section of the Employee Retirement Income Security Act and the Health Insurance Portability and Accountability Act.

Eligibility is further assessed through intake and follow-up screening that targets low-income children. Eligibility is based on the following:

- Age
- Income
- State residence (varies by state as to the actual requirements)
- Access to other coverage
- Periods without insurance (varies by state but some have no requirements and some require the child to have been uninsured for the previous 4 months)

The time from application to actual program enrollment ranges from a few days to approximately 30 days for processing plus an additional 30 days for payment of the premium. Some states have used presumptive eligibility as a strategy to reduce the waiting time between the point of application and enrollment in the program. Other states allow coverage to begin immediately for children who apply by phone because of presumptive eligibility rules. With presumptive eligibility, children are assumed to be eligible for a specific period until their eligibility can be verified. Once eligibility verification is completed, children are either officially enrolled in or disenrolled from the program. For recertification, many states require verification of eligibility every 12 months, with the parents notified by reminder letter a few weeks before the deadline.

The SCHIP law allows the Department of Health and Human Services to grant states a waiver for a Section 1115 demonstration project. These demonstration projects allow states to use strategies not otherwise allowable under the SCHIP statute. For example, a state takes a specific service or population it wishes to evaluate, establishes eligibility and other requirements as well as anticipated goals, and makes application to the federal government for the ability to operate or offer the service under a waiver or demonstration to the federal law. Participant outcomes are measured with findings reported. Key to any project studied under a waiver or demonstration will be the cost savings the program can bring as a whole. This waiver enables states to test new and innovative approaches to promote the objectives of SCHIP with the goal of expanded coverage and improvement in enrollment, health care outcomes, and access to health care services for children.

Enrollment and Reaching the Target Populations

States use a variety of mechanisms for enrollment such as (1) allowing mail-in applications versus face-to-face interviews; (2) offering presumptive eligibility until the final determination is made (this allows enrollment of a child on a temporary basis, making health care services available immediately); (3) allowing retroactive eligibility; and (4) providing continuous eligibility. These efforts are all important strategies for simplification of the enrollment process and for providing families with opportunities to apply and remain enrolled. Most states have accepted the option allowed under the Balanced Budget Act to enroll children in an SCHIP and a Medicaid program for up to 12 months, regardless of changes in income or family circumstances. Thus children do not lose coverage as a result of changes to the family's financial status or size.

Because schools are a natural conduit of information to parents, many states and their Medicaid programs and SCHIP use the schools as an avenue for identifying and enrolling uninsured children. Another avenue, which breaks the stigma associated with in-person encounters with the local welfare offices, is use of a variety of community centers as enrollment sites. These sites often include childcare centers, health centers, hospitals, various other health care service providers (e.g., WIC offices) or local clinics. Vulnerable populations often face a variety of socioeconomic, linguistic, cultural, literacy, and geographic isolation barriers, any of which have the potential to affect enrollment. Thus many states have adopted innovative and aggressive community-based strategies to assist in combating these barriers. Some strategies include the following:

- Development of all literature in specific languages for specific targeted geographic regions
- Participation in events such as health fairs, parades, and other local events where mass media messages appeal to specific audiences
- Use of flyers printed on grocery bags and stuffers included with local utility bills
- Sponsored public service announcements

Another way that states help reach families with uninsured children is through the outreach efforts of several agencies such as the Department of Health and Human Services, the National Governors' Association, private foundations and businesses, and other federal agencies. Many of these efforts include what is termed *Insure Kids Now campaign*. As part of this campaign, the National Governors' Association has established a national toll-free number (877-KIDS-NOW) that automatically directs callers to their state's program. In addition, a national website has also been created: www.insurekidsnow.gov. This website provides links to eligibility and contact information for each state, U.S. territories, and the District of Columbia.

Traditional Benefits of SCHIP

Traditional SCHIP benefits include the following:

- Inpatient hospital services
- Outpatient hospital services
- Transplant services
- Emergency and urgent care services
- Skilled nursing facility services
- Physician services
- Surgical services
- Clinic services (including health center services) and other ambulatory health care services, including well-baby and well-child care services and immunizations
- Prescription drugs and biologic agents and the administration of such drugs and biologic agents if not furnished for the purpose of causing or assisting in causing the death, suicide, euthanasia, or mercy killing of a person
- Over-the-counter medications
- Laboratory and radiology services
- Prenatal care and prepregnancy family planning services and supplies
- Inpatient mental health services, including services furnished in a state-operated mental hospital and residential or other 24-hour therapeutically structured services

- Outpatient mental health services furnished by a state-operated mental hospital, including community-based services
- Durable medical equipment and other medically related or remedial devices (such as oxygen, prosthetic devices, implants, eyeglasses, hearing aids, dental devices, and adaptive devices)
- Disposable medical supplies
- Home- and community-based health care services and related supportive services (e.g., home health nursing services, home health aide services, personal care assistance with activities of daily living, chore services, day-care services, respite care services, training for family members, or minor modifications to the home)
- Nursing care services in a home, school, or other setting (e.g., nurse practitioner services, nurse midwife services, advanced practice nurse services, private duty nursing care, pediatric nurse services, and respiratory care services)
- Abortion, only if necessary to save the life of the mother or if the pregnancy is the result of an act of rape or incest
- Dental services
- Inpatient and residential substance abuse treatment services
- Outpatient substance abuse treatment services
- Case management services
- Care coordination services
- Physical therapy, occupational therapy, and services for individuals with speech, hearing, and language disorders
- Hospice care
- Any other medical diagnostic screening, preventive, restorative, remedial, therapeutic, or rehabilitative services (whether in a facility,

home, school, or other setting) if such services are as follows:

- Recognized by state law
- Prescribed by or furnished by a physician or other licensed or registered practitioner acting within the scope of practice as defined by state law
- Performed under the general supervision or at the direction of a physician
- Furnished by a health care facility that is operated by a state or local government or that is licensed under state law and operating within the scope of the license
- Premiums for private health care insurance coverage
- Medical transportation
- Enabling services (e.g., transportation, translation, or other outreach services) only if designed to increase access to primary and preventive health care services

Case managers interested in learning more about SCHIP can obtain information from children's medical services. The Centers for Medicare & Medicaid Services (CMS) maintain information on every state's SCHIP program, including eligibility and enrollment information, approval letters, amendments, and contact information. For more information, see the CMS's website at www.cms.hhs.gov/schip.

Personal Responsibility and Work Opportunity Reconciliation Act of 1996

The Personal Responsibility and Work Opportunity Reconciliation Act of 1996 is an act that separated Medicaid and welfare eligibility for the first time. With this new act, families who lose eligibility for cash assistance are allowed to continue to qualify for Medicaid under other eligibility categories because states are required to make a separate determination about Medicaid eligibility when a family no longer qualifies for cash assistance. Unfortunately, many parents do not know about the possibility of continued Medicaid and their potential ongoing eligibility.

Under this act, the definition of disability for children in the SSI program was also changed (Box 7-4).

SUPPLEMENTAL SECURITY INCOME FOR CHILDREN

Although it is believed that the SSI program only serves adults, this is not true. SSI is a federal program that is administered by the Social Security Administration. The program is designed to provide monthly payments to individuals with low incomes who are elderly, blind, or disabled, regardless of age. A primary criterion for ongoing coverage is that the person must meet the federal definition of disabled. In addition

---

BOX 7-4
The Law's New Definition of Disability for Children

- Requires a child to have a physical or mental condition or conditions that can be medically proven and that result in *marked and severe* functional limitations
- Requires that the medically proven physical or mental condition or conditions must last or be expected to last at least 12 months or be expected to result in death
- Says that a child may not be considered disabled if he or she is working at a job that can be considered to be substantial work; however, the law did not change the rules that allow certain children already on the rolls to continue to receive SSI, even though they are working.

to the monthly payments, recipients of SSI are automatically eligible for Medicaid benefits. A family's income is not counted if the person is an inpatient in a nonfederally supported facility for 1 full month. Application for benefits is made to the local Social Security office.[2]

Children may be eligible for SSI in three ways:

1. **SSI Benefits For Children**—This program is for children who come from homes with limited income or resources, and benefits can be paid if the child is younger than 18 years.

2. **Social Security Dependents' Benefits**—This is a program for children who are (1) dependents of a parent who is collecting disability retirement benefits or (2) recipients of survivor's benefits from Social Security because they are younger than 18 years and are collecting Social Security benefits based on the record of a parent (the age limit can be extended to 19 years if the child is a full-time student in an elementary or high school).

3. **Social Security Benefits for Adults Disabled Since Childhood**—Normally, dependent benefits stop when a child reaches age 18 years, or if he or she is a full-time student, age 19 years. However, if the child is disabled and the disability was diagnosed before the age of 22 years, benefits can continue into adulthood. To qualify for these benefits, the person must have been eligible as a child or as a dependent of a disabled person, if the benefits were based on the parent's Social Security earnings record.

SSI Benefits for Children with Disabilities

As the name implies, SSI is a supplement to a person's income. The intent is to bring the income up to a certain level. Unfortunately, the level varies from state to state and is an amount that is adjusted annually and based on cost-of-living increases. For children younger than 18 years, the parent's income and assets are taken into consideration for the initial determination and ongoing eligibility. This rule applies to all children, regardless of whether they live at home or are away at school but return home occasionally, and as long as they are subject to parental control. Social Security terms this process *deeming* of income and assets.

As indicated previously, benefits generally cease for children who receive their SSI based on the fact that they are dependents or survivors at age 18 years. However, benefits can continue as follows:

- Until the child reaches age 19 years and remains enrolled as a full-time student in an elementary or high school
- Into adulthood if the child continues to meet disability guidelines

When a child turns 18 years old and remains disabled, the parent's income and assets are no longer taken into consideration for the child's eligibility. Thus a child who was not eligible for SSI before his or her 18th birthday because the parents' income or assets were deemed "too high" may become eligible at age 18 years based on "his or her own" income and assets. If a disabled child receiving SSI turns 18 years old and continues to live with his or her parents but is incapable of paying for food or shelter, he or she will remain eligible for SSI, but the rate will be lower than if the child were able to live alone.

SSI Disability and Eligibility Determination

The process for establishing disability for a child is no different from the determination process for older persons. The parents must bring not only information regarding their assets and income but also any documents that support or medically justify the disability. The review process can be expedited if case managers tell parents to assemble and bring to their eligibility screening interview:

- Any medical records they have that justify the request (if they do not have records, the disability unit can request the records)
- Names, addresses, and phone numbers of any physicians and other health care providers (e.g., clinics, hospitals, specialists)
- Any school records, including names, addresses, and phone numbers of schools, teachers, or day-care providers

As the family's income and assets are evaluated, the child's medical documents are submitted to the state's disability determination service (DDS) unit. The DDS evaluation unit comprises a team of health care professionals that includes a disability evaluation specialist and a doctor. If the available medical records do not provide sufficient information for the DDS team to make a determination, the child will be required to undergo a medical examination that has been arranged and paid for by Social Security. As with the disability laws for adults, a child is considered disabled if any of the following is established:

- The child has a physical or mental condition (or a combination of conditions) that results in "marked and severe functional limitations."
- The condition lasts or is expected to last at least 12 months or is expected to result in the child's death.
- The child is not able to hold a job that is considered gainful employment or substantial work.

To determine whether the child's impairment causes "marked and severe functional limitations," the DDS team obtains evidence from a wide variety of sources who have treated or who have knowledge of the child's condition and how it affects his or her ability to function on a day-to-day basis and over time. These sources include, but are not limited to, physicians and other health care professionals who have treated the child and the child's teachers, counselors, therapists, and social workers. Consequently, a finding of disability is not based solely on a parent's statements or on whether the child is enrolled in special education classes.

Presumptive Eligibility

Because the disability evaluation process generally takes several months, the law allows special provisions for people (including children) signing up for SSI disability whose condition is so severe they are "presumed" to be disabled. In cases such as these, SSI benefits are paid for up to 6 months while the formal disability decision is being made. Examples of presumptive disabilities are as follows:

- HIV infection
- Blindness
- Deafness (in some cases)
- Cerebral palsy (in some cases)
- Down syndrome
- Muscular dystrophy (in some cases)
- Significant mental deficiency
- Diabetes (with amputation of one foot)
- Amputation of two limbs
- Amputation of leg at the hip

Continuing Disability

The law requires that children with an ongoing disability have the disability verified at regular intervals to ensure that the child remains eligible for SSI. The actual frequency of the review depends on whether the individual's disability is expected to improve, might improve, or is not expected to improve. As a rule, continuing disability reviews are done for the following:

- Babies whose disability is based on low weight, not later than 12 months after the birth

- Children younger than 18 years whose condition is anticipated to improve (the review is conducted every 3 years)
- Children who will turn 18 years old (the re-review is done in the month before they turn 18 years old)

Medicaid and Medicare

In most states children who receive SSI benefits automatically qualify for Medicaid. In other states the parents must complete the Medicaid application process for eligibility as well. Although Medicare is a federal health insurance program for persons older than 65 years and the disabled younger than 65 years, most children are not entitled to any Social Security Disability Income until they turn 18 years old or to any Medicare benefits until the age of 20 years. The only exception made to this rule is for children who have been diagnosed with end-stage renal disease and require either a kidney transplant or maintenance dialysis. Children in this category can qualify for Medicare if a parent is receiving Social Security or has worked enough to be covered by Social Security.

APPEALS—ALL PROGRAMS

Because the rights of children are highly protected (e.g., Federal Rehabilitation Act of 1973, Titles VI and VII of the Civil Rights Act of 1964, and the Americans with Disabilities Act of 1990), anyone not in agreement with an agency's decision on eligibility, benefits, or other issues has the right to file an appeal. In most cases the appeal request must be in writing and done within a specific time frame.

SUMMARY

To create and implement successful case management plans, case managers working with children must have a basic knowledge of public funding programs and the many programs and services available to children. This is important because many times the services or items a child requires will be limited or excluded from private insurance coverage, since they may be deemed to be not medically necessary or for convenience or may be classified as educational.

Chapter Exercises

1. Research the IDEA, the Rehabilitation Act of 1973, the Civil Rights Act of 1964, and the Americans with Disabilities Act of 1990: report findings on how these acts are related and describe the primary focus of each as it pertains to children with special needs.
2. Contact the local state office designated to assist children with special needs and report your findings as they relate to types and scope of diagnoses covered and not, as well as the services provided and those excluded, the referral and eligibility determination processes and finally, how the program, if applicable, interfaces with any private health care insurance the child may have.
3. Contact the local school district to ascertain what services are provided for children with special needs.

Suggested Websites and Resources

www.ssa.gov/—Social Security Administration
www.acf.dhhs.gov/—Department of Developmental Disabilities
www.ed.gov/—Special Education
www.cms.hhs.gov/schip/default.asp—Centers for Medicare & Medicaid Services—information about every state's SCHIP programs including eligibility and enrollment information, approval letters, amendments, and contact information

www.insurekidsnow.gov—Consumer-
oriented information about each state's
SCHIP plan

www.nwica.org/—WIC

www.cms.hhs.gov/schip/default.asp—Centers
for Medicare & Medicaid Services

www.ichp.edu/schip/materials/893253826—
Institute for Child Health Policy

www.apha.org/ppp/schip—American Public
Health Association

www.ahcpr.gov/chip—Agency for
Healthcare Research and Quality

REFERENCES

1. Sacramento County Department of Education: Sacramento County SELP presents a parent's guide to special education, Sacramento, CA, 1993, The Department.
2. United States Code Service: Social Security Act Title XVI: supplemental security income for the aged, blind, and disabled (42 USCS 1381-1385). Washington, DC, 1993, The Service.

Department of Defense Health Care and Veterans' Benefits

Peggy A. Rossi, BSN, MPA, CCM, CPUR

OBJECTIVES

- To be able to identify the managed care and triple-option plans now offered by the Department of Defense (DoD) and describe the basic structure of each and how they compare
- To be able to identify two new programs now offered by the DoD for retirees
- To identify the core eligibility requirements of TRICARE and the enrollment system that tracks all eligible military persons
- To be able to describe a veteran's entitlement to the scope of services based on his or her military history, classification of the discharge, and his or her disability rating
- To describe the act that changed the Department of Veterans Affairs (VA) system and created a uniform benefit structure
- To describe the seven priority categories
- To list the basic benefits allowed
- To describe The Civilian Health and Medical Program of the Department of Veterans Affairs (CHAMPVA), who is entitled to care, and how it compares to standard VA benefits

TRICARE

TRICARE is the DoD's worldwide health plan for eligible military families, both active-duty and retired. In addition to the services previously available at military treatment facilities (MTFs), hospitals, and clinics, the DoD has contracted with managed care organizations (MCOs) to offer managed care and a triple-option plan to persons eligible for military health care benefits. TRICARE has undergone multiple revisions since the mid-1980s and now replaces the old CHAMPUS programs.

Not only has the name changed, so have many of the features. Eligible persons now have a "triple option" for selecting their health care coverage and the ability to select a point-of-service option. The triple option includes a health maintenance organization (HMO) model called *TRICARE Prime*, a preferred provider organization model called *TRICARE Extra*, and an indemnity option called *TRICARE Standard*.

Who Is Eligible for Benefits

The TRICARE program is the program that provides health care benefits to the seven branches of the uniformed services:

- Army
- Navy
- Marine Corps
- Air Force
- Coast Guard
- Public Health Service
- National Oceanic and Atmospheric Administration

To receive TRICARE benefits, the person must be enrolled in DEERS and must meet one of the following additional eligibility requirements:

- A family member of an active-duty military personnel—if a newborn, the newborn is covered for the first 120 days of life under the mother's coverage; for continued enrollment, the baby must be enrolled under his or her own name and birth date
- A military retiree
- A military retiree's family member
- A surviving eligible family member of a deceased active-duty or retired service member
- A ward (an unmarried person younger than 21 years; an unmarried person younger than 23 years, if enrolled in college carrying 12 units; an unmarried person who is unable to support himself or herself because of a mental or physical handicap; or one who has been placed in legal custody or in the home of a TRICARE member); an adopted child; or a former spouse (must meet requirements for length of marriage) of an active-duty or retired service member
- Enrolled in the Defense Enrollment Eligibility Reporting System (DEERS)—DEERS is a government agency that maintains records on all active-duty and retired military per-

sons and their dependents; contact with DEERS can be made by calling the national toll-free number: 800-538-9552

The following persons are not eligible for TRICARE Prime:

- Dependent parents or parents-in-law
- CHAMPVA beneficiaries
- North Atlantic Treaty Organisation (NATO) family members (NATO dependents are eligible for civilian outpatient care under the TRICARE Extra or TRICARE Standard programs)
- Those participating in the Continued Health Care Benefit Program. This program is like the Consolidated Omnibus Reconciliation Act (COBRA) for civilians. The Continued Health Care Benefit Program provides health care benefits similar to those of COBRA from the TRICARE Standard program. Benefits are provided for a specific period (18-36 months) to former service members and their family members who enroll and pay quarterly premiums.

TRICARE Prime

TRICARE Prime is like an HMO model, and to date, this option is the most favored. TRICARE Prime features include the following:

- A primary care manager (PCM), which is the same as a primary care physician (PCP); in any case, the beneficiary has the option to chose a PCM from an MTF or select a PCP if he or she elects to use the HMO's panel of providers
- Priority status given at military hospitals and clinics for care
- No deductibles
- Active-duty service members pay no enrollment fee for their families (retirees and non–active-duty

beneficiaries do pay a set amount each year, e.g., $230-$460)

- Enrollment portability, should a move to another region be required and Prime coverage is available and the beneficiary can be transferred to a new MCO (means that the enrollment fees, anniversary date for enrollment, and any copayments made year to date that have been credited toward the catastrophic cap are transferred)
- Split enrollment, which allows one enrollment fee for coverage of those families with children in college, children living away, or children who live with a former spouse
- Pharmacy benefits—no cost if obtained from the MTF, low cost if obtained from one of the MCO's pharmacy network providers, or low cost if obtained from the MCO's mail-order prescription service
- Preventive care services, at no extra cost

TRICARE Extra

TRICARE Extra is similar to a preferred provider option but includes some of the benefits of both the Prime and Standard programs. The main difference is that although beneficiaries have the option of using any provider of their choice, they will pay about 5% less if they use one of the MCO's network providers. Under TRICARE Extra, the members are not enrolled, so there is no health care card; they merely use their military identification card when they need access to care. TRICARE Extra benefits include the following:

- No enrollment fee or application
- Lower out-of-pocket costs (cost shares based on military rank and status) when network providers are used
- Lower annual deductible ($50-300) per fiscal year (October 1 through September 30)

- Lower priority for MTF or clinics
- Reduced paperwork (if network providers are used, these providers submit the claims)

TRICARE Standard

TRICARE Standard is the old standard CHAMPUS program and is the basic program for military health care. TRICARE Standards benefits include the following:

- No enrollment fee or application
- Best choice of coverage for persons who travel frequently or those away from home for extended periods
- Freedom to select most any provider
- Deductibles ($50-300) per fiscal year (October 1 through September 30)
- Copayment of 20% to 25% after deductible is met
- Lowest priority for use of the MTF or military clinics

TRICARE Choice Comparison

Although it is best to have patients and families work directly with the MCO's staff (e.g., health care finders or beneficiary services representatives) or MTF personnel (health benefits advisors), the following comparison is a guide for case managers working with military families who might request additional help as they select a TRICARE option. See Table 8-1 for a comparison.

Even if a person is eligible for TRICARE Prime, he or she remains responsible for what is termed *a catastrophic loss protection limit* (or catastrophic cap) for health care costs. This means that there is a limit to out-of-pocket expenses a patient is required to pay for health care. Included in this cap are copayments, deductibles, and any cost shares paid for allowed charges or for point-of-service care. Examples of the caps are as follows:

- For active-duty family members, the cap is $1000 per fiscal year (October 1 through September 30)

- For retirees and others there are two caps:
  - An enrollment cap, which is set at $3000 per year for a 12-month period covering Prime enrollment
  - A fiscal year cap of $7500 (October 1 through September 30)

TABLE 8-1
TRICARE Comparison

Services	Prime	Extra	Standard
Out-of-pocket costs	Low	High	Highest
MTF care	First priority	Space available	Space available
Annual deductible	None	$50-$300 per fiscal year	$50-$300 per fiscal year
Annual enrollment fee	Active-duty family members: none; retirees and others: $230-$460 per year	None	None
Costs for care	Small copayment for many services (fixed amount per medical services used)	After deductible 15%-20% of the contracted fee if MCO network providers are used	After deductible 20%-25% of the maximum amount TRICARE normally reimburses
Other	Choice of high-quality providers and less paperwork when an MCO network provider is used	Less paperwork if the MCO provider network is used Good choice for travelers	More paperwork because beneficiary is often required to bill TRICARE Good choice for travelers
Doctors' office visits	No fees if MTF physicians and providers used; $6-$12 copayment if network providers used	15%-20% cost share after deductible	20%-25% cost share after deductible
ED services	$10-$30 copayments; if at MTF, no fees	15%-20% cost share after deductible	20%-25% cost share after deductible
Laboratory or radiology services	No fees if MTF physicians and providers used; $6-$12 copayment if network providers used	15%-20% cost share after deductible	20%-25% cost share after deductible
Hospitalizations	At MTF, $11.45 per day; civilian care, $11 per day ($25 minimum copayment)	At MTF, $11.45 per day; civilian care, $250 per day or 25% cost share of hospital costs (whichever is less) plus 20% copayment of professional charges	At MTF, $11.45 per day; civilian care, $401 per day or 25% cost share of hospital costs (whichever is less) plus 25% copayment of professional charges
Routine physical examinations	No copayments	Covered only as part of cancer screening; 15%-20% cost share after deductible	Covered only as part of cancer screening; 20%-25% cost share after deductible

Data from TRICARE (www.tricare.osd.mil/frequentlyaskedquestions.htm) and Health Net (www.fhfs.com).
ED, Emergency department; *MCO,* managed care organization; *MTF,* military treatment facility.

Continued

TABLE 8-1
TRICARE Comparison—cont'd

Services	Prime	Extra	Standard
Pharmacy	At MTF, no charge; at network pharmacy, $5-$9 copayment (30-day supply); mail-order, $4-$8 copayment (90-day supply)	At MTF, no charge; at network pharmacy, 15%-20% cost share (no deductible) for 30-day supply; mail-order, $4-$8 copayment (90-day supply)	At MTF, no charge; at network pharmacy, 20%-25% cost share (after deductible) for 30-day supply; mail-order, $4-$8 copayment (90-day supply)
Well-child care	No copayment	15%-20 % cost share after deductible	20%-25% cost share after deductible

Health Care Finders

As a TRICARE provider, the MCO uses registered nurses, called *health care finders*, to assist in many aspects of program administration. This may include assisting beneficiaries and providers in locating care or services from a military facility or from a civilian provider or community resource. A health care finder also explains the many health care programs offered by the DoD for its uniformed services personnel and serves as the point of contact when a prior authorization is required for services obtained from a civilian health care provider.

Health Benefits Advisors

The military has historically used personnel called *health benefits advisors* to explain the TRICARE program and assist with claims processing and other administrative tasks. Although the MCO is required to have both health care finders and beneficiary services representatives, health benefits advisors continue to play a vital role in assisting military beneficiaries in understanding all their health care benefit options (e.g., the TRICARE plan and dental care, as well as various services with out-of-pocket costs) and in linking beneficiaries to key military base–specific programs.

Beneficiary Services Representative

In the MCO and TRICARE programs, a third group of professionals is also available to assist beneficiaries with understanding the TRICARE programs. These professionals are called *beneficiary services representatives*. Their primary responsibilities are explaining the TRICARE programs; assisting beneficiaries in finding a PCM or PCP; making changes when beneficiaries wish to switch PCMs or PCPs; enrolling TRICARE-eligible persons in Prime; replacing lost TRICARE Prime cards; offering claims assistance to all TRICARE-eligible persons; and disenrolling members.

TRICARE for Life

In 2001, the DoD made sweeping changes to the TRICARE program and expanded coverage for military beneficiaries who are eligible for Medicare and have purchased Medicare Part B. This new program is termed *TRICARE For Life (TFL)*. If the beneficiary is enrolled in TFL, the program offers many benefits such as the following:

- TRICARE serves as a secondary payer to Medicare.
- Claims are filed automatically by providers (no paperwork).
- Other than a Medicare Part B premium (deducted automatically

from the Social Security check), there is no monthly premium.

■ Comprehensive health care is offered for eligible beneficiaries.

TFL Eligibility

Eligibility for TFL is also based on the fact that the person has (1) a valid military identification card and (2) is enrolled in DEERS and has a DEERS file that contains accurate information. Retirees are registered in DEERS through the Defense Finance Accounting Services, and TFL is open to the following:

■ Medicare-eligible military retirees, including retired guard members and reservists (aged 65 years and older)

■ Medicare-eligible family members and widows or widowers aged 65 years or older *(dependent parents and parents-in-law are excluded)*

■ Certain former spouses, if they were eligible for TRICARE before they turned 65 years old

TFL Benefits

Benefits are comprehensive and cover traditional health care services as allowed under the TRICARE and Medicare programs. Except for inpatient mental health care and inpatient substance abuse treatment programs, *there are no prior authorization requirements for use of TFL benefits.* If enrolled in TFL, the following apply to the beneficiary:

■ Has no annual fees to pay

■ Is entitled to care at the MTF and military clinics on a space-available basis

■ If also enrolled in the TRICARE Plus program, may be able to receive primary care at the MTF

■ During travel overseas, is only required to pay applicable deductibles and cost shares

As with all health care coverage, many services are considered excluded benefits and thus are not covered. Although the service member might have dual insurance coverage (e.g., Medicare and a supplemental policy), if he or she also has TFL, TFL will be the payer of last resort (Table 8-2).

For a full listing of benefits, see TRICARE's website at www.tricare.osd.mil, or beneficiaries can call 888-DoD-LIFE or 888-363-5433. For TRICARE Senior pharmacy questions, beneficiaries can call 877-DoD-MEDS or 877-363-6337.

TRICARE Pharmacy Programs

Pharmacy benefits are available for all active-duty service members and their dependents worldwide, as well as all TRICARE-eligible beneficiaries regardless of age. In addition to the benefits allowed by use of the MCO's network pharmacy providers or those available at the nearest MTF, the TRICARE pharmacy program offers the advantages of mail order for those beneficiaries who want it. As with most mail-order pharmacy programs, the program is not suited for all beneficiaries (e.g., those with acute episodic illnesses) (see Table 8-3 for a comparison). The availability of mail-order pharmaceuticals best suits persons with chronic disorders who take medications on a long-term basis for their disorders. To be eligible for the TRICARE mail-order pharmacy program, the person must be enrolled in DEERS. The benefits of mail-order pharmaceuticals for eligible beneficiaries are as follows:

■ Convenience

■ Copayments as follows:
   ■ Active-duty service members have no copayment
   ■ Active-duty family members and eligible retirees and their family members (includes Medicare beneficiaries eligible for Base Realignment and Closure [BRAC] benefits) have a copayment of $9 for nongeneric or brand-name medications and a copayment of $3 for generic medications

TABLE 8-2
TRICARE for Life and Medicare Comparison

Services		Medicare	TRICARE for Life	Patient Pays
Services outside MTF—Medicare Part A coverage				
Inpatient acute-care hospital	Days 1-60	100% after acute-care deductible met for the first 60 days	First 60-day deductible (i.e., $792)	Nothing
	Days 61-90	All but the daily deductible amount (i.e., $198 per day)	The daily deductible amount (i.e., $198 per day)	Nothing
	Days 90-150	All but the daily deductible amount (i.e., $198 per day)	The daily deductible amount (i.e., $396 per day)	Nothing
	Days 151+	Not covered	80% if MCO network hospital used	20% allowable charges if in net work hospital
			75% if nonnetwork hospital used	25% allowable charges if in non-network hospital
Inpatient mental health hospitalizations require prior authorization, and if >30 days, a waiver for secondary TRICARE coverage; if authorized, TRICARE pays cost shares and deductible	Days 1-60	100% after deductible (i.e., $792)	First 60-day deductible (i.e., $792)	Nothing for services payable by Medicare and TRICARE
	Days 61-90	All but the day deductible amount (i.e., $198 per day)	The daily deductible amount (i.e., $198 per day)	Nothing for services payable by Medicare and TRICARE
	Days 91-150	All but the day deductible amount (i.e., $396 per day)	The daily deductible amount (i.e., $396 per day)	Nothing for services payable by Medicare and by Medicare and
	Days 151-190	100% after another inpatient deductible paid (i.e., $792)	First 60-day deductible (i.e., $792)	25% of TRICARE allowable charges if in nonnetwork hospital
Requires a new benefit period before days 151-190 can be used	Days 191+	Not covered	75% if nonnetwork hospital used	Nothing for services payable by Medicare and TRICARE
Skilled nursing facility care	Days 1-20	100%	Remaining beneficiary liability if any	Nothing for services payable by Medicare and TRICARE
	Days 21-100	All but daily deductible (i.e., $99 per day)	Daily deductible (i.e., $99 per day)	Nothing for services payable by Medicare and TRICARE
	Days 101+	Not covered	75% allowable	25% of TRICARE allowable charges

Data from TRICARE (www.tricare.osd.mil/tfl/tfl_fact.html and www.tricare.osd.mil/factsheets/index.cfm?fx= showfs&file_name=TFL.htm).
ED, Emergency department; *MCO,* managed care organization; *MTF,* military treatment facility.

TABLE 8-2
TRICARE for Life and Medicare Comparison—cont'd

Services	Medicare	TRICARE for Life	Patient Pays
Hospice care	Medicare pays 95%	Remaining beneficiary liability or 5%	Nothing for services payable by Medicare and TRICARE
Outpatient Services—Medicare Part B			
Non-MTF physicians' visits	80%	20%	Nothing for services payable by Medicare and TRICARE
ED visits	80%	20%	Nothing for services payable by Medicare and TRICARE
Mental health outpatient visits	50%	50%	Nothing for services payable by Medicare and TRICARE
Laboratory services	100%	Remaining beneficiary liability if any	Nothing for services payable by Medicare and TRICARE
Radiology services	80%	20%	Nothing for services payable by Medicare and TRICARE
Home health care	100% of approved care	Remaining beneficiary liability if any	Nothing for services payable by Medicare and TRICARE
Durable medical equipment	80%	20%	Nothing for services payable by Medicare and TRICARE
Outpatient hospital services	80%	20%	Nothing for services payable by Medicare and TRICARE
Blood transfusions	100% after TRICARE pays 100% for the first 3 pints of blood	100% of the cost of the first 3 pints of blood	Nothing for services payable by Medicare and TRICARE
Chiropractic services	80%	Not covered	20% of Medicare cost share
Inpatient services outside the United States	Not covered	75%	25% of TRICARE allowable charges after the TRICARE annual deductible has been met and if care is received from an author ized provider

Continued

TABLE 8-2
TRICARE for Life and Medicare Comparison—cont'd

Services	Medicare	TRICARE for Life	Patient Pays
Outpatient services outside the United States	Not covered	75%	25% of TRICARE allowable charges after the TRICARE annual deductible has been met and if care is received from an authorized provider
MTF pharmacy	Not covered	100% for a 90-day supply	Nothing
National Mail Order Pharmacy	Not covered	All costs except for the generic or brand-name prescription drug copayment up to a 90-day supply	Copayment for generic drug (i.e., $3); copayment for brand-name drug (i.e., $9)
MCO network pharmacy	Not covered	All costs except for the generic or brand-name prescription drug copayment up to a 30-day supply	Copayment for generic drug (i.e., $3); copayment for brand-name drug (i.e., $9)
Nonnetwork pharmacy	Not covered	All costs except for the generic or brand-name prescription drug copayment up to a 30-day supply	Copayment for all drugs (i.e., $9) or 20%, whichever is greater; a yearly deductible of $150 per individual or $300 per family applies

TABLE 8-3
Pharmacy Out-of-Pocket Cost Comparison

Place of Service	MTF	Mail Order	Network Pharmacy	Nonnetwork Pharmacy
Generic drug (copayments apply to all beneficiaries)	$0	$3 for 90-day supply	$3 for 30-day supply	$9 or 20% of charges (whichever is greater) after annual deductible met (i.e., $150 per individual or $300 per family)
Brand-name drug (copayments apply to all beneficiaries)	$0	$9 for 90-day supply	$9 for 30-day supply	$9 or 20% of charges (whichever is greater) after annual deductible met (i.e., $150 per individual or $300 per family)

Data from Health Net (www.fhfs.com/pdf/BeneChartWEB.Pdf).

- Orders can be placed by phone, by mail, or on-line (www.merckmedco. com)
- Free shipping and handling
- No claims forms to file and no waiting for reimbursement
- Door-to-door delivery (normal delivery time is within 7-11 days from the date of order and expedited delivery is available for an additional fee); this mail-order convenience also includes those beneficiaries who have an army post office or fleet post office address or an overseas US embassy address
- One low copayment for either a 90-day supply of noncontrolled medications or a 30-day supply of a controlled substance
- Automated payment plan available
- Drugs as listed on the National Mail Order Pharmacy Program Formulary as developed by DoD's Pharmceutical & Therapeutic (P&T) committee
- Availability of a pharmacist 24 hours a day, 7 days per week, for emergency consultations (800-903-4680)

Another TRICARE program that began in April 2001 is the TRICARE Senior Pharmacy program. This program allows eligible uniformed services retirees and their eligible dependents or survivors aged 65 years or older to have pharmacy coverage. To be eligible, the person does not have to have Medicare Part B if they reached the age of 65 years before April 1, 2001. Persons who turned 65 years old after April 1, 2001 are required to have both Medicare Part A and Part B.

Base Realignment and Closure

The BRAC program pharmacy benefit ensures that Medicare-eligible beneficiaries, who previously relied on an MTF pharmacy for their medications, can continue to receive the drugs they need after a military base has been realigned with another base or closed. BRAC pharmacy services are provided through the use of mail order or from a local retail pharmacy when a facility has closed. To be eligible for the program, beneficiaries must be older than 65 years and live within a 40-mile catchment area of the closed MTF. If beneficiaries live outside the catchment area, they are eligible if they used the MTF pharmacy at least once within 1 year of the facility's closing.

Beneficiaries affected by BRAC have the same pharmacy benefits as those who use TRICARE Extra. In the National Mail Order Pharmacy program, beneficiaries are allowed to receive up to a 90-day supply of medication for an $8 copayment. If they use a TRICARE retail network pharmacy, they can obtain a 30-day supply for a 20% copayment. In this program there are no deductibles.

TRICARE Plus

TRICARE's newest option for care is called *TRICARE Plus*. TRICARE Plus is open to persons eligible for care in MTFs and not enrolled in TRICARE Prime or a commercial HMO. The Plus program allows some military health system beneficiaries to enroll with the military PCM. Enrollees in this program are provided access to primary care on the same basis as those enrolled in TRICARE Prime. Unfortunately, the program is not available at all MTF sites.

The new TRICARE Plus program differs from both TRICARE Prime and TRICARE Senior Prime in the following ways:

- TRICARE Plus is not a comprehensive health plan because it is intended to provide primary care only and it has no effect on an enrollee's use of or payment of civilian health care benefits (thus TRICARE Standard, TRICARE Extra, or Medicare may pay for civilian health care services obtained by a TRICARE Plus enrollee).

- TRICARE Plus does not lock beneficiaries into "managed care." They may seek care from a civilian provider but are discouraged from obtaining nonemergency primary care from sources outside the MTF where they are enrolled. In addition to providing access to primary care, this plan enables beneficiaries' physicians to coordinate health care more effectively.
- TRICARE Plus does not guarantee enrollees access to specialty providers at the MTF where they are enrolled.
- TRICARE Plus is not portable. TRICARE Plus beneficiaries cannot use their enrollment at another facility.

The availability of TRICARE Plus is location-specific and region-specific. Also, the actual number of enrollees eligible to participate is based on the local MTF commander's determination of enrollment capacity.

PROGRAM FOR PERSONS WITH DISABILITIES

The Program for Persons with Disabilities (PFPWD) was formerly known as *the Program for the Handicapped*. This is a program established by Congress for active-duty families who have family members with a qualifying disability. The program offers not only some financial assistance to families but also another mechanism for receiving services, equipment, and supplies necessary for the diagnosis, treatment, habilitation, and rehabilitation of persons with disabilities. Eligibility is determined on a case-by-case basis. The PFPWD is not a stand-alone benefit; therefore, family members are also entitled to other TRICARE health care benefits.

Advantages and Disadvantages of the Program for Persons with Disabilities

- The PFPWD provides a source of financial relief and another mechanism through which to receive needed services, equipment, or supplies when such are not available from public agencies or community programs.
- PFPWD is available only for active-duty family beneficiaries and children who meet specific diagnostic categories.
- The cost share for services in any month is a fixed amount and is based on the active-duty member's rank (cost shares range from $25 to $250 per month).
- The maximum allowable monthly benefit is $1000 regardless of disability.
- There are no deductibles.
- Amounts for services that exceed the limit may not be cost shared through the other TRICARE options and are the financial responsibility of the family, unless more than one family member receives services through the PFPWD in any given month, in which case, the $1000 cap applies only to the family member with the lowest reimbursable services.
- The family has the option to determine and select the most cost-beneficial program through which to receive services.
- Preauthorization is required; authorizations are valid for a period of up to 6 months (can be reauthorized every 6 months).
- High-cost items may be prorated over several months such that the prorated amount does not exceed the maximum $1000 monthly benefit.
- To the extent adequate and available, services from other public resources must be used first. However, the Individuals with Disabilities Act was amended in 1997 to clarify that the DoD health care system is the primary payer before services from a school district can be used.

- PFPWD also shares in the cost of some additional benefits not available through the traditional TRICARE health programs. Some of these are as follows:
    - Equipment that does not qualify as durable medical equipment
    - Unique adaptive training
    - Special education or instructions or programs or tutors
    - Adjunct services, such as a reader for a blind beneficiary
    - Medical attendant during transport to receive PFPWD services
    - Transportation

EXCEPTIONAL FAMILY MEMBER PROGRAM

Another program offered by the DoD is the Exceptional Family Member Program. This program is designed to (1) identify the military service member's family members with special needs and (2) as the sponsor is reassigned, take the person's special needs into consideration to ensure linkage with either the MTF or nearby civilian community resources.

Identification of family members with special needs is a mandatory process for all four branches of the military services. Therefore military sponsors with family members who have special medical and/or educational needs must be enrolled in the Exceptional Family Member Program immediately on identification of special need. Early identification of the needs ensures that these needs and the resources necessary to treat them are considered early in the reassignment process. This allows a better match between medical and/or educational needs and the required resources.

INDIVIDUAL CASE MANAGEMENT PROGRAM FOR PERSONS WITH EXTRAORDINARY CONDITIONS

This program is designed to offer individual assistance to certain military beneficiaries who meet criteria for case management. If case management services are offered, the program allows waivers to traditional services that are limited by the design of the health benefits under TRICARE, including custodial care services for persons with exceptional conditions.

OFFICE OF CIVILIAN HEALTH AND MEDICAL PROGRAM OF THE UNIFORMED SERVICES

The Office of Civilian Health and Medical Program of the Uniformed Services (OCHAMPUS) is under the authority, direction, and control of the Assistant Secretary of Defense (Health Affairs). This office is primarily responsible for administering the civilian health and medical programs for retirees and for spouses and children of active-duty, retired, and deceased members of the uniformed services (the Army, Navy, Air Force, Marine Corps, Coast Guard, the Commissioned Corps of the National Oceanographic and Atmospheric Administration, and the Public Health Service). This office is the primary office where health care policies and procedures and regulatory requirements are developed. OCHAMPUS is also responsible for ensuring that contractors adhere to the requirements of the DoD and its medical readiness posture; for executing, administering, and monitoring contracts for the delivery and financing of civilian health benefits; for providing utilization control, peer review, and quality assurance of health care received by eligible beneficiaries; and for conducting studies, demonstrations, and research activities—including contract studies in the health care area—with a view to improving the quality, efficiency, convenience, and cost-effectiveness of the OCHAMPUS programs and the DoD health care delivery system.

GRIEVANCES AND APPEALS

As in all health care plans, the TRICARE program allows dissatisfied beneficiaries to file a grievance or appeal an issue (standard or expedited). The beneficiary has 90 days from the date of a denial to file an appeal. An appeal is related to dissatisfaction with payment or a coverage determination for services, and a grievance is dissatisfaction with an issue (e.g., quality or timeliness of care).

Both the appeal and grievance processes require the beneficiary to put the issue in writing to start the process. If the beneficiary is unhappy with the results of the appeal, he or she is allowed a second-level appeal, as well as another level of appeal by means of a hearing at the final level. In most cases, if services are denied, the denial ruling is final.

VETERANS' BENEFITS

The VA is responsible for overseeing and administering its available programs to eligible veterans. Approximately one of every three persons living in the United States is a potential VA beneficiary.

The VA operates health care facilities in 50 states and in the District of Columbia, Puerto Rico, and the Philippines, making it the nation's largest health care system network and the fifth largest insurance program. Almost all of the VA's medical centers are affiliated with medical schools. In addition to the medical centers, the VA's health care system includes nursing homes, domiciliary care facilities, readjustment counseling centers, outpatient clinics, and contracts with specific agencies for home health care and other services.[1]

Entitlement to the scope of services is based on a veteran's military history, the classification of the discharge, and the veteran's disability rating. Further information about benefits can be obtained by writing or calling any VA regional or service office. All 50 states have toll-free numbers for their regional VA offices.

Entrance of a veteran into a VA hospital is based on the veteran's service disability rating, regardless of whether he or she may also be entitled to the military's TRICARE benefits or private insurance. Many patients with a disability rating of less than 100% are medically retired from military service and are thus entitled to both TRICARE and VA benefits.

Referrals

The VA changed its eligibility rules with the passage of the Veteran's Health Care Eligibility Reform Act of 1996. This act mandated the VA to establish and implement a national enrollment system to manage the delivery of health care services to veterans. This legislation also created the Uniform Benefits Package. The Uniform Benefits Package standardized the health plan for most enrolled veterans and for certain other groups of veterans who are not required to enroll. Veterans may apply for enrollment at any time during the year. The following groups of veterans are not required to enroll, because they are automatically eligible for benefits:

- Veterans who need treatment for a VA-rated service-connected disability
- Veterans who are VA-rated as service-connected and the rating is 50% or more
- Veterans who have been released from active duty within the previous 12 months because of a disability incurred or exacerbated in the line of duty

The law also simplifies the rules for providing health care to veterans in the following ways:

- Eliminating the distinction between outpatient care and hospital care (a significant aspect of the old eligibility system)

- Permitting the VA to provide health care services in the most clinically appropriate setting
- Giving the VA the authority to furnish health promotion and disease prevention services and primary care
- Allowing greater flexibility in applying state-of-the-art health care techniques and more efficient use of VA resources

On-Line Enrollment

Veterans can now enroll on-line. The VA website is www.va.gov/health/elig/benefits. If the veteran does not have a computer or access to the Internet, he or she can obtain the necessary forms by contacting the nearest VA health care facility, county veterans' service office, or the Veterans' Service Organization or by calling the VA at its toll-free number 877-222-VETS.

Filing Claims or Making Referrals

To file a claim or make a referral for veterans' services, the patient or family must contact the nearest VA office. The patient or family will identify the veteran by submitting his or her full name, date of birth, and Social Security number. If the person has ever filed a VA claim, he or she will have an identification number on file. The identification number is key to expediting requests for VA services. To further expedite services, the veteran or his or her family is advised to keep the following information in a safe and convenient location for easy retrieval and use:

- Birth certificate
- Discharge papers
- Marriage license or certificate (if applicable)
- A statement regarding burial preferences
- Death certificate (if applicable)

Veterans who are disabled by injury, disease, or a condition exacerbated during active duty, whether during wartime or peacetime, and who have been honorably discharged, may be eligible for service-connected disability benefits. Disabilities are classified in terms of percentages and range from 0% to 100%. Monetary compensation is based on this disability rating. Veterans who are classified as 30% or more disabled are entitled to additional dependent allowances. Veterans with the same classification are entitled to further allowances if they have a spouse in need of aid and attendant care. Veterans aged 65 years or older, whether working or not, must meet income criteria and be classified as totally disabled to be granted a pension.

Because a veteran is allowed a variety of options for health care (e.g., private health care insurance, VA benefits, and possibly TRICARE), case managers must familiarize themselves with VA and other military benefits to ensure the right insurer is paying for care.

Eligibility

Once the VA is notified that a veteran has applied for benefits, eligibility is determined. Eligibility is based on specific assigned priority groups. The groups are then allowed benefits according to the Uniform Benefits Package.

Before a veteran can receive VA medical care, he or she must be evaluated, and his or her service-connected disability must be rated. Case managers working with patients who might be eligible for VA benefits must encourage veterans to list all disabilities that occurred during their terms of active duty. This helps to establish a formal record from which the VA can make a determination.

The basic eligibility requirements are based on the veteran's service record and whether he or she actively served in the Army, Navy, or Air Force, as well as whether he or she was discharged or released under honorable conditions. Under the Veterans Health Care Eligibility Reform Act of 1996, the law establishes two eligibility categories.

The first category includes veterans to whom VA shall furnish needed hospital and outpatient care and may furnish nursing home care, but only to the extent of costs allowed by Congress to provide the care. Veterans in this category include those with compensable service-connected disabilities, former prisoners of war, World War I veterans, low-income veterans (based on legally established VA income threshold), veterans exposed to environmental contaminants for conditions related to such exposure, and 0% service-connected veterans for the treatment of their service-connected disability.

The second group includes veterans to whom VA may furnish needed hospital care, outpatient care, and nursing home care. However, the restriction is that care can only be provided to the extent that resources and facilities are available and only if the veteran agrees to pay his or her VA copayment in exchange for the care. This group includes those veterans not listed previously.

If veterans or their families need help in establishing eligibility or if they have other questions, they should be encouraged to contact a benefits counselor at the nearest VA regional office serving their area, or they can obtain information by calling the VA's toll-free number: 800-827-1000. Websites that might be helpful include www.va.gov/vso/view.asp, which is the website for the various VA organizations, and www.va.gov/faq/show.asp, which is for frequently asked questions about VA benefits. The National Personnel Records Center (NPRC) Military Personnel Records (MPR) at www.nara.gov/regional/mpr.html serves as the repository for millions of military, personnel health, and medical records of discharged and deceased veterans of all services during the 20th century. The National Personnel Records Center also stores medical treatment records for retirees from all services, as well as records for dependents and other persons treated at Navy medical facilities. Information from the records is made available on written request (with signature and date) to the extent allowed by law.

Eligibility for VA health care depends on a number of variables, all of which may influence the final determination of the services for which the veteran might qualify. These factors include the following:

- The nature of a veteran's discharge from military service (i.e., honorable, other than honorable, or dishonorable)
- Length of service
- The level that the VA assigns to the VA-adjudicated disability (historically termed *service-connected disability*)
- The veteran's income level and available VA resources among others

If the veteran is to receive benefits he or she must enroll. The only veterans exempt from this rule are as follows:

- Veterans with a VA rating of 50% or more for a service-connected disability
- Veterans discharged from military service for less than 1 year with a disability incurred or exacerbated in the line of active duty, as deemed by the military, who have not yet been assigned a VA rating
- Veterans who are seeking care from the VA for a service-connected disability only

If the veteran is enrolled, he or she remains enrolled for 1 year. Depending on the priority group (there are seven) and the veteran's financial resources, enrollment is generally reviewed and renewed annually. The eligibility groups are divided into seven categories:

- Priority Group 1—This is the highest rating and veterans in this category are those with a service-connected disability rating of 50% or more. Service-connected veterans rated 50% or more or non–service-connected veterans who meet the low-income criteria are exempt from the prescription copayment.

- Priority Group 2—This is for those veterans with a service-connected disability rating of 30% or 40%.
- Priority Group 3—This is a category for veterans who are former prisoners of war; veterans whose discharge was for a disability that was incurred or exacerbated in the line of duty; veterans with a service-connected disability rating of 10% or 20%; and veterans awarded special eligibility classification who receive "benefits for individuals disabled by treatment or vocational rehabilitation."
- Priority Group 4—This is for veterans who are receiving aid and attendance or housebound benefits or veterans who have been determined by the VA to be catastrophically disabled.
- Priority Group 5—This is a category for non–service-connected veterans and service-connected veterans with a rating of 0% for disability but whose annual income and net worth are below the VA's established dollar threshold.
- Priority Group 6—This is for eligible veterans who are not required to make copayments for their care, including World War I and Mexican Border War veterans; veterans receiving care solely for disabilities resulting from exposure to toxic substances or radiation or for disorders associated with service in the Gulf War; or for any illness associated with service in combat in a war after the Gulf War or during a period of hostility after November 11, 1998; or those known as compensable 0% service-connected veterans.
- Priority Group 7—This is for veterans with non–service-connected disabilities and veterans with non-

compensable 0% service-connected disabilities whose needed care cannot be provided by enrollment in any of the other groups and who agree to pay specified copayments.

All veterans seeking care must do so at a VA facility. If services are not available at a VA center, the VA can authorize care in the private sector at the VA's expense. The VA only pays for private medical care services when they are authorized by a VA official under any one of the following circumstances:

- Treatment was provided for an adjudicated service-connected disability, for any condition for a permanently and totally disabled service-connected veteran, or for a non–service-connected disability associated with and exacerbating a service-connected disability.
- The medical care and services were provided in a medical emergency.
- A VA or other federal medical facility was not available

In the absence of any one of these three conditions, the VA cannot assume responsibility for the payment or reimbursement for the cost of non-VA care if it was not authorized. Therefore if a veteran is hospitalized in a non-VA facility, the case manager or discharge coordinator must make contact with the nearest VA facility for an authorization or directions for ongoing care or transfer. If the patient is too medically unstable for discharge, the case manager or discharge coordinator must obtain a continued stay authorization for the veteran's care; otherwise, the inpatient care can be denied in retrospect when the claim is submitted.

Enrolled veterans are entitled to urgent and limited emergency care services at a VA health care facility or non-VA health care facilities with which the VA has contracts for care and services. Veterans classified as having special eligibility can obtain emergency care at the VA's expense in a non-VA health care facility without a VA contract.

UNIFORM BENEFITS PACKAGE

Before 1996, VA benefits varied from region to region. However, with the passage of the Veterans' Health Care Eligibility Act of 1996 (Public Law 104-262), the Uniform Benefits Package was created. Basically, this standardized and enhanced the health benefits and made them available to all veterans enrolled. The law also simplified the process by which veterans could receive their care; introduced quality and timeliness standards; and placed an emphasis on preventive and primary care, as well as enhanced outpatient and inpatient services.

For qualified veterans, the VA is required to provide "needed" inpatient care in any hospital setting, as well as for any outpatient services the veteran requires. Needed care is that required to promote, preserve, and restore health. This includes a full range of treatment procedures, supplies, and services. The decision for needed care is based on the medical. judgment of the health provider who prescribes the services and on whether the services requested are those recognized to be in accordance with generally accepted standards of clinical practice. Should the VA not be able to provide the services, contracts with non-VA health care facilities and providers are in place to ensure that the appropriate level of care is provided.

Services Covered Under the Uniform Benefits Package

- Drugs, biologicals, and medical devices that are approved by the Food and Drug Administration and are used in conjunction with the VA treatments ordered
- Elective sterilization (tubal ligation or vasectomy)
- Emergency care in VA facilities

- Home health care
- Hospice care
- Hospital or medical center and outpatient care, including diagnostic services without a limit on days
- Maternity benefits and care
- Medical and surgical care
- Mental health care and substance abuse treatment
- Palliative care
- Preventive care and services
- Prosthetic and orthotic devices
- Rehabilitation care and services
- Respite care

Services Not Covered Under the Uniform Benefits Package

- Abortions as well as abortion counseling
- Drugs, biologicals, and medical devices not approved by the Food and Drug Administration
- Gender alterations
- Memberships to health clubs, gyms, and spas
- Private duty nursing
- Services not ordered and not provided by a licensed and/or accredited professional staff
- Cosmetic surgery
- In vitro fertilization and similar procedures, unless related to a service-connected condition

Services Covered Under Special Authorities

- Adult day health care
- Dental care
- Domiciliary care
- Emergency care in non-VA facilities
- Homeless programs
- Non-VA care
- Nursing home care
- Readjustment counseling services provided in VA centers
- Sensory-neural aids (e.g., eyeglasses, contact lenses, and hearing aids)
- Sexual trauma counseling

Despite the changes in the Uniform Benefits Package, little actually changed for veterans' care related to the following needs:

- The Home-Based Primary Care Program and its services and admissions are governed by clinical admission standards. This program was formally called *Hospital-Based Home Care*. Home health care services are restricted to skilled services, and the cost of home care cannot exceed the cost of care in a nursing home.
- Nursing home care eligibility remains basically the same, except that noncompensable 0% service-connected veterans receiving care at VA expense are required to make copayments for any non–service-related injury or disability.
- The VA continues to offer programs (either operated by the VA or by means of contracts with community programs) for adult day health care. Again, costs of care cannot exceed the cost of care in a nursing home.
- Domiciliary care eligibility was not changed and remains an option for those veterans who do not require hospital or nursing home care but are unable to live independently because of medical or psychiatric disabilities.
- Emergency care in a non-VA facility is limited to those veterans who are classified as having special eligibility. The VA does allow emergency care to be provided to enrolled veterans in non-VA facilities through a sharing agreement or contract.
- The homeless veterans' programs were not changed.
- Eligibility for readjustment counseling services was changed to include any veteran who served in the military in combat operations.

- Hearing aids and eyeglasses are generally not provided to non–service-connected veterans for naturally occurring hearing or vision loss (e.g., farsightedness, nearsightedness, and minor hearing loss) unless the condition is related to a service-connected disability.
- The sexual trauma counseling program (counseling required as a result of sexual harassment, sexual assault, rape, and other acts of violence) was not changed. Some veterans receiving these services are subject to a means test to determine copayment requirements if the sexual trauma counseling is not related to their military exposure or experience.
- Dental care eligibility was not changed. VA dental benefits include examinations and the full spectrum of diagnostic, surgical, restorative, and preventive services.

OTHER HEALTH INSURANCE AND THE VA

Although a veteran may have other health insurance, his or her eligibility for VA health care benefits is not affected. Although the VA allows hospitalization for non–service-connected care, if the veteran is hospitalized for such care, the veteran's private health insurance must be billed (the only exception to this rule is Medicare: the VA cannot bill Medicare). The VA is responsible for any VA-adjudicated service-connected disabilities. An adjudicated service-connected disability is one that the VA has determined was incurred or exacerbated in the line of active duty.

Thus should a veteran be hospitalized in a civilian hospital for care (usually as a result of an emergent condition), case managers must make every attempt to contact the VA to ascertain the veteran's priority rating. If the reason for civilian care is related to an active-duty service-connected disability, the VA remains responsible for the costs of care until the veteran can be moved, if authorization for his or her stay in the civilian facility has been sought.

If the veteran is also eligible for TRICARE, he or she is required to pay applicable copayments for care for all non–service-connected conditions according to his or her VA priority rating. If the veteran has both private insurance and TRICARE, the private health insurance is always the primary payer, and TRICARE is the secondary payer.

Copayments

The VA's copayments and deductibles depend on the veteran's priority group rating. In many cases the VA waives the copayments and deductibles, but some veterans are required to pay copayments for care or medications. If the veteran is classified as a non–service-connected veteran or as a noncompensable 0% service-connected veteran, he or she is required to complete an annual means test (income test based on family income and net worth). If the veteran does not complete the means test, he or she must agree to pay the applicable copayment for care and services. If the veteran is required to pay copayments, the copayments are as follows:

- Medication—The prescription copayment is $2 for each 30-day or less supply of medications provided on an outpatient basis for the treatment of non–service-connected conditions. Service-connected veterans rated 50% or more or non–service-connected veterans who meet the low-income criterion are exempt from the prescription copayment.
- Outpatient services—The outpatient copayment is 20% of outpatient costs of an average outpatient visit.
- Inpatient services—The inpatient copayment is the same as the cur-

rent year's Medicare inpatient deductible rate, plus $10 per day for the first 90 days.
- Nursing home care—The nursing home copayment is the same as the current year's Medicare skilled nursing facility deductible rate plus $5 for each day.

If a veteran cannot afford to make his or her copayments, the VA allows two options for waiving the requirements. The veteran may request a waiver for paying the current debt or medical care charges. If a waiver is requested, the veteran must submit sufficient proof that he or she cannot afford the payments. The veteran may request a hardship determination so that he or she can avoid future debts. If this type of waiver is requested, the veteran must submit specific financial information that supports the claim of hardship (Box 8-1).

Means Test

If a veteran is classified as a non–service-connected veteran, he or she is required annually to fill out a financial worksheet and submit any supporting documents validating the prior year's income and assets. From this information the VA then determines the veteran's priority group and whether he or she will be required to pay any copayments for care and services. A veteran claiming a financial hardship must submit documents that validate that his or her income was below the income threshold (threshold changes annually). A hardship determination is made when a veteran can demonstrate that his or her financial situation changed. Changes are often due to loss of employment, bankruptcy, or out-of-pocket medical expenses.

VOCATIONAL REHABILITATION AND EMPLOYMENT PROGRAM

The VA offers a vocational rehabilitation and employment program. This program

---

BOX 8-1

Payments for Services Obtained Through the VA System When the Veteran Has Private Insurance

- **Priority Group 1**—If veteran requires care and care is for a non–service-connected condition, the VA bills the private health insurance company.

- **Priority Groups 2, 3, and 4**—If the veteran is less than 50% service-connected disabled, he or she is required to pay a prescription copayment when the medication is for a non–service-connected condition. The VA will bill the veteran's health insurance company, if the treatment is for a non–service-connected condition.

- **Priority Group 5**—The VA bills the veteran's private insurance company when treatments are related to a non–service-connected condition.

- **Priority Group 6**—World War I and Mexican Border War veterans and compensable 0% service-connected veterans are required to pay a prescription copayment for non–service-connected conditions, unless they meet the means test or the medication is for a service-connected condition. If care is provided to these veterans and it is related to a non–service-connected condition, the VA bills the veteran's private health insurance company. If a veteran in this category receives care for military exposure–related disabilities, he or she is required to pay prescription copayments unless treatment is for a service-connected condition. If care is provided for a non–service-connected condition, the VA will bill the veteran's private health insurance company. Veterans are assessed all applicable copayments when the care they receive is for a condition not related to their exposure or experience.

- **Priority Group 7**—This group of veterans is required to pay copayments for inpatient hospitalizations, outpatient services, prescriptions, and nursing home care. If the veteran has private health insurance, the VA bills the insurance company for the copayments for any services rendered.

Data from the Department of Veterans Affairs Washington, DC (www.va.gov/elig/page.cfm?pg=1).

---

is designed primarily for assisting veterans with service-connected disabilities in obtaining employment, enhancing their functional abilities, and achieving as much independence as possible at home or in the community.

Like any vocational rehabilitation program, the VA's program is designed to help eligible veterans obtain meaningful and gainful employment. Severely disabled veterans are given assistance to achieve some functional level that will allow independence in their daily living.

Vocational Rehabilitation Eligibility

Vocational rehabilitation eligibility is based on the following four criteria:

1. The veteran served in the armed forces on or after September 16, 1940.
2. The service-connected disability rating is at least 20% (can be waived to 10% if the veteran has a serious employment handicap).
3. The veteran requires vocational rehabilitation to overcome an employment handicap.
4. It is less than 12 months since the VA notified the veteran of his or her eligibility to participate in the program (can be extended if the veteran's condition prevented him or her from applying for or participating in the training).

If a veteran is deemed eligible for vocational rehabilitation, he or she participates in a program that lasts at least 48 months, with the VA paying all training costs. These costs can include tuition and fees, books, supplies, equipment, and other specialized services. During training, the VA also pays a monthly benefit to the veteran to assist with living expenses (subsistence allowance), as well as the cost of any medical or dental care required.

On-line Application for Vocational Rehabilitation

The VA maintains an on-line application for its Vocational Rehabilitation and Independent Living Services program. Case managers working with veterans who want to learn more about the VA's program can encourage potential applicants to apply on-line. The VA website for this is www.vabenefits.vba.va.gov/vonapp/.

The VA considers the following persons candidates for vocational rehabilitation:

- A veteran or a service member awaiting a disability discharge
- A person with a VA-rated service-connected disability rating of 10% or more
- A person who believes he or she is disabled as a result of military service, who has an application pending an evaluation for rating the disability, or who has filed an application with his or her vocational rehabilitation claim

Veterans needing help or additional information can call a VA regional office toll-free at 800-827-1000.

Vocational Rehabilitation Services

Once the veteran is accepted into the program, the program offers traditional vocational rehabilitation assistance, which include the following:

- Helping the person find and maintain suitable employment
- Evaluating the person's employment abilities, skills, interests, and needs
- Providing vocational counseling and personal planning
- If needed, providing employment training or placement in a position for on-the-job training that constitutes unpaid work experience
- If needed, providing educational training, such as that found in a certificate or 2- or 4-year academic program

- Assisting with job placement
- Providing supportive rehabilitation services and additional counseling

Independent Living Services

In addition to vocational rehabilitation and educational guidance and counseling to assist service members, veterans, and certain dependents of veterans in selecting appropriate career goals and training institutions for use of their VA educational benefits, the VA also offers independent living services for certain eligible veterans. If a veteran is accepted into the independent living services program, the program offers the following:

- An evaluation to determine the person's independent living needs
- Training in activities of daily living
- Guidance and support throughout the rehabilitation program
- Technological assistance
- Personal adjustment counseling
- In some cases, training to improve the veteran's ability to reach a vocational goal
- In some cases, vocational training for Vietnam veterans' children with spina bifida

The Civilian Health and Medical Program of the Department of Veterans Affairs

The Civilian Health and Medical Program of the Department of Veterans Affairs (CHAMPVA) is a medical benefits program through which the VA helps to pay for medical services and supplies obtained from civilian sources for eligible dependents and survivors of certain veterans. CHAMPVA eligibility is restricted to the following:

- Persons not eligible for TRICARE or Medicare Part A as a result of reaching age 65 years
- Spouses and children of veterans rated by the VA as having a permanent and total service-connected condition

- Surviving spouses and children of veterans who died as a result of a VA-rated service-connected condition or of veterans who, at the time of death, were rated permanently and totally disabled from a service-connected condition
- Surviving spouses and children of a person who died in the line of duty whose death was not due to any misconduct that occurred within 30 days of entry into active military service

If a dependent or survivor is eligible for CHAMPVA medical care, care is normally provided in civilian facilities. In general, the program covers most health care services and supplies considered to be medically or psychologically necessary. VA facilities are used only when they are equipped to provide such care or when the use of these facilities does not interfere with the care and treatment of veterans. In the program, special rules or limitations apply to certain services. Clarification of what is and what is not covered can be obtained by calling the toll-free number for the CHAMPVA office located in Denver, Colorado, or by contacting a social worker at any VA medical center. Persons eligible for CHAMPVA are not eligible for the TRICARE PFPWD, nor can they receive care in an MTF.

CHAMPVA Administration

Although CHAMPVA and CHAMPUS have similar names, they are two totally different programs, administered by two different agencies. The CHAMPVA program, including all policies and procedures, is administered from the CHAMPVA Center in Denver, Colorado. CHAMPUS (now called TRICARE) is handled by the DoD and the Office of CHAMPUS (OCHAMPUS), operated out of Aurora, Colorado.

VA APPEALS

Claimants have 1 year from the date of notification of a denial of care to file an appeal if they disagree or are not satisfied with a decision on their case. An appeal is initiated by filing a notice with the VA facility responsible for issuing the determination. The appeal is filed with the Board of Veterans' Appeals (also known as the *BVA*). The Board of Veterans' Appeals is a part of the VA located in Washington, DC, and comprises attorneys experienced in veterans' law and in reviewing benefit claims. The Board of Veterans' Appeals can be accessed through the VA website at www.va.gov/vbs/bva/. Further information about the appeals process and the relevant time frames can be obtained by contacting any VA regional office.

SUMMARY

TRICARE is the DoD's health care program for all uniformed services personnel. Over the past few years, the old CHAMPUS has undergone major changes and is now known worldwide as TRICARE. The TRICARE program offers beneficiaries the ability to select from a triple-option plan—TRICARE Prime, TRICARE Extra, and TRICARE Standard. In addition, the DoD recently implemented a new plan for persons older than 65 years, TFL, and an expanded pharmacy program. For active-duty families, in which a dependent or dependents might have special needs, the DoD offers two programs to assist the sponsors—the PFWPD and the Exceptional Family Member Program.

Although not all patients will be eligible for VA benefits, many will be. Unfortunately, many veterans use their private health care insurance for services that should be covered by the VA because the condition is actually related to a service-connected disability. Case managers should always investigate, early in the course of a case, the person's entitlement to other insurance and eligibility for specific programs; the VA is one such program that should be explored for both men and women.

Chapter Exercises

1. Identify the three options now offered by the DoD, list the basic structure of each, list the copayments and deductibles, and describe how each program compares with the others.
2. Discuss the DoD's newest programs and compare the benefits now allowed to Medicare-eligible beneficiaries and show the differences between the programs.
3. List the core eligibility requirements for participation in TRICARE and identify the primary enrollment system used to track eligible persons.
4. Describe the VA system and how eligibility is determined.
5. Compare the VA system before the Veterans' Health Care Eligibility Act of 1996 (Public Law 104-262) and describe the differences now found.
6. Describe how the priority categories for disability affect a veteran's benefits.
7. List the basic benefits allowed, as well as those excluded.
8. Describe the CHAMPVA system, those entitled to care, and how the program differs from the VA's Uniform Benefits Package and the TRICARE program.

Suggested Websites and Resources

TRICARE Websites

www.tricare.osd.mil/tricaremanuals—TRICARE policy manuals and other manuals and documents.

www.mfrc.calib.com/snn/resources/index.cfm—Special needs resources

www.tricare.osd.mil/pharmacy/brac.htm—Pharmacy information for bases that have closed (Base Realignment and Closure)

www.mfrc.calib.com/snn/ed/sped.cfm—Military information on persons needing special education

www.nichcy.org/states.htm—Fact sheets on special education for each state developed by the National Information Center for Children and Youth with Disabilities (NICHCY)

www.ideapractices.org/lawandregs.htm—Individual with Disabilities Education Act (IDEA) website

www.usdoj.gov/crt/ada/adahom1.htm—Americans with Disabilities Act (ADA) website

www.access.gpo.gov/nara/cfr/waisidx_99/34cfr104_99.html—Act website

www.tricare.osd.mil/DEERSAddress/—Website for Defense Enrollment Eligibility Reporting System (DEERS)

www.tricare.osd.mil/claims/—Military claims website

www.tricare.osd.mil/pharmacy—TRICARE pharmacy website

www.tricare.osd.mil/Plus—TRICARE Plus website

www.merckmedco.com—TRICARE national mail-order pharmacy website

www.pec.ha.osd.mil/nmop/nmorphome.htm—Department of Defense National Mail Order Pharmacy Formulary website

www.ha.osd.mil—Health Affairs website for information from the Office of CHAMPUS.

www.ochampus.mil/ClaimForms—Website from which to download claim forms (e.g., TRICARE Standard)

TRICARE Regions

TRICARE Northeast

Service area: Maine, New Hampshire, Vermont, Massachusetts, Connecticut, Rhode Island, Delaware, Maryland, New Jersey, New York, Pennsylvania, District of Columbia, Northern Virginia, and the northeast corner of West Virginia

Toll-free number: 888-999-5195

Website: *www.140.139.13.36/region01/index.htm*

TRICARE Mid-Atlantic
Service area: North Carolina, and most of
   Virginia
Toll-free number: 800-931-9501
Website: *www.tma.med.navy.mil*

TRICARE Southeast
Service area: South Carolina, Georgia, and
   Florida (excluding
the panhandle)
Toll-free number: 800-444-5445
Website: *www.humana-military.com*

TRICARE Gulf South
Service area: Florida panhandle, Alabama,
   Mississippi, Tennessee, and eastern
   third of Louisiana
Toll-free number: 800-444-5445
Website: *www.humana-military.com*

TRICARE Heartland
Service area: Michigan, Wisconsin, Illinois,
   Indiana, Ohio, Kentucky, and West
   Virginia (excluding the northeast cor-
   ner)
Toll-free number: 800-941-4501
Website: *www.dodr5www.wpafh af mil*

TRICARE Southwest
Service area: Oklahoma, Arkansas, western
   two thirds of Louisiana, Texas (exclud-
   ing southwest corner)
Toll-free number: 800-406-2832
Website: *www.tricaresw.af.mil*

TRICARE Central
Service area: New Mexico, Arizona (exclud-
   ing Yuma), Nevada, Southwest corner
   of Texas (including El Paso), Colorado,
   Utah, Wyoming, Montana, Idaho
   (excluding northern Idaho), North
   Dakota, South Dakota, Nebraska,
   Kansas, Minnesota, Iowa, and Missouri
Toll-free number: 888-874-9378
Website: *www.web01.region8.tricare.osd.mil*
   or *www.triwest.com*

TRICARE Northwest
Service area: Washington, Oregon, and
   northern Idaho
Toll-free number: 800-404-0110
Website: *www.tricarenw.mamc.amedd.
   army.mil*

TRICARE Golden Gate
Service area: Northern California
Toll-free number: 800-242-6788
Website: *www.fhfs.com/tricaregoldengate.htm*

TRICARE Southern California
Service area: Southern California and
   Yuma, Arizona
Toll-free number: 800-242-6788
Website: *www.fhfs.com/tricaresouthernca.
   htm*

TRICARE Alaska
Service area: Alaska
Toll-free number: 888-777-8343
Website: *www.fhfs.com/tricarepacificalaska.
   htm*

TRICARE Hawaii
Service area: Hawaiian Islands
Toll-free number: 800-242-6788
Website: *www.fhfs.com/tricarepacifichawaii.
   htm*

TRICARE Latin America
Service area: Panama, Central America,
   and South America
Toll-free number: 888-777-8343   for
   Puerto Rico and 800-444-5445 for the
   Virgin Islands
Website: No specific website; for general
   information, visit *www.ochampus.mil*

TRICARE Europe
Service area: Europe, Africa, Middle East,
   Azores, and Iceland
Toll-free number: 888-777-8343
Website: *www.webserver.europe.tricare.osd.mil*

TRICARE Pacific
Service area: Western Pacific
Toll-free number: 800-777-8343
Website: *www.tricare-pac.tamc.amedd.army.
mil*

VA Websites

www.va.gov/health/elig/—VA health
benefits website

www.va.gov/seniors/health/—VA listing for
seniors

*www.va.gov/seniors/health/domlist.htm and
www.va.gov/seniors/health/
domcare.htm/*—VA domiciliary websites

www.va.gov/seniors/health/gem.htm—VA
website for geriatric services

www.va.gov/seniors/health/hospice.htm—VA
website for hospice services

*www.va.gov/seniors/health/homehealthcare.
htm*—VA website for home health
services

*www.va.gov/seniors/health/residentialcare.
htm*—VA website for community
residential care

*www.va.gov/seniors/health/nursinghome.
htm*—VA website for skilled nursing
facility care

www.va.gov/seniors/health/alzheimers.htm—
VA website for dementia services

*www.va.gov/seniors/health/adulthealthcare.
htm*—VA website for adult day health
care

www.va.gov/seniors/health/respite.htm—VA
website for respite services

www.va.gov/seniors/health/state.htm—VA
website for state VA homes

www.va.gov/vbs/bva/—VA website for
appeals

www.va.gov/health/elig/benefits—VA website
for benefit information

www.vabenefits.vba.va.gov/vonapp/—
Website at which veterans can apply on-
line for VA benefits

www.vba.va.gov/bin/vre/vbsvre.htm—VA
website for eligibility for VA's vocational
rehabilitation programs

www.va.gov/vso/view.asp—Website for the
various VA organizations

www.va.gov/faq/show.asp—For frequently
asked questions about VA benefits

www.nara.gov/regional/mpr.html—The
National Personnel Records Center
(NPRC) Military Personnel Records
(MPR), which serves as the repository
for millions of military personnel
health and medical records of
discharged and deceased veterans of all
services during the 20th century

REFERENCE

1. VA website: www.VA.gov.

BIBLIOGRAPHY

TRICARE beneficiary benefit information: www.
tricare.osd.mil/beneficiary/.

TRICARE benefits: www.tricare.osd.mil/.

TRICARE brochures for all the many programs offered
by the military personnel and their beneficiaries as
well as telephone numbers of the key programs if
additional information is needed: www.tricare.osd.
mil/TAAGBrochure/index.html.

Other Insurance, Funding, and Health Care Services

Peggy A. Rossi, BSN, MPA, CCM, CPUR

OBJECTIVES

- To distinguish the types of patients who might be eligible for Consolidated Omnibus Reconciliation Act (COBRA) or Tax Equity and Fiscal Responsibility Act (TEFRA) benefits
- To relate how the Mental Health Parity Act (MHPA) affects the benefits and treatments of those with mental health illness
- To identify the key elements a child needs to meet TEFRA eligibility criteria
- To describe the Social Security Disability Income (SSDI) process and how it differs from Supplemental Security Income (SSI)
- To define disability according to Social Security
- To describe the categories of eligibility for both SSDI and SSI and how they differ
- To know which offices to call if help is needed in educating patients and families about medigap policies
- To know the one plan code that must be offered in all states to allow the sale of medigap plans
- To describe the services of the Indian Health Service (IHS) and the populations it serves
- To know what agency is the lead agency for IHS and list the goals of the agency
- To identify some of the many free services for which a patient might be entitled when funds are limited or benefits are exhausted

Many cases served by case management will be those in which a covered employee has lost health care coverage (i.e., COBRA) or will have his or her health coverage provided by both a group health insurer and Medicare (i.e., TEFRA). Thus the patient served by case management might be the employee, the employee's spouse, or a dependent child. It is therefore important for case managers to understand the basics of COBRA and TEFRA and how these programs benefit coverage and, at times, the ongoing case management plan. Because new mental health laws have been enacted, it is also important to understand how the MHPA affects mental health benefits and treatments.

COBRA

The Consolidated Omnibus Reconciliation Act (COBRA) was passed in 1986. For the full text of the act, see www.cobrainsurance.com/COBRA_Law.htm. This act allows terminated employees or those who lose health coverage because of a reduction of work hours to purchase group coverage for themselves and their families for limited periods of time. COBRA amended the Employee Retirement Income Security Act, the Internal Revenue Code, and the Public Health Service Act to allow continuation of group health coverage that otherwise would be terminated. COBRA laws apply to group health plans maintained by employers with 20 or more employees for the prior year. Although COBRA does not apply to plans sponsored by the federal government and certain religious organizations, it does apply to health care plans in the private sector and those sponsored by state and local governments.

The Family and Medical Leave Act (FMLA), which became effective in 1993, requires employers to maintain group health plan coverage for an employee at the same level as would have been provided if the employee had not taken the leave. However, FMLA is not COBRA, and the use of FMLA does not constitute a qualifying event for COBRA. A qualifying event can occur when an employee covered under FMLA notifies the employer of his or her intent to not return to work.

Qualifiers

When employees are terminated or lose eligibility for health care benefits because of a reduction in hours, they can elect continued health care coverage under COBRA for themselves, their spouses, or dependents. The covered beneficiary is considered a qualified beneficiary if he or she was covered by the health plan on the day before the "qualifying event." A qualified beneficiary can be the employee, spouse, or dependent child; in some cases the beneficiary might be a retired employee, spouse, or dependent child.

Qualifying events are "certain types of events that would normally cause an individual to lose his or her health coverage."

Qualifying events for an employee or the subscriber are as follows:

- Voluntary or involuntary termination of employment for reasons other than gross misconduct
- Reduction in the number of hours of employment

Qualifying events for a spouse are as follows:

- Termination of the covered spouse from his or her employment for any reason other than for gross misconduct
- Reduction in the hours worked by the covered spouse
- The covered spouse's entitlement to Medicare
- Divorce or legal separation from the covered spouse
- Death of the covered spouse

Qualifying events are the same for dependent children, with the following addition:

- Loss of "dependent child" status according to the plan's rules (child turns 19 years of age but is not enrolled in school full time, is not disabled, and is not fully dependent on the covered parent for financial support)

If the employee is eligible for COBRA election, he or she has the right to elect to continue coverage that is identical to the health care coverage at the time of termination, change, or reduction in hours. Unfortunately, although the person's health coverage can continue at the out-of-pocket amount for group health rates, health coverage under COBRA is usually more expensive than health coverage for active employees. Because the employer is no longer obligated to pay any premium costs, the employee is responsible for his or her share of the premium cost as well as the costs previously paid by the employer. Fortunately, although COBRA premiums costs may seem high, they are generally less expensive than individual health care coverage.

Election Period

The election period is the time frame in which the qualified beneficiary has to elect continued health care coverage from the employer's group health plan through COBRA. Beneficiaries have 60 days from either the coverage loss date or the date of the notice to elect COBRA coverage. If coverage is not elected, the person loses all rights to benefits. COBRA rules also allow a covered employee or spouse to elect COBRA coverage on behalf of any other qualified beneficiary; each qualified beneficiary may independently elect COBRA coverage if desired. Parents or legal guardians have the right to elect COBRA coverage on behalf of a minor child. Once COBRA coverage is chosen, the person is required to pay privately for the coverage. If payments are not received by a specific due date, benefits are terminated.

Covered Benefits

A qualified beneficiary must be offered health care coverage identical to that received immediately before qualifying for COBRA. For example, if an employee was entitled to medical or hospitalization benefits as well as dental, vision, and prescription benefits before the qualifying event, he or she has the right to elect to continue identical coverage under COBRA. Most COBRA coverage includes the following:

- Inpatient and outpatient hospital care
- Physician care
- Surgery and other major medical benefits
- Prescription drugs
- Other medical benefits such as dental or vision care

Duration of Coverage

Once covered by COBRA, qualified beneficiaries may continue to pay for group coverage for a maximum of 18 months. Depending on the situation, a second qualifying event that occurs during the ini-

tial period of coverage may permit continuation of coverage for a maximum of 36 months. COBRA coverage ends when any of the following occurs:

- Premiums are not paid on a timely basis
- The last day of maximum coverage is reached
- The employer ceases to maintain group health benefits or the exact health plan for employees
- The employer changes group health plans and the new plan does not contain any exclusion or limitation regarding any preexisting condition clause
- The covered qualifying beneficiary is entitled to Medicare benefits

Disabled Qualified Beneficiaries

If the qualified beneficiary meets Social Security's definition of disability at the time of a termination of employment or reduction in hours of employment, it is imperative that the beneficiary notify the employer or the group health plan administrator of the determination by Social Security. This will automatically extend the 18-month period to a maximum of 29 months. The disabled beneficiary has 60 days from Social Security's determination to notify the group health plan administrator. This notice must also be submitted before the expiration of the 18-month period allowed for COBRA coverage.

Paying for COBRA

Under COBRA, the employee or his or her qualified beneficiaries are required to pay the entire premium and a small percentage for administrative costs.

To be covered, the initial premium payment must be made within 45 days after the qualified beneficiary elects COBRA. This payment covers the first month of coverage and a retroactive amount extending back to the date of the qualifying event. Ongoing premiums are due within 30 days after the due date. If premiums stay current, the qualified beneficiary remains entitled to benefits allowed by the plan. COBRA beneficiaries remain subject to all rules of the health plan and are responsible for all insurance copayments and deductibles. Case managers must educate patients of the importance of COBRA and prompt payment of premiums to maintain health care coverage. Patients must also be advised to set up a reminder system for premium payments due dates because health plans offering COBRA benefits are not obligated to send monthly premium notices.

COBRA Appeals

Qualified beneficiaries are allowed appeal rights if they are dissatisfied with a coverage determination. As with most appeal rights, the beneficiary has 60 days to file an appeal and must follow the health plan's appeal processes.

TEFRA

The Tax Equity and Fiscal Responsibility Act (TEFRA) has been amended by both the Deficit Reduction Act and COBRA. For case managers and their patients, the effects of TEFRA can be divided into three categories:

1. Payer status of persons older than 65 years covered by both a group health plan and Medicare
2. Certain categories of disabled children
3. Payment methods for health care facilities

TEFRA and Those Older Than 65 Years

TEFRA amended the Age Discrimination in Employment Act of 1967 so that employers are required to offer active employees aged 65 years and older and their spouses aged 65 years and older the same group health care plans offered to younger work-

ers. TEFRA affects health care coverage for these employees (often called the "working aged") who work for employers with more than 20 employees.

Under TEFRA persons older than 65 years can continue to work while receiving both Medicare and group health benefits. Persons older than 65 years can also remain covered by group health insurance because of a working spouse. In either case, for the person older than 65 years who is covered by Medicare, the health care plan is the primary insurer and Medicare is the secondary insurer.

TEFRA and Certain Children with Disabilities

TEFRA also allows states to extend eligibility for medical assistance to certain disabled children. Under this provision a child can be considered for medical assistance without considering the parents' income. This TEFRA option is often referred to as the "Katie Beckett program." The goal of this provision is to provide care for children in their own homes rather than in institutions. If a child is institutionalized, he or she is not eligible for benefits under TEFRA. To be eligible for medical assistance under TEFRA, a child must satisfy all the following rules:

- Be younger than 19 years
- Meet SSI disability standards
- Meet the medical necessity requirements of a hospital, nursing facility, or intermediate care facility for persons with mental retardation
- Be appropriately cared for at home
- Have home care medical assistance costs no greater than those in an institutional setting

Medical assistance is always the payer of last resort; any available health insurance benefits must be used first. In most cases medical assistance pays very little of the costs of health care but does pay for services not covered by traditional health insurance benefit packages.

TEFRA and the Prospective Payment System (PPS)

TEFRA was a key act that changed reimbursement methods for hospitals. One intent of TEFRA was to develop a payment method to control health care costs. General acute-care facilities have been paid by a diagnosis-related group and PPS method since 1983, and until the Balanced Budget Act, TEFRA had not been used to reimburse specialty hospitals and outpatient services. As PPS is implemented in all layers of health care, case managers will find it more difficult to discharge patients with multiple specialty needs. PPS diagnosis-related groups often do not accurately account for the resource costs of this patient category.

Facilities typically excluded from PPS are known as TEFRA facilities and include rehabilitation, psychiatric, children's, cancer, and long-term care facilities as well as distinct units of hospitals, Christian Science sanatoriums, and facilities located in other U.S. territories (e.g., Virgin Islands, American Samoa, Guam). Since the inception of TEFRA, physician practice and business patterns have changed and weakened the effectiveness of TEFRA and hindered its ability to control costs (e.g., attempts by providers to maximize payments by discharging patients to other settings to avoid exceeding their TEFRA cost limits).

MENTAL HEALTH PARITY

The Mental Health Parity Act (MHPA) is a federal act designed to create parity between mental health benefits and medical and surgical care benefits. The law prevents a group health plan from placing annual or lifetime dollar limits on mental health benefits when these limits would be lower or less favorable than annual or lifetime dollar limits allowed for medical and surgical care offered under the same plan.

Although the law requires equivalence regarding dollar limits, MHPA does not require group health plans and their health insurance issuers to include mental health coverage in their benefits package. The requirements do apply to group health plans with mental health benefits offered as part of the health benefit package. MHPA applies to most employers who have more than 50 workers and offer group health plan coverage. Unfortunately, MHPA does not apply to persons with individual health care coverage.

Thirty-one states currently have mental health parity statutes. For further information, see the National Institutes of Mental Health website at www.nimh.nih.gov/parity/appende.cfm. This website also provides the following information on state parity statutes:

- Definitions of broad-based mental illness
- Definitions of biologically based mental illness
- Definitions of serious mental illness
- Health plan definitions of mental illness coverage
- Variations in state mental health parity

DISABILITY AND LONG-TERM CARE INSURANCE

Disability Income

As case managers assist their disabled clients in evaluating financial resources, one of the first areas to explore—if the client's medical expenses and income will not be covered by workers' compensation—is the contribution the client may have made to either a state disability or private insurance program. Although neither of these programs covers medical expenses, they might replace income during the time off from work, especially if the disability is expected to be long term. Healthy people can obtain disability insurance from two major sources:

1. Participation in an employer's disability insurance plan, if offered
2. Purchase of a personal disability insurance policy

If disabled, he or she can draw benefits from the policy and possibly one of the following as well:

- Participation in a state disability program, if applicable (not all states have a disability program)
- Social Security, if the person has contributed to and has applicable work quarters on file and meets Social Security's definition of disabled
- SSI, if the person has low income and is disabled or blind

Long-Term Care Insurance

For those who can afford it, long-term care insurance has become popular in recent years. If participants are eligible and premiums are kept current, participants can draw up to the amount purchased and for the appropriate level of care to cover costs (e.g., $4000 per month multiplied by 4 years for either in-home care or facility care). This program is an income program because it pays the amount purchased each month. To draw from this policy, the participant is required to undergo an evaluation by an insurance company case manager. To determine eligibility, the case manager uses findings from this evaluation along with any medical records or information supplied by the participant's physician.

Social Security Benefits

A disabled person who is incapable of substantial gainful employment might be eligible for one or both of Social Security's programs: SSI or SSDI. Both programs pay money to disabled persons if they meet Social Security's definition of disability. Although SSDI offers nationally consistent benefits, SSI is fundamentally a state-run program. SSI benefits vary by state.

SSDI

SSDI is an income and insurance program available to disabled workers, the blind, and certain dependents younger than 65 years who meet Social Security's or the Railroad Retirement System's criteria for total disability. In some cases, government employees and certain members of their families can obtain benefits if they have been disabled for a specific period of time. Information about this category of disabled persons can be found at the Social Security Administration website at www.ssa.gov.

A person who qualifies for SSDI and receives income must receive SSDI for 2 years before being eligible for Medicare. The only exception to this rule is for a few specific categories of diagnoses (e.g., quadriplegia, amyotrophic lateral sclerosis, end-stage renal disease).

Social Security's Definition of Disability

The law defines disability as the inability to engage in any substantial gainful activity because of any medically determinable physical or mental impairment that can be expected to result in death or that has lasted or can be expected to last for a continuous period of not less than 12 months. The law defines a child who is younger than 18 years to be disabled if he or she has a medically determinable physical or mental impairment or a combination of impairments that causes marked and severe functional limitations that can be expected to cause death or that has lasted or can be expected to last for a continuous period of not less than 12 months.

A medically determinable impairment is defined as a physical or mental impairment that results from anatomic, physiologic, or psychological abnormalities that can be shown by medically acceptable clinical and laboratory diagnostic techniques. A physical or mental impairment must be established by medical evidence consisting of signs, symptoms, and laboratory findings—not merely by the individual's statement of symptoms.

In addition to meeting one of the definitions of disability, the individual applying for SSDI must have worked and paid into Social Security for the minimum number of required work quarters. If the person is to draw from his or her own Social Security account, the minimum number of quarters is determined by age and number of years worked before becoming disabled. If an individual is to draw from a parent's account, the disabled person's work record is not applicable. Thus the final amount of SSDI received is based on work history and the number of years worked as well as what was paid to Social Security, the rate of the person's pay, and the age at which he or she became disabled. Although both SSI and Medicaid use a process called "deeming" (proof of assets such as bank accounts, savings bonds, etc.) to ascertain qualification for the program, SSDI does not.

To receive SSDI a person must be totally disabled as defined in the Social Security Act (Box 9-1) as opposed to the definitions accepted by state disability programs, which are established to provide benefits to persons temporarily disabled from an illness, injury, or pregnancy. The following people are eligible to enroll in SSDI:

- Disabled workers younger than 65 years
- Unmarried children younger than 18 years (Medicare is not available to this group)

- Unmarried persons older than 22 years, if the disability occurred before the age of 22
- Disabled widows or widowers
- Disabled divorced spouses, if the marriage lasted more than 10 years

Disabling conditions must be supported by documented medical evidence and must result in significant loss of function, cognitive abilities, or judgment. The most frequently recognized disabilities are as follows:

- Diseases of the heart, lungs, or blood vessels
- Severe arthritis
- Brain abnormalities
- Cancer that is progressive and not under control or cured
- Diseases of the digestive system that result in serious weight loss or malnutrition
- Loss of motor function
- Serious loss of kidney function
- Total inability to speak
- Legal blindness

Application Process

Application should be made as soon as possible after the disabling condition has been diagnosed. The application and determination process takes approximately 5 months, the longest processing required for any Social Security program. Benefits start after the sixth full month of disability if the person is approved and meets eligibility criteria. To assist in expediting the application, case managers should inform the patient or family that the following are required at the intake appointment:

- Social Security number

BOX 9-1
SSDI's Definition of Diability

Social Security's definition of disability is related to work. People are considered disabled only if they are physically or mentally impaired, or both, and as such (1) will be prevented from obtaining gainful employment for at least one year or (2) the condition is expected to result in death.

- Proof of age of the disabled person (original birth certificate or a certified copy of the original)
- Names, addresses, phone numbers, and dates of treatment of all physicians, hospitals, clinics, or institutions
- Work history, summary of duties, and all jobs held during the past 15 years
- Copy of W2 form (or federal tax return if self-employed)
- Dates of any military service
- Dates of divorce if previously married
- Copy of death certificate and proof of marriage if widowed
- For a divorced spouse, proof that the marriage lasted 10 years or more
- For persons disabled before age 22 years, proof that disability started before age 22 years
- For stepchildren, proof of the parent's marriage
- Any supporting medical records

Once the application has been completed and the person meets the requirements of the law, the packet is forwarded to the Disability Determination Services unit. This unit, composed of a physician and a disability evaluation specialist, reviews the records, considers the medical facts, and issues a determination. If the information is incomplete or inadequate the team will request that the applicant undergo further testing. Further testing and any transportation costs are paid for by the Social Security Administration. Once a determination is made, Disability Determination Services issues a written notice of the decision.

The actual amount of the monthly cash benefit is based on the worker's earnings covered by Social Security before the disability. The benefit therefore varies significantly from person to person. Benefits continue indefinitely or until the patient can perform substantial gainful employment. To ensure continued payment, periodic evaluations are required.

During the initial coverage period by SSDI, health care expenses are paid by the patient's private insurance, Medicaid, or the patient's own funds. If the person receives SSDI for 24 months, he or she becomes entitled to Medicare.

SSI

A comparison of SSDI and SSI is shown in Box 9-2. SSI is a program that pays a monthly income to low-income persons who are elderly, blind, or disabled. Because eligibility is based on income and the cash benefits are paid from the general state and federal tax fund and not the federal Social Security trust fund, benefits vary from state to state. When a person is eligible for SSI, he or she will likely also be eligible for Medicaid. Eligibility is based on the following:

- Income assets and resources
- Blindness (20/200 vision or less in the better eye with best correction or visual field 20 degrees or less even with a corrective lens)
- Disability (if an adult, unable to work because of a disability; if a child of a qualifying adult, younger than 18 years, or if older than 18 to 22 years, a full-time student; if a disabled child, younger than 18 years with a medically proven physical or mental condition that results in marked and severe functional limitations; if aged 18 to 22 years, the adult disability definition applies or the condition or conditions must have lasted or be expected to last at least 12 months or end in death)
- American citizenship or lawfully admitted alien status
- Willingness to accept vocational rehabilitation, if offered

SSI Income Requirements

SSI requires the person to be disabled and incapable of gainful employment with very little income and few resources.

BOX 9-2
Differences Between SSDI and SSI

SSDI	SSI
Payments and eligibility are based on prior work history and contributions to the Social Security trust fund.	Payments are not based on an individual's or a family member's prior work.
Income and assets are not used for the evaluation process.	The person must have limited income and resources.
Until eligible for Medicare (generally 24 months), the person must use private health care insurance, Medicaid, or private funds to pay for health care. Once eligible for Medicare, Medicare pays for medically necessary care according to guidelines.	In most states, SSI recipients also can receive Medicaid (medical assistance) to pay for hospital stays, physician bills, prescription drugs, and other health care costs.
Because income is not counted, the person could also be eligible for a state Medicaid program and food stamps.	Recipients may also be eligible for food stamps in every state except California.
A person can be younger than age 65 years to qualify if they have a qualifying medical condition that prevents gainful employment.	A person must be at least 65 years old, blind, or disabled younger than 65 years old (for full listing of impairments see www.ssa.gov/OP_Home/cfr20/404/404-ap09.htm).
The person must be a citizen and resident of the United States.	The person must be a citizen or a lawful and qualified alien (very specific rules apply) and must live in the United States (including the District of Columbia and the Northern Mariana Islands); a child living with a parent in the military service assigned overseas to permanent duty ashore; or a student temporarily abroad for the purpose of conducting studies. There are special rules for children of active duty military personnel who can continue to receive SSI payments while overseas: ■ They must be a citizen of the United States. ■ They must be living with a parent who is a member of the U.S. armed forces assigned to permanent duty ashore anywhere outside the United States. ■ They must have been eligible to receive SSI in the month before the parent reported for duty overseas.
The person must be willing to accept vocational rehabilitation if offered.	The person must be willing to accept vocational rehabilitation if offered.

Qualifying individuals are generally allowed the following resources:

- Savings accounts to a maximum of $2000 for a single person or $3000 for a couple
- Life insurance with a face value of up to $1500
- Burial plots for the person and his or her immediate family members
- Burial funds up to $1500 for the person and spouse
- A car if the maximum fair market value is less than $4500, if it has

been adjusted to accommodate a disability, or if it is needed for employment purposes

- Medical treatment of a specific problem or for essential daily activities
- Furniture and household goods worth up to $2000 fair market value for a single adult or child or $3000 for a couple
- A home, regardless of value if the person resides there and it is not used as a source of income

SSI does not count the following income in deciding eligibility:

- The first $20 per month of most income from any source
- The first $65 per month of most earned income and half of any earned income more than $65 per month
- Food stamps
- Home energy assistance under certain conditions
- Food, clothing, and shelter from certain private nonprofit organizations that have met Social Security's approval as a nonprofit agency

SSI also considers impairment-related work expenses. These expenses are the costs for services and items that a person needs in order to work. The cost of these items and services must be paid by the disabled individual and not be an expense that is reimbursable by Medicare, Medicaid, or private insurance. Examples of impairment-related expenses are as follows:

- Attendant care services
- Transportation costs
- Medical devices
- Prostheses
- Work-related equipment (e.g., typing aids, page-turning devices, telecommunications devices for the deaf, guide dogs, and medical supplies such as elastic stockings, catheters, and incontinence pads)

SSI is designed to encourage blind or disabled recipients to work. Allowances are therefore given for certain expenses that permit the person to work. Examples of such expenses may include the following:

- Attendant care to provide assistance in getting to and from work
- Readers for the blind or interpreters for the deaf
- Special devices such as telecommunication equipment or braille reading materials and writing devices

- Residential modifications that improve mobility
- Cost of procuring and keeping guide dogs
- Special transportation arrangements or modified vans

Application

Applications for SSI should not be delayed if the required information is not readily available; Social Security representatives may be able to assist in obtaining some information. However, eligibility cannot be determined until all information is available; patients and families must be apprised of this fact. Application should be made as early as possible to the local Social Security office. To expedite the process the family or patient should expect to supply the following:

- Social Security number
- Birth certificate (original or certified copy of the original or evidence of lawful admission for permanent residence)
- Property tax records or mortgage or rent receipts
- Records that show amounts spent for food and utilities, if sharing a household
- Payroll slips, bank books, tax returns, car registration, and any other information about income or resources
- Medical records and names and addresses of physicians, hospitals, or clinics that have treated the disabling condition

Case managers must also be aware that persons eligible for both Aid to Families with Dependent Children and SSI cannot receive both. Families must decide which program offers better benefits or greater income for their situation.

The maximum federal payment for SSI changes annually. However, as of 2001 the SSI rates were $530 for an individual and $796 for a couple. Some states add to the federal SSI payment. Payment amounts vary based on the person's income, living arrangements, and other factors. The following states do not offer additional payments:

- Alaska
- Arkansas
- Delaware
- Florida
- Georgia
- Indiana
- Kansas
- Maryland
- Mississippi
- Missouri
- Northern Mariana Islands
- Ohio
- South Carolina
- Tennessee
- Texas
- West Virginia

Other SSI Caveats

Because the recipient of SSI benefits may also be eligible for Medicaid, he or she is often eligible for other social services offered by local social service or welfare departments. Services such as these may include food stamps, worker services (often called in-home supportive services) meal preparation, shopping, as well as transportation. Referrals are also made to other appropriate agencies within the community for counseling, job training and placement, or training for independent living.

Disabled drug addicts or alcoholics are referred to appropriate agencies for treatment. However, if they do not cooperate or undergo the recommended treatment or comply with the terms and conditions of the program, they are not eligible for SSI. SSI payments made to eligible drug addicts or alcoholics are often made to a representative payee and not directly to the addict or alcoholic.

Certain other conditions dictate which patients must have a representative payee.

The local Social Security Administration office assists in this determination. If the person does not have a family member or friend who can assume this responsibility, the Social Security office will make the necessary arrangements with an appropriate community agency or designee.

LONG-TERM CARE INSURANCE

Long-term care insurance has increased in popularity as more people become concerned about outliving their savings. However, if a person can afford the payments and meet the health assessment and other qualifications to be a long-term care insurance policyholder, they can continue to maintain a savings account while paying for expensive long-term care. Case managers working with older clients should therefore always ask about any possible long-term care insurance policies they might own.

Many people incorrectly believe Medicare and private health care insurance or even the Medicare supplement insurance policies will pay for long-term care. Medicare and health care insurance are for episodic acute care. Medigap or Medicare supplement policies are designed to pay gaps in coverage for hospital deductibles, physician office visit deductibles, and coinsurance payments—not the costs of long-term care.

Medicare and traditional health care policies do not pay for the long-term, chronic, or custodial care many elderly people need. If the client is fortunate enough to have a long-term care policy, this insurance does cover care beyond traditional insurance. Premiums must be current, however. A long-term care insurance policy, at a minimum, covers services such as housekeeping, private duty nursing, and home health assistance up to the policy limit. Some policies will also cover custodial care in a skilled nursing, residential care, or assisted-living facility.

Long-Term Care Statistics

According to statistics from the Health Insurance Association of America, by the year 2005 the number of older persons needing long-term care will be nearly 9 million. By the year 2020, 12 million older Americans will need long-term care. Most will be cared for at home; family members and friends are the sole caregivers for 70% of the elderly.

A similar study by the U.S. Department of Health and Human Services indicates that people aged 65 years face at least a 40% lifetime risk of entering a nursing home. Of this percentage, approximately 10% will stay there 5 years or longer. The American population is growing older, and the age bracket 85 years and older is now the fastest growing segment of the population. The odds of entering a nursing home and staying for longer periods increase with age. In fact, statistics show that 22% of those aged 85 years and older are in a nursing home. Because women generally outlive men by several years, they face a 50% greater likelihood than men of entering a nursing home after age 65 years.[1]

Long-term care, whether provided in the home or elsewhere, is expensive. The national average cost for nursing home care is approximately $46,000 per year. Assisted-living facility costs run approximately $30,000 to $42,000 per year, and "board and care," even at the lowest level, averages approximately $24,600 per year. Home care can be even more expensive than facility care. The cost for personal care is easily $15 per hour for an attendant, and many agencies set a minimum visit limit of 2 to 4 hours. Thus, at $15 per hour and for 2 hours per day, families can easily spend $1000 per month. Medicare only pays for at-home care that is skilled and if the patient's medical condition is unstable and he or she is "homebound" and unable to safely obtain the care from an outpatient setting. If not covered by insurance private nursing care costs average $100 per hour,

or $10,000 to $20,000 per month. In many regions of the country costs are twice these amounts.

According to the Health Insurance Association of America, approximately one third of all nursing home costs are paid out of pocket by individuals and their families. Medicare pays for only about 2% of the tab and only if care is short term and skilled. Most of the balance of the nation's long-term care bill—almost half of all nursing home costs—is picked up by Medicaid either immediately for people meeting federal poverty guidelines or after nursing home residents "spend down" their own savings and become eligible. Many patients who begin privately paying for nursing home care find their savings soon disappear and are not sufficient to cover the lengthy confinements necessary for long-term, custodial, or chronic care. If the person becomes impoverished after entering a nursing home, often their only option is to turn to Medicaid to pay the bills.[2]

Policy Coverage

Long-term care plans vary according to benefits offered, the amount and type of coverage, and the level of care provided. A limit on either the maximum dollar amount or day limit is typical. Some policies also have a deductible period or elimination period as well as separate benefit limits for nursing home, assisted-living facility, and home health care. For example, a policy may offer 5 years of nursing home coverage and 2 years of home health care coverage. However, all contain specific limitations and exclusions that differ from policy to policy. Many policies automatically exclude the following:

- Preexisting conditions (some might be included but require a waiting period)
- Some mental and nervous disorders
- Alcoholism and drug abuse
- Care necessitated by an act of war or an intentionally self-inflicted injury

MEDIGAP POLICIES

Medigap insurance is designed to supplement Medicare's benefits and is regulated by federal and state laws. Medigap policies must be clearly identified as a Medicare supplement and must provide specific benefits that fill the gaps not covered by Medicare. To make it easier for consumers to shop for a medigap policy, most states limit the number of available medigap policies to no more than 10. For specific information on a state's medigap policies, contact the local Health Insurance Counseling and Advocacy Program (HICAP) or the state insurance commissioner.

Medigap policies are developed by the National Association of Insurance Commissioners and have been incorporated into state and federal laws. There are 10 standardized medigap policies—identified as A through J—that are sold by private insurance companies. All states that allow the sale of medigap policies must ensure that at least policy version A is offered. Federal law allows insurers to add new and innovative benefits to standardized plans. However, to do so, any benefits added must be cost-effective and not otherwise available in the marketplace. They must also be offered in a manner consistent with the goal of keeping the medigap selection process simple.

To assist consumers in purchasing a policy, insurance companies must use the same format, language, and definitions. They are also required to use a standard chart that outlines the coverage or summarizes the benefits allowed. Case managers working with patients who might be contemplating the purchase of a medigap policy must encourage them to review several policies so they can adequately compare benefits, limitations, and premiums. An excellent resource for assistance in medigap insurance selection is the local HICAP office.

Medigap Coverage

Medigap policies pay most, if not all, Medicare coinsurance amounts; many also provide coverage for the Medicare deductible. The plan may cover services not covered by Medicare, such as outpatient prescription drugs, preventative health care services, and emergency medical care when traveling outside the United States. Unlike some health insurance plans that restrict where and from whom care can be received, medigap policies generally pay the same supplemental benefit regardless of the health care provider used. If Medicare pays for a service that is included in the patient's medigap plan, the medigap policy must pay its regular share of the costs for care. Some medigap policy benefits have dollar or day limits as well as a yearly maximum.

For patients who are disabled and eligible for Medicare Part B benefits before they turn age 65 years, federal law guarantees them access to the medigap policy of their choice when they do reach age 65 years. If the policy is selected during the first 6 months after they turn age 65 years, they cannot be refused the policy because of their disability and they cannot be charged more than other applicants for premium costs. Some medigap policies, however, impose a 6-month waiting period for any preexisting condition. State laws vary, so clients should contact the state's insurance commission or HICAP if they have questions.

INDIAN HEALTH SERVICE

The provision of health services to members of federally recognized tribes grew out of the special relationship between the federal government and Indian tribes. This relationship, established in 1787, is based on Article I, Section 8 of the Constitution and has been given form and substance by numerous treaties, laws, Supreme Court decisions, and executive orders. The Indian Health Service (HIS) currently provides comprehensive health services to approximately 1.5 million American Indians and Alaska Natives who belong to more than 550 federally recognized tribes in 35 states.[3] The goals of the program are as follows:

- To ensure comprehensive medical services
- To provide services in a culturally acceptable manner
- To ensure that personal and public health services are available and accessible

IHS is an agency of the U.S. Department of Health and Human Services that strives to:

- Assist tribes in developing their own health programs through health management, training, technical assistance, and human resource development
- Assist tribes in coordinating health planning and obtaining health resources available through federal, state, and local programs
- Provide comprehensive health care services, including hospital and ambulatory medical care, preventative and rehabilitative services, and development of community sanitation facilities
- Serve as the principal federal health care advocate for tribes to ensure comprehensive health services for American Indians and Alaska Natives

Health Care Delivery

The IHS health care delivery system is a single health care system. The system is a combination of preventative measures that involve environmental, educational, and outreach activities as well as therapeutic modalities. Within each category are special initiatives in areas such as injury control, alcoholism, diabetes, and mental health. Most IHS funds are appropriated for American Indians who live on or near reservations.

IHS services are provided directly and also through tribally contracted and operated health care programs. Health services also include health care purchased from more than 2000 private providers. In addition, IHS health care services are provided by a network composed of the following:

- **Contract health services**—health services purchased under contract from community hospitals and practitioners
- **Health centers**—facilities physically separated from a hospital that offer a full range of ambulatory and outpatient services available at least 40 hours a week, including primary care physicians, nursing, pharmacy, laboratory, and radiology
- **Health stations**—facilities that are physically separated from hospitals and health centers but offer primary care physician services on a regularly scheduled basis no less than 50 hours a week

Almost all IHS provider facilities are fully accredited.

IHS Headquarters and Area Offices

IHS headquarters are located in Rockville, Maryland. Some headquarters functions are conducted in IHS offices in Phoenix and Tucson, Arizona, and Albuquerque, New Mexico. Case managers can obtain information about IHS services by calling a regional administrative unit in their area (Box 9-3).

CLINICAL TRIALS

Definition

Clinical trials are research studies that rely on patient volunteers to test medicines, devices, procedures, or other new treatment options. The purpose of clinical trials is to find new and improved methods of treating different diseases and special con-

BOX 9-3
IHS Area Offices

Location	Phone No.
Aberdeen, South Dakota	605-226-7581
Anchorage, Alaska	907-257-1153
Albuquerque, New Mexico	505-248-5429
Bemidji, Minnesota	218-759-3412
Billings, Montana	406-247-7248
Nashville, Tennessee	615-736-2441
Oklahoma City, Oklahoma	405-951-3820
Phoenix, Arizona	602-640-2052
Portland, Oregon	503-326-2020
Sacramento, California	916-566-7001
Tucson, Arizona	520-295-2406

ditions. In most cases the trial includes treatment protocols (written guidelines) or medicines that are considered experimental and have not been deemed by the medical community to be efficacious for the condition studied. The National Cancer Institute defines a cancer clinical trial as "an organized study conducted in people with cancer to answer specific questions about a new treatment or a new way of using an old treatment."[4]

Many participants in clinical trials do so through private practitioners involved in clinical research, and just as many are healthy individuals who are recruited for a study by a newspaper advertisement or poster.

Before a new drug, device, or procedure is approved for marketing and use by the general public, it must undergo studies that show evidence of its safety and effectiveness. this evidence generally comes first from tests with laboratory animals and then proceeds to clinical trials in human volunteers. The AIDS epidemic radically changed approval times in clinical trials. What used to take years of research to bring something from test phase to a standard of care can now be done in months.

Phases of Clinical Trials

Most clinical trials are carried out in phases. Each phase is designed to find different information, and each new phase builds on the information obtained from the earlier phases. Depending on general condition, type and stage of disease, and what therapy may have been received, patients may be eligible for studies in different phases. Some patients might not be appropriate for one phase but may be appropriate for another. Larger numbers of people become involved as a trial progresses into later phases. At each phase, researchers review the accrued results and continue to observe unusual or adverse effects of the drug, device, procedure, or treatment being studied. Patients are examined regularly throughout the study to evaluate the effects of what is being tested. If severe side effects or complications are discovered, the study could be terminated.

The clinical trial is generally divided into four phases. Patients may be eligible in different phases of a trial depending on their overall condition. Most clinical trial participants will be in phases 3 or 4. The following is a brief explanation of each phase.

Phase I

Phase I clinical trials are primarily intended to test drug safety and toxicity and often use a small number of healthy volunteers (20-100) who do not receive any clinical care.

Phase II

Phase II trials focus on demonstrating the efficacy of a drug or intervention and identifying side effects. Phase II studies typically involve up to several hundred patients and are conducted as randomized trials. Only about one third of experimental drugs successfully complete both phase I and phase II studies.

Phase III

Phase III trials are used to clarify benefits and risks and to establish optimum dosage rates. They may also compare the efficacy of new therapies with that of standard treatments. In a phase III study, a drug is tested in several hundred to several thousand patients. Most phase III studies are randomized and blinded trials. Once a phase III study is successfully completed, a pharmaceutical company can file a new drug application (NDA) to request Food and Drug Administration (FDA) approval for marketing the drug.

Phase IV

In late phase III and phase IV studies, pharmaceutical companies have several objectives:

- To compare a drug with other drugs already on the market
- To monitor a drug's long-term effectiveness and impact on a patient's quality of life
- To determine the cost-effectiveness of the drug relative to other treatment or traditional or new therapies

Adjuvant Therapy

Adjuvant therapy trials are conducted through each phase of the clinical trial. The intent is to evaluate if additional treatment, in addition to the standard of care, will improve the chance for cure in patients. With adjuvant therapy, the study could involve one group of patients receiving the standard care (e.g., surgery) while the second group receives a combination of the standard therapy plus other therapies (e.g., chemotherapy and surgery). If the study shows that one group has better results than the other, the one with the best results could become the new standard therapy.

Neoadjuvant Studies

In neoadjuvant studies the subject matter is again progressed through phases I, II, and III of the trial. However, in neoadjuvant studies the patient receives treatments considered to be the standard of care for the disorder (e.g., radiotherapy and surgery) as well as additional therapies (e.g., chemotherapy, radiotherapy, and then surgery).

Supportive Care Studies

In addition to a clinical trial seeking better ways to treat a disease, clinical trials also may be used to study better ways of treating the side effects of specific treatments (e.g., nausea, vomiting, and hair loss) or the side effects of the disorder itself (e.g., pain or mental confusion). Supportive care studies follow the same phases as those in any clinical trial. However, the intent of supportive care studies centers on issues such as what other drugs or therapy might be needed to treat side effects or ease the discomfort of the family or survivor. Supportive care studies are also used to find better ways to help the patient or family cope with the illness.

Prevention and Early Detection Studies

Studies undertaken for prevention or detection involve groups of people who might be at high risk of a disease, possibly because they have had family members with the same disease. Prevention studies compare one group of patients against another. Although one group may receive special treatments, the other will not. Early detection studies examine groups of people to assess methods of screening for the disease. The intent is to find the disease in its early stages and offer treatments to increase chances of survival. Studies done for these purposes often take years.

Group C and Treatment Referral Center Studies

Group C studies often include studies in which drugs or a specific therapy is made available to some physicians who specialize in the disease. If a specific drug or treatment is offered, it has already been through the first stages of the clinical trial.

However, by offering the drug or treatment through physicians or centers that specialize in the disease, a wider group of patients can be studied.

Sponsors of Clinical Trials

Most clinical trials are sponsored by a pharmaceutical company, research institution, or other health organization that provides the funding as well as the design or protocol.

OVERSIGHT OF THE CLINICAL TRIAL PROCESS

Oversight of clinical trials is usually conducted by a group known as the institutional review board. This board is a committee of experts and laypeople who also review the research as it progresses through the various phases. Clinical trials are also watched by such agencies as the FDA, National Cancer Institute, National Institutes of Health (NIH), Centers for Disease Control and Prevention (CDC), and other federal agencies that protect patients who take part in medical research.

An institutional review board must be composed of at least five people with varying backgrounds. At least one person must come from a nonscientific profession, and at least one must not be affiliated with the research institution. All others must have knowledge through training or experience in the research areas likely to be considered.

Many managed care organizations (MCOs) and other organizations use Hayes, Inc., for assistance as they review, approve, or deny a request when a specific treatment, drug, device, or procedure is in question. Hayes, Inc., produces medical technology assessment reports and publications and specializes in evidence-based analyses of health care technologies.

Hayes, Inc., identifies, analyzes, and reports on emerging medical technology. Their extensive team of professionals in clinical research, medicine, and law works with experts from national and federal organizations such as the FDA and National Cancer Institute to evaluate and rate scientific research as it relates to procedures, drugs, medical devices, and equipment. Their ratings are A, standard of care; B, almost approved as a standard of care; C, experimental; and D, not efficacious. Hayes, Inc., also publishes legal and medical reports that analyze the legal status of medical technologies and managed care issues specific to insurance coverage, medical malpractice, and legislative trends. Their team of experts can also be used for an organization's third-party outside review process. Their review process offers a wide variety of specialists who can be used when independent medical review is required on a issue in debate. Contact Hayes, Inc., through their website at www.hayesinc.com.

FDA

The FDA is a government agency that enforces laws on the testing and use of drugs and medical devices. Before the general public can use them, the FDA must approve all drugs and medical devices. Before 1992 and the passage of the Prescription Drug User Fee Act, the approval time for new drugs took many years. Since 1992, the drug approval time has averaged less than 12 months. The FDA uses the following as a guide:

- **Priority NDA**—These drugs have a 6-month performance goal for FDA review because the product being tested is designated as one that could provide significant therapeutic or public health benefit.
- **Standard NDA**—These drugs have a performance goal of 10 to 12 months for FDA review because the product being tested is not designated as a priority NDA.[5]

The FDA website (www.fda.gov) maintains a link to clinical practice, clinical trials, and numerous websites at www.fda.gov/oc/ohrt/irbs/websites.html.

Informed Consent

All clinical trial participants in the United States are required to sign a consent form that indicates they agree and understand that they are participating in a clinical trial or human experimentation. For informed consent, researchers must give participants adequate information from which to make an informed decision. They must also allow participants adequate time and an opportunity to ask questions before making a decision. In all cases, participation must be voluntary. Informed consent is very specific and informs patients of:

- Which treatments they will receive
- What side effects to expect
- The costs covered by the study and those excluded and possibly owed by the patient
- The risks and responsibilities that participation entails
- Treatment alternatives and options along with the advantages and disadvantages of the subject being studied by the clinical trial

If the case manager is working for an MCO and receives a request for a service for which the standard of care is unknown, the best and easiest way to validate if the treatment is linked to a clinical trial is to have the provider fax or mail a copy of the informed consent.

Medicare's Approach to Clinical Trials

Medicare has covered the routine costs of clinical trials since September 2000. To be covered, the clinical trial must be qualified. If it is, Medicare covers certain costs (listed below) and any reasonable and necessary items or services used to diagnose and treat complications arising from participation. Routine costs of a clinical trial include all items and services that are otherwise generally available to Medicare beneficiaries (there is a benefit category; it is not statuto-

rily excluded from Medicare regulations; the clinical trial is efficacious and judged to be safe for the condition at hand; and the medical community accepts it as a treatment for such). The following costs are excluded:

- The investigational item or service itself
- Items and services provided solely to satisfy data collection and analysis needs and that are not used in the direct clinical management of the patient (e.g., monthly computed tomography scans for a condition usually requiring only a single scan)
- Items and services customarily provided by the research sponsors free of charge for any enrollee in the trial

The following routine costs are covered:

- Items or services typically provided outside a clinical trial (e.g., conventional care)
- Items or services required solely for the provision of the investigational item or service (e.g., administration of a noncovered chemotherapeutic agent)
- Clinically appropriate monitoring of the effects of the item or service or the prevention of complications
- Items or services needed for reasonable and necessary care arising from the provision of an investigational item or service, in particular for the diagnosis or treatment of complications

Medicare only allows coverage for treatment of any complications that arose from the delivery of the noncovered item or service and unrelated reasonable and necessary care. If the item or service is not covered by an existing Medicare noncoverage policy (see Medicare's Coverage Issues Manual) and the item or services are the focus of a qualifying clinical trial, the routine costs of the clinical trial are covered but not the item or services classified as noncovered.

As part of their contractual agreements with the Centers for Medicare & Medicaid Services (CMS), Medicare regulations require Medicare + Choice organizations to follow CMS' national coverage decisions for a clinical trial. This national coverage decision raises special issues that require some modification of most Medicare + Choice organizations' rules governing provision of items and services in and out of network. The items and services covered under the national coverage decision are inextricably linked to the clinical trials with which they are associated and cannot be covered outside the context of those trials. Medicare + Choice organizations must cover these services regardless of whether they are available through in-network providers. Additionally, Medicare + Choice organizations have reporting requirements when enrollees participate in clinical trials to track and coordinate their members' care but cannot require prior authorization or approval.[6] Because of these requirements, most Medicare + Choice contracts have a carve-out for beneficiaries participating in a clinical trial. If this is the case, these clients will have their clinical trial covered by fee-for-service Medicare and not the Medicare + Choice organization.

Medicare Requirements for Participation and Coverage

The following three requirements must be met to be considered for coverage of routine costs for the clinical trial:

1. The subject or purpose of the trial must be to evaluate an item or service that falls within a Medicare benefit category (e.g., physicians' services, durable medical equipment, diagnostic tests) and is not statutorily excluded from coverage (e.g., cosmetic surgery, hearing aids).
2. The trial must be based on therapeutic intent and not exclusively designed to test toxicity or disease pathophysiology.

3. Trials of therapeutic interventions must enroll patients with diagnosed disease rather than healthy volunteers. Trials of diagnostic interventions may enroll healthy patients to have a proper control group.[6]

The previous three requirements are insufficient by themselves to qualify a clinical trial for Medicare coverage of routine costs. Clinical trials must have the following desirable characteristics to receive Medicare coverage:

- The principal purpose of the trial must be to test whether the intervention potentially improves the participants' health outcomes.
- The trial is well supported by available scientific and medical information or it is intended to clarify or establish the health outcomes of interventions already in common clinical use.
- The trial does not unjustifiably duplicate existing studies.
- The trial design is appropriate to answer the research question being asked.
- The trial is sponsored by a credible organization or individual capable of successfully executing the proposed trial.
- The trial is in compliance with federal regulations relating to the protection of human subjects.
- All aspects of the trial are conducted according to the appropriate standards of scientific integrity.[6]

CERTIFICATION OF TRIALS

CMS requires that all clinical trials be certified before beneficiaries are allowed to participate. This certification is done by a multiagency federal panel. This panel assists the Agency for Healthcare Research and Quality (AHRQ) in certifying the trials for coverage and is composed of representatives from agencies such as:

- Department of Health and Human Services
- NIH
- CDC
- FDA
- The research arms of the Department of Defense (DOD) and the Department of Veterans Affairs (VA)

Although the panel does not review or approve individual clinical trials, one of its primary tasks is the development of qualifying criteria that indicate whether a trial will exhibit desirable characteristics. An additional task of the panel is to review and evaluate the trial periodically and make recommendations as necessary to CMS. As the panel develops criteria, the goal is to keep criteria easily verifiable and, when possible, dichotomous. Trials that meet the panel's qualifying criteria are eligible to receive Medicare coverage for their routine associated costs.

If AHRQ and its multiagency panel deem that the clinical trial will likely meet the desirable characteristics, some trials are automatically qualified to receive Medicare coverage of their routine costs. Clinical trials that are deemed to be automatically qualified are as follows:

- Trials funded by NIH, CDC, AHRQ, CMS, DOD, and VA
- Trials supported by centers or cooperative groups that are funded by the NIH, CDC, AHRQ, CMS, DOD, and VA
- Trials conducted under an investigational NDA reviewed by the FDA
- Drug trials exempt from having an investigational NDA status (unless the qualifying criteria has not been developed; if it has not, the principal investigators must certify that the trials meet the qualifying criteria)

The only exceptions to these rules are if CMS' chief clinical officer subsequently finds a clinical trial does not meet the qualifying criteria or the trial jeopardizes the safety or welfare of Medicare beneficiaries. If an item or service is considered noncovered or statutorily prohibited by Medicare, Medicare can only cover the costs of treatments that are reasonable and medically necessary or those related to any complications that arose from the delivery of the noncovered item or service. However, if the item or service is not covered by a national noncoverage policy in Medicare's Coverage Issues Manual and is the focus of a qualifying clinical trial, the routine costs of the clinical trial will be covered, but the noncovered item or service itself will not.[6]

If CMS finds a trial's principal investigator misrepresented the trial and certified that the trial met the necessary qualifying criteria to gain Medicare coverage of routine costs, Medicare coverage of the routine costs would be denied and serious consequences would result. If this occurs, the participants enrolled in the trial would not be held liable and would be held harmless from collection of any costs associated with their care or treatment while involved in the trial. However, the billing providers and the trial's principal investigator would be held liable for costs and consequences of any fraud investigation.

MEDICARE + CHOICE OBLIGATIONS FOR COVERAGE

Because Medicare now covers the costs of qualified clinical trials, Medicare regulations require Medicare + Choice organizations to likewise follow CMS' national coverage decisions on the issue. Medicare + Choice organizations are required to cover such trials and services regardless of whether they are available through the organization's network provider panel. A further requirement is that although the Medicare + Choice organization has reporting requirements for members who participate in clinical trials—and they may want to track and coordinate the members' care while in a clinical trial—they cannot require prior authorization or deny the trial.

Medicare's rule on clinical trials is binding and applies to all Medicare carriers, fiscal intermediaries, peer review organizations, health maintenance organizations, competitive medical plans, health care prepayment plans, and Medicare + Choice organizations. Additionally, Medicare does not allow an administrative law judge to disregard, set aside, or otherwise review a national coverage decision issued under section 1862 of the Social Security Act.

Although Medicare + Choice organizations are required to cover clinical trial costs for Medicare beneficiaries, other persons insured by the organization may have their clinical trials excluded. Thus case managers must be astute to standard medical practices for conditions as well as clinical trials and various categories of enrolled members affected by this legislation.

WORKING WITH PATIENTS IN CLINICAL TRIALS

Because many patients receiving case management are in clinical trials or might be considered as a trial candidate, case managers must be familiar with clinical trials. Case managers must understand what a clinical trial is, how information can be located, and what the requirements are from an MCO or Medicare if a trial is to be considered for approval.

Helping patients prepare questions to ask during evaluations and visits with the different professional disciplines associated with the trial may be necessary. Some questions they may want to ask are include the following:

- What is the purpose of the trial and how will it benefit their condition?
- How will the trial affect their life as well as that of their loved ones?

- If the center of excellence is a distance from their home, can their family members be nearby?
- What arrangements have been made for housing and transportation and what are the costs?
- What are some of the adverse outcomes or side effects that can be anticipated?
- Will they be hospitalized? If so, for how long and how often?
- How long will the trial last?
- What other tests and procedures will they be required to endure, are these considered part of the trial, and will any out-of-pocket costs be the their responsibility?
- What other out-of-pocket costs can be anticipated?

FREE SERVICES

Free Medications

Nearly every major pharmaceutical company offers a program to provide free pharmaceuticals to people who cannot afford to buy the drugs they need. Each company has its own program with special requirements, forms, and procedures. Some companies have different programs for different drugs. Unfortunately, no central clearinghouse exists for obtaining up-to-date information about these programs, available drugs, or a standardized process. Drug manufacturers develop the free drug programs voluntarily and set their own eligibility criteria.

Some companies publicize their programs, but others do not. In some cases, the application forms are sent only to a physician's office after physician request. The physician is often the one to determine that the patient cannot afford the drugs prescribed. Most programs do require financial screening (the patient must meet income and asset criteria); this is especially true when expensive drugs are required. In all cases, if the patient has insurance (private health insurance, Medicaid, or Medicare) he or she may be disqualified from an indigent patient program. Although a large number of medications may be prescribed, not all medications are available through these programs. More important, any drug release of prescription drugs is subject to applicable federal and state laws. When working with patients who cannot afford their medication, the following steps should be taken:

- Consult the drug maker directly
- Call the FDA
- Contact *Indi*Care, the preferred provider for U.S. public health services
- If the patient is Medicare eligible, contact Medicare at www.medicare.gov/Prescription/Home.asp
- Review drug companies and phone numbers as listed in the *Physician's Desk Reference* and then query these companies for the programs they offer
- Contact Pharmaceutical Research and Manufacturers of America (PhRMA) about free medications at www.phrma.org
- For VA patients, call the nearest VA office
- For military patients, call the nearest military treatment facility to inquire about a TRICARE program

PhRMA

A growing number of programs are available for needy patients, especially if the drug manufacturer is a member of the PhRMA. PhRMA has created a directory that lists companies that offer drugs to physicians whose patients cannot otherwise afford them.

Unfortunately, if a drug manufacturer is not a member of PhRMA, the information about the drug and any indigent program requirements must be obtained directly from the manufacturer. If a partic-

ular drug is not listed by PhRMA, the drug may not be available or may not be manufactured by a company that belongs to PhRMA. Eligibility criteria are listed in the directory, but case managers may need to contact the drug company directly. The drug companies that frequently have programs available can be found at www.phrma.org/whoweare/members.

Making Use of Websites

Case managers must advise their patients to follow FDA warnings and suggestions when using websites to order drugs or other health products:

- Patients should check with the National Association of Boards of Pharmacy (www.nabp.net or call 847-698-6227) to determine whether websites are licensed pharmacies in good standing.
- Patients should be aware that medications purchased from an illegal website might put them at risk. They might receive a contaminated or counterfeit product, the wrong product, an incorrect dose, or no product at all.
- Patients should be aware that taking an unsafe or inappropriate medication puts them at risk for dangerous drug interactions and other serious health consequences.
- Patients should know that getting a prescription drug by filling out a questionnaire without seeing a doctor poses serious health risks. A questionnaire does not provide sufficient information for a health care professional to determine if that drug is appropriate, safe, whether another treatment is more beneficial, or if an underlying medical condition may make that drug harmful. The American Medical Association has determined that this practice is generally substandard medical care and the FDA agrees.

- Patients should not buy from websites that offer to prescribe a prescription drug for the first time without a physical examination, sell a prescription drug without a prescription, or sell drugs not approved by FDA.
- Patients should not do business with websites that have no access to a registered pharmacist to answer questions.
- Patients should avoid websites that do not identify with whom they are dealing, and they should not use one if it does not provide a U.S. address and phone number to contact if there is a problem.
- Patients should not purchase drugs from foreign websites because (1) it might be illegal to import the drugs bought from these sites, (2) the risks are greater, and (3) there is very little the U.S. government can do if patient gets cheated.
- Patients should beware of sites that advertise a "new cure" for a serious disorder or a quick cure-all for a wide range of ailments.
- Patients should be careful of sites that use impressive-sounding terminology to disguise a lack of good science or those that claim the government, the medical profession, or research scientists have conspired to suppress a product.
- Patients should steer clear of websites that include undocumented case histories claiming "amazing" results.
- Patients should talk with their physicians before using any medications for the first time.[7]

SHRINERS HOSPITALS AND ST. JUDE CHILDREN'S RESEARCH HOSPITALS

Case managers not traditionally assigned to children should be aware of two valuable programs that offer free services to children with orthopedic and spinal cord injuries, burns, and cancer. These programs are offered by the Shriners and their network of hospitals located in North America as well as St. Jude Children's Research Hospitals.

Shriners Hospitals

Shriners Hospitals for Children is a network of pediatric specialty hospitals founded and run by the Shrine of North America fraternal organization. These hospitals provide free medical care (there is never a charge to the patient, parent, or third-party insurer) to any child younger than 18 years regardless of race, sex, religion, or relationship to a Shriner. The primary referral criteria is the need of orthopedic, burn, or spinal cord injury care and services.

The Shriners Hospital network consists of 22 hospitals, 20 in the United States and one each in Mexico and Canada. Of the 18 orthopedic hospitals, three hospitals (Chicago, Philadelphia, and Sacramento) offer special programs dedicated to caring for children with spinal cord injuries. The Shriners Hospitals in Boston, Cincinnati, Galveston, and Sacramento also treat children with acute fresh burns; children needing plastic reconstructive or restorative surgery as a result of "healed" burns; children with severe scarring resulting in contractures or interference with mobility of the limbs; and children with scarring and deformity of the face.

All hospitals are considered centers of excellence, serve as major referral centers for children with complex orthopedic or burn problems, and are equipped and staffed to treat children with congenital conditions and orthopedic problems resulting from injuries and diseases of the musculoskeletal system. Parents of Shriners Hospital patients are given free housing and clothing, if needed, as well as transportation.

Applications or additional information on eligibility for Shriners Hospitals services can be obtained by calling any local Shrine Temple or Shrine Club; writing to Shriners Hospitals at PO Box 31356, Tampa, FL 33631; or calling the Shriners Hospitals toll-free referral line at 800-237-5055 (in Canada, call 800-361-7256). Applications can also be downloaded from the Shriners website at www.shrinershq.org/Hospitals/eligible.html. Completed applications should be returned to the nearest Shriners Hospital.

For a full listing of Shriners Hospitals (addresses and phone numbers), see the Shriners website at www.shrinershq.org/shc/index.html. The Shriners website also links to many additional health and medical resources and websites devoted to children (www.shrinershq.org/hospitallinks.html).

St. Jude Children's Research Hospitals

St. Jude Children's Research Hospital, located in Memphis, treats and conducts research on cures for children with catastrophic illnesses. In addition to the Memphis site, St. Jude also has affiliate hospitals at the following sites:

- Our Lady of the Lake Regional Medical Center, Baton Rouge, Louisiana
- Johnson City Medical Center, Johnson City, Tennessee
- St. Jude Midwest Affiliate, Peoria, Illinois
- Louisiana State University Department of Pediatrics, Shreveport, Louisiana

Admission to St. Jude is based on the patient's eligibility for treatment under research (this includes disorders such as cancer, blood diseases, genetic syndromes, infectious diseases, and immunodeficiency disorders as well as specific conditions such as leukemia, lymphoma, solid tumors, sickle cell disease, osteogenesis imperfecta, and AIDS).

Referrals are accepted from physicians and admission is not based on race, sex, ethnicity, religion, nationality, or ability to pay. To be eligible the child should be between birth and 18 years old. If the child needs diagnostic surgery he or she can be accepted with a presumptive diagnosis of cancer. Final acceptance occurs when the patient is deemed eligible and is enrolled on a protocol. Referring physicians can call the toll-free physician referral line at 888-226-4343 or they can fax information to 901-525-2720. Parents or case managers can obtain additional information about referrals, consultations, and treatment policy by calling the toll-free number 888-226-4343 or by visiting the St. Jude website at www.stjude.org. Additional websites include the American Cancer Society (www.cancer.org), NIH (www.nih.gov), National Organization for Rare Disorders (www.rarediseases.org), and the Index of the Pediatric Internet (www.pedinfo.org).

Although most children are treated in an outpatient setting, the hospital does have 56 beds for children who require hospitalization during treatment. Patients are accepted for treatment at St. Jude based on their eligibility for treatment protocols. No child is turned away because of the parents' inability to pay.

The American Lebanese Syrian Associated Charities (ALSAC) is the fundraising arm of St. Jude and covers all costs of treatment and supportive care beyond those reimbursed by third-party insurers. When no insurance is available, all treatment costs are covered by ALSAC. ALSAC also provides travel expenses for the patient and one parent as well as assistance with local living expenses (housing and meals) while the child is hospitalized. If housing assistance is needed, case managers or parents can call the Patient Services Department at 901-495-2909 or 901-495-3340. The Department of Patient Housing works with Patient Services to provide three unique residence facilities: Target House, Ronald McDonald House, and Wyndham Garden House. Housing is based on the patient's expected length of stay.

Other Fraternal and Charitable Organizations

Although some free services can be obtained from other fraternal and charitable organizations, they are community and organization specific. The most common organizations that assist persons and families in need include local churches, ethnic-specific groups, The Salvation Army, Volunteers of America, Lutheran Family Services, Catholic Charities, and the like.

At times, a fraternal or other organization will hold a community fund-raising drive, purchase one-time items, assist with the building of ramps, or perform other charitable projects.

The best way to locate resources in a community is through the telephone directory or by calling a local information and referral line.

FREE TRANSPORTATION

AirLifeLine, a national nonprofit organization of private pilots, donates time, skills, aircraft, and fuel to fly ambulatory patients to receive medical care. AirLifeLine transports patients of all ages with medical conditions ranging from severe burns or trauma to terminal cancer. Case managers needing additional information can call 800-446-1231 or visit their website at www.airlifeline.org.

Children's Angel Flight and the National Patient Travel Center

Children's Angel Flight functions as a charity in full cooperation with the Angel Flight America Network of charitable medical air transportation. These flights provide medical air transportation at no cost or reduced rate for needy patients and their families. This network cooperates with and uses the services administered through the National Patient Travel Center (NPTC) and the Angel Flight regional flight operations. The mission of the organization is to ensure that financially needy patients are not denied access to long-distance specialized medical evaluation, diagnosis, or treatment because they cannot pay for medical air transportation. To locate the many charities to which the Angel Flight America Network is linked, see their website at www.angel-flight.org/air_transportation_charities.htm.

NPTC exists to facilitate patient access to appropriate charitable medical air transportation resources in the United States. NPTC also develops, administers, and consolidates airline patient ticket programs and operates various Special-Lift and Child-Lift programs on behalf of special disease organizations and clinical research centers in the United States. NPTC also brings ambulatory patients from overseas locations to the United States for treatment. Services offered by NPTC include:

- **National Patient Travel HELPLINE Program**—This line helps coordinate the most appropriate Angel Flight America Network program in the United States. Their phone number is 800-296-1217.
- **Airline tickets for patients and escorts**—This service refers patients to the most appropriate charitable airline ticket program. Many programs offer free and highly discounted tickets, even for last-minute medically related long-distance travel. Their phone number is 800-325-8909.
- **Special-Lift and Child-Lift programs**—These programs offer a single point of contact for the administration of patient air transportation for special disease organizations and clinical research centers. Their phone number is 888-675-1405.

- **Airline program development—** This service offers no-cost consulting to airline executive staff developing charitable or reduced-rate patient ticket programs. Their phone number is 757-318-9175.
- **Airline ticket program management—**This service offers staff and volunteers to administer charitable airline ticket programs on behalf of individual airlines. Their phone number is 800-325-8908.[8]

Air Flight for Veterans

Angel Flight for Veterans is a flight service dedicated to helping veterans and active duty military personnel and their families in need of medical or compassionate air transportation. The mission and purpose of this system is to ensure that a financially needy veteran or active duty military person or family members are not denied access to distant specialized medical evaluation, diagnosis, treatment, or rehabilitation because of an inability to pay for long-distance medical air transportation. For further information on Angel Flight for Veterans, see their website at www. veterans-aeromedical.org.

Military Aeromedical Evacuation System

The military offers their active personnel and retirees, as well as their dependents, free civilian air transportation if the patient needs assistance in getting to a center of excellence. Although active duty personnel and their dependents have first priority for use of the system, it may be available to anyone eligible for benefits under TRICARE. The aeromedical evacuation system is based at Scott Air Force Base in Illinois. One primary duty of this base is managing the domestic aeromedical evacuation system. Further information about aeromedical evacuation can be obtained by calling the closest military base and ask-

ing for the health benefits advisor, personnel from the Patient Administration Office, a TRICARE health care finder, or beneficiary service representative.

FREE HOUSING

Caregivers have discovered the importance of the total family as part of the care plan. A plan involving the family achieves more satisfactory outcomes for patients. The National Association of Hospital Hospitality Houses has developed a program to care for the forgotten patient—the family or caregiver who attends to the person receiving medical care. When such houses are not available, families are forced to spend countless hours in hospital waiting rooms. Worse yet, many caregivers deny themselves basic necessities, such as meals and proper rest, to conserve financial resources when a long-term hospitalization is required. They must also bear the high cost of hotels or motels. To locate a Hospital Hospitality House, call 800-542-9730 or 317-288-3226 or visit their website at www.nahhh.org.

■ SUMMARY

The IHS health care delivery system is a single health care system. The system is combination of preventative measures that involve environmental, educational, and outreach activities as well as therapeutic modalities. Within each category are special initiatives in areas such as injury control, alcoholism, diabetes, and mental health. Most IHS funds are appropriated for American Indians who live on or near reservations.

Only a small percentage of the total costs for long-term nursing home care are covered by Medicare and private insurance. Over the past several years an influx of insurers have created long-term care policies. However, these policies are costly and not every patient or family can afford them. Thus the bulk of long-term care is covered by Medicaid.

For many patients, compliance with their medical program is based on their financial resources. Although some patients have private disability policies or supplemental insurance that may cover required care, the majority of patients do not. Case managers must be astute regarding the various public programs that offer income or financial support for disabled persons. Far too often the public and, at times, professionals are unaware of the benefits allowed for persons who meet disability guidelines for either SSDI or SSI. Although both are programs of the Social Security Administration, they are different programs—from the application process, eligibility requirements, and actual benefits received.

As technology advances the need for clinical trials and human subjects will also grow. Clinical trials are research studies designed to evaluate the safety and effectiveness of drugs, devices, treatments, and procedures. They are often key to understanding the appropriate use of medical interventions in many conditions and diseases. Although only a small percentage of people will be involved in clinical trials, case managers will likely have such patients. Thus case managers must be aware of the processes involved with clinical trials and their organization's requirements.

Insurance is only one funding program for which patients might be entitled. Consequently, case managers must learn all they can of the various funding programs available. This knowledge includes the basics of referral and what conditions might be eligible to receive the benefits offered. More important is knowledge of the appeal processes and when and to what level the patient can appeal if services are denied. This knowledge will be invaluable in the long run if benefits and resources are to be used wisely.

Chapter Exercises

1. List the differences between COBRA and TEFRA eligibility rules.
2. Research the Mental Health Parity Act, list the federal requirements, and compare them to your state program on parity.
3. List the TEFRA criteria for eligibility of a child.
4. Describe the SSDI and SSI programs and list their differences and similarities.
5. Using Social Security's definition, define disability and give several examples of patients who might be eligible.
6. Describe eligibility requirements for both SSDI and SSI and how they differ; if there are similarities, what are they?
7. To validate the statistics listed in the text, contact some of your areas nursing homes and speak with either the administrator or billing office and determine what percentage of their patients' care is covered by Medicare, private pay, or Medicaid.
8. Although there are many caveats and requirements to individual private policies for long-term care, list the common conditions long-term care insurers evaluate before their approval determination.
9. Call or visit the local HICAP office and discuss the various medigap policies offered with a representative. Ask the person to do a step-by-step comparison of the three plans as they would with a private consumer wanting help with the selection of a plan.
10. When contacting the local HICAP or insurance commissioner's office for your state, ascertain the types of plans offered and, at a minimum, discuss the benefits allowed by plan code A.

11. Discuss in a group the many services available to the American Indian and Alaska Native populations. If your area has an Indian Health Service branch, call or visit the center and discuss what types of services are in the immediate area and how patients are referred.

12. Discuss in a group the role and goals of the U.S. Public Health Service and the type of care IHS provides American Indian and Alaska Natives.

13. Describe the phases a clinical trial goes through to be considered a standard of care. Take one treatment recently approved and describe how long it took to go through the phases and how many people were involved in the study.

14. Describe the roles of the institutional review board and AHRQ in clinical trials.

15. Describe Medicare's new stance on clinical trials and interview a Medicare + Choice organization's compliance director or designee to ascertain his or her take on the new rule, how it will affect implementation processes and costs, and what mechanism is used to track such patients.

16. Discuss in a group some of the known free services in your area and share this information with your colleagues.

COBRA and TEFRA

www.dol.gov/dol/topic/health-plans/cobra.htm—Consumer information on COBRA through the U.S. Department of Labor

www.cobrainsurance.com/COBRA_Law.htm—Full information on COBRA

www.cms.hhs.gov/hipaa/hipaa1/content/mhpa.asp—Full text of MHPA through CMS

www.cms.hhs.gov/hipaa/hipaa1/default.asp—Information on HIPAA and the insurance reform through CMS

www.nimh/nih.gov/parity/appende.cfm—Lists states with mental health parity and contains other information on mental health, including definitions of broad-based mental health and serious mental health illness

Social Security

www.ssa.gov/notices/supplemental-security-income/#income—SSI information

www.ssa.gov/OP_Home/handbook/handbook.21/handbook-toc21.html—For a copy of the SSI handbook

www.ssa.gov/OP_Home/ssact/title16b/1600.htm—For a copy of the SSI law

www.ssa.gov/disability/professionals/bluebook—For information about Social Security's SSDI programs

Long-Term Care

www.hiaa.org/consumer/guideltc.cfm—Health Insurance Association of America

Indian Health Service

www.ihs.gov—Indian Health Service

www.ihs.gov/MedicalPrograms/Medical_index.asp—Indian Health Service, U.S. Department of Health and Human Services

Clinical Trials

www.clinicaltrials.com—Internet resource that allows on-line inquiry regarding clinical trials and requirements for participation

www.fda.gov/cder/ob/default.htm—Contains a wealth of information on approved drug products for both professionals and the public

www.fda.gov/cder—FDA website for its Center for Drug Evaluation and Research

www.cms.hhs.gov/coverage/default.asp—Medicare Coverage Policy, a national coverage policy based on the authority found in section 1862(a)(1)(E) of the

Social Security Act (section 1852(a)(1)(A) of the act)

www.clinicaltrials.gov—NIH website on clinical trials

www.nih.gov/sigs/bioethics—NIH bioethics information

www.nlm.nih.gov/medlineplus—Health information from NIH

www.nlm.nih.gov—NIH's National Library of Medicine

www.healthfinder.gov—Consumer guide to health

www.cms.hhs.gov/coverage/8d.asp—Medicare's coverage policy

www.clinicaltrials.gov and *www.nlm.nih.gov/pubs/factsheets/clintrial. html*—National Library of Medicine websites on clinical trials

www.nih.gov/health/infoline.htm—NIH toll free information listing of disease-specific agencies

www.rarediseases.info.nih.gov/ord—National Cancer Institute and NIH Office of Rare Diseases

www.fda.gov/cder/cancer/index.htm—FDA oncology tools

Free Services

www.nabp.net—National Association of Boards of Pharmacy

www.medicare.gov/Prescription/Home.asp—Medicare

www.airlifeline.org—AirLifeLine

www.angel-flight.org/air_transportation_ charities.htm—Angel Flight America Network website with links to affiliated charities

www.veterans-aeromedical.org—Angel Flight for Veterans

www.nahhh.org—National Association of Hospital Hospitality Houses

www.shrinershq.org—Shriners

www.stjude.org—St. Jude Children's Research Hospital

www.cancer.org—American Cancer Society

www.nih.gov—NIH

www.rarediseases.org—National Organization of Rare Disorders

www.pedinfo.org—PEDINFO, an index of pediatric websites

REFERENCES

1. Health Insurance Association of America: www.hiaa. org.
2. Health Insurance Association of America: www.hiaa. org/research/research_studies.cfm.
3. Indian Health Service: www.ihs.gov.
4. National Cancer Institute: www.nci.nih.gov.
5. Food and Drug Administration: www.fda.gov.
6. Medicare: www.medicare.gov.
7. Food and Drug Administration: www.fda.gov/oc/ buyonline/default.htm.
8. National Patient Travel Center: www.patienttravel. org/afas/nptc.htm.

Utilization Management Challenges

Sharon M. Reichle, BS, MA, URQAP

OBJECTIVES

■ To define the goals of utilization management as well as those of case management
■ To describe the processes associated with utilization management
■ To describe the common industry benchmarks for commercially insured and Medicare-insured populations
■ To describe at least three of the most common utilization management reporting requirements

---

UTILIZATION MANAGEMENT VERSUS CASE MANAGEMENT

Although many organizations consider case management to be synonymous with utilization management, the two are not the same. *On the whole, utilization management and case management are two completely different specialties; each has a different intent, and each requires different types of expertise.*

The purpose of any utilization management process is to establish eligibility, interpret covered benefits, and evaluate the medical necessity, appropriateness, and effectiveness of the delivery of health care. At the same time, all processes must ensure that services are performed by an appropriate health care provider at the appropriate

level of care, within a time frame that is consistent with the urgency of the patient's condition, and in compliance with the guidelines of federal, state, and accrediting agencies. As is well known by many professionals in case management, case management in some organizations and for some health care payers is really nothing more than intensified utilization management. In other organizations, the duties of utilization management and case management are combined. This combination is unfortunate and unproductive, because the functions of each process represent a separate and specialized field, and combining them compromises the effectiveness of both. The best outcomes are achieved when the functions of utilization management and case management are kept separate and are performed by different departments in the organization (Figure 10-1).

Worksheet for Determining Appropriate Levels of Health Plan Medical Management Staffing

This document gives suggested staffing ratios for the medical management positions of case manager, concurrent review nurse, and medical director, with additional calculations for discharge planning and the combined position of concurrent review/discharge planner. The ratios for each position are separated by commercial and Medicare populations. The range of ratios represents the minimum, midpoint, and maximum staffing levels. The appropriate staffing level is dependent on a number of factors including but not limited to budget limitations, characteristics of the health care delivery network and systems, membership demographics, extent of external and internal departmental support staff and systems, and education and experience of professional and clerical personnel.

The ratios are followed by a list of the characteristics that determine the actual recommended staffing levels within the given range that would be necessary to achieve "moderately managed" utilization benchmarks. The attributes do not address the budget limits, the competency of the staff, or an organization's philosophy as to the degree that medical care needs to be managed. The characteristics are presented in the same format as a starting point and adjusted based on the characteristics of a given attribute. The term *network*

refers to the provider delivery system including staff physicians, IPAs, and medical groups. No weight is given to the attribute categories.

Finally, there is a section that relates ratios to caseload levels and populations served. The ratios are given for pure commercial and Medicare populations as well as for combined populations based on the product mix. This will allow for further adjustment of the ratios based on caseloads, the percentage of the total management philosophy, and financial and strategic issues. This document is a guide and resource for determining an organization's staffing ratios. Management must arrive at the actual staffing levels on the basis of diverse factors including the local health care environment, management philosophy, and financial and strategic issues.

Case Management

The need for case management is driven by member needs rather than the characteristics of the delivery system. The staffing level is given for a health plan, but it can be applied to the provider organization (IPA/medical group) as well. The more knowledgeable and committed the providers are to managed care, the more likely they are to use case management resources.

	Maximum	Midpoint	Minimum
Medicare members	1,200	2,000	4,000
Commercial members	10,000	20,000	40,000

Attributes That Determine the Above Ratios

	Maximum	Midpoint	Minimum
Departmental attributes			
Clerical support	RNs do data entry	Some clerical support	1 clerk: 2 FTEs
Information systems	Completely manual system	Combined manual/ computer	Computerized tracking and reporting
Network attributes			
Primary care physician's relationship with health plan or network entity	Direct contract (IPA)	IPA with a single contract	Fully integrated group practice
Number of office sites	Patients served at single office site	4-8 office sites	>8 office sites
Geographic distribution of facilities	Within 10 miles	Within 10-15 minutes	>15 miles

Utilization Review Nurse and Medical Director

The staffing levels for these functions, as opposed to case management, are influenced significantly by the nature of the delivery system. The managed care sophistication of the physician network; the type of contracts and incentive programs in place, both within the network and with the health plan; and the medical management resources provided by the delivery system

all weigh heavily in the staffing levels required by the health plan.

The term *utilization review nurse* refers to all inpatient review functions. This combined role includes concurrent review and discharge planning and is the most common model currently used by health plans. The staffing levels required if the positions are separated are addressed in the final section. These figures include out-of-area utilization review.

Figure 10-1   Health plan medical management staffing. *IPA,* Independent practice association; *FTE,* full-time equivalent; *UM,* utilization management; *RN,* registered nurse; *DRG,* diagnosis-related group; *CM,* case manager.

Continued

Utilization Review Nurse (Includes Discharge Planning Function)—One FTE Per:

	Maximum	Midpoint	Minimum
Medicare members	2,000	3,600	10,000
Commercial members	8,000	25,000	50,000

Attributes That Determine the Above Ratios

Departmental attributes

	Maximum	Midpoint	Minimum
Clerical support	RNs do data entry	Some clerical support	1 clerk: 4 FTEs
Information systems	Completely manual system	Combined manual/ computer	Computerized tracking and reporting

Network attributes

	Maximum	Midpoint	Minimum
Degree of delegation of medical management activities to the provider organization	Health plan performs all functions	Some functions delegated	Most functions delegated
Primary care physician's relationship with health plan or network entity	Direct contract (IPA)	IPA with a single contract	Fully integrated group practice
Payment mechanism for specialty care	Discount fee-for-service	Global (case) rates	Risk sharing/ capitated
Provider organization's experience, commitment, and success with managed care	Minimal experience (<3 years)	Some experience (3-5 years)	Leaders in the field
Profits	Losses in the past	Break even—minimal profits	Meeting projected net income
Patients in managed care	<15%	15%-40%	>40%
Provider organization staff licensed staff committed to medical management	None	Part-time staff	Dedicated RNs for UR and CM
Hospital payment mechanism	DRG or global risk/ capitated	Per diem	Shared
Incentive potential for physicians as percentage of total reimbursement by the health plan	None (profit or loss)	<20% (profit or loss)	≥ 20% profit or loss
Geographic location of facilities	Patients primarily at a single facility	2-4 facilities	>4 facilities

Medical Director—One FTE Per:

	Maximum	Midpoint	Minimum
Medicare members	4,000	8,000	15,000
Commercial members	16,000	50,000	100,000

Attributes That Determine the Above Ratios

Network attributes

	Maximum	Midpoint	Minimum
Degree of delegation of medical management activities to provider organization	Health plan performs all functions	Some functions delegated	Most functions delegated
Primary care physician's relationship with health plan or network entity	Direct contract (IPA)	IPA with a single contract	Fully integrated group practice
Payment mechanism for specialty care	Discount fee-for-service	Global (case) rates	Risk sharing/ capitated

Figure 10-1, cont'd

Medical Director—One FTE Per:

	Maximum—Cont'd	Midpoint—Cont'd	Minimum—Cont'd
Provider organization's experience, commitment, and success with managed care	Minimal experience (<3 years)	Some experience (3-5 years)	Leaders in the field
Profits	Losses in the past	Break even—minimal profits	Meeting projected net income
Patients in managed care	<15%	15%-40%	>40%
Physician organization medical director activities	No medical director	Advisory or retroactive review only	Active in all management functions
Physician organization UM committee	None	Advisory or retrospective review only	Active in all UM functions
Department chair or other physician leadership (UM committee chair) involvement within the physician organization	None	Figure head only	Active involvement with all UM processes including determining incentive bonuses
Hospital payment mechanism	DRG or global	Per diem	Shared risk/capitated
Incentive potential for physicians as percentage of total reimbursement by the health plan	No profit or loss	<20% profit or loss	≥ 20% profit or loss

Additional Calculations for Determining Staffing Needs

	POPULATION SERVED		
Parameter	Medicare Only	Commercial Only	Total Population (Based on Mix)
Case Management			
Percentage of patient population	25%	75%	
Average length of time patient is in case management	72 days	80 days	78 days
% of members in case management in a given year	10%	1.00%	3.3%
Active patients per CM	50	50	50
Members per CM	2,500	22,000	7,200
Utilization Review			
Percentage of population	25%	75%	
Acute bed days per 1000 members per year	1,200	200	
Acute census per concurrent review RN	28	32	30
Members per concurrent review RN	6,800	52,000	41,000
Acute census per discharge planner RN	18	28	25
Member per discharge planner	4,500	45,000	35,000
Member per FTE if concurrent review and discharge planning done separately	2,700	24,000	19,000
Acute census for single position performing combined duties: concurrent review and discharge planning RN	15	25	20
Members per utilization review RN performing combined functions of concurrent review and discharge planning	3,500	30,000	23,000

Figure 10-1, cont'd

Table 10-1 shows the differences between utilization and case management processes in a managed care setting. The ultimate goal of utilization management is to maintain the quality of health care delivery by keeping the patient at the appropriate level of care, coordinating all existing health care policy benefits and community resources, and holding costs to a minimum.

"The overall goal of case management is to produce a service delivery approach to (a) ensure cost-effective care, (b) provide alternatives to institutionalization, (c) provide access to care, (d) coordinate service, and (e) improve the patient's functional capacity."[1] In addition, according to the American Nurses Association, among the goals of case management are to "provide quality along a continuum, decrease fragmentation of care across many settings, enhance the quality of life and contain cost."[1]

If the health care organization employs both a utilization management nurse and a case manager, it is very important for the two parties to spend time familiarizing each other with their respective job functions. (See job descriptions in Boxes 10-1 through 10-4.) This process not only helps

TABLE 10-1
Utilization Management Versus Case Management

Utilization Management	Case Management
Begins when the patient arrives for care.	Uses proactive screening to identify the high-risk patient *before* care is accessed.
Focuses on the care episode.	Focuses on the continuum of care.
Focuses on a large number of patients at a low level of intensity.	Focuses on a small percentage of high-risk/high-cost patients at a high level of intensity.
Assesses benefit eligibility, medical necessity, and level of care via prior authorization, concurrent, and retrospective reviews.	Collaborates with utilization management in case finding and facilitates the development and implementation of a comprehensive, interdisciplinary treatment plan focused on the ambulatory setting.

BOX 10-1
Job Description for Concurrent Review/Discharge Planning Case Manager

Position Objective and Purpose
The concurrent review/discharge planning case manager manages the inpatient utilization of health care resources and develops, coordinates, and implements the discharge plan in an effort to ensure that the coordination and continuity of care result in optimal patient outcomes.

Position Responsibilities
- Validates all inpatient admissions for appropriate level of care within 24 hours of admission
- Develops and documents a discharge plan for each inpatient within 24 hours of admission
- On a daily basis or as appropriate, concurrently reviews all inpatient care, on-site or telephonically, to validate appropriateness of services, lengths of stay, and levels of care, using nationally recognized guidelines, protocols, and critical pathways including, but not limited to, InterQual and Milliman and Robertson
- Develops, monitors, modifies, and implements individualized transfer or discharge plans to ensure a timely discharge between levels of care and between facilities

Continued

BOX 10-1

Job Description for Concurrent Review/Discharge Planning Case Manager—cont'd

- Communicates regularly with the attending physician/medical group/IPA/hospital staffs regarding the patient's status, any identified problems related to appropriateness of services, quality of care, or issues that may prevent a timely discharge
- Confers with the medical director daily regarding patient- and physician-related issues and refers appropriate problems to the medical director for intervention and resolution
- Performs concurrent quality review and reports identified quality issues to the health plan's and hospital's quality improvement departments
- Initiates immediate postdischarge referral authorizations for ambulatory care
- Initiates referrals to ambulatory case management using the health plan's criteria for referrals
- Researches community resources available to members, assesses the financial implications of a specific discharge plan, and develops a plan to most appropriately access those resources as well as covered benefits
- Identifies aberrant inpatient days and documents, codes, and reports the data to the utilization management data entry coordinator
- Captures required inpatient utilization data and forwards the information, on a daily basis, to the utilization management data entry coordinator

Minimum Position Qualifications

- Current in-state RN license
- Bachelor's degree in business or equivalent in a health care–related field
- Five years' clinical acute care hospital experience: intensive care unit, emergency department, surgical department
- One to 3 years' experience in a managed care, health services setting
- Strong interpersonal skills
- Excellent verbal and written communication skills
- Independence and ability to be a self-starter
- Ability to analyze and problem solve
- Familiarity with state and federal governmental regulations and national accrediting agency requirements
- Ability to work flexible schedules including weekends and holidays
- Current state driver's license and ability to commute to various facilities on any given day within 25 miles of the worksite office

to clarify roles but also assists these individuals in gaining an appreciation and understanding of each other, the duties required of each, and the daily problems encountered by each that present roadblocks to performing job responsibilities in a timely manner. Any such roadblocks can represent critical issues for the health plan and/or provider in terms of liability; compliance with the requirements of federal, state, and accrediting agencies; and implementation of an effective discharge or case management plan.

Utilization management has certain limitations, and it is these "limitations" that make it an efficient process. For instance, it would be inefficient to use one-to-one, labor-intensive case management in every case when "data show that even as far back as 1928, the top 5% of health spenders account for more than half of aggregate health expenditures; the top 30% account for 90% of expenditures. Consistently over the past 25 years, half of the U.S. population consumes only 3% of all health care resources"[2] and only "10% of the over 65 year olds account for 70% of the older population's total health care costs."[3]

Utilization management employs many tools to ensure that the majority of patients who receive health care services experience

BOX 10-2
Job Description for Ambulatory Case Manager

Position Objective and Purpose

The ambulatory case manager proactively identifies and assesses high-risk/high-utilization patients and develops and implements a coordinated treatment plan, in collaboration with the primary care physician, resulting in a documented cost-effective, quality treatment outcomes focused in the ambulatory setting.

Position Responsibilities

- Reviews screening tools, claims information, urgent and emergency department reports, acute inpatient census, referrals, and other appropriate data to initiate follow-up care and develop individualized treatment plans incorporating assessment, education, resource planning, and coordination of services for patients accepted into the case management program
- Facilitates the development and implementation of a multidisciplinary treatment plan and monitors the effectiveness incrementally with defined, measurable goals and cost-benefit documentation
- Performs a liaison function for the physician by consistently communicating any modifications to the treatment plan to all participating disciplines and coordinates appropriate information that must be communicated to the patient and family
- Maintains documentation of individual case management plans, interventions, cost-benefit analyses, and other statistics as needed, to demonstrate the clinical quality outcomes and cost-effective financial impact of case management
- Chairs meetings, as appropriate, with the multidisciplinary team, primary care physician, and other participating personnel to update all relevant team members regarding the patient's status and the need for any modification to the treatment plan
- Initiates case conferences with the patient and family as necessary and coordinates the participation of appropriate multidisciplinary team members
- Delegates and coordinates activities of the case management clerk
- Performs all other duties normally associated with this position or as defined by an immediate superior

Minimum Position Qualifications

- Current in-state RN license
- BSN (preferred) or equivalent experience in or related to case management in the acute, ambulatory, home health, or managed care setting
- Excellent verbal, written, and interpersonal communication skills
- Current state driver's license and vehicle available to drive for work between several locations
- Ability to work independently and make appropriate decisions within the realm of nursing practice and judgment
- Computer literacy with knowledge of Microsoft Word, Excel, and Access programs

optimal outcomes, and these tools should not be confused with case management itself. While these tools are also used by case managers, other members of the health care team may also employ them without referral to the case management department.

Examples of some effective utilization management tools that need to be distinguished from case management per se are the following: (1) referral to educational classes to teach patients to manage chronic illness (e.g., diabetes, asthma, hypertension); (2) authorization of alternative health care in the sense of coordinating and providing a noncovered benefit to prevent the need for a more expensive covered benefit (e.g., authorizing the use of a temporary caregiver in the home in certain instances to avoid admission to an acute-care hospital or skilled nursing facility for primarily "social" reasons); (3) referral of the frail elderly for an interdisciplinary geriatric assessment to assist in directing the care of these individuals, only a minority of whom will require ongoing formal case management; and (4) implementation of clinical tracking systems, which are

---

BOX 10-3
Job Description for Director of Ambulatory Case Management

Position Objective and Purpose

The director of ambulatory case management, in collaboration with the medical director(s) and the director of utilization, is responsible for the proactive identification and management of the high-risk population that uses the majority of health care services and dollars and for implementing programs and processes to manage this population's health care in the most cost-efficient manner, resulting in optimal quality treatment outcomes focused in the ambulatory setting. This includes all staffing and activities involved in the screening and identification of the high-risk membership, health care assessments, problem identification, treatment plan development and implementation, evaluation, report generation, and state and federal regulatory and accreditation program compliance.

Position Responsibilities

- Assumes a leadership role, in collaboration with the medical director(s), in the direction, monitoring, and support of the ambulatory case management staff
- Interviews, hires, evaluates, counsels, and terminates employees
- Identifies opportunities for improvement and provides additional orientation and skill development on an ongoing basis
- Ensures that all department functions are staffed appropriately and that all departmental processes are completed in a timely and accurate manner on a regular basis
- Develops and participates in the new employee orientation process internally and assists the provider relations person in the new and ongoing orientation of contracted vendors
- Maintains regularly scheduled meetings with the medical staff, including on-on-one scheduled, individual meetings with managers and supervisors
- Participates in all internal quality improvement plans, programs, and activities
- Along with the appropriate persons and committees, develops standards for quality of care and service and monitors and reviews statistical data to identify aberrant trends and coordinates and monitors corrective actions
- Oversees the generation of reports for submission to appropriate government agencies, health plan–participating providers, and internal management

Minimum Position Qualifications

- Current in-state RN license
- MBA or equivalent in a related field
- Case manager certification from the Case Management Society of America
- Five to 10 years' management experience in a managed care, health services setting
- Excellent verbal and written communication skills
- Ability to analyze and problem solve
- Familiarity with federal and state governmental health care regulations and accrediting agency requirements
- Ability to conduct departmental activities in a confidential, educational, and nonthreatening manner
- Current state driver's license and ability to commute to various facilities on any given day
- Computer literacy with knowledge of Microsoft Word, Excel, and Access programs

---

algorithms to respond to abnormal laboratory and radiographic findings (e.g., seeing a patient step by step through a timely and appropriate workup in response to an abnormal mammogram result).

All of these tools are very important in managing finite health care resources to meet the infinite needs of the patient population, but none in and of itself is case management. These tools support the process, however, and often obviate the necessity to resort to formal case management.

Historically, what we might call basic utilization management has been provided by the primary care physician and by the physician's team, traditionally the physician's office staff. The primary care

---

BOX 10-4
Job Description for Director of Utilization

Position Objective and Purpose
The director of utilization, in collaboration with the medical director(s), is responsible for planning, developing and implementing all medical management programs and processes and, in conjunction with the medical director(s), is responsible for daily medical management operations that are consistent with the strategic, operational, and budgetary goals approved by the board of directors. This includes all staffing and activities related to referral and prior authorization, concurrent review, discharge planning, retrospective claims review, report generation, and state and federal regulatory and accreditation program compliance.

Position Responsibilities
- Assumes a leadership role, in collaboration with the medical director(s), in the direction, monitoring, and support of the medical management staff
- Interviews, hires, evaluates, counsels, and terminates employees
- Identifies opportunities for improvement and provides additional orientation and skill development on an ongoing basis
- Ensures that all department functions are staffed appropriately and that all departmental processes are completed in a timely and accurate manner on a regular basis
- Develops and participates in the new employee orientation process internally and assists the provider relations person in the new and ongoing orientation of contracted vendors
- Participates in the development of all managed care contracts and service standards
- Maintains regularly scheduled meetings with the medical staff, including one-on-one scheduled, individual meetings with managers and supervisors
- Participates in all internal quality improvement plans, programs, and activities
- Develops, implements, and reviews the quality improvement and utilization management plans and programs annually and revises them as needed to ensure that all applicable governmental and accrediting agencies' regulations are met or exceeded.
- Coordinates the medical management governmental and accrediting agencies' on-site reviews
- With the appropriate persons and committees, develops standards for quality of care and service and monitors and reviews statistical data to identify aberrant trends and coordinates and monitors corrective actions
- Oversees the generation of reports for submission to appropriate government agencies, health plan–participating providers, and internal management
- Along with the medical director, co-chairs the utilization management committee and actively participates in the quality improvement committee.

Minimum Position Qualifications
- Current in-state RN license
- MBA or equivalent in a related field
- Five to 10 years' management experience in a managed care, health services setting
- Excellent verbal and written communication skills
- Ability to analyze and problem solve
- Familiarity with federal and state governmental health care regulations and accrediting agency requirements
- Ability to conduct departmental activities in a confidential, educational, and nonthreatening manner
- Current state driver's license and ability to commute to various facilities on any given day
- Computer literacy with knowledge of Microsoft Word, Excel, and Access programs

---

team, however, is appropriately focused on ordering diagnostic workups and prescribing treatments for the patient's medical problems, and not on addressing complicated issues of compliance and costs. The severity and complexity of both chronic and acute illnesses in an aging population have necessitated the development of a specialized body of knowledge in utilization and case management. These skill sets supplement those of the primary care team in accomplishing the best results for the patient, provider, and payer.

Patients requiring the one-to-one intensive services of a case manager fortunately constitute a distinct minority of any population—1% to 2% of those younger than 65 years and 5% to 10% of those older than 65 years, depending on the diagnosis, cost, and utilization triggers that are implemented as criteria for referral to case management. Other less needy patients can be given the extra boost they need by use of some of the tools of utilization management.

In summary, utilization management mobilizes the organization's available resources and coordinates them to ensure that eligible patients receive effective health care benefits in a timely manner by an appropriate provider in an appropriate setting.

Formalized case management, on the other hand, is an intensive resource employing the personal services of a case manager working individually with a physician or physicians, patient, and family. Both utilization management and case management support the patient so that the therapeutic regimen of the primary care team can be implemented.

CASE MANAGEMENT AS INTENSIVE CARE UNIT

As more health care organizations "down size," utilization management may be shifted to the case management department or vice versa. When this happens, little thought may be given to the qualifications and knowledge needed by case managers to function effectively. Unfortunately, when a shift in duties occurs, one or the other process may suffer.

True case management, if it is to achieve the outcomes desired, is a labor-intensive process. It requires a vast knowledge not only of clinical medicine and treatment modalities but also of commu-

nity resources, alternate funding programs, standards of care, and alternate treatment settings outside the acute-care hospital. In all cases, action must be taken immediately if problems arise; solution of these problems cannot wait until the hospital nurse case manager or utilization reviewer has completed his or her duties. In today's litigious society, too much is at stake for the case manager and the organization if problems are not dealt with immediately.

To understand the relationship between case management and utilization management, it may be helpful to compare these two functions with the different kinds of hospital nursing. In this comparison, case management is equivalent to the intensive care unit and utilization review to the general medical-surgical unit. As we know, each unit requires a different level of expertise, with medical-surgical nursing being more generalized and critical care nursing more specialized. Nurses in both areas function similarly, but they have different emphases. The same statement is true of utilization management and case management.

Senior managers of health care organizations, like those in hospitals, must realize that case managers must have more expertise if the goals of case management are to be reached and costs contained. To achieve these goals, case managers must have the ability and flexibility to see patients and to become involved with them as events unfold. Hospital general-duty nurses do not just read charts and talk on the phone without seeing the patient—they are actively involved with all aspects of care. The same thing occurs with case managers. Unlike hospital nurses, however, case managers are not providing hands-on nursing care and are frequently operating at "arm's length" in a health plan, independent practice association (IPA), or medical group. They must be able to visualize the actual care if the patient is to be linked appropriately with available resources. Therefore, on-site assessments are strongly advised unless the patient is well known to the case manager and is, or has recently been, part of an active case load.

In the absence of an on-site assessment, it is critical that the case manager have a collaborative working relationship with the hospital utilization review and discharge planning staff. An initial and ongoing accurate, detailed assessment of the patient's clinical progress and a comprehensive, well-understood and well-coordinated discharge plan must be communicated to all participants—the patient, family, physician(s), hospital, health plan, and any ancillary providers. Such communication will decrease the likelihood of the patient's returning to the emergency department shortly after discharge because services that were medically necessary were never received.

CASE MANAGEMENT INVOLVING TWO ENTITIES

When two entities are involved, one providing utilization management and the other case management, or when one case manager is facility based and the other is employed by a non–facility-based organization (e.g., health care payer, IPA or medical group, or home health agency), two major problems can occur. These are (1) lack of timely sharing of information, which results in delays in implementation of care, and (2) inappropriate delays in case identification or referral.[4]

The earlier the intervention occurs and the case is referred and opened to case management, the greater the opportunities for success. If more than one case manager and one utilization reviewer are involved, it is important for case managers to establish good working relationships with all team members and to educate the referral sources about the importance of early referral and timely sharing of information.

Referral Flags or Triggers

Most health care payers and case management organizations use some form of flagging system that triggers cases at any point in the review process for referral to case management. Depending on the type of case management organization, most referrals originate from several sources. Once the program education process is completed and there is a heightened awareness of its presence, the most common referral sources are primary care physicians and their office staff, utilization and quality management personnel, claims processing staff, hospital admission and discharge planning personnel, and home health agency staff.

These referral sources, as well as certain other key departments in the health care organization, must be educated about the following:

- What the referral or trigger flags are.
- How the referral information is to be communicated (formally or informally, by phone or in writing) and to whom.
- What type of information is required and how much time should elapse from the time of identification for referral and the resulting assessment by the case manager to determine whether the patient is accepted for case management; acceptance is based on whether the patient meets the diagnostic, cost, or utilization criteria as well as on whether the cooperation of the patient, family, and attending physician is obtained in the development and implementation of the treatment plan.

It is important to continue the internal and external education and awareness processes semiannually to ensure that referral sources are aware of the effectiveness of the case management program from the perspective of quality of care and financial savings, and to educate new personnel who are hired due to normal employee attrition.

If utilization management and case management are offered by the same organization, the various departments in that organization must be educated about the different goals and emphases of these two functions. This education should consist not only of basic knowledge regarding the job duties of each but also of information on typical cases, diagnoses, and costs, and the value of an integrated system and case management approach. Some of the best cases to present during such educational sessions are those that arrived at case management too late; examples of these case outcomes can be contrasted with the outcomes of similar cases that were managed successfully.

Just as important as early referrals and a flagging system is open, honest, and frequent communication between the utilization management staff, the case management staff, and the health care team. The simple task of communication is the critical link if all departments are to function as a team. To foster this process, weekly staff meetings in which all participants can compare notes and share pertinent information are an excellent modality. These meetings must include the patients' attending physicians, participating in person, by phone, or by e-mail or faxed report.

If communication is not open and frequent, disastrous outcomes and a crisis atmosphere can ensue. For example, the concurrent utilization review staff may not approve the extension of an inpatient stay, yet unforeseen barriers may surface that preclude a patient's safe discharge. What happens? The patient or family may receive an unnecessary letter of denial and file an appeal, whereupon the denial is overturned. Thus, the patient and family (and often the entire health care team as well) endure a crisis situation for nothing.

Although case management is a variant of utilization management, the processes are totally different, and each discipline requires different types of expertise. Utilization management is designed to monitor service delivery for benefit eligibility and to interpret benefits, medical necessity, and appropriateness of care. In contrast, case management is designed to coordinate the patient's care over the continuum with the appropriate providers and resources, and to monitor the patient's treatment plan to ensure that high-quality care with optimal outcomes is rendered. The processes are essential to one another, and the ultimate goal for both is high-quality, cost-effective care. The need for education, early referrals, and excellent communication cannot be overemphasized.

UTILIZATION MANAGEMENT PROCESSES

Although this manual is not intended for utilization reviewers, the various types of utilization review and some of the criteria used for such reviews are worth mentioning. In most organizations and regulatory and accrediting agencies, utilization management is closely related to quality improvement or performance. Both utilization management and quality improvement rely on review of individual medical records to evaluate and analyze the relationship between the patient's need for medical services and the services actually received. Whereas utilization management focuses on the appropriateness and efficiency of care and its costs, quality improvement focuses on the effectiveness of the services provided as well as on the qualifications of the providers who actually rendered the services. Three types of review function are included in utilization management:

Prospective (also known as precertification or prior authorization)—the review that occurs before elective or urgent services are rendered

Concurrent—the review that occurs while the services are being rendered

Retrospective—the review that occurs after the services or treatments have been rendered[5,6]

Utilization review can be broken down even further into four categories—what, when, where, and how much. For instance, when review is conducted (prospectively, concurrently, or retrospectively), the reviewer is looking for answers to the following questions:

- What type of care is or was required?
- Is or was the patient eligible for the care?
- Is or was the care a covered benefit?
- Is or was there a limitation or maximum to the benefit coverage?
- Where was or will the care be provided—does or did the patient require inpatient care or outpatient care, or care in an alternate setting? Also, for inpatient care, was the care provided (or will it be provided) in a general care facility or a center of excellence or tertiary care facility?
- When is or was the care provided? What are or were the dates of service?
- How much care is or was provided, and is it appropriate, as a covered benefit, for the diagnosis in terms of duration, types of care, and frequency? Also included in this category is an estimation of quality compliance in assessing whether services were overutilized or underutilized.

When an organization denies coverage on the basis of lack of medical necessity, the determination must be made by a physician who has expertise in the field of medicine that is appropriate for the services at issue but who need not, in all cases, be of the same specialty or subspecialty as the treating physician.[7,8] The rationale for the determination must be clearly documented and must be made available to the provider upon request in compliance with the requirements of federal, state, and accrediting agencies.

Prospective Utilization Review

Prospective utilization review for both inpatient and outpatient services is defined by contractual arrangements through benefit design. The request for authorization of services should clearly state the following:

- Patient's demographic information
- History and clinical findings
- Diagnosis
- Purpose of the requested service
- Results of diagnostic tests and evaluations conducted to date

The prospective review includes the following:

- Eligibility confirmation
- Benefit level interpretation and verification
- Coordination of benefits
- Identification of benefit limitations or exclusions
- Review of medical information by health care professionals using standard criteria, protocols, or guidelines as defined by the health plan and/or IPA or medical group
- Authorization and referral to an appropriate provider and/or facility within a period that is consistent with the urgency of the patient's condition in compliance with the requirements of federal, state, and accrediting agencies

Federal regulations specify that emergency services do not require any prospective authorization and that retrospective claims review for payment eligibility must use a "prudent layperson" definition of an emergency in the approval-denial process as specified by Medicare and many state regulatory agencies.

Concurrent Utilization Review

Concurrent reviews are performed to ensure the following:

- That the patient is admitted to an appropriate facility at an appropriate level of care using standardized criteria for intensity of service and severity of illness.
- That the treatment plan is appropriate.
- That the continued stay and level of care are appropriate.
- That discharge planning has begun within 24 hours of admission. Frequently, the positions of concurrent review specialist and discharge planning specialist are combined, and one person performs both functions (see Figure 10-1).

This review process also acts as a concurrent case-finding vehicle for quality-of-care issues that allows real-time intervention and corrective action. Acute-care hospital reviews to determine appropriate level of care and treatment plan should be initiated within 24 hours of admission. The discharge plan assessment should be completed within 24 hours of admission. Ongoing review should take place as frequently as the patient's condition dictates. The review is conducted by utilization review nurses with referral to the medical director or physician reviewer as necessary. Should a patient meet the case management criteria, a referral is made to case management and the utilization review and discharge planning nurse works collaboratively with the case manager in developing and implementing a comprehensive discharge plan. Upon discharge, the case manager continues coordinating the patient's care in compliance with the physician's treatment regimen and in concurrence with the patient and family.

The inpatient facility review should include, but is not limited to, the following:

- Verification of health plan and benefit eligibility
- Prospective authorization of elective admissions
- Where appropriate, communication of an estimated length of stay to the attending physician, facility, and patient prospectively or within 24 hours of admission
- Review of appropriate level of care within 24 hours of admission
- Completion of discharge planning assessment within 24 hours of admission
- Ongoing review for appropriate level of care congruent with the severity of the patient's condition using standardized intensity-of-service and severity-of-illness criteria
- Appropriate same-day intervention when an inappropriate level of care or service is identified
- Designation of an aberrant day when a lack of care or inappropriate level of care and/or service is identified (Figure 10-2)
- Issuance of a denial letter the same day when a specific level of care is deemed to be no longer justified
- Routing of patients inappropriately admitted through the emergency department to a skilled nursing facility, home health care, or observation as indicated
- Referral to an ambulatory case management program as appropriate
- Forwarding of the discharge plan to physician as appropriate

Out-of-Plan and Out-of-Area Requirements

The patient's care should be reviewed as frequently as the patient's condition dictates, over the phone or on site if the out-of-plan facility is within traveling distance and there are questions regarding the appropriate level of care. Level of care,

Patient name:_____ Patient ID:_____

No. of aberrant bed days:_____

Admission date:_____

Facility:_____

Authorization No.:_____ Physician:_____

UR nurse:_____ Case manager:_____

Comments:_____
_____
_____
_____

Aberrant day (date)	Aberrant reason code (A-C)	Actual level of care (1-8)	Level of care proposed (1-8)	Action code (A-K)
1.___	( )	( )	( )	( )
2.___	( )	( )	( )	( )
3.___	( )	( )	( )	( )
4.___	( )	( )	( )	( )
5.___	( )	( )	( )	( )
6.___	( )	( )	( )	( )

Physician related
A02—Patient not meeting SI/IS criteria
A03—SNF level of care
A04—Physican service delay
A05—On-call physician refuses to discharge patient
A06—Physician refuses to discharge patient

Action code: avoided aberrant day
A—Patient discharged home
B—Patient discharged to SNF
C—Patient discharged home with home health care
D—Transferred to appropriate level of care
E—Denial letter issued

Facility related
B01—Diagnostic service delay
B02—Discharge plan service delay
B03—Surgical service delay
B04—Transfer bed not available
B05—Preoperative days
B06—Benefits exhausted
B07—Noncontracted facility

Action code: did not avoid aberrant day
F—Denial letter issued
G—Physician determined patient meets acute or SNF criteria
H—Delay in determination by physician
J—No action
K—Attending physician did not agree with plan

Social issue related
C01—Patient homeless
C02—Patient refuses transfer discharge
C03—Patient refuses treatment
C04—Family unavailable

Level of care
1—ICU
2—Telemetry
3—Medical/surgical
4—Obstetrics
5—SNF
6—Rehabilitation
7—Home
8—Custodial

Figure 10-2 Aberrant day report. *UR,* Utilization review; *SNF,* skilled nursing facility; *SI/IS,* severity-of-illness and intensity-of-service; *ICU,* intensive care unit.

intensity of services, estimated transfer date, and transfer arrangements should be reviewed and documented with an appropriate time line.

Each organization that conducts utilization review has its own set of criteria and its own methods of conducting the review.[5] Many organizations perform reviews using on-site techniques and actual examination of the patient's medical records. Others conduct the review by telephone, requesting only selected portions of the patient's medical record when questions arise.

Although many organizations use review techniques such as those employed by Medicare, others use explicit criteria developed either internally in specific policies and procedures or by recognized experts in review techniques. Possibly the best-known and most widely used criteria are those developed by Medicare. Another source of nationally recognized, standardized criteria is InterQual, which developed the original criteria in 1978 and has revised them frequently since that time. Until recently, InterQual's criteria were designed strictly for inpatient services and left a void when it came to outpatient services and care. Fortunately, this void has now been filled, and InterQual offers level-of-care criteria for acute, subacute, skilled nursing, and long-term care, and for rehabilitation, home care, and behavioral health. Their care planning criteria cover procedures, imaging, specialty referral, workers' compensation, rehabilitation and chiropractic, and retrospective review.

The InterQual criteria are designed to determine whether the level of care is appropriate by evaluating the intensity of the services provided and the severity of the illness. If patient care fails to meet the relevant criteria, the reviewer moves to the criteria used for discharge. These criteria are referred to as intensity–severity–discharge appropriateness criteria. Basically, they pertain to the intensity of the service, the severity of the illness, the stability of the patient for discharge, and the appropriateness of the current or proposed level of care. If the patient meets the criteria for intensity of services and severity of illness, admission to or continued stay at a specific level of care can be approved. If not, the patient's admission or continued stay is denied, and discharge or transfer to an appropriate level of care is expected. In all cases, the appropriateness of the level of care (e.g., care in specialty units) continues to be assessed as frequently as the patient's condition warrants and/or available staffing levels allow (Figures 10-3 through 10-5).

Still another source of criteria is Milliman and Robertson's Healthcare Management Guidelines. In contrast to the InterQual criteria, Milliman Care Guidelines focus on the appropriate services for specific days of a hospital stay as defined by diagnoses and/or procedures. Such criteria are especially useful in training utilization review staff because they offer prompts regarding what should be happening clinically in a "best-case" scenario, on a daily basis, and focus inquiries about potential adverse outcomes or quality-of-care issues when specific services are not taking place within the specified time.

In some organizations, a combination of review techniques may be used. For example, the organization may use its own review techniques or criteria in combination with review criteria from various and specifically selected length-of-stay manuals.

In many organizations clinical pathways or "best practice guidelines" are taking on new importance as a review tool. Clinical pathways are very similar to Milliman Care Guidelines and are a management tool that proactively depicts important events and all the interdisciplinary aspects of patient care that should take place on a daily basis. Throughout the patient's entire stay, key events change daily, as the patient is moved toward discharge. The overall goal is to achieve high-quality care by paying continuous concurrent attention to variances, minimizing delays, and maximizing the use of resources. Departures from these standard events or aspects of patient care should be documented with a focus on the outcome of care, which is integral to the quality-improvement process when the pathways are evaluated and updated.

Regardless of the criteria used for review, the results of utilization review are contingent on such factors as the medical care process, patient variables, inaccuracies

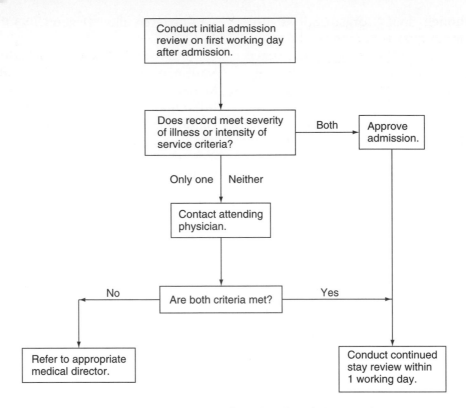

Figure 10-3 Cyclic review flow chart for admission review.

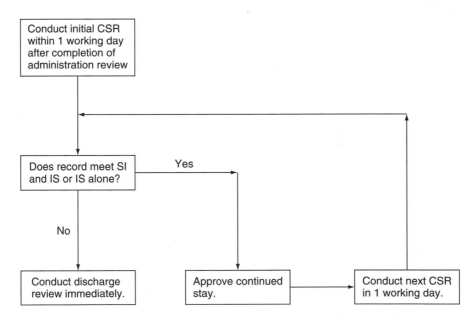

Figure 10-4 Cyclic review flow chart for continued stay review *(CSR)*. *SI*, Severity of illness; *IS*, intensity of service.

in the medical record, and differences in practice patterns of physicians in various regions. Results vary depending on the scope and depth of review performed and the availability and level of expertise of the staff.

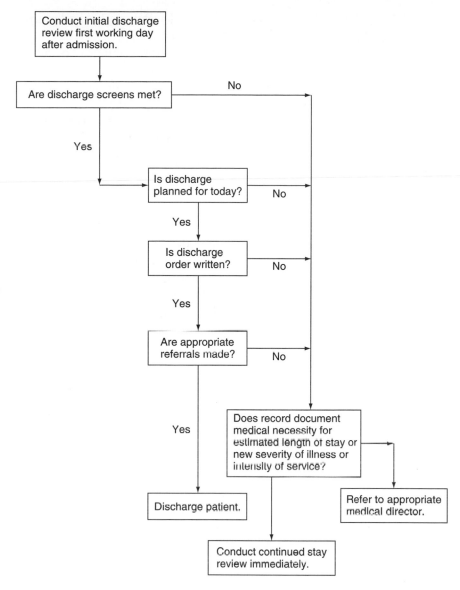

Figure 10-5   Cyclic review flow chart for discharge review.

Levels of Review

Utilization review, whether accomplished internally or externally, by telephone or outsourcing, is generally conducted by professional nurses using one or more set of criteria for review. This is called first-level review. The nurses review for benefit eligibility, medical necessity, appropriateness of care, place of service, quality of care, and overutilization or underutilization. Their job is to approve services and/or length of stay. Any review findings that do not meet criteria and require further review are forwarded to a physician who has "expertise in the field of medicine that is appropriate for the services at issue but need not, in all cases, be of the same specialty or subspecialty as the treating physician."[7,8]

EFFECTIVE INDIVIDUAL CASE UTILIZATION REVIEW FORMAT

There is nothing more unproductive or frustrating to a medical director or physician advisor than having to discuss an individual case with someone who is not prepared with the relevant details or who takes an inordinately long time to review the issues of a case. An effective individual utilization case review should take no longer than 1 to 2 minutes per patient. The following five pieces of information provide a standardized format that gives structure to the daily or weekly utilization report:

1. Patient's name, age, and gender
2. Date of and reason for admission to the facility
3. Rationale for *acute* level of care *today* (intensity of service)
4. Discharge plan and estimated length of stay
5. Appropriateness of a "yes" answer to the following question: "Is it unreasonable for anyone in this clinical situation to be cared for at a lower level of care or on an outpatient basis?"

Frequently, utilization functions such as utilization review, discharge planning, and case management are combined within a given facility, IPA or medical group or health plan. There are many factors that influence the staffing ratios when any or all of these positions are combined (see Figure 10-1).

Since federal and state regulations prohibit nurses from denying services, denials are always generated from a second-level review, and that review is normally conducted by the medical director (Box 10-5)

BOX 10-5
Job Description for Medical Director

Position Objective and Purpose
The medical director provides leadership and clinical expertise to the medical management department and is responsible for coordinating all aspects of the overall health services delivery system. The medical director also ensures optimal performance of the health care provider network in terms of quality of care and service by integrating the needs of the members and the providers into the vision, mission, and goals of the health plan.

Position Responsibilities
- Administers the medical management program as it relates to members and providers of health care and participates in ongoing program review and refinement, which includes precertification, concurrent and retrospective review, case management, and quality management and improvement processes
- Recruits and leads community providers in the development of clinical and service standards and "best practice" guidelines to foster continuous quality improvement in health care delivery
- Participates in the strategic planning and development of new programs, products, and services in the areas of health service delivery, member education, support services, quality improvement activities, marketing activities, and provider education
- Participates, on an ongoing basis, in the identification, development, and implementation of programs, processes, and systems to support the following:
  - Utilization/quality management
  - Provider performance profiling
  - Communication
  - Provider network development
  - Provider information and practice management
  - Medical criteria/guidelines/clinical pathways
  - Provider education

Continued

BOX 10-5
Job Description for Medical Director—cont'd

- Works collaboratively with team members and participates in necessary activities to meet regulatory and accrediting agency compliance requirements
- Manages all aspects of cost-efficient, quality health care through participative and active interventional utilization and quality management including but not limited to the following:
  - Inpatient utilization (on-site and by telephone)
  - Referral authorizations
  - Retrospective review of claims
  - Case management
  - Staff and network provider educational programs
- Administers credentialing program functions, processes, policies, and procedures
- Oversees provider performance and outcomes analysis, provides feedback, and initiates and monitors action plans congruent with the quality improvement process
- Oversees and facilitates medical criteria, guidelines, and clinical pathway development, implementation, and dissemination
- Participates in contract negotiations and provides medical expertise related to the understanding of contractual rates and nuances and their impact on health care costs
- Works with health care providers and medical management staff in the development of alternative, innovative, cost-effective treatment options and programs
- Identifies new technology and initiates a formal, multidisciplinary assessment to determine plan coverage
- Work collaboratively with the medical management and senior management staff
- Assists the provider relations department through active participation in all management functions, including but not limited to the following:
  - Recruiting
  - Educational sessions
  - Problem solving
  - Data analysis and interpretation
- In collaboration with provider relations, manages those aspects of health care delivery that affect member services, quality of care, cost-effectiveness, and community relations
- Ensures that provider educational needs are met in an organized and systematic manner
- Participates in committees as needed
- Participates in special projects and organizational activities as needed
- Coordinates schedules to ensure adequate support of the medical management program
- Pursues professional and personal educational enhancement for continuous improvement of managerial skills

Minimum Position Requirements*
- A thorough understanding of all aspects of managed care, including HMOs, PHOs, risk arrangements, capitation, peer review, performance profiling, outcome management, practice guideline development and application, pharmacy management, credentialing, and risk management, as well as a comprehensive background in utilization and quality management
- Excellent interpersonal, marketing, verbal, and written communication skills
- Proven ability in a medical leadership position possessing clinical credibility with peers and the ability to be a team player and a team builder
- Flexibility and ability to prioritize day-to-day position requirements including but not limited to the ability to drive a car and be mobile to deliver verbal presentations at various locations
- Continuous quality improvement experience demonstrating an ability to analyze physician profiles and outcome data and effectively communicate results, producing positive changes in physician performance
- Commitment to a successful long-term career in medical management with 3 to 5 years' experience as a medical director in an HMO setting preferred
- Experience with Medicare + Choice, commercial, and Medicaid products preferred
- Five years of nonsupervised clinical practice with 1 year of management training
- Board certification in a specialty primary care preferred

*The statements in this job description are intended to describe the general nature and level of work being performed by people assigned to this job. They are not intended to be an exhaustive list of all responsibilities, duties, and skills required of the incumbent in this position, and candidates should expect modifications as needed.

or by a selected panel of physician advisors.

Physician Advisors

If the medical director reviews the case and can reach no determination on coverage, he or she may request another opinion from a physician advisor. Physician advisors play a key role in utilization review and case management processes. As a rule, physician advisors review cases in their own specialties when questions arise. They also serve as an internal second opinion for the medical director. In general, physician advisors are used to resolve issues such as validation of the standards of care, recommendations for treatment alternatives, validation of denials made by the review organization's medical director, and evaluation of cases in which the patient's attending physician requests another review. Most review organizations require their physician advisors to be active practitioners in their specialties (local, statewide, or nationally), and these physicians agree (by contract or by a specific letter of agreement) to review questionable cases when they arise, before the final coverage determination is made.

If a determination still cannot be made, the case may require review by a committee of physician advisors (termed third-level review) or the health plan may elect to refer the decision to an independent review organization. Medicare and many states now require a review by an independent third party if the health plan cannot approve a service upon appeal in a timely manner, consistent with federal and/or state time lines, or if there is a full or partial denial of a service that has been appealed by a patient or by a physician representing a patient.

Second Opinions

One tool used frequently in both utilization management and case management when the current treatment program raises doubt is the second opinion. Case managers often obtain a second opinion to validate treatments before proceeding with the treatment course or allowing the present treatment course to continue.

A second opinion is a medical, surgical, or psychiatric consultation provided by a physician other than the attending physician (generally one with a similar specialty). His or her opinion is sought to validate the proposed treatment plan or recommend alternative methods. Although many health care organizations offering case management services delegate the authority to seek second opinions to their case managers, others allow second opinions to be obtained only at the order of the medical director.

Retrospective

Retrospective utilization review includes (1) the review of claims for services that have been prospectively reviewed and authorized by the utilization department as part of the provider profiling process, performed to identify underutilization and overutilization trends; (2) the review of claims for services that have been provided without prior approval, to make an organizational determination to authorize or deny payment, which is dependent upon the individual circumstance. Most often the unauthorized services are those believed to be emergent or urgent and are received in an out-of-plan, out-of-area setting. These are approved on the basis of medical necessity using standard criteria, protocols, and guidelines for inpatient and/or ambulatory review and the availability or unavailability of in-plan facilities at the time the service was rendered.

An appropriate licensed professional should review all cases when the possibility of denial is raised. In all cases, if criteria of appropriateness are not met, the case is referred to a medical director or physician advisor, and denial notification is sent to the patient and provider. In review of the appropriateness of medical claims, contractual agreement language and standardized criteria, protocols, and guidelines are used in making payment determinations. The rationale for the determination is clearly documented and made available to the provider upon request.

SYMBIOSIS OF QUALITY AND UTILIZATION

Overutilization and underutilization are two types of costly and inappropriate use of services that must be monitored and evaluated in compliance with the requirements levied by federal agencies and many state and accrediting agencies. Overutilization is best described as care that is of no benefit to the patient (e.g., excessive testing) or that could have been provided in a less costly alternative setting. In contrast, underutilization of services results in care or services that are inadequate to meet the medical needs of the patient. Underutilization is often found when one reviews the types of care provided and the location, duration, frequency, and intensity of care.

Whereas overutilization results in unnecessary expenditures, underutilization results in costly and inappropriate readmissions, deterioration of the patient's condition, or even death. Although underutilization may be intended as a means of saving money, it can actually be a doubleedged sword and has tremendous longterm cost implications with regard to not only financial outcomes but personal and social outcomes as well. Briefly, underutilization is directly related to the quality of care. Providers are monitored by comparing their performance with predetermined benchmarks for the utilization of health care services. When a variance toward either underutilization or overutilization is identified, it is incumbent upon the organization to implement, monitor, and evaluate a corrective action plan as part of the quality improvement process, in compli-

ance with the requirements of regulatory and accrediting agencies.

There are certain axiomatic principles involving utilization management that require explanation:

- Quality and effective utilization are symbiotic.
- An integrated health care delivery system, whether owned or contracted, is best positioned to succeed in delivering efficient health care.
- Integration implies coordination of services across disciplines throughout the health care continuum from doctors' offices through hospitalization and back to ambulatory care.
- Ideally, when a thoroughly integrated health care delivery system is harmoniously functioning, the result is the greatest value for the financial customer and satisfaction for the patient who is the consumer.

As the elements of health care coalesce, it is obvious that some organizations are "managers" of convenience rather than strategic alliances of excellence. The success of the resulting system will be limited by its least effective component. Every part of the integrated system must be genuinely interested in the quality of the contribution of each of the participants. An integrated system, whether owned or contracted, should control key elements of the continuum of care and provide a total coordination of all aspects of health care to payers and beneficiaries.

Professional integration may provide as great a competitive advantage as amalgamation of health care components. The Joint Commission on Accreditation of Healthcare Organizations (JCAHO) has taken the lead in "de-departmentalization" and emphasizing that all components of care affect the success in managing a patient's episode of illness. An integrated health care system must focus the whole system on the continuum of the patient's health. It is not enough for the doctor to be astute if the ancillary services are inadequate. It is not enough for the inpatient nursing services to be caring if the discharge planning is careless.

It is incumbent upon the integrated delivery system to ensure that every patient benefits from totally coordinated care.

The most notable among generally accepted misconceptions is that "high" quality and effective utilization are reciprocal elements. This assumption includes the concept that health care quality is incrementally quantifiable from "negligible" to "highest" with intermediate levels such as "minimal," "moderate," "high," and "higher." The fact is that either quality is present or it is absent. If that fact is doubted, a quick check with legal council will substantiate the contention. Second, it is assumed that intensifying utilization activities will not only decrease costs but also correspondingly diminish quality. This notion appears to be based on the belief that the more one spends, the higher the quality of the product one receives. In health care, quality actually exists only in a "window" on a services graph.

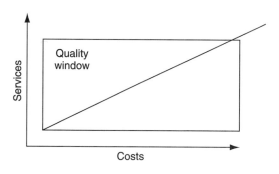

Efficiency, therefore, becomes a measure of quality. Effective utilization is the means by which efficiency is achieved. Prolonged hospitalization, unnecessary surgery, nonindicated procedures, and inappropriate medications all increase costs, add no benefits, and carry unacceptable risk of complications. Conversely, denying preventive health care, delaying indicated procedures, and failing to coordinate services not only are frustrating to customers but

will actually increase the consumption of health care resources. Effective utilization and maintenance of quality each require appropriate actions by an appropriate caregiver at an appropriate time in an appropriate facility that lead to prompt, accurate diagnosis and expeditious recovery.

MEDICARE BENEFICIARIES VERSUS COMMERCIALLY INSURED PATIENTS

Medicare beneficiaries have unique health care needs that require an entirely different and more complex type of medical management and health care delivery infrastructure, complete with new types of provider contracting models and health care provider networks. Increased services in the areas of rehabilitation and geriatric medicine, with a focus on early identification and management of high-risk patients, are critical to maintaining an optimal level of functioning in members and to ensuring the financial success of the health plan. "Persons identified as high-risk . . . have been found to use health care services in the future at twice the rate of their low-risk peers."[9] In addition, obtaining, managing, and retaining a government contract and satisfying federal regulations is a new type of business experience that should not be easily dismissed as requiring only minor operational adjustments. The health care delivery system must be transformed from a sickness-based system, which provides access and manages care to recipients only when they are sick, to one that emphasizes routine and appropriate primary and preventive care. This change optimizes the utilization of finite health care resources while ensuring positive health outcomes.

In general, a paradigm shift must take place in the medical management of the frail elderly. The focus must change from utilization management, which administers the health care of a high volume of patients at a low level of intensity on an episodic, reactive level at the time the patient arrives for service, to proactive utilization and quality management, which concentrates on a small percentage of high-risk, high-cost patients treated at a high level of intensity throughout the continuum of care. Consider, for example, the use of inpatient acute-care hospital services: the proactive process focuses on preventing the need for future hospitalizations, whereas traditional utilization management seeks to limit unnecessary inpatient services after the patient has come to the hospital for treatment.

ALIGNMENT OF UTILIZATION AND FINANCIAL GOALS FOR SUCCESS

To ensure that the provision of health care services is financially congruent with budgetary goals, utilization management develops and implements programs, processes, policies, and procedures for meeting the following objectives for all products within the health plan, IPA or medical group, or self-insured employer group:

1. To define inpatient and ambulatory utilization benchmarks that are congruent with membership and premium revenue, and result in projected net income
2. To develop benefit interpretations, clinical pathways, and referral protocols for standardized prospective, concurrent, and/or retrospective review and authorization of services in an effort to do the following:
   - Establish accurate accruals on a monthly, quarterly, and annual basis
   - Project financial outcomes
   - Identify overutilization and underutilization trends so that action plans can be developed for continuous quality improvement and regulatory compliance

   - Accurately estimate underwriting risk and establish benefit plan premiums
3. To implement standardized, disease-specific, "best-practice" treatment guidelines to achieve cost-efficient utilization of resources
4. To interpret provider profiling utilization data in an effort to contract with, refer patients to, and utilize the most cost-efficient providers whose care results in high-quality patient outcomes

BENCHMARKS

Benchmarking is a process, a structured approach or a discipline that is continuing or ongoing and involves measuring, evaluating, and comparing both results and processes that produce the best results. The actual measurement used to gauge the performance of a function, operation or relative business practice is a benchmark.[10]

A "best practice" is a service, function, or process that as been fine tuned, improved, and implemented to produce superior outcomes. *Best* is used in a contextual sense. It means "best for your patients or your community" in the context of your regional health environment, your health system's strategies and missions, your organizational or community culture, or your practice systems. Best practices are those practices that result in benchmarks that meet or set a new standard.[10]

Utilization benchmarks are a function of local and regional provider practice patterns, availability of local and regional health care delivery services and networks, mandated and optional benefit designs, premium revenue, negotiated contractual agreements, and the diversity and demographics of the population being served. Even in the absolute world of actuaries these projections are subject to the unanticipated and unpredictable aspects of disease processes. Therefore, one must use the best information available from all sources, including claims, finance, and actuarial and historical utilization data, and effectively manage the health care delivery process in a manner consistent with the financial goals of the health plan, IPA, and medical group, and the satisfaction of the consumer.

Current widely accepted industry benchmarks for well-established managed care plans (those that have operated for a minimum of 3 years and have achieved a membership of 25,000) are shown in Table 10-2.

These service benchmarks vary considerably by region, with the lowest utilization on the West Coast and the highest utilization on the East Coast. The table illustrates benchmarks for a moderately managed health care plan that would currently apply in most regions of the United States, for a sophisticated managed care model in which financial incentives for all participating entities are aligned.

Utilization and costs are best controlled when all participating entities have aligned financial incentives to deliver quality care in an efficient manner. Thus, difficulty in managing utilization and controlling costs is directly related to the financial model under which the health plan, IPA, or medical group operates. Fee for service or discounted fee for service is the most difficult environment in which to control utilization, because the provider has a financial incentive to provide as much service as possible at the highest cost possible. Per diem or global contracting (such as diagnosis-related group [DRG] reimbursement) is middle of the road because the incentive to provide more services remains. For example, in per diem arrangements, the more days a patient remains in a facility, the higher the reimbursement; in DRG-based systems, the more patients admitted to a facility, the higher the reimbursement; in global procedure contracting, the more procedures that are performed, the higher the reimbursement rate.

At the other end of the spectrum is risk-based contracting in which all dollars are prospectively divided by the participating entities for the provision of all health care services, and financial success is directly related to appropriate patient management and provider performance. Although allegations have been made that this type of contracting leads to underutilization, no credible studies have been done to validate this accusation, and in fact all regulatory and accrediting agencies require that health plans have ongoing monitoring processes that track and identify trends in underutilization or overuti-

TABLE 10-2		
Industry Benchmarks for Well-Established Managed Care Plans		
	Commercial (Non-Medicaid)	Medicare
Acute-care admissions/K	65	250
Acute-care bed days/K	200	1200
Skilled nursing admissions/K	<1	55
Skilled nursing bed days/K	15	800
Emergency department visits/K	75	150
Primary care physician encounters/K	1.5	4
Specialist encounters/K	<1	3
Home care admissions/K	6	150
Home care visits/K	66	2250

/K, Per 1000 members.

lization, and implement corrective actions should either be detected. When a utilization department is staffed, the contract models must be taken into consideration (see Figure 10-1).

"Increased provider leverage and a shift in consumer preference away from tightly controlled managed care products have significantly reduced risk-based contracting. Most providers view risk-based contracting as automatically leading to losses, and there is a trend back to per-diem or DRG payments for hospitals and to fee-for-service for physicians."[11] "As health plans move away from risk-based contracts toward discounted fee-for-service, employers give beneficiaries greater flexibility in health care decisions," and government mandates increase benefit coverage and attempt to direct the level of care, "holding the line on utilization will become more difficult."[12]

MINIMUM UTILIZATION MANAGEMENT REPORTING REQUIREMENTS

To manage utilization on a daily, weekly, monthly, and year-to-date basis (for seasonal trend comparisons) and to track and identify trends in utilization to project a company's success in meeting budgeted financial targets, capturing the following information, using reasonable facsimiles of the illustrated reports, is critical:

- **Encounter report**—month-to-date and year-to-date ambulatory and inpatient encounters by product line, defined by fund financial responsibility, provider, Current Procedural Terminology category, HCFA Common Procedure Coding System, DRG codes, type of service, cost, and per capita monthly and year-to-date claims cost (Figure 10-6)
- **Monthly bed-day utilization report**—inpatient days per 1000, admissions per 1000, and average

length of stay by IPA or medical group (Figure 10-7)
- **Length-of-stay comparison report**—average length of stay by IPA or medical group, by facility, by DRG code, and by month and year to date, with comparison of benchmark length of stay to average length of stay by facility (Figure 10-8)
- **Daily census report**—budgeted inpatient days per 1000, by IPA or medical group, compared to current inpatient days per 1000 with a 7- and 30-day trend (Figure 10-9)
- **Utilization formulas**—bed days, admissions, length of stay, readmissions, emergency department visits, denials, referrals (Box 10-6)
- **Daily inpatient detail by facility or product**—inpatient data by facility, patient, level of care, physician, and diagnosis (Figure 10-10)
- **Aberrant bed-day report**—aberrant bed-day data by patient, physician, facility, reason, and level of care (see Figure 10-2)

These reports should be used to proactively accrue reserves that reflect the plan's actual financial liabilities on a monthly basis and to project financial success or failure when combined with projected membership and premium revenue reports on a quarterly basis.

The data related to facilities and individual providers should be reported on a daily basis for ongoing utilization management and should be used annually in negotiating the contract with providers for health care delivery service rates and in underwriting to determine benefit designs and the associated premiums.

UTILIZATION MANAGEMENT REGULATORY AND ACCREDITATION REQUIREMENTS

Health plans and providers must adhere to federal and state regulatory requirements,

Text continued on p. 275

Fund responsibility code
1 = Hospital
2 = Group
3 = Shared risk
4 = Health plan

IPA/medical group (___)
Date of service ____ and ____

Enrollment
Commercial ____
Senior ____

Encounter (service description)	Fund responsibility	General ledger code	Types of service code	Month to date							Year to date						
				Cost	Commercial	Cost	$pmpm	Senior	Cost	$pmpm	Cost	Commercial	Cost	$pmpm	Senior	Cost	$pmpm
1. Family practice		FP..#..															
A. Consults			MD-1														
1. IP—Comprehensive	2																
2. IP—Follow-up	2																
3. OP—Comprehensive	2																
4. OP—Follow-up	2																
2. Internal medicine		IM..#..															
A. Consults																	
1. IP—Comprehensive	2																
2. IP—Follow-up	2																
3. OP—Comprehensive	2																
4. OP—Follow-up	2																
3. Pediatrics		PED..#..															
A. Consults																	
1. IP—Comprehensive																	
2. IP—Follow-up																	
3. OP—Comprehensive																	
4. OP—Follow-up																	
B. Procedure (IP-OP)																	
1. Other	2		Doc														
C. Facility component (check for OP)	1		Ofc														
4. OB/GYN		OB/GYN#															
A. Consults																	
1. IP—Comprehensive																	
2. IP—Follow-up																	
3. OP—Comprehensive																	
4. OP—Follow-up																	
B. Surgery/procedure IP/OP																	
1. Caesarean section			Sur														
2. Caesarean section (repeat)			Sur														
3. Vaginal delivery			Sur														
C. Facility component																	

Figure 10-6   Sample encounter report. *IPA*, Independent practice association; *IP*, inpatient; *OP*, outpatient; *$pmpm*, dollars per member per month.

Time period		
Begin 1/1/1999	End 1/22/1999	Total days 22

Acute hospital

Membership	Network A				Network B				Total network			
	Commercial 13,629		Medicare 2778		Commercial 6385		Medicare 592		Commercial 20,014		Medicare 3470	
	No. of days	Days/K/Y	No. of days	Days/K/Y	No. of days	Days/K/Y	No. of days	Days/K/Y	No. of days	Days/K/Y	No. of days	Days/K/Y
In plan												
ICU/CCU	0	0		0		0		0	0	0	0	0
Medical	244	297	247	1475	120	312	70	1578	364	302	317	1516
Surgical	0	0		0		0		0	0	0	0	0
Obstetrics	0	0		0		0		0	0	0	0	0
Psychiatric	0	0		0		0		0	0	0	0	0
Subtotal	244	297	247	1475	120	312	70	1578	364	302	317	1516
Percent	100%		100%		100%		100%		100%		94%	
Out of plan												
ICU/CCU		0		0		0		0		0		0
Medical		0		0		0		0		0		0
Surgical		0		0		0		0		0		0
Obstetrics		0		0		0		0		0		0
Psychiatric		0		0		0		0		0		0
Subtotal	0	0	0	0	0	0	0	0	0	0	0	0
Percent	0%		0%		0%		0%		0%		0%	
Rehabilitation	0	0	0	0	0	0	0	0	0	0	21	100
Total acute	244	297	247	1475	120	312	70	1878	351	302	338	1616
Budgeted acute	239	291	259	1647	112	291	65	1567	351	291	324	1547
SNF	0	0	0	0	0	0	0	0	0	0	0	0
Total SNF	0		0		0		0		0		0	
Budgeted SNF	0		0		0		0		0		0	
ED visits	Visits	Visits/K/Y	Visits	Visits/K/Y	Visits	Visits/K/Y	Visits	Visits/K/Y	Visits	Visits/K/Y	Visits	Visits/K/Y
In area	12	15	27	161	12	31	27	647	36	30	27	129
Out of area	8	10	8	48	8	21	8	192	24	20	8	38
TOTAL	20	25	35	209	20	52	35	839	60	50	35	167
Budget	25	30	17	100	12	30	4	100	36	30	21	100

Figure 10-7   Sample monthly utilization summary. /K, Per 1000 members; /Y, per year; *SNF,* skilled nursing facility; *ICU,* intensive care unit; *CCU,* critical care unit.

IPA/medical group:_____

Date:_____

Month:_____

Facility	DRG	Narrative description	No. of admissions	Benchmark LoS	Average LoS	No. of days under	No. of Days over	No. of admissions	Average LoS	No. of days under	No. of days over

(Columns No. of admissions, Average LoS, No. of days under, No. of days over grouped under "Year to date")

Figure 10-8 Length-of-stay (*LoS*) comparison report by independent practice association or medical group and by product. *IPA*, Independent practice association; *DRG*, diagnosis-related group.

Medical group	Enrollment	Budget BD goal/K	Current BD/K	Daily patient census goal	Status	1	2	3	4	5	6	7	8	9	10	11	12	13	14	15	16	17	18	19	20	21	22	23	24	25	26	27	28	29	30	31	7-Day trend	30-Day trend
TOTAL																																						

Plan is capitated   Status ⬆   R = Routine (40% over goal)   M = Moderate (10%–20% over goal)   C = Critical (20%–30% over goal)

Policy and procedure accompanying report should indicate management action based on status indicator.

Figure 10-9 Daily census report. /K, Per 1000 members; BD, bed day.

Date:
___/___/___

Admission date	Patient name	Contracted noncontracted	Health plan ID No.	Days of month																																C	M	T	P	S	N	O	RP	Narrative diagnosis
				1	2	3	4	5	6	7	8	9	10	11	12	13	14	15	16	17	18	19	20	21	22	23	24	25	26	27	28	29	30	31										
Facility				C	C	C	T	T	T																										Contracted									
																																			Noncontracted									
																																			Subtotal	3		3						
Facility																																			Contracted	3	2	1						
				C	C	C	M	M	T																										Noncontracted									
																																			Subtotal									
Facility																																			Contracted						4			
				N	N	N	N																												Noncontracted									
																																			Subtotal									
Facility																																			Contracted						2	0		
				N	N	O	O																												Noncontracted									
																																			Subtotal									

C, Critical care; *M*, medical; *T*, telemetry; *P*, psychiatric; *SA, s*ubacute; *N*, skilled nursing facility; *O*, other; *RP*, responsible physician.

Figure 10-10 Daily inpatient detail by facility and by product.

BOX 10-6
Utilization Formulas

Bed Days/K/Y

Instantaneous bed-day rate – (Current census as a bed-day rate BD/K/Y) (365/M) (H)

Total bed-day rate/K/Y – (for a specific reporting period; Current Day, Month to Date BD/K/Y)
(P/D) (365/M) (1000)

Admits/K/Y for a Specific Reporting Period

$$\frac{\text{(Total admissions [for reporting period]} \times 365)/(\text{Days in reporting period} \times 1000)}{\text{Member months (for the reporting period)}}$$

Average Length of Stay for a Specific Reporting Period

$$\frac{\text{Total bed days (for reporting period)}}{\text{Total discharges (for reporting period)}}$$

Readmissions/K/Y for a Specific Period

$$\frac{\text{(Total readmissions [for reporting period]} \times 365)/(\text{Days in reporting period} \times 1000)}{\text{Total admissions (in reporting period)}}$$

Total Emergency Department Visits/K/Y for a Specific Period

$$\frac{\text{(Total emergency department visits [for reporting period]} \times 365)/(\text{Days in reporting period} \times 1000)}{\text{Member months (for reporting period)}}$$

Referral or Claims Payment Denial Rate (% of Referral Requests Denied or % of Claims Denied) for a Specific Period

$$\frac{\text{Total referral or claims payment denials (for reporting period)} \times 100}{\text{Total Referral or Claims Payment Denials Processed (for reporting period)}}$$

Referral or Claims Turnaround Time (% Exceeding the Health Plans, State, Federal, or Accrediting Agencies' Standard) for a Specific Period

$$\frac{\text{Total referrals or claims payments exceeding the standard turnaround time (for the reporting period)} \times 100}{\text{Total referrals or claims paid processed (for the reporting period)}}$$

These formulas are generic. Use population-specific membership and utilization data where indicated.
BD, Bed days; *D,* number of days elapsed in the current month; *H,* current number of inpatients; */K,* per 1000 members; *M,* member months; *P,* patient days so far in the current month; */Y,* per year.

and many employers and payers must receive accreditation by an independent entity such as the National Committee for Quality Assurance (NCQA), American Accreditation HealthCare Commission (URAC), or JCAHO.

Accreditation organizations establish state-of-the-art, professionally based standards for the industry in key functional areas and evaluate the performance of health care organizations against these benchmarks on a regular basis.

Accreditation is recognized as a symbol of quality indicating that an organization meets certain performance standards that affect the quality of patient care.[13]

The NCQA is an organization that accredits managed care organizations (MCOs) by determining the degree to which the organization ensures consistent quality management and operational performance across all administrative and clinical functions and processes. The accreditation process examines the organization's structure, tests quality management and improvement processes, and looks for evidence that quality improvement activities have resulted in measurable improvement in the organization's performance in both clinical and service areas. Accreditation is offered for the following types of organization:

- MCOs
- Managed behavioral health care organizations
- New health plans
- Provider-sponsored organizations

NCQA offers the following certification programs:

- Credentials Verification Organization
- Physician Organization

"MCOs that contract with NCQA accredited or certified organizations can reduce the amount of delegation oversight required for MCO accreditation,"[14] although Medicare requires that the MCO obtain prior approval for this delegated status from the Centers for Medicare & Medicaid Services.

Many large employer groups currently require NCQA accreditation prior to contracting with an MCO, and it is strongly recommended that all providers obtain a copy of the NCQA accreditation manual and integrate its standards into their systems, policies, procedures, and work processes. Employers, to compare health plans in an objective and standardized evaluation process, have collaboratively joined health care providers, the Washington Business Group on Health, and the NCQA to establish HEDIS, the Health Plan Employer Data and Information Set. These employers expect that the utilization of health benefits will be reported in a standardized format that reflects services to their employees in the areas of preventive medical care, counseling, and early detection and treatment programs. The NCQA requires that health care providers' quality improvement efforts be driven by those data.

The NCQA requires that the HEDIS data that the MCO submits, as well as the results from the Consumer Assessments of Health Plan Survey, be audited by an NCQA-certified auditor.[14] The latter is "a consumer survey that provides information on a) Claims Processing, b) Courteous and Helpful Office Staff, c) Customer Service d) Getting Care Quickly, e) Getting Needed Care, f) IIow Well Doctors Communicate."[14]

"The American Accreditation HealthCare Commission (URAC) has developed a 'modular approach' to managed care accreditation programs by offering accreditation to HMO and non-HMO managed care systems."[14] URAC offers 10 different accreditation programs for MCOs:

1. Case Management
2. Credential Verification (CV0)
3. Health Call Centers
4. Health Networks
5. Health Plans
6. Utilization Management
7. Provider Credentialing
8. Workers' Compensation Networks
9. Workers' Compensation Utilization Management
10. External Review

The JCAHO is most widely known for accrediting inpatient facilities and improving the safety and quality of care provided. It develops standards that focus not simply on what the organization *has*, but on what it actually *does*. "Health care organizations seek JCAHO accreditation because a) it is frequently used to meet Medicare certification requirements, b) enhances medical staff recruitment, c) expedites third-party payment, d) fulfills state licensure requirements, e) may favorably influence liability insurance premiums, f) enhances access to managed care contracts, and g) may favorably influence bond ratings and access to financial markets."[14]

The JCAHO provides accreditation services for the following types of organizations:

- Acute-care, psychiatric, and rehabilitation hospitals
- Health care networks
- Home care providers
- Nursing homes and long-term care facilities
- Assisted living residences
- Behavioral health care organizations
- Ambulatory care providers
- Clinical laboratories

Although efforts are currently underway to standardize the requirements of various federal, state, and accrediting agencies, to date those of each entity remain separate and distinct. Frequently, vast differences are seen in agencies' requirements and standards, especially in the category of "timeliness of decisions." For example, for precertification of nonurgent care the NCQA requires that an organization's determination be made within 2 working days of obtaining all necessary information. Medicare requires that the determination be made within 14 calendar days, with a 14-day extension under certain circumstances. Individual states may have different time requirements. Therefore, it is incumbent upon the health plan to use the most restrictive time standards in implementing utilization management processes and in writing policies and procedures. This ensures that the health plan will subsequently meet all time requirements that may be mandated by federal, state, or accrediting agencies. Conversely, when some requirements are more comprehensive, such as by demanding a higher number of quality improvement studies annually, the health plan should adhere to the broadest provisions to meet all requirements.

Health plans are facing increasing pressure from external customers, including accrediting and governmental regulatory agencies, to provide clear evidence of health care utilization of the purchased services by a given population and of the health care status of that population prior to and subsequent to receiving those services. The evidence will have to confirm that the health interventions resulted in improvement in the health status of the population. Documentation will also be required that the health interventions utilized were continually evaluated, monitored, and modified to improve patients' treatment outcomes. Eventually, standard treatment guidelines for specific disease processes (disease management) may be mandated.

HEALTH INSURANCE PORTABILITY AND ACCOUNTABILITY ACT

The Department of Health and Human Services has released final regulations (the Final Rule) on the most significant legislation affecting health plans and providers since the Balanced Budget Act of 1997. "This 'Final Rule' implements the privacy provisions of HIPAA and generally prohibits health care providers, health plans and health care clearinghouses from using or disclosing individually identifiable health information except as authorized by the patient or as otherwise permitted by the regulations."[15] The specifics of these regulations continue to be clarified at this time, but they impose costly burdens on payers and providers, who must now designate a specific individual to be responsible for privacy policies, procedures, education, and training of staff and must identify appropriate ways to transfer patient information between providers and payers in a timely manner. These regulations will strongly affect the utilization department, which must coordinate care, both internally and externally, and transfer patient information among multiple inpatient, outpatient, and disease management providers on a daily basis. Updating the policies and procedures of the department to remain in compliance with ongoing regulatory refinements will be crucial to avoid the need for corrective actions at survey time. The Final Rule became effective February 26, 2001, but large health plans were given until February 26, 2003, and small health plans until February 26, 2004, to comply.

UTILIZATION MANAGEMENT PLAN

Because of the differences in the standards of the various regulatory and accrediting agencies, the information in this section is a *generic* summary of the structure and processes that are needed in the development and implementation of an effective utilization management plan that meets the majority of the utilization management program requirements issued by federal, state and accrediting agencies. For specific and comprehensive program requirements, see Suggested Websites and Resources at the end of this chapter.

The purpose of the utilization management plan, in conjunction with the quality management plan, is to ensure that payers and providers have a comprehensive, documented, strategic plan for health care delivery. The overall principle one must remember in developing this operational plan is that the delivery of medically necessary, eligible services at the appropriate level of care by the appropriate provider ensures optimal treatment outcomes and cost efficiencies while maximizing financial performance.

Scope

The utilization management plan must include the following provisions:

- An annual written program description of the utilization management structures and processes and the responsibilities assigned to specific individuals is prepared.

- A summary is provided of the standards, procedures, and methods to be used in evaluating proposed or delivered services.

- A work plan is developed that identifies specific time frames for the implementation and evaluation of identified quality improvement processes related to utilization management.

- Written criteria based on sound clinical evidence are applied in determining medical appropriateness and are presented in a format that clearly documents the rationale for employing the criteria in decision making.

- Procedures are developed for applying criteria based on the needs of individual patients and characteristics of the local delivery system.

- Actively practicing health care professionals are involved in the development and adoption of criteria, and in the development and review of procedures for applying the criteria.

- Criteria are reviewed at specified intervals, usually on an annual basis, and updated as necessary.

- Utilization criteria are available to practitioners upon request.

- At least annually, health care professionals are evaluated for their consistency in applying utilization review criteria in decision making (interrater reliability audits are performed for all licensed personnel, including physicians).

- Qualified health professionals assess the clinical information used to support utilization management decisions, and appropriately licensed health professionals supervise all review decisions.

- Denials are always generated from a review by a physician who has expertise in the field of medicine that is appropriate for the services at issue but who need not, in all cases, be of the same specialty or subspecialty as the treating physician.[7]

- Board-certified physicians from appropriate specialty areas are available to assist in making determinations of medical appropriateness.
- Reconsideration reviews are conducted by a person or persons who were not involved in making the original organizational determination to approve or deny a service.
- Precertification, concurrent, and retrospective review determinations are decided within the time period required by federal, state, and accrediting agencies as appropriate (includes standard and expedited reviews).
- When precertification of nonurgent or urgent care results in a denial, the member and practitioner receive written or electronic confirmation of the decision the time period required by federal, state, and accrediting agencies as appropriate (includes standard and expedited reviews).
- An enrollee or a physician may request an expedited organizational determination if adherence to the standard processing time would jeopardize the life or health of the enrollee or the enrollee's ability to regain maximum function.
- If a request for an expedited determination is denied, the request is automatically transferred for processing within the standard time period, and the enrollee is informed of the right to file a grievance if he or she disagrees with the decision not to expedite.
- A written description identifies the information that is collected to support utilization management decision making.

- The reasons for each denial, including specific utilization review criteria or benefits provisions, are clearly documented and communicated to the practitioner and patient.
- A physician reviewer is available to physicians to discuss by telephone determinations based on medical necessity.
- Information about the appeals process is included in all denial notifications.
- Member and provider satisfaction with the utilization management process is monitored through satisfaction surveys.
- Health care professionals who make organizational determinations affirm, in writing, that no financial incentives are present and that decision making is based only on appropriateness of care and benefit eligibility.

Utilization Management Committee

The utilization management committee (UMC) is responsible for oversight of the utilization management plan. The committee is composed of participating physicians, utilization staff members, the medical director, and any other interdisciplinary professionals who may be appropriate, such as medical records personnel, quality management or risk management personnel, and/or nursing personnel.

The UMC should meet at least monthly, and its topics of consideration should include, but are not limited to, (1) retrospective review of inpatient and ambulatory utilization trends, (2) utilization of emergency department and out-of-plan services, (3) trends in appeals and grievances related to the authorization and/or denial of services, (4) access and availability of care, (5) monitoring of compliance of utilization processes with regulatory requirements of accrediting and governmental agencies, (6) evaluation of provider profiling data identifying overutilization and underutilization, and (7) recommendations for and monitoring and evaluation of quality improvement action plans related to providers and/or utilization processes.

Methodology

To ensure the consistent application of criteria and guidelines in the utilization management process, all medical records and requests for medical services that require prospective, concurrent, and/or retrospective review and authorization should be analyzed using nationally accepted resources that *may* include but are not limited to the following:

- **InterQual level-of-care (intensity-of-service or severity-of-illness) criteria**—These criteria are the most effective in determining the appropriateness of a patient's admission and continuing care at a specific *level* of service and in determining the appropriate setting for those patients who do not follow a "routine, uncomplicated" course of treatment or who have multiple comorbidities. Thus, these guidelines are optimal for reviewing care of the elderly population and can be used in conjunction with Milliman Care Guidelines, which most commonly apply to the commercially insured population.
- **Health plan–specific clinical guidelines**—These guidelines are developed by participating providers using quality, utilization, and clinical outcome data, including documentation of cases in which the guideline was not followed and the resulting patient outcome with regard to utilization of services and quality of care.
- **Milliman Care Guidelines**—These guidelines provide an excellent educational tool for utilization review nurses because they delineate what services should be taking place on each day of a patient's hospitalization when a routine, uncomplicated individual case is treated efficiently and the level of care to which the patient should be transferred subsequent to discharge from the acute-care facility. The utilization review nurse may use these guidelines as prompts when discussing a case with an attending physician.
- **Federally approved or state-approved criteria mandated by Medicare and/or Medicaid nationally recognized specialty standards-of-practice criteria or guidelines**—These are published by specific specialty organizations such as the American Academy of Obstetrics and Gynecology or the Agency for Healthcare Research and Quality.

The structure described in the following sections has proven effective in the implementation of utilization management programs and processes.

Utilization Management Department

A utilization management department is required for implementation and operation of the utilization management program. The department provides leadership, support, and education to assure the success of the program and performs reviews of medical information to determine the appropriateness of the health services rendered and the providers involved in treating the health plan beneficiary. The reviews are performed on a prospective, concurrent, and retrospective basis and result in authorization of, denial of, or referral for health care services. Personnel may include, but are not limited to, physicians, nurses, analysts, and clerical staff.

Implementation of the policies and procedures used in making prospective, concurrent, and/or retrospective review decisions is supervised by a physician. In addition, (1) an appropriate licensed medical professional reviews all cases when the possibility of denial is raised during the review, (2) denials are always generated from a review by a physician with expertise in the field of medicine appropriate for the services at issue, and (3) board-certified physician consultants from the appropriate specialty areas advise as needed.

Medical Director

The medical director is most commonly the utilization department senior manager. Should the department report to another licensed professional, the medical director must have a matrix or advisory relationship to the department and should chair or be a member of the utilization management committee.

The individual filling this position provides medical management leadership and clinical expertise and is responsible for coordinating all aspects of the health services delivery system. "The Medical Director's role may be viewed as the hub around which the many spokes of the wheel of the health plan turn. This physician leader is responsible for integrating the needs of the patients and the physicians in the community into the vision, mission, and goals of the health plan. The critical skills of a successful medical director include: strong leadership, customer service, change management, education of providers, financial management and disease management."[16] This person is responsible for ensuring the optimal performance of the health care provider network and delivery system in terms of quality of care and service to members from the perspectives of both clinical and financial management (see Box 10-5).

Vice-President, Director, Manager, or Supervisor

Depending on the size of the organization and the complexity of the products offered, any or all of the positions of vice-president, director, manager, and supervisor may be present within the utilization department. The basic, *minimal* requirements for these positions are as follows:

- Current registered nurse, nurse practitioner, or physician assistant license in the state in which the person is employed by the health plan
- Bachelor's degree in business or a health care–related field; master's degree in business or a health care–related field preferred
- Two to 3 years (supervisor), 3 to 4 years (manager), 4 to 5 years (director), or 5 to 7 years (vice president) of supervisory experience in the medical management of an MCO, preferably in a staff, IPA, or medical group health care delivery model
- Familiarity with federal, state, and accrediting agencies' requirements for MCOs
- Ability to perform at the highest level in a continuously changing, crisis-oriented, high-stress environment managing multiple levels of licensed and nonlicensed personnel
- Ability to analyze financial and clinical data, to determine utilization benchmarks, and to implement best practices so that ongoing budgetary goals are met on a regular basis
- Ability to strategize, prioritize, and develop and implement effective utilization strategies, programs, and processes that deliver effective health care services to all members efficiently and within budgeted financial targets
- Ability to act as a change agent and to motivate staff to meet all utilization department goals and objectives on an ongoing basis with minimal turnover of personnel (see Box 10-4)

For all other professional staffing needs, refer to Figure 10-1.

SUMMARY

The purpose of any utilization management process is to establish patient eligibility, interpret covered benefits, and evaluate the medical necessity, appropriateness, and effectiveness of the delivery of health care services. At the same time, all processes must ensure that the services are performed by an appropriate health care provider, at the appropriate level, within a time frame that is consistent with the urgency of the patient's condition, and in compliance with the guidelines of federal, state, and accrediting agencies. Both utilization management and the case management component support the patient so that the therapeutic regimen of the primary care team can be implemented.

Three types of review function are included in utilization management:
1. **Prospective** (also known as precertification or prior authorization)—the review that occurs before elective or urgent services are rendered
2. **Concurrent**—the review that occurs while the services are being rendered
3. **Retrospective**—the review that occurs after the services or treatments have been rendered

Quality and utilization are symbiotic. Quality exists only in a "window." It is not incrementally quantifiable from "lowest" to "highest." Quality is either present or it is absent. Also, the notion that the more one spends, the higher the quality obtained is erroneous. Efficiency thus becomes a measure of quality. Effective utilization is the means by which efficiency is achieved.

To ensure that the provision of health care services is financially congruent with budgetary goals, utilization management must set benchmarks, implement best practices, and effectively manage the health care delivery process in a manner consistent with the financial goals of the health plan and IPA or medical group and with consumer and provider satisfaction. Utilization and costs are best controlled when the financial incentives of all participating entities are aligned to deliver quality care in an efficient manner.

Federal, state, and accrediting agencies require that the organization have a comprehensive, documented, strategic plan for health care delivery. The plan must incorporate specific structural, operational, and personnel requirements in implementing utilization programs, processes, policies, and procedures. The overall principle is that the provision of medically necessary, eligible services, delivered at the appropriate level of care by the appropriate provider, ensures optimal treatment outcomes and cost efficiencies while maximizing health plan performance.

Chapter Exercises

1. In a group setting describe the goals of utilization management and discuss how they compare with those of case management.
2. If a local HMO or other MCO is nearby, arrange to spend time with the utilization management department to watch firsthand the processes involved in making coverage determinations for a new referral, for a hospitalization, and for a case that requires retrospective review.
3. Describe the benchmarks used by the industry for both a commercially insured and a Medicare population. When you visit a local HMO or MCO, discuss with their personnel the benchmarks and other tools and reports they use to monitor their utilization rates and their successes in managing the care of the clients they serve.
4. Describe at least three of the common utilization management reporting requirements.

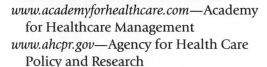
Suggested Websites and Resources

www.academyforhealthcare.com—Academy for Healthcare Management

www.ahcpr.gov—Agency for Health Care Policy and Research

www.urac.org—American Accreditation Healthcare Commission

www.cms.hhs.gov—Centers for Medicare & Medicaid Services

www.ahcpr.gov—Agency for Healthcare Research and Quality

www.jama.ama-assn.org—*Journal of the American Medical Association*

www.aishealth.com—*Managed Care Week*

www.aishealth.com—Managed Medicare and Medicaid

www.millerholguin.com—Miller & Holguin Health Care Update

www.aahp.org—On Managed Care

REFERENCES

1. Lyon JC: Models of nursing care delivery and case management, *Business and Health* 4(3):12-16, 1993.
2. Mucklo M: Charting health care expenditures, *On Managed Care* 6(6):2, 2001.
3. Crozier DA: DATAWATCH: National medical care spending, *Health Affairs* 3(3):108-127, 1984.
4. Mazoway JM: Early intervention in high cost care, *Business and Health* 4(3):12-16, 1987.
5. Boland P: *Making managed health care work: a practical guide to strategies and solutions,* Gaithersburg, Md, 1995, Aspen, pp 172-175.
6. Kongstvedt PR: *The managed care handbook,* ed 2, Gaithersburg, Md, 1993, Aspen, pp 182-188.
7. Rules and regulations, *Federal Register* 63(123):35111, June 26, 1998.
8. Quality Improvement System in Managed Care (QISMC), Domain 3: Health services management, Services authorization, 3.3.1.4, *Federal Register,* Part II, Department of Health and Human Services, 42 CFR, Part 400, Medicare Program Final Rule.
9. HMO Workgroup on Care Management, *Planning care for high-risk HMO members,* Unpublished manuscript, July 1997.
10. Carneal G, D'Andrea G: Defining the parameters of case management in a managed care setting, *Manag Care Q* 9(1):58, 2001.
11. Lesser C, Ginsberg P: Back to the future? New cost and access challenges emerge, *Healthcare Leadership Review* 20(5):1, 2001.
12. Royce P: New M&R benchmarks reveal HMO industry trends, *Healthcare Leadership Review* 20(4):13, 2001.
13. The Joint Commission on Accreditation of Healthcare Organizations, available on-line at www.jcaho.org, accessed Aug 15, 2001.
14. National Committee for Quality Assurance, available on-line at www.ncqa.org/definitions.asp, accessed July 15, 2001.
15. Miller O, Holguin H: Health information privacy standards impose new burdens on healthcare providers and plans, *Health Care Update,* pp 1-3, Feb 5, 2001.
16. Killian R: The adaptive role of the medical director is critical to a health plan's success, *Managed Health Care Executive,* pp 38-40, July/Aug 2001.

BIBLIOGRAPHY

Rules and regulations, *Federal Register* 63(123):35111, 1998.

InterQual clinical support criteria, Marlborough, Mass, 2001, InterQual.

M+C contractor performance monitoring system, Section IX: Medicare organization determination and appeals, Final, Washington, DC, May 21, 2001, Health Care Financing Administration.

Healthcare management guidelines, San Diego, 1999, Milliman & Robertson.

Powell SK: *Nursing case management: a practical guide to success in managed care,* Philadelphia, 1996, Lippincott, pp 77-142.

Quality Improvement System of Managed Care: *Domain 3: Health services management, 3.3.1.4 Service authorization,* Washington, DC, 2000, Centers for Medicare & Medicaid Services.

PART

III

Legal and Legislative Issues

CHAPTER
11

Introduction to Legal and Legislative Issues

Peggy A. Rossi, BSN, MPA, CCM, CPUR

OBJECTIVES

- To understand the importance of standards of care and practice in protecting oneself from litigation
- To list the key standards of practice as outlined by one's professional organization

Over the past several decades case management has evolved from a grassroots organization of professionals filling similar roles into a recognized new discipline in health care. Over these same years, Americans have begun to view health care as a right. When they feel this right has been violated, lawsuits are filed. Although many lawsuits have proved warranted, with millions of dollars awarded to the plaintiffs or their representatives, others have been dismissed as frivolous. Because many case managers work with patients who have catastrophic illnesses at the time the case is referred, and because they also work for large organizations that are viewed as having deep pockets, not only the organization but also the case manager may be sued if things go wrong. Likewise, because legislation affects the way health care organizations do business, the case manager must know the basic provisions of the many statutes that have either a direct or an indirect impact on the success of a patient's care while that care is being overseen by a case manager. This chapter focuses on some of the many laws and regulations that affect how health care professionals conduct their business in today's world.

STANDARDS OF CARE AND PRACTICE

First and foremost, as case managers ready themselves for practice, a critical step is to understand the importance of adhering to general standards of care and to the standards that pertain in one's specific area of professional practice. The basic purpose of standards of care is to protect not only patients but health care professionals as well. Although over the years standards of care have evolved to help patients avoid substandard care, they have also evolved to serve as a tool or guideline for professionals.

Standards of care are broken down into four categories:

1. **External**—the rules, regulations, and guidelines established by state boards, professional organizations, and federal organizations

2. **Internal**—the rules or guidelines used by individual health care professionals or institutions, which often include job descriptions as well as organizational policies and procedures
3. **National**—the practices followed by other professionals in the same specialty, which are based on reasonableness and reflect the average degree of skill, care, and diligence exercised by members of that profession throughout the country as a whole
4. **Local**—the practices followed by other professionals of the same specialty, which are based on reasonableness and reflect the average degree of skill, care and diligence exercised by members of that profession within the local geographic area

Not only does every specialty in health care have its own set of standards for the given area of practice, but there are also general health care standards established by review and regulatory agencies such as the Case Management Society of America, the American Nurses Association, the National Committee for Quality Assurance, the Joint Commission on Accreditation of Healthcare Organizations, the Centers for Medicare & Medicaid Services, and state departments of health and human services.

BEST DEFENSES FOR PROTECTION FROM LAWSUITS

That our society is becoming more litigious is well known. Although some lawsuits may focus on areas such as lack of proper diagnosis or lack of an expeditious coverage determination, many are due plainly and simply to the failure to follow established standards of practice or standards of care. In other cases, the lawsuits result from a lack of information, documentation, and communication, which often leads to lack of understanding, frustration, and anger on the part of the patient. Not enough can be said about the importance of documentation. In most states the statute of limitations is very short (2 years for adults). Because few people remember details for any length of time, documentation of key case events plays a critical part in one's defense should a lawsuit be filed, and often the deciding factor in a case will be the on or lack thereof.

Of all the activities performed by any health care professional, the most important probably is documentation. This one key area cannot be overlooked. The patient's medical record, if compiled correctly, represents a history that spans specific time periods—and even, at times, a lifetime, if records are moved as providers are changed. The same is true of the case management chart and any case management plan. Consequently, confidentiality of medical information is important: first and foremost because patients expect it, and second because legislation requires that personally identifiable information be protected. Greater protection is mandated for information in some areas than in others.

Unfortunately, in today's technological era, many organizations continue to use a paper system for their charting. Depending on the charting standards implemented, many organizations require staff to use organizationally approved forms, standardized charting language, and a standardized filing system within the chart or record. In addition, many organizations allow automated clinical documentation of the key activities most common in treating the patients they serve. In some organizations, staff may be allowed to document using any piece of paper handy, and there is no system for how documents are filed. The following are some of the major problems with handwritten notes:

- Handwriting may be illegible.
- If information is transferred to a more formal charting system later, data can be lost.
- When there is no official form to prompt health care personnel as they complete the charting, duplication of effort, redundancy, fragmentation, and failure to capture key information in the notes are common.

As with documentation, not enough can be said about the need to draft an adequate case management plan. Nursing care plans have existed for decades. Over the past several years, however, clinical pathways and care maps have become the documents most widely used in clinical settings. Although clinical pathways are important tools for hospital-based case managers, most external case management organizations continue to allow their nurses to document treatment details in a care plan or case management plan.

Regardless of the format used, it is critical that the documentation describe the plan for patient care at all levels at which care is given, as well as the linkages to community resources, services, and care. At a minimum the plan must include the types of services required with details on both scope and frequency. In some care plans it is also important to include the costs of services and to identify which source is paying for which services. In today's health care atmosphere, with a strong focus on costs, cost containment, and length of stay, one must not lose sight of the need to ensure that a safe and effective plan is in place. If safety cannot be assured or the patient refuses the recommended plan of care, documentation of the reasons is vital to protect against litigation.

ETHICAL DILEMMAS

Although some nurses feel that ethical issues are someone else's responsibility and that specialized expertise is required to deal with them, this is not true, for the American Nurses Association has established standards for ethical practice to which they hold all nurses accountable.

Because of the nature of the job, case managers often walk a fine line when it comes to ethics, and for this reason they are frequently confronted with ethical dilemmas. Some dilemmas can be handled individually, whereas others may require a team approach. In some cases, resolution of the ethical dilemma may require a committee review of the issues at hand. Because of the position and authority given to them, case managers assist in promoting and safeguarding patient autonomy. In all instances, case managers play a key role in educating patients and their families and in helping them understand the options available.

INFORMED CONSENT

Long gone are the days when a handshake between doctor and patient was all that was needed to proceed with a treatment or patient care. In today's technologically advanced health care arena, obtaining informed consent for certain procedures and following advance directives are not only desirable but are mandated by law. Again, because case managers often assume the role of advocate, they are in a position to help those patients with decision-making capacity to explore treatment options and make wise decisions. Lack of decision-making capacity does not negate the right of self-determination, but in cases such as this, the case manager must proceed cautiously to ensure that appropriate documentation is present should questions arise at a later date.

LAWS AND REGULATIONS

Because laws change and vary by state, leaders in case management strongly recommend that, to be effective, case managers familiarize themselves with some of the many federal laws influencing health care as well as the relevant statutes of at least their own states.

SUMMARY

Until consumers, health care purchasers, providers, and health care insurers come to a consensus on health care issues, legislative initiatives can be expected at both the state and federal levels. With each new law comes a myriad of mandates and processes that must be followed. Depending on their scope, many laws will have little direct impact on case management processes; however, others will. When legislation affects health care, especially resources and services, case managers must stay informed about the implications of the laws' provisions so that patient needs can be handled appropriately.

Chapter Exercises

1. Research the standards of practice of your professional organization (e.g., for registered nurses, social workers) and ask yourself if you are practicing as the standards dictate. If you work for an organization that has standards of care, review these standards and identify key ones that relate to your area of responsibility.

2. In the standards of practice for your professional organization, identify the key standards that apply directly to your role and identify means to help protect yourself against litigation.

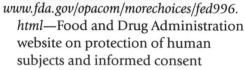

Suggested Websites and Resources

www.fda.gov/opacom/morechoices/fed996. html—Food and Drug Administration website on protection of human subjects and informed consent

www.medrecinst.com/media/document/ summary.shtml—Medical Records Institute

www.ahcpr.gov/data/hcup/—Agency for Healthcare Research and Quality

www.jcaho.org/accredited+organizations/ standards+faqs.htm—Accreditation information, Joint Commission on Accreditation of Healthcare Organizations

www.nursingworld.org/ancc/—American Nurses Credentialing Center

www.cmsa.org/—Case Management Society of America

www.ncqa.org/—National Committee for Quality Assurance

BIBLIOGRAPHY

Cohen EL, Cesta TG: *Nursing case management: from essentials to advanced practice applications,* ed 3, St Louis, 2001, Mosby.

Cohen EL, DeBack V: *The outcomes mandate case management in health care today,* St Louis, 1999, Mosby.

O'Keefe ME: *Nursing practice and the law: avoiding malpractice and other legal risks,* Philadelphia, 2001, FA Davis.

CHAPTER
12

Protecting Oneself from Malpractice

Peggy A. Rossi, BSN, MPA, CCM, CPUR

OBJECTIVES

- To identify the four reasons a patient might file a malpractice claim and at least six measures a case manager can take to protect himself or herself from malpractice
- To identify the agency that disseminates the state's nurse practice act and obtain access to a copy for personal use
- To be able to access at least one clinical practice guideline from the Agency of Healthcare Research and Quality (AHRQ) website
- To identify the most important component in case management for protection from malpractice

As health care costs skyrocket and society demands a reduction in these costs, case managers have become more closely involved in managing health care benefits through or for third-party payers. Case managers thus find themselves in a dichotomous situation. On the one hand, they are patient advocates, and on the other, they must also serve as their organizations' advocates and ensure that care is provided in the most cost-effective manner. Because there are no national standards, outcome criteria, or clear guidelines for such dual advocacy roles, the case manager is placed at risk of liability. To reduce this risk, case managers must understand their role and practice in a manner that is consistent with their obligations.

Case managers have chosen a calling that directly affects patients' lives. Consequently, the entities that license health care professionals have established rules, regulations, procedures, criteria, complaint processes, and standards for disciplining licensees. Patients who believe they have been harmed at the hands of their health care providers can bring suits against those they believe harmed them. Thus although a health care professional's primary duty is to the patient, every act of providing health care is done in a much broader context of licensure, ethics, and the law. Often the health care professional's first introduction to the legal system is being handed papers stating that he or she is being sued. This is an unpleasant, confusing, and often frightening experience.[1]

Malpractice occurs when a health care professional fails to do what a reasonable prudent peer would do under the same or similar circumstances. The person making the claim of malpractice is required to prove the following:

- The existence of the duty, in a patient–health care professional relationship, to conform to a recognized standard of care
- A failure to conform to the required standard of care
- Actual injury
- A reasonable close causal connection between the professional's conduct and the patient's injury

Once the existence of a legal duty is established in a malpractice claim, the plaintiff must prove the breach of duty. Breach of duty can be proven by showing that conduct fell below the applicable standard of care.

Although the following list refers to failures that lead to liability for case managers working with elderly clients, these breaches of duty can occur with any patient followed up by case managers[2]:

- Failure to adopt a care plan specific to the needs of the patient
- Failure to adequately assess and implement a care plan
- Failure to evaluate the patient's condition and modify care to prevent deterioration and maintain health
- Failure to ensure that medications are administered in a timely and proper manner
- Failure to observe and detect multiple interactions of drug therapy
- Failure to document in a timely and proper manner the patient's condition, care and treatment rendered, and the patient's response to such
- Failure to follow the facility's or organization's policies and procedures
- Failure to document appropriate teaching, including patient's responses and evidence of his or her understanding
- Failure to adequately protect a patient who is sedated, confused, or disoriented

- Failure to go through hierarchy to provide appropriate and timely treatment
- Failure to recognize the need for restraints or improper use of restraints
- Failure to provide or recognize the need for timely and proper skin care to prevent decubitus ulcers that can lead to amputation, sepsis, and death
- Failure to properly assess and monitor patients and failure to implement safety measures to prevent falls and injuries
- Failure to protect patients from burn injury
- Abandonment of patients

The risk of medical liability can also be reduced through such practices as the following[3]:

- Working closely with the legal department of the organization to prevent patient care problems from escalating into a medical liability
- Immediate investigation and resolution of patient care problems
- Constant review to ensure that only current revisions of policies and procedures and standards of care and practice are used
- Compliance with managed care contracts and ensuring that care is precertified if this is a requirement and that the care is provided according to these contracts
- Use of appropriate resources
- Timely dissemination of information to key players and decision makers

Wise case managers will always make every effort to protect their licenses as they take action that could have a negative impact.

STANDARDS OF CARE

The basic purposes of standards of care are to protect and safeguard not only patients but also health care professionals. Over the years, standards of care have evolved to help patients avoid substandard care and to give guidance to professionals. Standards of care describe the minimal requirements that define an acceptable level of care, which is the provision of ordinary and reasonable care to ensure that no unnecessary harm comes to a patient.[4] However, standards are not absolute because they depend on subjective determinations.

Standards of care, clinical guidelines, and *standards for professional performance* are terms that are often confused and used interchangeably. The confusion often centers on the fact that standards of care involve standards for the process, whereas standards of professional performance relate to the behavior. Various organizations have established standards, and it is imperative that professionals know their specialty organization's standards. Standards of care are authoritative statements promulgated by a profession from which the quality of practice, service, or education can be evaluated and are considered to be the minimum requirements for health care activities. Standards are not absolute because they depend on subjective determinations about minimum acceptable behaviors.

Standards of care are broken down into four categories—external, internal, national, and local (Box 12-1). Internal standards are those set by the role and education of the health care professional or by individual institutions. Internal standards include job descriptions, education and expertise, and policies and procedures. External standards are the rules and regulations and guidelines established by state boards, professional organizations, and federal organizations. National standards are based on reasonableness and are the average degree of skill, care, and diligence exercised by members of the same profession. Local standards of care are judged by the skill, care, and diligence of members of the same profession within that geographic area. As a rule, national standards of care are the recognized authority. Basically, a standard of care is what a reasonable and prudent professional would do in the same or similar circumstances.

BOX 12-1

Guidelines for Standards of Care

- Recognize that all professionals have standards of care. Standards are the minimal level of expertise that must be delivered to the patient. Standards of care are the starting point for greater expectations.
- Standards of care may be either externally or internally set. The health care professional is responsible for both categories of standards: those set on a national basis and those set by the role of their profession.
- Standards of care for nursing, for example, can be found in the following:
  - The state nurse practice act
  - Published standards of professional organizations and specialty practice groups
  - Federal agency guidelines and regulations
  - Hospital or a health care organization's policy and procedure manuals
  - An individual's job description
- Health care professionals are accountable for all standards of care as they pertain to their profession. To remain competent and skillful, the professional is encouraged to read professional journals and to attend pertinent continuing education and in-service programs.
- Standards of care are determined by the judicial system by expert witnesses. Such persons testify to the prevailing standards in the community—standards that the specialty's professionals are held accountable for matching or exceeding. Adherence to such standards ensures that patients receive quality and competent care.[4]

The Joint Commission on Accreditation of Healthcare Organizations (JCAHO) is an independent nonprofit entity that may be the most widely known organization that establishes standards for the delivery of health care from multiple health care organizations. Because members of the JCAHO believe that standards are the backbone of nursing, they have established parameters for nursing activities. The JCAHO's standards are patient-centered, performance-focused, and organized around functions common to all health care organizations. A process for evaluation of the standards is required, and the JCAHO surveys each organization to ensure that it adheres to the standards.

Another entity that establishes standards for nurses is the American Nurses Association (ANA). The ANA has its standards of nursing practice divided into two categories: standards of care and standards of professional performance. The ANA standards of care involve the nursing process and activities directly related to patient care and are as follows:

- Assessment
- Diagnosis
- Outcome identification
- Planning
- Implementation
- Evaluation

The ANA standards of professional performance involve professional nursing behavior, and nurses are expected to engage in these activities as appropriate according to their education and position:

- Quality of care
- Performance appraisal
- Education
- Collegiality
- Ethics
- Collaboration
- Research
- Resource utilization

All 50 states, the District of Columbia, and the five United States territories have their own nurse practice acts. In general, the nurse practice acts are designed to protect the public from incompetent practitioners, determine the scope of practice issues, and define and set standards for nursing practice within the state. Each state's nurse practice act has been established by legislation, and a state's nurse practice act is by far the most definitive piece of legislation regulating nursing.[5] Nurses should familiarize themselves with their state's nurse practice act because of its overriding effect on all nursing practices: neither physician orders nor institutional policy can override a state's nurse practice act.

States differ as to which designated regulatory board or agency enforces the act, but in most states it is the board of nursing. It is the regulatory board's duty to issue the rules and regulations and oversee specific practices. This same board is often the state's designated regulatory agency for establishing requirements for licensure application, ongoing professional licensure, and disciplinary actions and for regulation, to some degree, of the schools of nursing within the state. Although the ANA provides guidelines (structure and function) to each state's board of nursing, each board has the power to act independently and accept or reject the ANA's recommendations as it sees fit.

Most state boards set and approve the standards for undergraduate and graduate programs, as well as continuing education and refresher courses. The standards are set to ensure a consistent and educationally sound nursing curriculum in an attempt to produce competent practitioners by using minimum competencies based on the state's nurse practice definition of nursing. For formal accreditation of schools of nursing, states rely on the National League of Nursing.

For licensed nursing professionals, knowledge of their state's regulations (or if they practice in multiple states, each state's regulations), requirements for licensure, and standards defined by the nurse practice act is imperative. This is necessary to prevent falling victim to a state board's investigation or disciplinary actions on the basis of perceived shortcomings of practice as they relate to the state's nurse practice act. Likewise, all professionals have an obligation to report a peer who appears to be in violation of the act.

CLINICAL PRACTICE GUIDELINES OR BEST PRACTICES

Clinical guidelines are the recommended clinical practice for patient management. Clinical guidelines are patient-focused and are based on diagnoses, procedures, or clinical conditions. They are viewed as a means of controlling costs while providing continuity and quality of care. Facts about clinical practice guidelines include the following:

- They provide research-based information and a wide range of acceptable practice options, which can be modified or adapted to specific patient clinical needs.
- They do not take the place of standards of care but provide a researched-based option for decisions.
- They must be updated regularly, and updates must be based on valid review and opinion.
- Once they are in place, the clinician must be cognizant of the need to document any deviation from the guidelines and the clinical rationale for the deviation.

The most widely known agency used for the development of clinical practice guidelines is the Agency for Health Care Research and Quality (AHRQ), formerly the Agency for Healthcare Policy and Research. The AHRQ was established in 1989 under the Omnibus Reconciliation Act as a division of the Department of Health and Human Services. The AHRQ's prime missions are to compile and provide health care providers and consumers with research information and clinical practice guidelines. The AHRQ's current clinical guidelines can be found on their website: www.ahrq.gov.

Best practices are those practices that result in benchmarks that meet or set a new standard. Benchmarking is a process, a structured approach, or a discipline that is continuing or ongoing and involves measuring, evaluating, and comparing the results and processes that produce the best results. The actual measurement used to gauge the performance of a function, operation, or relative business practice is benchmarking. An objective of benchmarking is to help an organization set higher goals and improve performance, and the overall goal of benchmarking is to identify best practices that can be implemented to produce improvements. Learning how to adapt best practices that are learned through the benchmarking process promotes breakthrough process improvements and builds healthier communities.[6]

EVIDENCE-BASED MEDICINE

Evidence-based medicine is now being used as a standard for making informed medical care decisions, developing practice guidelines, and evaluating the efficacy of alternative treatments. Outcomes researchers, practice guideline developers, and health care professionals are more frequently basing decisions on evidence found by taking the best from practice patterns of specific specialty providers who have the necessary clinical expertise and applying it to the delivery of health care. The concept of evidence-based medicine gained momentum in the late 1980s and early 1990s as a response to both a new opportunity and a tough challenge. The opportunity was provided by better, less costly information systems that could gather research data and then disseminate the findings for decision making. The challenge was to apply the most effective modalities of treating patients at the least cost and risk, while still maintaining quality of care and reaching treatment goals.

This new technology made the rewards of evidence-based medicine more attainable. At the same time, the increased demands on limited health care resources prompted a search for more effective care and for ways to reduce inappropriate care. The result was that the Agency for Health Care Policy and Research (now the AHRQ) launched an initiative that created 12 evidence-based practice centers. The purpose of these centers was to provide a scientific foundation for public and private organizations to use as they developed and implemented their own practice guidelines, performance measures, and other tools needed to improve quality and make decisions related to the effectiveness or appropriateness of specific health care challenges.[7]

Evidence-based medicine is the conscientious, explicit, and judicious use of current best evidence by physicians in making decisions about the care of individual patients. In the practice of evidence-based medicine, individual clinical expertise (the proficiency and judgment acquired through clinical practice) is integrated with the best available external clinical evidence (clinically relevant research not necessarily restricted to randomized trials) obtained from systematic research of available treatment options. The practice of evidence-based medicine gives clinicians the benefit of others' expertise and results in more efficient diagnostic techniques and encourages more thoughtful identification of individual patient needs and preferences in making clinical decisions about care.

Good doctors use both individual clinical expertise and the best available external evidence, and neither alone is enough. Without current best evidence, practice may become rapidly outdated, often to the detriment of patients. Evidence-based medicine is not cookbook medicine. It requires an approach that integrates the best external evidence with individual clinical expertise and patient choices. External clinical evidence can inform but never replace individual clinical expertise, and it is this expertise that is used to determine whether the external evidence applies to the patient at all and, if so, how it should be integrated into a clinical decision. Similarly, any external guideline must be integrated with individual clinical expertise in determining whether and how it matches the patient's clinical state, predicament, and preferences, and thus whether it should be applied.[8]

CRITICAL PATHWAY, CLINICAL PATHWAY, MULTIDISCIPLINARY PLAN, MULTIDISCIPLINARY ACTION PLAN, AND ACTION PLAN

The critical pathway was first introduced in 1985 by the New England Medical Center in Boston. It was the first system that attempted to incorporate expected outcomes within specific time frames. The term *critical pathway* means that the plan defines critical or key events expected to happen each day of the patient's hospitalization for a specific diagnosis or procedure.[3] Efforts to reduce expenditures are a continual battle. Therefore many organizations are directing efforts specifically toward procedures and diagnoses that consume relatively large amounts of resources. It has been found that outcomes, cost, and process are related and that one factor cannot be altered without affecting the other two. However, by standardizing patient care and caregiver techniques, if positive outcomes are the end results, these outcomes can play a part in improving quality of care for others with the same diagnosis or medical condition. One approach to meeting these objectives is the use of critical pathways. Critical pathways have been described as time-specific blueprints for diagnosis or for planning a patient's treatment during hospitalization. The pathway should focus on key events and interventions that are made by health care personnel focusing on achievement of predetermined outcomes in an effective time frame and using appropriate resources.[9]

Since their inception, critical pathways have also been referred to as *clinical pathways, multidisciplinary plans, multidisciplinary action plans*, and *action plans*. In essence, each, although titled differently, is the same in theory. Each attempts to outline expected outcomes of care for each professional discipline during each day of hospitalization. A critical pathway or plan is defined as "a structured, multidisciplinary patient care plan in which diagnostic and therapeutic interventions performed by nurses, physicians and other team members for a particular diagnosis or procedure are sequenced on a timeline."[1] Although the pathway or plan emphasizes nursing planning and the medical plan of care, it must also incorporate all disciplines, taking into account the unique contributions of each. Such plans are the driving force behind case management because they help determine the plan of care and arrange the plan around the expected length of stay or time frame for reaching goals.

Critical pathways are developed for patients, procedures, or symptoms associated with high volume, high cost, or high risk and should identify specific diagnoses and recommended interventions. Pathways have four major features: patient outcomes, a timeline, collaboration, and definitions of comprehensive aspects of care. With a critical pathway, all interventions, actions, and services are graphically depicted and planned for the patient along the continuum of care. When a critical pathway is used, a form is used to document findings that vary from those expected. When variances from the determined goals and timeline are observed, an

explanation is required.[9] The design of any critical pathway or plan begins with a strategic planning process. In planning one must decide the following:

- Who are the stakeholders and which disciplines are important?
- What criteria will be used?
- What outcome goals are expected?

Pathways should be built around the types of cases that are seen most often or those that have unacceptable rates of complications or variances from the expectations of customers (providers, patients, payers).[11] When pathways are developed, specific elements must be considered and selected before any form is created. Factors that affect the design and content of the form include the complexity of care, the extent to which the plan will include other disciplines, and whether the form will include nursing documentation. Once the form has been created and approved, the organization must decide which diagnoses or procedures will be planned first.

In designing pathways, several factors must be considered, including the number and type of patients that will be served, issues that affect length of stay and other time frames, and health care disciplines to be involved.

Because not every patient will fit exactly into a projected pathway, pathways must be tailored to the individual. Projected pathways are designed for the average patient within the category chosen. Unusual or aberrant conditions or circumstances must be taken into consideration. Once the projected pathway is completed, it must be reviewed and approved by a representative of each discipline that participated in its development.

When pathways are developed, it should be kept in mind that reimbursement will play a role and will differ by payer source. Thus it is important to determine an average length of stay or time in which to achieve specific goals. The pathway should be designed so that time frames are shorter than the reimbursable length of stay to allow for a "margin of error." This allows additional time should the patient require it. For assistance in planning projected time frames, case managers my refer to national guidelines such as those of Milliman and Robertson or diagnosis-related groups, which are good resources for benchmarking. Use of national guidelines such as these provides not only length-of-stay expectations but also alternative settings and options for managing the length of stay or time to reach goals.

Guidelines for the development of critical pathways or plans include the following:

■ Identify the high-volume case types of the organization.
■ Validate issues that affect length of stays and time frames through chart reviews of the selected high-volume cases (this means random selection of charts for patients with the same diagnosis or procedure), because the issues identified are the drivers of the clinical content of the plan.
■ Determine which physicians or other members of key health care disciplines who work with these patients are willing to help write and adopt the case management plan (this will depend on the diagnosis or procedure).
■ Determine time frames (hours might be representative of emergency department cases; days, of surgery cases; weeks, of diagnoses or procedures for which longer time frames are common; and months, of plans for neonates or persons in long-term care facilities).
■ Determine variance time frames. Typical variances categories include the following:
  ▪ Operational problems (e.g., breakdown of equipment or inability to perform a task because of inability to locate an appropriate postacute-care setting)

  ▪ Use of varying practice patterns by health care provider
  ▪ Patient refusal or a change in status
  ▪ Unmet clinical indicators (e.g., patient has not reached expected outcome)
■ Determine demographic and clinically specific information for the diagnosis or procedure.

For a series of on-line clinical practice guidelines developed with the support of the former Agency for Health Care Policy and Research (the AHRQ), see the AHRQ website at www.info@ahrq.gov.[12]

Case managers are the driving force behind the success of most pathways: they check on variances related to both cause and remedy. Key to any pathway is documentation of variances to events or variances necessary to support actions. Using the pathway as a guide, case managers are responsible for ensuring the following:

■ Patients' continued success in moving through the system
■ The process is a collaborative (team) effort
■ Patient teaching is accomplished if a need is identified
■ The patient and family are involved to achieve the best outcomes
■ Other resources are coordinated when identified (e.g., social services or community resources for postacute care)
■ Communication occurs with all internal disciplines, as well as with all community care providers involved
■ All other health care disciplines are kept focused on achieving expected and timely outcomes of care

The health care team can use an in-depth, detailed pathway, and the same pathway can be modified for use by the patient and family. If a modified pathway is to be used by the patient and family, it must be in language that can be understood by a layperson. The patient's pathway should not be too clinically specific; it does not need to contain the details included in the health care team's pathway. However, it should contain specific information that is relevant to the patient's needs. Benchmarks, milestones, or goals for each identified task should be included in the patient's pathway.

DOCUMENTATION

The importance of documentation in case management is clear because it is an essential component and tool of assessment, planning, communication, evaluation, and monitoring of patient care outcomes, resource utilization and management, clinical progress, and quality of care. Regardless of his or her field, the case manager must document the essential components to tell the story. Documentation must be clear and concise. It is critical to an effective case management practice. During documentation, the following questions should be asked. Who is the audience? What is the objective? What information must be told? Case managers should keep in mind that most states require case management agencies and providers to retain patient files for 5 to 7 years. Thus records can be subpoenaed if a legal situation arises, underscoring that case management documentation must be accurate and objective without mention of suspicions, opinions, or allegations.[13]

From a legal standpoint, documentation is often the deciding factor in a case. The JCAHO manual gives an excellent overview of the main points that should be included in documentation. Although it was originally written for staff nurses, much of it also applies to case managers. For example, the JCAHO mandates that documentation should do the following:

- Be pertinent and concise and reflect the patient's current status

- Identify the patient's needs, problems, capabilities, and limitations
- Indicate nursing interventions and the patient's responses
- Indicate the patient's status at the time of any transfer or discharge
- Indicate when individual discharge counseling has occurred and the patient requires ongoing care; included should be descriptive documentation that the patient or family has an understanding of what was taught

The statute of limitations (time frame in which to file a lawsuit) varies from state to state and also varies with the age of the patient (i.e., an adult has 2 years, whereas a minor has until the age of 21 years).[14] Therefore because few people can remember events for a long period, documentation becomes the critical defending factor when a lawsuit is filed. The case manager should keep in mind that documentation in medical records and e-mails is discoverable, which means that it must be disclosed before a trial. Therefore the importance of documentation and the contents and location of documents cannot be emphasized enough.

Should the patient's medical record require alteration or correction, this can be done if it is for valid purposes, such as transcription errors, changing erroneous date, and notation or clarification of any new information that is relevant to that aspect of the patient's care. If changes are made, they must be noted clearly by making a single line through the portion of the record to be altered, corrected, or appended; and the date of the change and the person's signature must be noted conspicuously. Also, if a change is made, there must be an explanation in the chart as to why the alteration occurred. State statutes, medical bylaws, or both dictate which changes can be made to a medical record. Changes to a medical record for purposes of fraud or intent to deceive are subject to criminal penalties and could result in loss of licensure.

Guidelines for documentation include the following:

- Keep it accurate and concise; chart only the facts in chronological order. A case manager should ask whether this is what he or she would want presented if the case went to court.
- Chart as objectively as possible. Although subjective charting can be done, state the facts as related by the patient.
- Chart information that communicates the patient's progress and/or potential problems.
- Document informed consent pertaining to medical procedures.
- Document information regarding transfers of patients to other facilities (e.g., permission obtained from the patient or family, others spoken with, who made the decision to transfer, when the transfer took place, and the mode of transportation).
- Document communications and all efforts made for communication between team members and physicians regarding specific incidents.
- Record all procedures, treatments, medications, and teaching.
- Chart information about the patient's assessments or any reactions to treatments, procedures, medications, or teaching; patient noncompliance or concerns; and any actions taken and names of persons contacted.
- Use only abbreviations accepted by the organization or the JCAHO and do not use labels, derogatory comments, personal opinions, or unfamiliar medical terms.
- Write neatly and legibly.
- Record events as promptly as possible after they occur. Actual findings, responses, and dates and times must

be included on all entries. Document all follow-up events.

- If changes are needed, follow the organization's guidelines for changes; or if a mistake is made, draw a line through the entry, mark "error," make the new entry, and sign the record with first initial and last name and title.
- Do not destroy any parts of the chart.
- Date, time, and sign all documentation.

Documentation for case management, as with all health care disciplines, should be an ongoing procedure. Documentation should be done at the frequency dictated by case events, each event should be summarized concisely. By their very roles, case managers are reporters and analyzers, and effective case management documentation is important in telling the patient's whole story.

TELEPHONIC CASE MANAGEMENT

Although telephone technology is wonderful, it carries with it a significant barrier: persons speaking by phone cannot see one another. In some cases when talking with a patient, a case manager may not have the patient's chart handy (e.g., when a cell phone is used). Also, sometimes automated telephone systems leave patients angry and frustrated. As a result of the rise in telephonic case management (e.g., telephone advice lines or actual case management services), there is a growing trend by organizations to protect their staff from litigation. The following techniques are helpful for anyone who spends a great deal of time on the phone talking with patients or providers:

- Never leave a client or patient on hold for more than 2 to 3 minutes.
- Prepare for accidental disconnection by making sure that each party has the other's name and telephone number.

- Always follow written protocol of the organization.
- Comply with the Americans with Disability Act: ensure that services designed to assist the hearing impaired (telecommunication devices for the deaf [TDD]) are available or, if there is a language barrier, that American Telephone and Telegraph (AT&T) interpretive services are available.
- Keep telephone communications as confidential as written ones.
- Avoid allowing inappropriate personnel to give advice on the telephone.
- Keep hard-copy manuals and records on hand.
- Companies must ensure that 24-hour maintenance is available.
- Be prepared for emergencies (e.g., difficult situations such as suicide threats, obscene phone calls, difficult callers, or callers in distress).
- Try not to hang up on angry callers or transfer them to another party; this only makes the situation worse, so try to stay calm.[15]

INFORMED CONSENT

The right to informed consent mandates that adequate information about the procedure at hand be provided in the patient's primary language at a level appropriate for the patient's understanding Informed consent is the process by which a health care provider communicates and discusses the risks and benefits of each diagnostic or treatment alternative that a reasonable provider in similar circumstances would give, including doing nothing, for the patient's disease state in a manner that the patient can comprehend.[16] Finalization of informed consent occurs when the patient signs a document acknowledging that he or she understood all the information provided. The consent document must be witnessed, dated, and timed to be valid.

Managed Medicaid takes the informed consent process a step further when it comes to many procedures. For example, in the case of sterilization procedures, Medicaid requires not only that the discussion occur in the patient's own language or through an interpreter who can explain medical aspects of the discussion, but also that the consent form be signed at least 30 days before the actual procedure. The final step is that for claims payment to occur, the consent form must be attached to the claim.

Before a patient can be informed, it must be determined that the patient is capable of comprehending what is said. An incompetent person must be deemed so by a court of law. Consequently, an incompetent person cannot provide informed consent, and an agent must be appointed to act on his or her behalf. Although informed consent documents are used primarily when an invasive procedure is to be performed or the topic of the consent has potentially dangerous side effects or complications, they are not restricted to this use.

For minors, informed consent documents must be signed by the parent(s) or a legally appointed guardian. If the patient is considered an emancipated minor, some states allow the patient to sign. In the Medicaid managed care arena, informed consent documents can be signed by minors for several treatments, emancipated or not. Treatments in this area include such services as testing and treatment for human immunodeficiency virus (HIV) infection or sexually transmitted disease, abortions, and family planning.

Refusal of Care

Lack of information may hamper a patient's decision-making capabilities. Health care professionals must take every opportunity to educate patients and correct any misunderstandings about their illness or the proposed care. Health care professionals may try to persuade patients to accept treatments without first ascertaining the reason they refused. Refusal of care is often a result of poor communication, emotional factors, and cultural or religious differences. At times patients may feel intimidated; or patients may believe that their views are being ignored or that their opinions are not considered important. Also some patients may base their decisions on previous personal experiences or the experience of friends or relatives in similar situations. If professionals visibly react to a refusal, this may exacerbate an already tense situation. As a result, the patient becomes more anxious and adamant. Therefore do the following to allow a patient to make an informed decision:

- Remain calm (a sense of crisis will only make matters worse).
- Use open-ended questions to engage the patient in the discussion.
- Do not use medical jargon or terms that are incomprehensible to a layperson.
- Provide information in an understandable way.
- Allow patients to ask about alternatives to the proposed treatment.
- Explain adverse consequences if the proposed treatment is refused.
- Make every effort to clarify what is going to happen.
- Present rational reasons as to what is believed to be best in the circumstances, taking into account the patient's values and preferences.

Use of such an approach fosters patient autonomy, and patients are more likely to make informed decisions if they truly understand the reasons for treatment, what will happen during treatment, alternatives, and consequences of refusal.

Implied Consent in Emergencies

Implied consent is often used to prevent delays in treatment in an emergency when informed consent may be impossible to obtain because the patient is comatose or delirious. In these cases the delay caused by trying to obtain informed consent might jeopardize the patient's life or health. Implied consent is recognized in life-and-death situations when it is considered appropriate to presume that the patient in question would consent.

Implied consent should not be used when informed consent is feasible or when it is known that the patient does not want treatment. Also, a general consent form signed at the time of admission to a hospital should never be used as implied consent for all treatments and procedures. If specific invasive interventions are to occur, the patient or his or her legal representative must sign an informed consent document for each intervention.

Although a consent form is a means to document that the patient agrees to treatment, it does not address the issue of whether a provider's disclosure was adequate. Therefore because case managers often serve as patient advocates, it is both their ethical and legal responsibility to protect patients from misinformation, omissions, and errors. If, as an advocate, the case manager detects that a misunderstanding has occurred, the physician must be notified and actions must be documented (Box 12-2).

ADVANCE DIRECTIVES

The Patient Self-Determination Act was enacted in 1991 as part of the federal Omnibus Reconciliation Act of 1990 and became law in 1992. The act was developed to ensure that health care organizations (hospitals, home health agencies, skilled nursing facilities, hospices, and health maintenance organizations) receiving federal money from Medicare and/or Medicaid informed patients of their rights to use an advance directive and to refuse or accept care. It also ensures that organizations follow their state laws related to advance directives, directs the Centers for

---

BOX 12-2
Basic Guidelines for Informed Consent

- Before a patient can be informed, it must be determined that the patient is capable of comprehending what is said. If it is determined that the patient is too confused or will not understand what is said, it may be necessary to have him or her evaluated for competency.
- Adequate information must be relayed to the patient about the procedure at hand, and it must be provided at the level appropriate for the patient's understanding. Information must also be given in the patient's primary language. If the patient does not speak the case manager's language, an interpreter must be used.
- For minors, informed consent documents must be signed by the parent(s) or a legally appointed guardian. If the patient has been declared an emancipated minor, some states allow the patient to sign. Case managers must know what their state allows for consent services pertaining to minors. Finalization of informed consent occurs when the patient signs a document acknowledging he or she understood all the information provided. The consent document must be witnessed, dated, and timed to be valid.
- If the patient refuses the proposed treatments, the case manager should remain calm and engage the patient in open-ended questions to ascertain perspectives and reasons for refusal.

Medicare & Medicaid Services (CMS) to determine compliance with the law, and prevents discrimination against a patient on the basis of whether an advance directive has been signed. Health care organizations are mandated to provide the following advance directive information[16]:

- Provide all adult patients, residents, and enrollees with written information on their rights under state law to make decisions regarding health care and their right to execute these wishes in an advance directive.
- Maintain policies and procedures with respect to how advance directives are to be implemented.
- Document in the medical record whether the person has an advance directive on file.
- Educate the organization's staff and community about advance directives.
- Ensure compliance with state laws regarding advance directives.

An advance directive is a legal document that states the person's wishes regarding future health care and specifically his or her desires regarding life-and-death situations, and terminal illness is not required for the document to be applied. An advance directive also allows the person to designate another person to make his or her health care decisions. Advance directives must be drawn up while the person is competent. They can only be used when the person becomes incapacitated or incompetent and is unable to make his or her own medical decisions. With an advance directive, the person has the ability to direct care in advance of need. Without a written, signed advance directive, a person's wishes cannot be honored.

Although the law applies to institutions and does not cover individual health care professionals or emergency teams, the law and a condition of accreditation by the JCAHO do require providers to supply information as follows:

- Hospitals or skilled nursing facilities must provide the information at the time of admission.
- Home health agencies and hospices must provide it before rendering care.
- Health maintenance organizations must provide it at the time membership becomes effective.

The ANA position statement on nursing and the Patient Self-Determination Act of 1991 can be used by case managers as they conduct initial assessments. The ANA recommends that the following questions be asked in a nursing assessment[5]:

- Do you have basic information about advance care directives including living wills and durable power of attorney?
- Do you wish to initiate an advance care directive?
- If you have an advance care directive, can you provide it now?
- Have you discussed your end-of-life choices with your family and/or designed surrogate and health care worker?

Durable Power of Attorney

Durable power of attorney is another written advance directive that designates a person as an attorney-in-fact (also known as *a surrogate*) to make health care decisions for the patient (known as the principal) when he or she is no longer able to make decisions. In addition to naming a person to be his or her attorney-in-fact, the patient may also name an alternate party should the specified attorney-in-fact not be available or be unwilling to make decisions.

Living Will

The most common advance directive is a living will. This document indicates the patient's wishes when specific clinical situations occur and whether the patient wants his or her life sustained through specific medical treatments. A living will can be as broad or as narrow as the executing individual wishes.

Most states have living will statutes that indicate the acceptable form of the living will and the specifics under which the living will is recognized. The major disadvantage of the living will is that it has limited clinical use because it may not be specific enough for a person's current clinical circumstances, it may contain ambiguous language, and it only applies to an incurable injury, disease, or illness. If ques-

tions related to the living will's directives arise, often the only recourse a provider has is to bring the case to court. The court will decide whether the specific withdrawal of medical intervention is covered by the living will in question.

Choosing a Surrogate

Despite the availability of the foregoing documents, the majority of individuals do not complete an advance directive. As a result, many states have enacted surrogacy laws under which patients without an advance directive who become incapacitated may have a decision maker appointed for them. The decision maker might be a spouse, family member, or other person as outlined by the state's statute. Fortunately, the ability to use surrogacy laws gives legal recognition to a process that many physicians used in the past when no one had been appointed as the guardian, that is, turning to the person most likely to be recognized as the appropriate representative for the patient. In states that do not have surrogacy laws, physicians are often required to await the formal appointment of a conservator before continuing treatments.

Determining and Declaring Decision-Making Incapacity

Determining whether a patient is competent to make his or her own health care decisions is one of the most difficult areas of medicine. Very few patients with life-threatening illnesses or injuries retain decision-making capacity until the end of life. Likewise, many patients not declared incompetent by a court of law may nonetheless have problems with their capacity to make health care decisions. If this occurs and there is a question of a patient's competency, family members and the physician must be consulted before the patient's health care decision is considered. If not satisfactorily determined, competency may have to be determined through the court. Competency often fluctuates, and proving incompetence is a difficult task to execute because unless deemed legally incompetent by a court, a person is presumed to be competent to make his or her own health care decisions.

Case managers, as members of a health care team, have a primary responsibility to promote informed decision making that includes decisions related to advance directives. Individuals with an intact decision-making capacity have the right to consent to and to refuse all medically indicated therapy. Because those who know patients best should ideally make judgments about decision-making capacity, it is very important for health care professionals to participate in efforts to determine and document capacity. Criteria for decision-making capacity include the following:

- The ability to comprehend information relevant to the decision at hand.
- The ability to deliberate in accord with a relatively consistent set of values and goals.
- The ability to communicate preferences.

In some cases a declaration of incapacity is made when a primary physician and a psychiatrist conduct evaluations and document their findings in the patient's medical record. The recorded evaluation documents the basis for declaring the patient incapacitated.[13]

There are also times when a patient's lack of decision-making capacity must be determined before a power of attorney for health care can be activated. In cases such as this, two physicians must attest to the patient's mental capacity and document their evaluations in the medical record.

When asking patients to make decisions related to their care, the wise health care professional will evaluate three primary elements of the patient's capacity to make health care decisions. The three elements are as follows:

1. The patient must possess the ability to understand the information given about the medical problem, the impact of the disease, and the consequences of the various options for treatment.
2. The patient must possess the ability to evaluate the options by comparing benefits and risks and to make rational choices.
3. The patient should be able to communicate his or her choice.

A lack of decision-making capacity (i.e., the inability to understand, to reason and evaluate, or to communicate a decision) can be presumed for the following groups of patients:

- Patients in a coma
- Infants and young children
- Patients with profoundly mental disabilities
- Patients at the end of life
- Patients with significant metabolic or physical abnormalities that limit reasoning or thinking abilities
- Patients with confusion, disorientation, or dementia (they may retain some degree of decision-making capacity but must be evaluated for their ability to make *informed* decisions)

Guidelines for decision making are listed in Box 12-3.

Do Not Resuscitate

DNR (do not resuscitate) orders are another form of an advance directive. A DNR order indicates the patient's wishes, at a minimum, that no cardiopulmonary resuscitation be provided. When DNR wishes are expressed, it is imperative that the health care professional discuss, communicate, and clarify with the patient the limits of the order and his or her expectations. This is necessary because what a patient or layperson may perceive as no resuscitation may be contrary to what a professional knows will be the case.

BOX 12-3
Guidelines for Decision Making

The patient or family opposes a treatment favored by the health care team.	Competent adults have the right to refuse treatment, but the case manager should review all options should be and ensure that the patient and family understand the prognosis and options. If the patient has an advance directive, this must be reviewed. All discussions must be clearly documented in the patient's chart.
The patient is not competent, and the family opposes a treatment favored by the health care team.	The case manager should review information carefully, identify a primary decision maker, and ensure that the family has a full understanding of the patient's prognosis, condition, and options. At times, it may be necessary to consult the organization's ethics committee.
There is disagreement between the patient and family regarding health care treatment decisions.	A competent adult has the right to refuse care. If an advance directive is not available, the patient should be encouraged to complete one. In cases such as this, the family may need counseling to be supportive of the patient's decision.
The patient or family wants treatments, despite the fact that the health care team does not support them.	The health care team should consider a second opinion and provide the option of transfer to another practitioner. In cases like these, the ethics committee might play a critical role.
The family is in disagreement and the patient is incompetent.	The case manager should attempt to identify one primary decision maker while making every attempt to bring the family into agreement. In cases like these, the ethics committee might play a critical role.
The health care team is in disagreement (e.g., one physician against another; physician against discharge plan).	Every attempt should be made to reconcile the differences. A second opinion should be sought if the patient is in favor of it.
Health care team and family favor treatment for an incompetent patient but patient is opposed.	A court must prove incompetence and a legal guardian or conservator must be appointed.
Competency is not clear.	The patient's mental status and capacity for decision-making must be assessed. At some point, a psychiatric evaluation might be required or the ethics committee might be consulted. However, until the patient is declared incompetent, he or she has the right to make his or her own health care decisions—right or wrong.[18]

PATIENT RIGHTS AND CONFIDENTIALITY

Confidentiality

Confidentiality of medical information is important because, first and foremost, patients expect it. Other reasons confidentiality is important are that it protects privacy, fosters trust in provider-patient relationships, and prevents harmful consequences, particularly discrimination based on the illness. Confidentiality also encourages people to seek health care if their condition is one of stigma (e.g., substance abuse, sexually transmitted diseases, or mental illness). The patient's medical record represents a history that spans specific periods, and at times, a lifetime if records are moved as providers are changed.

Although hospitals as a rule have been subject to specific requirements regarding patient medical records through the years, the requirements are no longer specific to hospitals alone. Both private accrediting organizations and public law mandate standards for record keeping. Their standards are similar to federal regulations for organizations serving the Medicare program. State laws vary, but as a rule, medical records should be kept for up to 10 years, and the legal mechanisms for enforcing confidentiality are also state-specific.

Regardless of how confidentiality is regulated, under the law there are two general tort theories. The first is an obligation to keep medical record information confidential, and unauthorized disclosure is considered a violation of privacy. The second is called *a breach of fiduciary duty of confidentiality*. This occurs when a provider discloses to a third party personal information obtained during the course of treatment and the patient has not signed a release for such information to be shared.

In today's health care environment, maintaining confidentiality is becoming increasingly more difficult. It seems that everyone has access to medical records. "One physician-ethicist estimated about 75 people have legitimate reason to access medical records because they are providing direct or supportive services to the person."[19] Breaches of confidentiality occur every day in a number of ways, for example, mentioning a patient by name in an elevator or cafeteria or during conversations at parties or with spouses or other family members.

Although medical records are the property of the entity that created them, patients are considered to have some ownership of their own records.[16] Health care professionals are obligated to keep the information within a person's medical records confidential as dictated by professional ethics, formal court decisions, legislative means, and state statutes. The legal mechanisms enforcing confidentiality are state-specific, but under common law, providers are obligated to keep medical record information confidential. If patient information is released without a person's knowledge or permission, the release of such information constitutes an invasion of privacy. Unless the disclosure is justified, the patient or another person is not in danger, or the patient approves the release of the information, another breach of the confidentiality law occurs. This is termed *breach of fiduciary duty* and occurs when a health care provider discloses, to a third party, patient information obtained during the course of treatment or a provider-patient relationship.

Federal laws are specific when dealing with confidentiality as it pertains to substance abuse and HIV or acquired immunodeficiency syndrome (AIDS). There are strict rules and requirements for maintaining confidentiality of patient records, and this includes hospitals or other facilities that provide substance abuse diagnostic treatments or treatment referrals or receive federal funding (e.g., Medicare or Medicaid) reimbursement. These rules prevent disclosure and even acknowledgment of a patient's presence in a facility. These regulations preempt state laws, even if state laws are as stringent. The consent to disclose information is only valid if the patient or legal representative consents to disclosure to a particular agency or party and the consent is in writing. If information is revealed without written consent, this is an invasion of privacy.

In cases of treatment for substance abuse, information can be released if the patient or his or her legal representative has signed a consent form. Even with a court order or subpoena, release of information cannot occur if the following elements are not contained in the consent. In cases of child abuse, reports may be made under state law without a parent's consent or court order, but release of a child's medical records to the abuse agency must have a consent form or order for their release. The consent form must be written and contain all the following elements:

- Name of the patient
- Purpose of the disclosure
- The case manager's name and organization responsible for disclosure of the information
- Name of the organization or person who will be receiving the information
- What kind of information and how much will be disclosed
- Patient's signature
- Date of signature
- A statement that the consent can be revoked at any time by the patient
- The date when the consent will automatically expire[4]

For HIV and AIDS information, many states have adopted a variety of legislative and administrative approaches for handling the release and disclosure of information, while still protecting the patient's confidentiality and right to privacy. All 50 states require that cases of AIDS be reported, without patient consent, to the Centers for Disease Control and Prevention and to the state's health department for epidemiologic purposes.

Many states also require reporting of all persons who are HIV-positive. Many states also allow the disclosure, at least to health care professionals who are involved in the treatment of the patient, of information about the person infected with HIV or AIDS. Not all states allow this same protection for caregivers. States also vary in how they handle HIV and AIDS testing, any mandatory testing requirements, needle exchange programs, and contact tracing or partner identification. For case managers involved with patients in substance abuse treatment programs or patients with HIV or AIDS, it is imperative to know state laws on release of information, the reporting of such patients, and the state's statutes as they pertain to HIV and AIDS.

General Release of Information

As new patients are referred for case management, it is wise to have the patient sign a general release of information form. This is necessary because there will be occasions when a patient's medical information must be revealed to other providers if they are to accept the patient and provide ongoing care without fragmentation or duplication. For the release of information, the form must be in writing and should contain the following elements:

- Name of the patient
- Purpose of the disclosure
- The case manager's name and organization responsible for disclosure of the information
- Name of the organization or person who will be receiving the information
- Type of information that will be disclosed
- Patient's signature
- Date of signature
- A statement that the release of information can be revoked at any time by the patient

Patient Rights

In 1997 President Clinton established an Advisory Commission on Consumer Protection and Quality in the Healthcare Industry to study patient rights and responsibilities. Although it is still undergoing much change, a basic consumer bill of rights was formulated by this commission. Patient rights are not fully enforced federally, but many states have passed legislation in an attempt to address patient rights. Also, as a result of the commission's recommendations, many large health purchasers require health plans to adopt the following for their members:

- Information disclosure—Consumers have the right to receive accurate information and if necessary assistance in making informed health care decisions about their health plans, professionals, and facilities.
- Choice of providers and plans—Consumers have the right to a choice of health care providers that is sufficient to ensure access to appropriate high-quality health care. Public and private group purchasers should, whenever feasible, offer consumers a choice of high-quality health insurance products. Small employers should be provided with greater assistance in offering their workers and their families a choice of health plans and products.
- Access to emergency services—Consumers have the right to receive emergency health care services when and where the need arises. Health plans should provide payment when a consumer presents to an emergency department with acute symptoms of sufficient severity—including severe pain—such that a "prudent layperson" could reasonably expect the absence of medical attention to result in placing that consumer's health in serious jeopardy, serious impairment to bodily function, or serious dysfunction of any bodily organ or part.
- Participation in treatment decisions—Consumers have the right and the responsibility to fully participate in all decisions related to their health care. Consumers who are unable to fully participate in treatment decisions have the right to be represented by parents, guardians, family members, or other conservators.
- Respect and nondiscrimination—Consumers have the right to considerate, respectful care from all members of the health care system at all times and under all circumstances. An environment of mutual respect is essential to maintain a quality health care system. Consumers must not be discriminated against on the basis of race, ethnicity, national origin, religion, sex, age, mental or physical disability, sexual orientation, genetic information, or source of payment in the delivery of health care services consistent with the benefits covered in their policy or as required by law. Consumers who are eligible for coverage under the terms and conditions of a health plan or program or as required by law must not be discriminated against in the marketing and enrollment practices based on the preceding discrimination factors.
- Confidentiality of health information—Consumers have the right to communicate with health care providers in confidence and to have the confidentiality of their individually identifiable health care information protected. Consumers also have the right to review and copy their own medical records and request amendments to their records.
- Complaints and appeals—All consumers have the right to a fair and efficient process for resolving differences with their health plans, health care providers, and the institutions that serve them, including a rigorous system of internal review and an independent system of external review.
- Consumer responsibilities—In a heath care system that protects con-

sumers' rights, it is reasonable for a health plan to expect and encourage consumers to assume reasonable responsibilities.

In 1999 the Health Care Financing Administration (now CMS) also adopted new standards for patient rights for hospitals that participate in federal funding and reimbursement from Medicare and Medicaid. These new standards became effective August 2, 1999, and include the following:

- Notification of rights—Patients must be informed about their rights in advance of furnishing or discontinuing patient care. Also a procedure for prompt resolution of patient grievances must be established.
- Exercise of rights in regard to care— This allows a patient to formulate an advance directive, as well as to participate in the development and implementation of the plan of care, and to make informed decisions about care issues.
- Privacy and safety rights—These allow patients the right to personal privacy and care in a safe place, free from all forms of abuse or harassment.
- Confidentiality of records—This allows a patient access to his or her medical records.
- Freedom from restraints that are not clinically necessary—Restraints, whether chemical or physical, can be applied according to a standing or as-needed order and are to be used only if needed to improve the patient's well-being and if less restrictive interventions have proved ineffective.
- Freedom from seclusion and restraints used in behavior management unless clinically necessary— This allows a patient to remain free of restraints when imposed as a

means of coercion, discipline, convenience, or retaliation by staff members. CMS requires hospitals to report all deaths that occur when there is reason to believe that seclusion or restraint of person may have been a contributing factor.

MANDATORY REPORTING

Most states have a listing of mandated reportable conditions, which may vary by state. These conditions include specific infectious diseases, deaths, and elder and child abuse. Case managers must be knowledgeable about their state's mandated reportable conditions. In most states the following will be included in a list of conditions that must be reported:

- Abuse—child/adult/elder
- Communicable/infectious diseases (such as hepatitis, typhoid, tuberculosis, AIDS and HIV infection, sexually transmitted diseases) and these reporting requirements will be state-specific
- Violent injuries (gunshot wounds, stab wounds, and other miscellaneous wounds caused by fights, robbery, assault, or any unlawful act)
- Coroner's cases—any death for which the cause is not clear
- Impaired drivers (includes people with epilepsy, dementia, and other disorders that affect or impair consciousness)

Child and Elder Abuse

Although specific laws for reporting abuse vary by state, as do the resources for handling the caseloads, most states require health care workers to report cases of child and elder abuse, and in many states, domestic violence is also a mandated reportable event. These reports are made to a county's adult protective services agency, or in the case of domestic violence, to the local law enforcement authorities. In most states the indication for reporting abuse merely consists of reasonable cause to suspect abuse, and definite proof is not required. Health care workers, unlike laypersons, are required to report abuse if abuse is suspected during the course of treating a patient. To encourage reporting, even from a layperson, most states grant immunity from civil or criminal liability when reports are made in good faith.

A means for elder abuse reporting is necessary because many elderly patients are incapable of seeking assistance or may be unwilling, unable, or afraid or may feel too intimidated to complain about physical, psychologic, or financial abuse or neglect. Patients often believe that if they complain, they will be worse off; receive worse care; be further neglected; or if at home, be sent to a nursing home. Family members commit most elder abuse. Many abusers are overwhelmed by the responsibility and daily pressures of providing care to an elderly patient. In cases of financial exploitation, a family member sees an opportunity to gain access to money or other assets.

The same is true for child abuse. Children are often too young or are afraid or unwilling to report abuse, and they may not realize that they are being abused.

CAUSES OF MALPRACTICE, LIABILITY, AND NEGLIGENCE

Courts are increasingly holding nurses liable for malpractice and negligence in part because of increased nursing responsibilities but also because of increased individual malpractice insurance coverage. Malpractice is defined as the failure of one rendering professional services to exercise that degree of skill and learning, commonly applied under all the circumstances in the community by the average prudent reputable member of the profession, with the result of injury, loss, or damage to the recipient of those services or to those enti-

tled to rely on them.[1] Negligence is defined as conduct that falls below an accepted standard of care and causes harm or damage.[1]

Most nursing malpractice is due to failures to assess, plan, implement, evaluate, and adhere to the standards of care, as detailed in the following[1]:

- Failure to assess (i.e., this is a fundamental responsibility of nursing)
- Failure to plan (i.e., clinical decision making is an integral part of nursing)
- Failure to create a plan of care based on the patient's condition (i.e., the patient has specific care needs that are ignored because there is not a plan to address how care will be rendered to prevent complications)
- Failure to implement the plan based on the patient's condition (i.e., a plan is in place for a specific issue but is not implemented)
- Failure to follow organizational policies and procedures (i.e., not following established policies and procedures for the unit or organization)
- Failure to implement a plan of care (i.e., not performing appropriate interventions and harm results)
- Failure to advocate for the patient through organizational hierarchy (i.e., going to the administrator or physician, or if the nurse is uncomfortable with a physician's order, he or she must advocate for the patient until appropriate resolution)
- Failure to administer medication properly (i.e., give the right drug in the right dose to the right patient, by the right route and at the right time)
- Failure to implement specific actions (i.e., responses to patient/family complaints or inadequate staffing or conditions that endanger patient safety, monitoring, or special care needs)

- Failure to perform care according to the standard of care (i.e., making sure there is an informed consent for a procedure and then performing treatments safely and according to established standards of care)
- Failure to educate the patient (i.e., another fundamental of nursing, teaching)
- Failure to adequately supervise care (i.e., a supervisor does not respond when an issue is identified)
- Failure to adhere to the standard of care in specific instances (e.g., using restraints inappropriately)
- Failure to evaluate, observe, monitor, communicate, and follow up (i.e., another fundamental duty of nursing—observe changes, recognize when they are significant, report them to appropriate persons, and follow up if the response is not sufficient)
- Failure to observe a significant change or condition (i.e., knowing what the condition has been, what it is now, and what it should be, according to a patient's history or progression)
- Failure to appreciate the significance of a change or condition (i.e., knowing the significance of the observation and doing something about it other than documenting the observation)
- Failure to report or document a significant change or condition (i.e., reporting a change of condition to the appropriate provider and documenting the event accurately)
- Failure to document follow-up care (i.e., follow-up does not confirm the initial assessment and reasons were not explored)

To prevent malpractice, nurses should follow the steps in Box 12-4.

E. Hogue, in her article, "Are Case Mangers Liable?" declared, "Case man-

---

BOX 12-4
Proactive Steps to Prevent Malpractice

1. Respond to the patient
2. Educate the patient
3. Comply with standards of care
4. Supervise care
5. Adhere to the nursing process
6. Document
7. Follow up[20]

---

agers beware! Patients' attorneys are increasingly focusing attention on case mangers as defendants in lawsuits involving negligent premature discharge of patients or negligent denial of payment for services."[21] To hold case managers responsible, patients must prove all three of the following statements, and if patients fail to prove even one, they may not win[21]:

1. Case managers owed a duty to patients to make reasonable decisions.
2. Case managers breached this duty when they failed to authorize payment for appropriate services.
3. The case managers' failure to authorize payment for care caused injury or damage to patients.

Therefore the best protection is to follow basic good practices of case management, which include the following:

- Act first for patient safety. Always take into consideration the safety of the patient in light of the patient's condition and needs. Whenever in doubt as to what is best for the patient, the case manager should always advocate for the patient, as well as protect his or her license. If in doubt, consult a supervisor, physician, or other medical consultant. Likewise, if care is found to be compromised, the case manager must take action, and if necessary, move the patient to another location.

- Obtain signed medical releases of information and keep them filed in the patient's chart to reinforce to the patient that confidential and private information will be protected.
- Operate in an advisory role as plans are developed and implemented. Do not be dictatorial or issue ultimatums.
- Be savvy when it comes to conflicts of interest and learn to be open, honest, and willing to reveal contractual relationships with referral sources and the case manager's organization.
- Be savvy when it comes to contractual arrangements with vendors and providers. Be open and honest with patients when options are limited to contracted providers. If a contracted provider is found to be at fault for poor-quality care or services, be diligent about reporting such incidents.
- Obtain all relevant information without necessarily having to resort to costly expenditures to do so.
- Make use of a physician advisor in the appropriate specialty when questions arise or communicate or negotiate with the attending physician when issues arise.
- Consult with the treating physician and team as much as needed to present options and promote discussions that ensure an informed decision. Keep in mind that the treating physician is the one who ultimately makes the final decision.[22]
- Follow procedures: this cannot be stressed enough. To this end, the case management organization must ensure that policies and procedures are current and follow nationally and local recognized practice guidelines and any state laws.
- Act promptly. Unnecessary delays cause conditions to worsen, com-

promise quality of care, and often cause increased financial expenditures.

WHEN A PATIENT NO LONGER NEEDS ACUTE CARE

There will be times in the course of treatments that patients no longer need the acute care setting. A question that plagues any discharge planner or case manager in these situations is "When is it appropriate to discharge the patient who no longer needs the care but an appropriate postacute-care setting cannot be found, or in some extreme instances, the patient who has no home or has inadequate support systems at home?" These cases all require special handling and discussion with senior management to determine the steps necessary to protect not only the organization but also the case manager and the patient. In all cases, documentation of events is critical.

HOMELESS PEOPLE

At times a homeless person may enter a hospital and require ongoing care on discharge. In cases such as this, the discharge nurse or case manager must take reasonable steps to ensure that the necessary services are established. However, in most instances, the homeless person will have no postacute-care needs. If this is the situation, it is okay to allow the person to be discharged back to the street. The person has the right to make his or her decisions, no matter how bad the decision seems to be or seems to go against moral obligations or logical reasoning.

Many case managers take the homeless a step further by making sure the person has a ride to the nearest shelter. This often means the hospital pays for the taxi ride. A process such as this must be used wisely, because if not, the hospital is setting up the expectation that every patient who needs a ride home will have it paid for by the hospital.

UNABLE OR UNWILLING CAREGIVER

There will be situations when a patient's family is unable or unwilling to care for him or her. If the patient is medically stable, is competent to make his or her own decisions, and has no postacute-care needs at the time of discharge, then discharge is appropriate. However, if the patient is medically stable and ready for discharge but needs ongoing care and the caregiver is unable or unwilling to provide that care, the case manager must make all reasonable efforts to offer services and options for ongoing care that is necessary to prevent reasonably foreseeable harm. If this occurs, the discharge must be delayed until it can be done as safely as possible. Again, document all case events.

LESS THAN IDEAL HOME ENVIRONMENT

If the patient does not require ongoing care but the home environment is less than ideal, as a health care professional, there is nothing that a case manager can do to send the patient to an alternate setting. If there is evidence of possible abuse, exploitation, or other reportable issues, then the appropriate authorities for researching such issues should be contacted. This will mean a report to either Adult Protective Services or Child Protective Services. At the same time the patient should be referred to the institution's social services staff.

When a patient requires ongoing care on discharge and it is known that the home environment is less than ideal, the case manager or discharge planner will need to explore alternatives to acute care. Often this means keeping the patient in the hospital until appropriate postacute-care alternatives can be established. If the less than desirable environment is known at the time of admission and Adult

Protective Services or Child Protective Services is involved, this may mean keeping the patient hospitalized until clearance is given from the agency. Again, case events should be documented.

PATIENT PRESENTS A FORESEEABLE RISK OR HARM TO SELF OR OTHERS

Depending on the circumstances of the event and state laws (e.g., those pertaining to psychiatric commitment, guardianship, conservatorship, and disclosure of confidential information), the hospital and its personnel have the following obligations:

- To warn third parties of the foreseeable danger of the person's discharge (the breach of confidentiality may be outweighed by a duty to protect the patient or others)
- To inform other members of the health care team and/or law enforcement personnel (the breach of confidentiality may be outweighed by a duty to protect the patient or others)
- To restrain and detain the patient until there is no longer a risk to either himself or herself or others (the patient should be kept in the least restrictive environment that is consistent with his or her needs)
- To discharge the patient into the custody of persons or institutions that will protect the patient and prevent harm to others
- To consider formal conservatorship actions, if needed
- To begin involuntary commitment proceedings

PATIENTS WHO REFUSE TO BE DISCHARGED OR ACCEPT THE DISCHARGE PLAN

When a patient refuses to be discharged, events surrounding this must be clearly and concisely documented in the patient's chart. Documentation by the physician must clearly indicate that the patient is medically stable for discharge and list the requirements for postacute care. Discharge planners must also document the efforts made to discharge the patient. There will be times when the patient or family believes that the patient is not ready for discharge, or in many cases, the patient may merely be waiting for a ride. In cases such as this, it is permissible to inform the patient of the hospital's admission agreement that he or she signed (in most cases this will list the time of discharge and indicate that the patient will be billed if the discharge does not occur at the time a physician discharges him or her). Most hospitals allow their discharge planners to also verbally inform patients of costs for room and board should they refuse discharge and elect to stay. This alone is often the biggest impetus to move patients (i.e., if patients know that the cost will be $2000 day and that they will be billed for this amount and that their insurance will not cover such costs, plans are often made very quickly).

For patients who refuse discharge and any alternate plans, it may be necessary to ensure that they are competent to make such decisions. If this is the case, the discharge might need to be delayed until a competency evaluation can be done. The best protection if the patient or family refuses discharge and the alternate plans is to have plans in place that can qualitatively meet the patient's care needs. Then if the patient and family continue to refuse discharge, they can be held accountable for the costs of care until discharge actually occurs.

CMS and many managed care organizations address this issue by allowing the patient or their family to file for an expedited appeal. The patient or family calls a specified phone number (operational 24 hours a day, 7 days a week) and gives pertinent information on the case. It is then up to the hospital to submit the patient's medical records for an independent review of the situation. In the interim, the patient is not held accountable for any charges until an independent party reviews the details of the case and renders a decision.

PATIENTS LEAVING AGAINST MEDICAL ADVICE

Any person who is not deemed incompetent has the right to refuse care or to seek discharge that might be contrary to his or her physician's medical judgment. The hospital and hospital personnel cannot force a patient to accept a particular treatment or discharge plan. If the patient insists on leaving or refusing care, the health care team members can discuss the issue with the patient, but again, they cannot force the patient to do anything. In cases such as this, all events including the proposed discharge plan must be documented in the patient's medical record. Additionally, the patient should be asked to sign a form indicating that the risks of discharge and the benefits of continued stay have been explained and that he or she is voluntarily accepting the risks and releasing the hospital from liability. If the patient refuses to sign such a form, this should be documented in the patient's medical record.

Although many hospitals may not have policies and procedures in place to handle these situations, wise case management organizations will protect their workers by having their own policies and procedures in place. *The key is to document all events clearly in the chart.* It is not the responsibility of the hospital or its personnel to provide the ideal discharge, but steps must be taken to ensure discharge was reasonable under the circumstances and that risks that may have a foreseeable negative impact on the patient's health and medical status were eliminated.

PATIENTS FORCED TO BE DISCHARGED BECAUSE OF A REVIEW DECISION

A patient might be denied further inpatient care because he or she no longer meets criteria for such care. However, if the patient has ongoing skilled care needs, which can be performed at a lower level of care, the patient should not be discharged until an appropriate care setting can be located. In cases such as this, the patient or family must be notified of the denial for continued care and must be informed of their appeal rights. Until a ruling on an appeal is issued, the patient has the right to remain an inpatient until the appropriate care can be arranged.

FRAUD AND ABUSE

The Health Insurance Portability and Accountability Act is bringing new meaning to fraud and abuse. This new law requires organizations to have a functional compliance department for the development of applicable policies and procedures and internal monitoring of fraud and abuse activities at a minimum. In addition, the new law established the Office of the Inspector General to oversee, monitor, and implement actions on fraud and abuse. For more information on the Office of the Inspector General's projects, please see their website at www.os.dhhs.gov/oig. Fraud is generally defined as intentional deception or misrepresentation by an individual who knows the information he or she is giving to be false and knows that the deception could result in some unauthorized benefit to himself or herself or some other person.

The most frequent kind of fraud arises from a false statement or misrepresentation made or caused to be made that is material to entitlement or payment. In most cases violators include both internal and external perpetrators (e.g., physician or other practitioner, hospital or other institutional provider, clinical laboratory or other supplier, an employee of any provider, billing service, the patient or any person in a position to file a claim for benefits). Under a broader definition of fraud are other violations including the offering or acceptance of kickbacks and the routine waiver of copayments.

Fraud schemes range from those perpetrated by individuals acting alone to broad-based activities perpetrated by institutions or groups of individuals, sometimes with the use of sophisticated telemarketing and other promotional techniques to lure consumers into serving as the unwitting tools in the schemes. Seldom do such perpetrators target only one insurer or the public or private sector exclusively. Rather, most are found to be defrauding several private and public sector agencies, such as Medicare, simultaneously.

According to a 1993 survey of private insurers' health care fraud investigations conducted by the Health Insurance Association of America, overall health care fraud activity can be broken down as follows:

- 43% fraudulent diagnosis
- 34% billing for services not rendered
- 21% waiver of patient deductibles and copayments
- 2% other

In Medicare the most common forms of fraud include the following[23]:

- Billing for services not furnished
- Misrepresenting the diagnosis to justify payment
- Soliciting, offering, or receiving a kickback
- Unbundling or "exploding" charges
- Falsifying certificates of medical necessity, plans of treatment, and medical records in order to justify payment
- Billing for a service not furnished as billed (i.e., upcoding)

CORPORATE COMPLIANCE

Having and enforcing a corporate compliance plan is critical for all organizations, and case management is not exempt. To ensure compliance, a case manager must be cognizant of the requirements of his or her organization's compliance plans for several reasons. There are several benefits to a corporate compliance plan[24]:

- Potentially reduces civil or criminal wrongdoing
- Potentially reduces administrative or civil penalties if a violation occurs
- Provides a more accurate view of employees' behaviors
- Identifies and eliminates criminal and unethical conduct
- Provides a means for efficient dissemination of information relating to changes in government requirements
- Establishes a structure that encourages employees to deal with concerns internally, which reduces the potential for Qui Tam actions and government investigations
- Ensures that accurate claims will be submitted to government and private payers.
- Enables the hospital or facility to fulfill its caregiver mission.
- Assists the hospital or facility in identifying any weaknesses in internal systems and management.
- Demonstrates a strong commitment to honest, responsible provider and corporate conduct.
- Improves quality of care.
- Develops a procedure that allows for prompt, thorough investigations of alleged misconduct by corporate officers, managers, employees, independent contractors, physicians, other health care professionals, and consultants.
- Initiates immediate and appropriate corrective action.

- Minimizes the loss to government from false claims and thereby reduces the hospital's or facility's exposure to civil damages and penalties, criminal sanctions, and administrative remedies

In the development of a corporate compliance program, there are three critical steps. The first step is performing a baseline assessment to determine responsibilities and existing processes for compliance, focusing on the most common compliance programs. Additionally, the federal sentencing guidelines must be referred to and used. Common areas that must be assessed because they are generally considered high risk include billing for services not provided, plan-of-are documents not signed by the physician, falsification of physicians' signatures, backdating physicians' signatures, physicians' consultation and administrative fees, kickbacks, and cost report fraud. As guidelines are developed, the following must be included[24]:

- Compliance standards and procedures
- Overall compliance program oversight by high-level personnel
- Due care delegating authority
- Employee education and training
- Monitoring, auditing, and reporting systems
- Consistent enforcement and discipline
- Response and corrective actions

The second step needed in compliance development is establishing a code of conduct that applies across the board. A code of conduct should include the following[24]:

- Ethical principles
- Explanation of laws
- Schedule for amending the code
- A vehicle to report potential compliance issues
- A nonretaliation policy for whistleblowers
- Description of disciplinary measures

The third step is oversight of the compliance plan. Oversight must be delegated to a high-level person in the organization. Just as oversight is critical, so is the need to ensure that what is written in the corporate compliance documents is truly functional and complies with the Federal Sentencing Guidelines, which are as follows[25]:

- The organization must have established compliance standards and procedures to be followed by its employees and other agents that are reasonably capable of reducing the prospects of criminal conduct.
- Specific individuals among high-level personnel within the organization must have been assigned overall responsibility to oversee compliance standards and procedures.
- The organization must have used due care not to delegate substantial discretionary authority to individuals whom the organization knew, or should have known through the exercise of due diligence, had a propensity to engage in illegal activities.
- The organization must have taken steps to effectively communicate its standards and procedures to all employees and agents.
- The organization must have taken reasonable steps to achieve compliance with its standards.
- The standards must have been consistently enforced through appropriate disciplinary mechanisms, including responsibility for an offense as a necessary component of enforcement; however, the form of discipline that will be appropriate will be case-specific.
- After an offense has been detected, the organization must have taken all reasonable steps to respond appropriately to the offense and to prevent further similar offenses, including

any necessary modifications to its program to prevent and detect violations of law.

SUMMARY

Case managers have significant legal liability when it comes to their roles as decision makers, and liability crosses all types of case management, regardless of payer or provider.

It is imperative that documentation contain a summary of the events of the case, but more importantly, events must never be falsified.

Chapter Exercises

1. In a group discuss the key reasons a patient might sue for malpractice and then identify the ways a case manager can protect himself or herself from malpractice. Then take a chart of a patient that is under case management and review it with your organization's legal counsel to ensure that appropriate steps have been taken on all actions and you feel comfortable that you and your organization are protected from malpractice.

2. Conduct your own research in your local community to ascertain which agency is responsible for the dissemination of your state's nurse practice act. Call the agency, request a copy, and review it. If time allows, discuss your state's requirements in a group, taking a case or two and reviewing case actions against the acts requirements or mandates.

3. Go to the AHRQ's website and pull up at least one guideline for a current case on which you are working. If your organization uses guidelines, is the AHRQ's guideline similar to yours? If your organization does not use guidelines or critical pathways, make contact

with an organization you know does and ask whether you can sit in on a committee meeting during which a guideline or pathway is being developed.

4. In a group setting, discuss why and how documentation is to be used as the key component for protection against malpractice. Using several charts, conduct some peer audits to ensure personnel are documenting events appropriately.

Suggested Websites and Resources

www.ussc.gov/2000guid/—Federal sentencing guidelines

www.info@ahrq.gov—Clinical practice guidelines produced by the Agency for Health Research and Quality

www.os.dhhs.gov/oig—Department of Health and Human Services, Office of Inspector General

REFERENCES

1. O'Keefe ME: *Nursing practice and the law: avoiding malpractice and other legal risks*, Philadelphia, 2001, FA Davis.
2. Aiken TD: Here's how to reduce your liability, *Case Management Advisor* 9 (7):120–121, 1998.
3. Cohen EL, Cesta TG: *Nursing case management from essentials to advanced practice applications*, St Louis, 2001, Mosby.
4. Wacker G, Guido JD: *Legal and ethical issues in nursing*, ed 3, Upper Saddle River, NJ, 2001, Prentice Hall.
5. Missouri Department of Health & Senior Services: *Standards of nursing practice*, available on-line at http://www.dhhs.state.mo.us/publications/200-05.html.
6. Hamill CT: Best practices & accreditation extravaganza, *Care Manag J* 6 (4):18, 2000.
7. Fitzgerald P: Making the case for evidence based medicine, *Healthplan* 39 (3):88–94, 1998
8. Lee PR, Estes CL: *The nation's health*, ed 5, Sudbury, Mass, 1997, Jones and Bartlett.
9. Bloyd B, Faimon C: Finding a direction, *Continuing Care* 6 (6):24–30, 1997.
10. Newell M: *Using nursing case management to improve health outcomes*, Gaithersburg, Md, 1996, Aspen.
11. Agency for Healthcare Research and Quality website at info@ahrq.gov.
12. Franzee T: Telling the whole story, *Advance for Providers of Post-Acute Care* 4 (1):34–35, 2001.
13. Powell SK: *Nursing case management: a practical guide to success in managed care*, Philadelphia, 1996, Lippincott-Raven.
14. Stock C: Breaking down barriers to CM by telephone, *Case Management Advisor* 8 (10):172–173, 1997.
15. Liang BA: Health law and policy: a survival guide to medicolegal issues for practitioners, Woburn, Mass, 2000, Butterworth-Heinemann.
16. Taylor C: Ethical issues in case management. In Cohen EL, Cesta TG, editors: *Nursing case management from essentials to advanced practice applications*, St Louis, 2001, Mosby.
17. Reference deleted by author.
18. Lo B: *Resolving ethical dilemmas: a guide for clinicians*, Baltimore, 1995, Williams and Wilkins.
19. Hogue EE: Are case managers liable? *J Care Management* 1(2):35, 1995.
20. Siefker JM, Garrett MB, Van Genderen A, et al: Fundamentals of case management: guidelines for practicing case managers. St Louis, 1998, Mosby.
21. Kaiser Permanente's Compliance Basics for Managers Workshop. June 2001.
22. Cady RF: Compliance and regulation. In Cohen EL, Cesta TG, editors: *Nursing case management: from essentials to advanced practice applications*, St Louis, 2001, Mosby.
23. Federal Sentencing Guidelines 2000 from website: www.ussc.gov/2000guid/.

BIBLIOGRAPHY

Annas GJ. *The rights of patients: the basic ACLU guide to patient rights*, ed 2, Totowa, NJ, 1992, Humana Press.
Beckmann JP: *Nursing negligence: analyzing malpractice in the hospital setting*, Thousand Oaks, Calif, 1996, Sage.
Evidence-based medicine: www.herts.ac.uk/lis/subjects/health/ebm.htm#def.
Evidence-based medicine on-line: www.ebm.jjournals.com.
Hamill CT: Creating best practices in case management, *Continuing Care* 18(7):22–24, 1999.
Ignatavicius DD, Hausman KA: *Clinical pathways for collaborative practice*, Philadelphia, 1995, WB Saunders.
La France AB: *Bioethics: health care, human rights and the law*, New York, 1999, Matthew Bender.
Lee S: Clinical pathways for case management, *Continuing Care* 14 (6):14–16, 1995.
Milliman and Robertson: www.milliman.com.
Poirier GP, Oberleitner MG: *Clinical pathways in nursing: a guide to managing care from hospital to home*, Springhouse, Pa, 1999, Springhouse.
White BC: *Competence to consent*, Washington, DC, 1994, Georgetown University Press.

Legislative Issues Affecting Health Care

Peggy A. Rossi, BSN, MPA, CCM, CPUR

OBJECTIVES

- To identify at least one key health care act for every decade and recite the impact the act has had on health care in general
- To identify how these acts have affected the community and what changes had to occur within the community agencies or health care organizations to implement and meet the requirements of the acts
- To identify which department within a given organization handles that organization's preparation and readiness for the implementation of an act

Federal and state legislation and laws as well as events of a specific time period have influenced health care through the years. Case managers must know and understand the laws and events that shape the health care system—especially those that affect not only the processes and requirements of health care but also financing and resource allocations and limitations.

Case managers affiliated with managed care organizations (MCOs) frequently have an advantage over their peers because their organizations have legal staff available to summarize state and federal legislation yearly. Many health plans have their legal or compliance staffs define not only the scope of impact of the individual legislation on the health plan's processes and financial reserves but also the extent to which their insured employer groups will

be affected. Having documents prior to any final enactment of a law allows the staff to have a "heads-up" view of the departments or areas that will be affected and to have policies and procedures readied for the law's implementation date.

The following listing certainly does not include all the many health care laws enacted over time. Nevertheless, it is important to note that many of the laws and events that have helped shape the U.S. health care system date back to the early 1900s.

1863

The Federal False Claims Act was signed into law by Abraham Lincoln to encourage private persons to report fraud against the Union, particularly by those who wished to profit from the war.

EARLY 1900s

In the early 1900s Montgomery Ward was the first employer to offer health care benefits to its employees.

- **1901**—The American Medical Association (AMA) was formally organized.
- **1906**—The name of the Association of Hospital Superintendents was changed to the American Hospital Association (AHA).
- **1910**—Worker's compensation was first recognized by New York. The new worker's compensation program required employers to contribute to a fund. This fund provided prompt medical care to a worker injured on the job and also replaced a portion of the wages lost while the injured worker was out of work.
- **1913**—The American College of Surgeons (ACS) was formed to improve the quality of care of surgical patients. The ACS also developed minimum standards for hospitalized care of surgical patients as well as for surgical education and practice.
- **1918**—The Ontario Medical Association and the Hospital Standardization Committee developed a survey process to evaluate hospital standards of care.
- **1918**—The Hospital Standardization Committee developed a survey process to evaluate standards of care.
- **1921**—The principal legislation allocating federal funds for health services to recognized Indian tribes is the Snyder Act of 1921. This act authorized funds for use for health care for American Indians in the United States.
- **1929**—Baylor Hospital in Dallas, Texas, offered the first prepaid health plan to teachers for care at Baylor. The plan was known as the Hospital Insurance Plan and later became the basis for the Blue Cross hospital insurance plans.

1930s

The 1930s saw the start of ongoing congressional efforts to enact various forms of health care coverage, the first of which were voluntary hospital insurance plans for people who could afford them. This changed attitudes toward hospital care. Hospitals were no longer a place to die but a place to receive complex treatments and services. Also, for those people who could afford insurance, direct payments by patients to physicians diminished, and patients could rely on their third-party payer for payment of bills related to their care during hospitalization.

- **1930**—The National Institutes of Health was created. Here the focus would be on the following:
  - Research and treatments for major medical conditions
  - Activities that promoted health planning through developing and providing opportunities for Americans to receive better health care services
  - Provision of grants to schools of medicine, nursing, pharmacy, and dentistry
  - Provision of financial aid to students pursuing health-related professions
  - Lobbying of Congress for increased health care regulation
  - Promotion of consumer protection
- **1935**—Congress passed the Social Security Act of 1935. The act achieved the following:
  - Provided old age retirement benefits for industrial and commercial occupations

- Became the basis for and principal source of federal aid to states for programs such as public health initiatives, welfare assistance, maternal and child health services, and disability programs
- Became the basis for Medicare and Medicaid
- 1937—The AHA established the following:
  - Standards of care for acute-care hospitals as well as some outpatient services
  - Guidelines for what insurance companies should cover
- 1937—This was also the year the first Blue Cross plan was established, and under this type of insurance hospitals billed Blue Cross directly for inpatient care and the patient had no responsibility to pay. Outpatient services were still not covered.
- 1937—This was also the year Henry Kaiser and Sidney Garfield established the first Kaiser Foundation of Health Plans. The Kaiser plan was the forerunner of today's prepaid health maintenance organizations (HMOs) because workers paid in advance for health care services.
- 1939—Blue Shield emerged offering the first reimbursement system for payment of physician care outside the hospital setting.

1940s

- 1943—The McCarran Act was passed. This act decreed that emerging health insurance companies be controlled by the states in which they provided coverage.
- 1944—The Public Health Service Act was passed. This act not only strengthened the Office of the Surgeon General but also placed public health services into four subdivisions—the National Institutes of Health, the Office of the

Surgeon General, the Bureau of Medical Services, and the Bureau of State Services.

- 1946—The Hill-Burton Act was passed. This act funded the expansion and modernization of hospitals, significantly increased the number and size of hospitals, and became a major influence in the expansion of the hospital industry. In exchange for funding, hospitals had to provide a percentage of medical services at no cost or reduced cost to patients who had difficulty paying.
- 1948—After the 1946 Nuremberg trials of those conducting experiments on concentration camp inmates, the Nuremberg Code, a formal statement on medical ethics, was developed and serves as the standard used in the United States and elsewhere to protect human research subjects.

1950s

- 1950—The Social Security amendments of 1950 established the programs of Aid to Families with Dependent Children (AFDC), Old Age Assistance (OOA), Aid to the Blind (AB), and Aid to the Permanently and Totally disabled (APTD).
- 1951—The Joint Commission on Accreditation of Hospitals (JCAH) was established. It has expanded through the years and now has 10 accreditation programs for different types of facilities
- 1951—The ACS, the AMA, and the American College of Physicians joined together to form the JCAH.
- 1953—The JCAH published new minimum health and safety standards for accreditation of acute-care hospitals, which quickly became the industry standard.

1960s

- 1962—Informed consent was a requirement of the 1962 Kefauver-Harris amendments to the federal Food, Drug, and Cosmetic Act, and while the act did not require a signed consent document, it did require a chart notation that verbal consent had been obtained. By 1967, the Food and Drug Administration (FDA) outlined the consent process and required that consent be obtained in writing from participants in early stages of research.

- **1963**—The Health Professions Education Assistance Act was passed. This act created the opportunity for physicians and other health care professionals to receive training through government-sponsored grants and loans.
- **1963**—The Social Security amendments of 1963 improved crippled children's medical services (Title V) and added provisions for mental retardation care planning.
- **1964**—The Civil Rights Act, which prohibited discrimination and ensured constitutional rights, was passed.
- **1964**—The Older Americans Act of 1964 established the Administration on Aging and helped to develop services for gerontology and care of the aged.
- **1965**—Medicare or Title XVIII of the Social Security Act was passed. This amendment to the act provided the following:
  - Health insurance for people aged 65 years or older.
  - Coverage for hospitals, known as Part A and funded through Social Security payroll taxes.
  - Coverage for physician and other outpatient services, known as Part B. Part B is a voluntary insurance program that is funded not only by payments from the insured but also by payments from the government.
- **1965**—Medicaid or Title XIX of the Social Security Act was passed. This is a mandatory federal and state program that shares funding based on a state's per capita income. Medicaid provides

basic medical and dental services to the poor. Under this amendment, the federal government instituted broad national guidelines under which each state had to do the following:
  - Establish that state's eligibility standards
  - Determine the type, amount, duration, and scope of services
  - Administer that state's program
- **1965**—The Public Health Services Act was amended to establish a nationwide network of programs to address the leading causes of death due to heart disease, cancer, and stroke. The amendment focused on ensuring that physicians were provided with the latest clinical information to enable them to better treat their patients.
- **1966**—The implementation of not only Medicare and Medicaid but also the Medicare Conditions of Participation (COP) began. The COP (a minimum set of health and safety standards) focused on evaluation and determination of appropriateness of care for Medicare beneficiaries. If hospitals were to receive Medicare reimbursement, they first had to meet the COP. Hospitals could meet the COP (known as achieving "deemed status") by complying with the requirements of their state's survey agencies or by receiving accreditation from the JCAH.
- **1966**—The Comprehensive Health Planning Act was instituted to improve or equalize national and regional distribution of services and personnel in health care.
- **1966**—The U.S. Public Health Service (PHS) defined the right of research subjects to be told about the benefits, risks, and purpose of the research for which they are volunteering. It made this "informed consent" a condition of PHS funding for research grants.
- **1967**—The Social Security amendments of 1967 consolidated all maternal and

child health services and crippled children's services under one authority.

The term *cost shifting* was introduced in the 1960s. Hospitals were prospering, and they justified the costs of new technology, equipment, and increased staffing by maintaining high patient occupancy rates. They also began to shift the cost of providing care to the elderly and poor to private insurers, since the Medicare and Medicaid programs had standardized reimbursement rates and private insurers did not.

1970s

The first attempts at cost containment occurred in the 1970s. This was necessary because health care costs were skyrocketing and employers were seeking ways to decrease the significant costs of providing health care benefits. At the same time, the government provided funding to the AMA to develop criteria of appropriateness for physicians and hospitals, and those who did not comply were excluded from the program due to potential conflict of interest.

- 1970—The Federal Occupational Safety and Health Act was passed and provided law and subsequent legislation requiring employers to establish occupational safety and health programs to ensure safe and healthful working conditions for employees.
- 1972—A further amendment was added to the Social Security Act (the Bennett amendment). This amendment established professional standards review organizations (PSROs) and marked the beginning of utilization review (UR). PSROs were nonprofit organizations comprised of physicians who were responsible for monitoring services and making determinations of medical necessity and appropriateness for care pro-

vided to Medicare beneficiaries. One of the first PSROs in California was the Medical Care Foundation of Sacramento. Here nurse reviewers, using a patient's actual medical record, performed concurrent review to establish the medical necessity of hospital admissions and continued stays related to provision of medical and surgical services. Chart reviews were conducted using mandated reference criteria and length-of-stay guidelines, with the nurse looking at quality-of-care issues, as well as medical necessity, for inpatient care. Care that fell outside of the criteria was then reviewed with the PSRO's physician medical director and a final coverage determination was made.

- 1972—The Bennett amendment also further extended Medicare coverage to persons aged 18 years or older who had been disabled for at least 24 consecutive months and to persons with end-stage renal disease who had been on peritoneal dialysis for 3 months or longer. This amendment also established the Supplemental Security Income program to replace the OOA, AB, and APTD programs.
- 1973—The Rehabilitation Act was passed. This legislation established vocational rehabilitation services.
- 1973—The Health Maintenance Organization Act of 1973 (Public Law [PL] 93-222) was passed. Employers, who had increasing concern over the rising cost of employee health benefits, drove establishment of this act. The act was a multipurpose act that did the following:
  - Established loans and grants for planning, developing, and implementing combined insurance and health care delivery organizations called HMOs

- Required that HMOs have access to the employer-based insurance market
- Required that employers with 25 or more employees offer HMO options when available in addition to any other health plans they may offer
- Required that employers contribute to the HMO premium an amount that is equal to what they contributed to indemnity premiums
- Required that disincentives (e.g., rate increases) be applied to employers if the volume of health care services to enrollees increased

- 1974—The Uniform Hospital Discharge Data Set (UHDDS) was implemented. Under the UHDDS, hospitals began collecting standardized discharge data on Medicare and Medicaid patients. The Department of Health and Human Services (DHHS) used these data in comprehensive studies that identified trends in Medicare and Medicaid data nationwide. These data tracked trends in areas such as diagnosis, procedures implemented, discharges, and deaths, and were organized by age, sex, and religion. The identification of these trends was the first attempt to develop regional and national length-of-stay norms based on admission and discharge dates.

- 1974—The National Health Planning Act of 1974 was also passed. Under this act, states defined which state health service agency would be responsible for administering the Certificate of Need (CON) programs. CONs document a community's need to increase health care expenditures, and they also limit the investment in and expansion of hospitals, nursing facilities, and technologic services.

- 1974—The Employee Retirement Income Security Act (ERISA) was also passed. Under the 1974 provisions, ERISA regulated the corporate use of pension funds, empowered the federal government to enact any laws or regulations that related to employee-sponsored benefit plans (e.g., retirement, health, or pension), required commercial health insurance plans to meet state regulations, and allowed large employers to establish self-insured health plans that were not subject to state regulations on health plan rates or benefits, or other protective provisions. For example, ERISA established uniform national standards to protect the health and pension benefits that employers voluntarily provide to their workers. If employers operate across state borders, ERISA preempts state regulations on these plans. It also focused on pension abuse. Under ERISA, employees and their families are entitled to receive a summary of plan benefits that spells out information about the plan, the benefits available, the rights of participants under the plan, and the way the plan works. This summary also must explain how plan benefits might be obtained and the process for appealing denial of benefits. Originally, ERISA shielded HMOs from liability for questionable health care. States are now active in promoting greater accountability on the part of HMOs toward their patients, and several states have passed legislation that allows managed care providers to be held legally responsible for adverse medical decisions that cause damage to patients. The Pension and

Welfare Benefits Administration of the Department of Labor is responsible for administering and enforcing the fiduciary, reporting, and disclosure provisions of Title I of the 1974 ERISA.

- **1974**—The Privacy Act of 1974 was also passed. This act established guidelines for the protection of personal information that is released between parties.
- **1975**—The Education for All Handicapped Children Act mandated that all children from birth to age 21 years are entitled to a free public school education, despite any handicapping illness or injury.
- **1978**—The Social Security Medicare amendments of 1978 relating to end-stage renal disease established improvements in renal and kidney disease treatment and services.
- **1979**—The National Committee for Quality Assurance (NCQA) was formed by the Group Health Association of America (GHAA) and the American Managed Care Association. GHAA is now the American Association of Health Plans.

1980s

The 1980s marked a period during which health care finances were heavily monitored and attempts were made to control the growth and proliferation of medical facilities, equipment, and personnel.

- **1981**—The Boren amendment to Title XIX (Medicaid) of the Social Security Act was passed. This amendment required states to provide assurances that their inpatient rates met certain specified standards of adequacy, that there was reasonable and adequate reimbursement to efficiently and economically operate facilities, and that there was reasonable access to facilities that provided adequate quality of care for Medicaid beneficiaries.
- **1981**—This was also the first year the Omnibus Budget Reconciliation Act (OBRA or PL 97-35) was passed. OBRA is a term applied by Congress to the many annual tax and budget acts. OBRA is important to health care because many of the acts contain provisions that relates to managed care. Under the 1981 act, the PSROs were allowed to delegate to hospitals the PSRO review function. This act allowed provision waivers to Medicaid for a variety of home care services.
- **1981**—The FDA revised its regulations and expanded the requirement for obtaining subjects' written informed consent to all studies of products regulated by the FDA.
- **1982**—The Tax Equity and Fiscal Responsibility Act (TEFRA) was passed. Under this act, the basis for hospital reimbursement under the Medicare program was dramatically changed. Prior to TEFRA, hospitals billed to cover costs. Under TEFRA, a cost-per-case reimbursement method is paid for each admission. Hospitals reacted by enhancing their UR programs, decreasing patients' lengths of stay and ancillary services, beginning to unbundle service charges, and encouraging earlier discharge to alternative, lower-cost care settings. TEFRA also established, at the state level, peer review organizations (PROs) to replace the PSROs and carry out Medicare UR for hospitals. In addition, the act also required employers to offer workers over the age of 65 years the same health plan as workers under the age of 65 years,

thus making the employer's plan the primary insurer and Medicare the secondary insurer.

- **1983**—The Social Security amendments of 1983 (PL 98-21) established the prospective payment system (PPS). Under PPS, hospital reimbursements were changed from a retrospective to a prospective payment system for given diagnoses. Under PPS, major diagnostic categories (MDCs) were developed. These categories defined major organ systems, demographic characteristics, and relevant clinical data, and they were further subdivided into diagnosis-related groups (DRGs). A DRG is a means to determine the resource consumption that is required to treat disorders with specific diagnoses. With the establishment of DRGs, a proliferation of cost-accounting systems for hospitals became necessary because hospitals were now being reimbursed by one fee for all services required to treat a specific diagnosis group.

- **1983**—Uniform Bill 82 (UB-82) was created. UB-82 allowed for standardization and uniformity in all patient billing. The form was later expanded to UB-92, which used the UHDDSs as its basis and increased the availability of standardized billing codes. Another method of billing developed in 1983 by the Health Care Financing Administration (HCFA) (now the Centers for Medicare & Medicaid Services [CMS]) was the Ambulatory Patient Group (APG). The APG method established fixed reimbursements for outpatient procedures.

- **1984**—Hospitals were required to contract with a PRO for their reviews.

- **1984**—The Developmental Disabilities Act of 1984 required states to provide services to developmentally disabled persons whose disability occurred before the age of 22. It also required states to meet minimum requirements of care so that the disabled person could live in the least restrictive environment.

- **1986**—The Consolidated Omnibus Budget Reconciliation Act (COBRA) of 1985 (PL 99-272) was passed. Under COBRA, employers were required to offer to employees who resigned or whose employment was terminated the ability to continue their health insurance coverage at the employer's group rate for a limited period. Under COBRA, employees or their families who may lose coverage due to termination of employment, death, divorce, or other life events may continue their coverage by the group health plan for a limited period. Employees have up to 60 days to choose to continue their benefits, and once COBRA coverage is selected, employees or their families must pay the premiums for continued coverage.

- **1986**—The Health Care Quality Improvement Act was passed and was intended to provide protections for all health care organizations and individual participants engaged in formal peer review activities. This act provided immunity to peer reviewers, established mandatory reporting of specific data on health plan activities, and contained prescribed penalties for not reporting. The act also established a national practitioner data bank that contains the history of clinical privileges and professional liability claims for all licensed individual practitioners and is used by organizations as they credential practitioners.

- **1986**—The False Claims Amended Act allowed any citizen to file suit in federal court against anyone who knowingly presents a false or fraudulent claim to the federal government. This act basically allotted the private citizen filing suit a percentage (15% to 25%) of the recovered funds when the government intervenes in any litigation for falsified claims. If the government does not intervene and there is a judgment or settlement, the individual is entitled to 25% to 35% of the amount recovered.

- **1986**—The Emergency Medical Treatment and Labor Act (EMTALA) — this Act established the right of access to medical care regardless of one's ability to pay for the care. This law was enacted to prevent patient *dumping* (mainly from emergency departments) based solely on the patient's ability to pay for health care. The law mandated the following:
  - Examination and treatment must be provided for individuals with emergent medical conditions and women in labor.
  - Any patient coming to an emergency department must be provided with an appropriate medical screening examination (within the facility's capabilities) to determine whether or not an emergency condition exists. This screening examination must occur regardless of the patient's ability to pay, and the hospital or provider must not allow a denial of payment or uncertainty of payment to interfere with or influence the physician's obligation to evaluate the patient or provide treatment.

- MCOs or health insurers cannot impose a prior authorization requirement if it will prevent or delay the performance of the medical screening examination or the initiation of necessary stabilizing treatment once it is determined that a medical emergency exists. Concurrent contact can be made with the MCO or insurer as long as it does not interfere with the course of evaluation or treatment.

- If the patient has been determined to have an emergent medical condition or to be in active labor, the facility either must provide available treatment within the hospital or must transfer the patient to a facility that can treat the patient.

- Transfer is restricted until the patient is medically stable unless the patient or a legally appointed representative requests in writing a transfer to another facility or a qualified medical person has signed a medical certificate attesting that the patient is stable for transfer and there is an accepting physician and hospital who are willing to receive the patient and provide the treatment required.

- Providers that have a Medicare provider agreement in effect are required do the following:
  - Offer examination and treatment for emergency medical conditions to women in labor
  - Offer appropriate medical screening (within the facility's capability) whenever a patient comes to the emergency department to determine whether or not an emergency exits
  - Either provide necessary stabilization treatment within the

hospital or transfer the patient to another facility capable of providing the treatment required

- Restrict any transfer of a patient until the patient has been deemed medically stable; the patient or the patient's legal representative, after being informed of the hospital's obligation to treat and the risk associated with the transfer, requests in writing that the transfer occur; or a qualified medical person signs a certificate of transfer after consultation with an accepting physician
- Provide an appropriate transfer—a transfer in which the transferring hospital provides treatment within its capabilities and in which the receiving hospital has available space, has personnel qualified to perform the treatment, and has agreed to accept the patient and provide the care needed

- **1987**—The JCAH recognized other health care organizations and changed its name to the Joint Commission on Accreditation of Healthcare Organizations (JCAHO).

- **1988**—The Medicare Catastrophic Coverage Act (MCCA) of 1988, designed to expand the Medicare program, was repealed. A part of the act remains in effect, however; it expands Medicaid eligibility rules for spouses of nursing home residents. Under this rule, called the spousal impoverishment rule, the MCCA requires states to permit the at-home spouse to retain a "maintenance needs allowance," and spouses of nursing facility residents are protected from spousal impoverishment.

- **1988**—The Family Support Act of 1988 extended Medicaid coverage to more low-income Americans who have jobs without health coverage. The act provided for a 12-month extension of Medicaid benefits to families losing AFDC benefits because of increased earnings. The law also expanded coverage for two-parent families whose principal earner became unemployed.

- **1988**—The Clinical Laboratory Improvement Act of 1988 was passed but did not become effective until 1992. Both hospital and independent laboratories, including reference laboratories, are affected. The act established specific standards and requirements that must be met (e.g., certification, accreditation) in conformity with specific DHHS regulations and mandated proficiency standards for staff testing for most procedures performed.

- **1989**—The Omnibus Budget Reconciliation Act (OBRA) of 1989 (PL 101-239) established the Resource Based Relative Value Scale (RBRVS) as a means of reimbursing physicians who provide services to Medicare beneficiaries. The RBRVS system was implemented over a 5-year period, and payments were determined based on measures of work performed and recognition of the unique medical skills required by physicians to perform their specialties. Allowances were created to help offset the cost of a physician's medical practice expenses and to help defray the cost of medical malpractice insurance. OBRA helped to address the long-standing imbalances in Medicare payments between rural and urban practitioners and between primary care physicians and certain specialists.

OBRA also mandated the Early and Periodic Screening, Diagnosis, and Treatment program. This act required that more preventive screenings be made available to children and that any federally allowable diagnostic and treatment service determined to be medically necessary be provided, regardless of whether the state otherwise covers the service.

1990s

- **1990**—The Americans with Disabilities Act was passed to guarantee the rights of the disabled and ensure equal access and opportunity. The act is closely related to the Civil Rights Act of 1964 and to the Rehabilitation Act of 1973 because it incorporates the antidiscrimination principles of both.
- **1990**—The Ryan White Comprehensive AIDS Resource Emergency Act was passed to provide emergency assistance to localities that had a disproportionate number of persons infected with the human immunodeficiency virus in their communities.
- **1990**—The American Accreditation Healthcare Commission (URAC) was founded. URAC established UR accreditation standards.
- **1990**—The National Committee for Quality Assurance (NCQA) was founded. The NCQA assesses and reports quality-of-care outcomes for MCOs and serves as the accrediting agency for MCOs and HMOs.
- **1991**—The Patient Self-Determination Act of 1991 mandated that all hospitals, home health agencies, and skilled nursing facilities counsel patients of their right to accept or refuse treatment and of their right to an advanced directive.
- **1991**—The Individuals with Disabilities Education Act of 1991 replaced the Education for All Handicapped Children Act of 1975.

- **1992**—President Clinton announced widespread plans for health care reform. While health care reform as envisioned never occurred, many changes did take place at the state level, such as the following:
  - Purchasing cooperatives were introduced that allowed small business owners options for obtaining health services for their employees at reduced costs.
  - Medical savings accounts were introduced that allowed individuals to save pretax earnings to offset medical expenses.
  - States were allowed to enroll Medicaid beneficiaries into managed care plans and expand Medicaid eligibility to a larger number of low-income and uninsured residents.
- **1993**—The Family and Medical Leave Act (FMLA) became effective. Under FLMA, employers are required to maintain coverage under any "group health plan" for an employee on FMLA leave under the same conditions under which coverage would have been provided if the employee had continued to work. FMLA is not COBRA, and FMLA leave is not a qualifying event under COBRA.
- **1994**—The Section 1115 waivers to Medicaid were enacted. These allowed states to redesign their Medicaid programs, develop managed care plans for Medicaid beneficiaries, and expand enrollment criteria and benefits.
- **1994**—The Family and Medical Leave Act of 1994 entitled employees up to 12 weeks of unpaid leave for the care of an ill child, parent, or spouse or for birth or adoption, and guaranteed protection of employment and health benefits during this leave period.

- **1996**—The Health Insurance Portability and Accountability Act (HIPAA) of 1996 was passed as an amendment to ERISA and the Public Health Services Act. HIPAA is also referred to as the Kassebaum-Kennedy legislation. HIPAA was a multiprovisional act that improved the portability and continuity of health insurance coverage in group health and individual markets to combat waste, fraud, and abuse in health insurance and health care delivery; to promote the use of medical savings accounts; to improve access to long-term care services and coverage; to simplify the administration of health insurance; and to fulfill other purposes. The act applied to both group and individual health insurance because it allowed individuals to keep their insurance coverage regardless of preexisting conditions if they leave or lose their jobs.
  - Under HIPAA, there was also a new federal law which prohibited inappropriate disclosure of information that could be used to identify a person, including any information about a person's physical or mental health, the care received, or the payment mechanism for health care. Under this law, a fine of up to $50,000 and/or imprisonment can be imposed, and penalties increase if the perpetrator acts under false pretenses for commercial purposes, personal gain, or malicious harm. The only exceptions to this provision are disclosures for provider referrals and research.

    HIPAA also established the Medicare Integrity Program. This program contracts out to private organizations the responsibility for audits, medical and URs, and fraud reviews by external entities, replacing the carriers and intermediaries who traditionally performed these roles. In addition, the act allows the DHHS to pay individuals who report health care fraud to the Office of Inspector General. Under this statute, a new health care fraud and abuse database, the Healthcare Integrity and Protection Data Bank, will archive information regarding final adverse actions against any health care provider, including any criminal convictions, provider exclusions from programs, and other actions taken when fraud or abuse has been proven.

- **1996**— Newborns' and Mothers' Health Protection Act of 1996 was passed. This act ensured that health plans that cover hospital stays for childbirth and HMOs provide coverage for minimum stays. For a vaginal delivery the minimum stay is 48 hours, and for a cesarean delivery the minimum is 96 hours. If the mother and newborn are doing well and the physician agrees, they may choose to leave the hospital early.

- **1996**—Congress passed the Indian Self-Determination and Education Assistance Act (PL 93-638, as amended) to give tribes the option of either assuming from the Indian Health Service (IHS) the administration and operation of health services and programs in their communities or remaining within the direct IHS health system.

- **1996**—The Veterans' Health Care Eligibility Reform Act of 1996 created the Uniform Benefits Package. This act standardized health benefits plans available to all enrolled veterans, simplified the process for veterans to receive services, introduced improvements in the quality and timeliness of care, and with the

Uniform Benefits Package placed new emphasis on preventive and primary care and enhanced outpatient and inpatient services.

- **1996**—The Mental Health Parity Act (MHPA) was passed as federal law. This law helped prevent group health plans from placing annual or lifetime dollar limits on mental health benefits that are lower (less favorable) than annual or lifetime dollar limits for medical and surgical benefits offered under the plan. Although the law required "parity," or equivalence, with regard to dollar limits, MHPA did *not* require group health plans to include mental health coverage in their benefits package. The law's requirements apply only to group health plans and those health insurance issuers that include mental health benefits in their benefits packages, and parity covers only very specific diagnoses.

- **1997**—The Balanced Budget Act (BBA) of 1997 was another multi-provisional act. Under the BBA, Medicare Risk programs were replaced with the new Medicare + Choice (M+C) program. The M+C program established new rules for beneficiary and plan participation, along with a new payment methodology. The M+C program was designed to expand the availability of health plans in markets where access to managed care plans was limited or nonexistent and to offer new types of health plans in all areas. Under the BBA, several rules also were established regarding posthospital discharge to home health agency providers. For example, if the patient is a Medicare beneficiary, the hospital must notify the patient of the availability of home health services that participate in the Medicare program in the area. In addition, if the hospital has a financial interest in the home health agency, the hospital must disclose to the Secretary of Health and Human Services information on the nature of the financial interest, the number of patients discharged from the hospital who required home health agency services, and the percentage of individuals who received such services from the home health provider in which the hospital has a financial interest. The BBA also prohibited MCOs from imposing prior authorization requirements for patients seeking emergency medical care, whether an emergency exits or not. The BBA also established Title XXI—the States' Children's Health Insurance Program. It also gave the HCFA the authority to establish and oversee a deeming program in two MCO performance areas: (1) quality assessment and improvement, and (2) confidentiality and accuracy of enrollee records.

- **1997**—The Consumer Bill of Rights and Responsibilities (drafted by President Clinton's Advisory Commission on Consumer Protection and Quality in the Health Care Industry in 1997) was defined. It included the following:
  - **Information disclosure**—Consumers have the right to receive accurate information, and some require assistance in making informed health care decisions about their health plans, professionals, and facilities.
  - **Choice of providers and plans**—Consumers have the right to a choice of health care providers that is sufficient to ensure access to appropriate high-quality health care. Public and private group purchasers should, whenever feasible, offer consumers a

choice of high-quality health insurance products. Small employers should be provided with greater assistance in offering their workers and their families a choice of health plans and products.

- **Access to emergency services**—Consumers have the right to access emergency health care services when and where the need arises. Health plans should provide payment when a consumer comes to an emergency department with acute symptoms of sufficient severity—including severe pain—that a "prudent layperson" could reasonably expect the absence of medical attention to result in placement of that consumer's health in serious jeopardy, in serious impairment of bodily function, or in serious dysfunction of any bodily organ or part.
- **Participation in treatment decisions**—Consumers have the right and the responsibility to fully participate in all decisions related to their health care. Consumers who are unable to fully participate in treatment decisions have the right to be represented by parents, guardians, family members, or other conservators.
- **Respect and nondiscrimination**—Consumers have the right to considerate, respectful care from all members of the health care system at all times and under all circumstances. An environment of mutual respect is essential to maintain a high-quality health care system. Consumers must not be discriminated against in the delivery of health care services consistent with the benefits covered in their policy or as

required by law based on race, ethnicity, national origin, religion, gender, age, mental or physical disability, sexual orientation, genetic information, or source of payment. Consumers who are eligible for coverage under the terms and conditions of a health plan or program or as required by law must not be discriminated against in marketing and enrollment practices based on the preceding discrimination factors.
- **Confidentiality of health information**—Consumers have the right to communicate with health care providers in confidence and to have the confidentiality of their individually identifiable health care information protected. Consumers also have the right to review and copy their own medical records and request amendments to their records.
- **Complaints and appeals**—All consumers have the right to a fair and efficient process for resolving differences with their health plans, health care providers, and the institutions that serve them, including a rigorous system of internal review and an independent system of external review.
- **Consumer responsibilities**—In a heath care system that protects consumers' rights, it is reasonable to expect and encourage consumers to assume reasonable responsibilities.
- **1997**—The 1997 amendments to the Individuals with Disabilities Education Act required early intervention services for children with disabilities or developmental delays from birth until 3 years of age and special education for children with disabilities from age 3 years through age 21 years.

- 1997—The Indian Health Care Improvement Act (PL 94-437) was passed. The goal of this act was to provide the quantity and quality of health services necessary to elevate the health status of American Indians and Alaska natives to the highest possible level and to encourage the maximum participation of tribes in the planning and management of those services.
- 1998—The Omnibus Consolidated and Emergency Supplemental Appropriations Act of 1998 amended the BBA of 1997.
- 1999—The HCFA enacted new standards for hospitals that participate in federal programs such as Medicare and Medicaid. These new standards, intended to ensure a minimum level of protection of patient rights, include the following:
  - Notification of rights—Health care providers are to inform patients of their rights in advance of furnishing or discontinuing care.
  - Establishment of a grievance procedure for prompt resolution of patient grievances.
  - Exercise of rights in regard to care—A patient is allowed to make informed decisions and participate in the development and implementation of his or her plan of care and to formulate advance directives.
  - Privacy and safety rights—A patient is ensured freedom from all forms of abuse as well as personal care provided in a safe setting in which the person's privacy during personal care is preserved.
  - Confidentiality of records—The patient is given the right to access his or her medical record.
  - Freedom from restraints (chemical or physical) that are not clini-

cally necessary—The use of restraints is restricted to only those that are required on a regular basis (use cannot be from a standing or "as needed" order) to improve the patient's well-being and when less restrictive methods have been determined to be ineffective.
  - Freedom from the use of seclusion and restraints for behavior management unless clinically necessary—The patient is allowed to be free of restraints for any use such as discipline or convenience; any deaths that occur while a patient is in seclusion or is restrained must be reported.
- 1999—The Ticket to Work and Work Incentives Improvement Act of 1999 created two new optional categories of needy Medicaid eligibility groups: (1) the basic coverage group, and (2) the medical improvement group. The definition of the basic coverage group does away with the stipulation of a percentage of the federal poverty level for family income and an age is applied (at least 16 years but not more than 64 years). In addition, under these new group definitions, states are free to establish their own income and resource standards, or to have no income and resource standards if they choose.
- 1999—The Balanced Budget Refinement Act of 1999 (BBRA) gave the HCFA the authority to establish and oversee a program that allows private, national accreditation organizations to "deem" that an M+C organization is in compliance with certain Medicare requirements. The BBRA of 1999 further amended the BBA by expanding the scope of deeming to include four additional areas: antidiscrimination,

access to services, advance directives, and provider participation rules.

THE NEW MILLENNIUM

- **2000**—Medicare's Benefit Improvement and Protection Act (BIPA) of 2000 contained a wide variety of information on new and expanded benefits, reimbursement, access, and demonstration projects. The legislation also extended bonus payments set by the BBRA of 1999 over a period of the next several years. BIPA also invited M+C organizations that had given notice of their intent to terminate coverage for Medicare beneficiaries to rescind that decision by January 18, 2000. Finally, the BIPA legislation contained a provision that phased in risk adjustment payments over the next 7 years. Risk adjustment pays health plans more for treating beneficiaries who are sicker and therefore more costly to treat.

- **2000**—The Breast and Cervical Cancer Prevention and Treatment Act of 2000 gave states the option to provide medical services to certain women who have been found to have breast or cervical cancer or precancerous conditions.

- **2000**—Public Law 106-265, the Long Term Care Security Act, was signed into law in September 2000. This act provided for the establishment of a program under which long-term-care insurance is made available to federal employees, members of the uniformed services, and civilian and military retirees.

- **2000**—The National Defense Authorization Act was signed into law on October 30, 2000. This act entitled uniformed service retirees and their spouses and survivors who are over age 64 to participate in a program called TRICARE for Life. This program is a supplement to Medicare that offers additional TRICARE benefits, including

coverage for pharmaceuticals. The program became effective on October 1, 2001.

- **2001**—The Patient Rights Act was passed. This legislation granted all Americans with private or public insurance the following:
  - The right to access emergency care without prior authorization.
  - The right of access to medical specialists and routine care during clinical trials.
  - The ability to sue insurers in state courts over denials of care that are based on medical judgment once the patient has exhausted outside appeals; however, patients with terminal illnesses or in immediate danger of permanent injury may sue immediately.
  - The legislation further covered the following:
    - Class action lawsuits are addressed, and such lawsuits are restricted to employees of one company or health plan.
    - Private dues-paying membership organizations now receive the same treatment as employers under federal pension law in offering their members and workers health insurance.
    - All patients can now participate in a previously limited program that allows consumers to use tax-free medical savings accounts to pay for their health expenses.
- **2001**—President Bush approved the use of stem cells in research, allowing federal funds to be used for research when (1) there is informed consent of the donors, (2) only stem cells from excess embryos created solely for reproductive purposes will be used, and (3) there are no financial inducements to the donors. Federal funds cannot be used for

(1) the derivation or use of stem cell lines from newly destroyed embryos, (2) the creation of any human embryo for research purposes, or (3) the cloning of human embryos for any purpose.

The foregoing listing of legislative events is by no means inclusive. In addition to the many federal laws in effect or under review, each state also has a myriad of laws either similar to the federal ones or specific to that state regarding how the law will be implemented, what the population focus will be, and which agency will be used for monitoring for compliance.

SUING HEALTH PLANS

Of the newest laws for 2001, the ones allowing patients to sue health plans have the potential for the greatest impact on case managers working for MCOs because such case managers can likewise be sued by an unhappy patient. "With the new trend toward allowing patients to sue their health plans, insurance companies and HMOs a health professional while working for a health plan, insurer or HMO and following its rules can commit malpractice and can be sued along with the health insurer, health plan or HMO if the health plan falls below acceptable professional standards. States have been active in promoting greater accountability on the part of HMOs to their patients."[1]

For health plans to be financially successful, they must restrict patient choices and redirect health care away from high-cost alternative treatments and nonnetwork providers. Two modalities have historically been used: the gag rule and end-of-year profit sharing. Under the gag rule many health plans prevented their providers from offering more costly therapies as options or they restricted service for a medical condition to their network of providers. Under end-of-year profit sharing or performance bonus plans, an incen-

tive is given to providers for keeping costs at a minimum or within budget. Under this rule a certain percentage of the profits is distributed at the end of the year to health providers. Often, the more money saved during the year, the higher the bonus. Both means of keeping costs low contribute to substandard care. Because of the potential harm that can be caused by such methods, most states have outlawed both practices.

DOCUMENTATION TO MEET REGULATIONS

As stated earlier, a primary key for case actions is documentation. Documentation of medical events originated in an initiative of the ACS. The objective was to use written documentation of medical interventions to help improve the standards of surgery. There are specific purposes for the medical record (at all levels, not just at the hospital level) that support the need for documentation. These include the following:

- Patient focused:
  - Justifies admission
  - Justifies continued stay
  - Supports the diagnosis
  - Supports and defends the treatment modalities
  - Describes the patient's progress and responses to interventions
  - Justifies discharge
- Medical practice centered:
  - Provides a teaching vehicle for the education of health professionals
  - Provides information for research
  - Provides evidence of quality performance
- Business related:
  - Supports claims for the costs of care
  - Defends reimbursement requests
- Ethical and legal:
  - Defends ethical practices
  - Provides evidence that legal duties were met

- Provides evidence that accreditation standards were met[2]

What and how much to document are questions frequently asked as managers attempt to control the amount and quality of information generated. When one is determining this need, the use of the following questions might be helpful:

- **Case finding and screening**—How are patients who do or do not need discharge planning or case management interventions identified? When a patient is identified through a referral, the who, what, when, and why should be included in the note. If the patient refuses any intervention, this refusal must also be documented.
- **Assessment**—How was the assessment done, who did it, and what have other health care professionals contributed? When and under what circumstances will the patient need to be reassessed? What is the overall health history, and does it include any chronic illnesses that have an impact on the current medical condition? What are the elements of the psychosocial history that may have an effect on the outcome of the plan? What services were used prior to admission, and how and at what level was the patient functioning with these services?
- **Problem identification**—What problems are present that need to be solved before the patient is moved to the next level of care?
- **Planning**—Was there adequate involvement of the patient, family, and entire multidisciplinary team serving the patient in the planning process? Is documentation from personnel in any of these disciplines present? Has the case manager taken the lead in documenting the overall process of planning and taken into account the information provided by the team?
- **Implementation**—Is a rationale included in the implementation note as to why one plan was chosen over another? Was the implementation of the plan documented after it was completed? Is it clear who did what and what else needs to be done? Has the referral process, as outlined in any policies and procedures, been followed? Was adequate medical information sent to the referral agency? Is the patient's agreement or understanding of the implemented service indicated?
- **Monitoring**—Is the patient's progress toward discharge being monitored throughout the hospital stay? Is reassessment performed based on evidence of changes in the patient's condition or in the availability of resources?
- **Evaluation**—While it is not part of a medical record, evidence should be present in committee notes or other documents that evaluations have occurred and their results recorded.[3]

It is reported that health care professionals—nurses and physicians in acute-care hospitals—spend 36 minutes on paperwork for every hour of care; in skilled nursing facilities 30 minutes of paperwork was required for every hour of patient care! In home health care every hour of patient care results in 48 minutes of paperwork! In an emergency department every hour of patient care is matched by an hour of paperwork, including compliance with the vast array of federal, state, and local health regulations!

While much of the paperwork does provide necessary documentation of important clinical information, a significant increase in paperwork has resulted from the demands made in the area of regulatory compliance. Since 1997, more than 100 regulations affecting health care have officially come on the books. The AHA requested PricewaterhouseCoopers to conduct a survey of hospitals to assess the paperwork burden. Based on this survey, many regulations were promulgated, a number of which do not apply directly to organizations but more to the regulators who issue new mandates. The single recommendation for organizations and the one organizations struggle with continually is to limit the collection and reporting of patient assessment data to *useful* information and to develop a common form to eliminate duplication and inconsistent requirements.[4]

SUMMARY

Keeping abreast of regulatory laws and legislation is a must in case management. This is necessary because so many actions taken by nurses in various organizations are affected by or are the result of legislation. While certainly the nurse case manager is not required to recite the many legislative mandates, an astute case manager will be familiar with the ones that have the greatest impact on how business is conducted and why.

Chapter Exercises

1. From either a state library or the website for the law, research at least one act from each decade. Be prepared to discuss the act in a group setting and describe how you feel the act has affected care within your organization or community.
2. Taking these same acts, discuss in your same group how these acts have affected your community and what changes had to occur in the agencies and health care organizations to implement the requirements of the acts.
3. Contact your organization's legal, regulatory, or compliance department and discuss with a representative the steps the department takes to keep on top of

new and proposed laws and regulations as well the actions they expect departments to take to be prepared for the impact of a new law.

Suggested Websites and Resources

www.urac.org/—URAC or the American Accreditation Healthcare Commission

www.access.gpo.gov/su_docs/aces/aces140. html—*Federal Register* database

www.gpo.gov/nara/cfr/index.html—Code of Federal Regulations

cms.hhs.gov/schip/kidssum.asp—Balanced Budget Act and the State Children's Health Insurance Programs

www.cms.hhs.gov/healthplans/bba/—Balanced Budget Act and HMOs

www.cms.hhs.gov/hipaa/hipaa1/content/mhpa .asp—Mental Health Parity Act

www.hhs.gov/ocr/hipaa/—U.S. Department of Health and Human Services and Office of Civil Rights

www.cms.hhs.gov/hipaa/—Health Insurance Portability Accounting Act (HIPAA)

www.eeoc.gov/laws/rehab.html—U.S. Equal Employment Opportunity Commission and the Rehabilitation Act of 1973

www.access-board.gov/508.htm—The 508th amendment to the Rehabilitation Act of 1973, which added electronic and information technology accessibility standards

www.ssa.gov/OP_Home/ssact/title18/1867. htm—Social Security Act and Emergency Medical Treatment and Active Labor Act

www.dol.gov/esa/regs/statutes/whd/fmla.htm —U.S. Department of Labor and the Family Medical Leave Act of 1993

www.ncld.org/advocacy/fedlaws.cfm—National Center for Learning Disabilities and the various laws that pertain to children with disabilities and their education

www.thelaughtongroup.com/pddsupport/idea/ ideatext.htm—Full text of the Individuals with Disabilities Education Act (IDEA) of 1991

www.eeoc.gov/laws/vii.html—U.S. Equal Employment Opportunity Commission on the Civil Rights Act of 1964

www.icanonline.net/news/fullpage.cfm/article id/6CAEB15E-3A1A-4743-8BCCD55D82731B98/cx/issues.stay_infor med/article.cfm and *www.usdoj.gov/crt/ada/adahom1.htm*—Both websites give information about the Americans with Disabilities Act

www.ssa.gov/history/law.html—Social Security Administration on the history of the Social Security Act

www.harp.org/hmoa1973.htm—U.S. Public Health Code and the Health Maintenance Act of 1973

www.acf.hhs.gov/programs/add/DD-ACT2.htm—U.S. Department of Health and Human Services and Administration on Developmental Disabilities

REFERENCES

1. Wacker G, Guido JD: *Legal and ethical issues in nursing,* ed 3, Upper Saddle River, NJ, 2001, Prentice Hall.
2. Birmingham J: Discharge planning—charting patient progress, *Continuing Care* 16(1):13-14, 1997.
3. Birmingham J: Discharge planning—patient documentation, *Continuing Care* 16(2):9,25, 1997.
4. Regulatory issues—new report assesses amount of time nurses and physicians spend on health care regulations, *Care Management* 7(3):60, 2001.

Complex Care

CHAPTER
14

Introduction to Complex Care

Peggy A. Rossi, BSN, MPA, CCM, CPUR

OBJECTIVES

- To identify what field of medicine is best suited for case management and list at least two reasons why
- To identify at least four other types of patient management that health plans and health systems are using as they try to contain costs for various client populations
- To identify at least two competencies now required, especially by accreditors such as Joint Commission on Accreditation of Healthcare Organizations (JCAHO) and National Committee for Quality Assurance (NCQA), in addition to case management and professional competencies
- To identify at least two assessments that should be performed as a new case is opened and to explain their importance for case management

As we prepare to manage complex cases, this chapter will cover the key elements necessary for case management. While each section and its contents can be a complete chapter in itself, the contents only briefly summarize some of the many issues that must be addressed as the case management plan is developed and implemented. Thus, sections covered in this chapter include the following:

- **Section I**—General overview of case management, new modalities for case management, and the case management processes
- **Section II**—Discharge planning
- **Section III**—Shifts of care
- **Section IV**—Special complexities
- **Section VI**—Caregivers, training, and other pointers
- **Section VII**—Transportation, travel, and other activities
- **Section VIII**—Other planning needs
- **Section IX**—Providers of care
- **Section X**—Durable medical equipment, supplies, and devices
- **Section XI**—Alternate funding

SECTION I—GENERAL OVERVIEW OF CASE MANAGEMENT, NEW MODALITIES FOR CASE MANAGEMENT, AND THE CASE MANAGEMENT PROCESSES

Which Profession Dominates in the Role of Case Manager?

Today's health care system is complex, diverse, fragmented, and heavily dominated by managed care, capitation, and risk agreements. However, frequently interchanged case management is not the same as managed care. Managed care is a system of cost-containment strategies designed to enhance cost-effectiveness by eliminating inappropriate services. In contrast, case management is a process. The National Case Management Task Force states the following:

Case management is a collaborative process that assesses, plans, implements, coordinates, monitors and evaluates options and services to meet an individual's health needs, using communication and available resources to promote quality, cost-effective outcomes.[1]

Through the years, case management has been performed by a variety of health care professionals. Social workers and nurses dominated the field. However, as the health care system of today is struggling with how to handle an older, sicker, more technology-dependent population with a variety of comorbid diagnoses, nurses as case managers (CMs) are taking the lead.

Much of the literature written on case management supports the fact that nurses make the best CMs. A host of case management writers feel that if professionals other than nurses offer case management, they are often neither prepared nor capable of providing the direct care activities required by today's clients. It further supports the fact nurses are better prepared to assume case management roles as their clinical expertise gives them an added benefit that ensures better coordination of services to meet the total needs and concerns presented by patients and their families. Nurses also have the skills and knowledge that extends beyond the biophysical and pathologic aspects of care and as such bring a holistic perspective and knowledge base to the care of case-managed clients.[2]

While the literature is clear on nurses as CMs, the big question that remains basically unanswered for many organizations is what criteria should be used to select the best nurse CMs. Many of the criteria used concentrates on the educational preparation of nurses, their communication skills, leadership skills, clinical knowledge, and expertise. Additionally, as CMs are selected, interview questions often center on personality traits and previous successes to serve as an interdisciplinary team player, care negotiator, and patient and family advocate.

Tahan (1993) conducted a study on selection criteria for nurse CMs. Twenty-six nursing administrators of case management systems were surveyed on their preferences and perceptions of the criteria that make a successful CM. The following results were found[2]:

- 40% recommended a BSN as the minimum requirement for the role.
- 48% recommended 4 to 6 years of nursing experience, and 38% recommended 2 to 4 years.
- 38% did not approve of the clinical ladder as a requirement for the role.
- 61.9% did not have a preference for generalized versus specialized nursing experience.
- 28.6% preferred specialized practice.
- Communication skills and certification in area of practice or specialty were recommended as prerequisites for the role.

Characteristics of a CM

While an organization will make every attempt to locate CMs meeting any predetermined criteria, the following characteristics are important in selecting candidates:

- Ability to be a change agent
- Level of clinical knowledge and previous experiences conducive to the role of a CM
- Astuteness and ability from previous job to keep abreast on current advances in clinical care as well as resources
- Ability to serve in a consultant role and guide the multi/interdiscipli-

nary team through case management processes

- Ability to coordinate and facilitate care and resources as well as collaborate and seek help from the multi/interdisciplinary team to ensure patient needs and treatment goals are met
- Ability to serve as an educator of both the patient and family (and at times the multi/interdisciplinary team members) to ensure the teaching plan meets the needs of the patient and family
- Ability to serve as a manager for patient care needs and allocation of available resources
- Ability to assume the role of lead negotiator for the plan of care, acceptable rates, length of stay, acceptable resources, approval of care, or to improve the productivity of the team
- Ability to serve as a patient and family advocate when applicable
- Ability to serve as the quality improvement coordinator and assure the quality of patient care is maintained or improved at all times
- Ability to serve as a researcher to gather data to support the care plan and recommendations or data for other organizational needs
- Ability to serve in the role of risk manager and identify issues that place an organization at risk for litigation (Figure 14-1)

Experience validates the fact that case management is not a job for all persons, especially those who have meek or nonassertive personalities. The ability to assert oneself must rank among the top skills on the list of assets. The need for this skill will become apparent as one reads this chapter and understands the intensity and complexity of the services and care necessary for many patients. Other skills required of CMs are basic business management techniques. These include the ability to prioritize, organize, and manage activities and people (which involves delegation, conflict resolution, crisis intervention, collaboration, consultation, and negotiation).

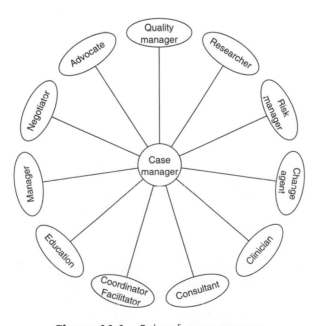

Figure 14-1   Roles of a case manager.

New Modalities for Case Management

Historically, case management has been used to link clients to applicable resources, and in more recent years it is viewed as a primary means for cost containment. Thus, as health care costs continue to rise, health care organizations and large employer health care purchasers have demanded and organizations have responded through the development of a variety of techniques in the quest to contain costs. Although many types of cost-containment strategies are being used for case management in health care today, some newer processes and methods include a variety of different approaches, such as the following:

- Disease management
- Demand management
- Resource management
- Care management
- Outreach care management
- Drug state management
- Disability management
- Life care planning

Organizations can use the following approaches separately or in any combination. Each approach is only briefly discussed in this section, as each can be a text of its own. The approaches are discussed to give a flavor of common methodologies used today for cost containment, as well as to ensure quality of care to specific segments of care.

Disease Management

This is a population-based approach to management of specific diseases identified at risk of being costly both economically and in human terms. Disease management programs have proliferated since 1992 and have been driven primarily by health care organizations and their desires to contain costs and improve the quality of life for specific diseases. Disease management is an evolving concept in which a coordinated proactive disease-specific approach to care is undertaken. Goals are designed to produce the best clinical outcomes in the most cost-effective manner.

Disease management can be defined in a variety of ways. However, a general operational definition of this type of case management is "a systematic proactive approach to the prevention of or treatment for chronic illnesses across the continuum of care." Its primary challenge is to encourage health wellness, self-management, and promotion of activities for individuals with both early-stage as well as chronic stages of the illnesses, teach prevention for these illnesses, provide advocacy and support, and reduce the numbers of acute and chronic episodes as well as complications and hospitalizations that will occur during the illness duration.[3] Disease management goes beyond case management because it features earlier intervention and an element of demand management, steering patients toward preventive practices and more efficient and effective therapies and away from costly and less useful care.[4]

In most disease management programs, diseases are selected on the basis of chronicity, high costs of care over time, high patient volume for the particular disease, treatments offered by primary and specialty providers, and the wide variation in practice patterns and the potential for patient involvement for improved self-care. If a disease management program is offered, the CM works with the patients within the specific disease population to educate, monitor, and ensure compliance. As this training is done, assessments and profiles of the patients are maintained to document any changes.

Many programs include the use of practice guidelines and clinical pathways; patient, family, and provider education; outpatient drug management; physician buy-in and support; triage protocols; patient survey tools; and by all means a way to measure outcomes. Education is enhanced through the use of newsletters and educational material relevant to the disease, health promotion programs, and informational services, especially when the disease in not yet in the chronic stages. The traditional modes of education are either through working closely with the patients via the telephone or in class-type settings. The structure of a disease management program establishes linkages between clinical and nonclinical services, care delivery locations and products, or other medical devices applicable for use with the disease.

Demand Management

Demand management is another process that is used by many managed care organizations (MCOs) as they try to contain costs. For example, MCOs now offer advice lines in which demand management is used for decisions and behavior support systems to appropriately influence patient and family decisions on whether, when, where, and how to access medical services. In most programs, MCO members can call a toll-free number 24 hours a day, 7 days a week. The demand program uses a variety of tele-service technologies with triage and algorithm-driven care guidelines and provider databases from which free medical advice and directions for care or triage can be obtained.

Triage is accomplished through the use of trained demand management nurses who use trigger information prompted by a computer screen's questions to direct the caller to appropriate care. Advice often includes preapproved basic medical interventions or directions, or triage to a level of care appropriate for the situation at hand. In all cases, the MCO's medical director must approve scripts used. Another form of demand management is the use of call-back programs designed to manage patients who overuse or misuse health care services such as emergency department (ED) care.

Demand management uses a variety of tools in order to be effective, many of which are also predeveloped computer-prompted questions. However, the programs also make use of easy-to-access health education resources, self-care booklets, and classes on lifestyle and stress management. The overall programs are designed to help the caller and health care organization focus on topics such as the following:

- Prevention and wellness programs
- Patient education and self-care models and programs
- Chronic disease management programs
- Risk assessments and early intervention programs
- Health screening and immunization programs

The ultimate goals of demand management are as follows: empowerment of patients to provide self-care and make health care decisions, creation of a partnership between patient and provider, and the ability to provide information to members/clients on demand. Common goals of any demand management program are as follows: prevention of unnecessary ED visits and appropriate utilization of health care resources, improved access to care, linkage of callers to appropriate information and care options, appropriate triage of patients to clinicians, improvement in health behaviors, increased access to preventive services, provision of better self-care and an understanding of the appropriate use of treatment options, and enhanced relationships among the MCO, its policyholders, and members. Demand management can also be used as an effective trigger for assigning case management when chronic cases are developing or before costs spiral.[5]

Resource Management

This is the process of identifying, confirming, coordinating, and negotiating benefits for a patient when the benefit dollars allocated do not cover necessary medical care. It also surfaces when aligning benefits with post-discharge needs or when negotiations are necessary.

Public health professionals have always been trained in resource management, but the majority of coordination is performed from within the health care organization. In undertaking resource management, the CM assesses the multifactorial problems impeding a plan holder's ability to maintain and achieve wellness and then identifies a care plan utilizing available community resources. Factors hindering wellness can be episodic or continual.[5]

Care Management

This type of management is independent of case management and has a different focus. Its clinical algorithms are diagnosis-specific rather than patient-specific, and all patients with the same disease are eligible. With care management, the practice takes place with a specific setting rather than across the continuum and is designed to promote quality outcomes for all patients. This is in contrast to case management as it focuses on cases that tend to be outliers that center on patient and family and are designed for only a small percentage of patients.

With care management, all patients with the specific disease are linked to the same sequence of care activities despite the fact the patient might not be a good fit. Care management unfortunately assumes that all patients uniformly fit its classification even though real-life situations can only approximate this orderly arrangement. It also requires the gathering and tracking of data and focuses on the care process. Teams using a care process treatment work out the most efficient and effective pathway for each diagnosis for patients that can remain compliant and stay on track with the goals and treatment regimen. Care management focuses also on biometric or biologic measures of treatment outcomes that are defined by the provider and not the patient.[6]

Outreach Care Management

This type of management is considered one of the most aggressive and compre-hensive links among health care organizations and the communities in which they serve. Outreach care management transplants organization-based CMs into the heart of the community and throughout the continuum of care. This model uses both an interrelated and interdisciplinary care management approach and bridges the community via a nurse CM or social worker that manages and follows patients across the continuum.

The overall goal of outreach care management is to enhance quality and maximize the maintenance of one's health status while providing cost-effective care through service coordination and improved access to appropriate services. The focus is on identified high-risk participants and community clusters of members of the health care organization.

The high-risk groups often targeted for care management include members with chronic heart failure, high-risk pregnancy or risk of prematurity, pediatric asthma, mental illness, substance abuse, diabetes, chronic obstructive pulmonary disease, uncontrolled hypertension, and end-stage cancers. Once identified, the patient is contacted via phone and an on-site interview is scheduled. As one plans the interview, the appropriate health assessment screening forms must be used. Separate forms are used for pediatric and adult patients; all forms are individually designed to capture physical and psychosocial events that affect a case.

Health screening tools are organization-specific. They must have the ability to assist the care manager in determining the patient's level of functional status, perceived health status, likeliness of medication compliance, status of home care assistance, financial limitations, and health educational needs. From these assessments, the outreach care manager designs a care plan that has mutually agreed-upon goals. The plan is then shared with other CMs to ensure concurrent tracking and review of requests for authorization purposes. The implementation, coordination, documentation, and monitoring of the care plan, as well as any cost savings reporting, remain the responsibility of the outreach care manager. It is a well-known fact that when patients are faced with depression, caregiver problems, financial challenges, or care and medication issues, many of them traditionally fall through the cracks of our health care system. However, an outreach care manager can help such patients bridge the care continuum more easily.[6]

Drug State Management

This mode of management offered by some MCOs is fairly new to the United States and is the result of spiraling drug costs. Through drug state management, CMs can create patient/family educational material and perform telephonic or on-site self-care education with the patient and family. Educational materials developed for a drug state management program are designed to improve patient medication compliance. The material takes into consideration factors such as age, cultural diversity, and educational level of the readers.

While an MCO may offer drug state management, the real drivers of such programs are the pharmaceutical companies. This is because they have found the value of direct consumer and case management education to be an invaluable resource. The same companies are providing CMs with assessment tools, clinical literature, defined nonpharmaceutical interventions, systems for outcomes documentation, and other pertinent information. Additionally, these companies are also providing consumers with user-friendly educational materials, personal diaries, and other tools to maximize their medication management and self-care.[7]

Effective drug state management programs offer sound pharmaceutical interventions, improve patient medication adherence, build patient empowerment, and offer a systematic approach to documenting and monitoring patient outcomes. CMs working in such a program may be given the autonomy to recommend drugs that may be at first glance more expensive. However, cost-benefit analysis has shown that these drugs prevent more expensive care costs. As one analyzes drugs and their costs, there are four distinct pharmacoeconomic analysis categories[8]:

1. **Cost-minimization analysis**—This is the simplest form of analysis used to compare two or more treatment options whose outcomes are accepted as being identical. It is most often used to compare two drugs in the same therapeutic class or a branded drug and its generic equivalent. Cost related to preparation, administration, and monitoring is measured to determine which agent produces the outcome less expensively.

2. **Cost-effectiveness analysis**—This is possibly the most common form of analysis used as it measures both the clinical outcomes and costs associated with two or more interventions. Outcomes are measured in natural units such as decreased length of hospital stay (in days), reduced levels of cholesterol (in micrograms per liter), or decreased blood pressure (in millimeters of mercury). Results are presented as a cost-effectiveness ratio—the cost required to produce a unit of outcome. Cost-effectiveness studies that are conducted in tightly controlled settings are sometimes distinguished as cost-efficacy analyses.

3. **Cost-utility analysis**—This process closely resembles a cost-effectiveness study. The difference is that the cost-utility study attempts to measure subjective humanistic variables

such as well being or quality of life, along with costs and clinical outcomes. Results are adjusted to include patient-assessed outcomes that are usually expressed in form of quality adjusted life years.

4. **Cost-benefit analysis**—This type of study differs from other pharmacoeconomic analyses in one key way: Both outcomes and costs are measured in monetary units. Cost-benefit analysis attempts to put a dollar value on the health benefits of a given intervention. Because outcomes are converted to a simple common denominator, cost-benefit analysis allows for broad comparisons of widely divergent interventions across a variety of settings.

If a drug state management program is not available, due to the continual rise in prescription costs and the ever challenging increase in poly pharmacy usage, CMs must make every effort to include a pharmacist in the overall case planning. It is equally important to educate patients and families about the value of using one pharmacy so that they can discuss medications and interactions with a professional who should be a supportive resource team member.

Disability Management

Disability management programs have their roots in workers' compensation. These programs are part of the rehabilitation and return-to-work processes used by employers in attempt to return injured workers to their job as quickly as possible. The goal of the program is to minimize the overall effect of disabilities in terms of psychologic, social, and economic costs to the individual worker, the company, and society.

To reach goals, disability management programs are designed to use specialists (referred to as disability managers or coordinators) who are specially trained to work primarily with injured employees. The specialist's goals are to ensure the injured worker is provided with timely and necessary services that accommodate the his or her medical and vocational needs while minimizing the cost impact of the disability and absence of the employee. To reach program goals, this form of case management provides services to the injured worker as well as the employer or union. To do this, the specialist works with the following:

- The employer or union to develop a disability management program at the worksite
- The disabled worker through activities such as coordinating medical and rehabilitation services
- Both the employer and the worker in designing return-to-work programs to facilitate the early return of a disabled worker

Using such laws as the Americans with Disabilities Act (ADA), the Family and Medical Leave Act (FMLA) and other disability discrimination regulations, the disability specialist's primary job duties are to identify essential job functions performed by the injured worker prior to the injury and make reasonable accommodation recommendations and, when possible and applicable, to assist the injured worker in a return-to-work program. Other job duties often include the following:

- Communicating with the employee as soon as possible after the injury or onset of illness to keep the employer apprised of expected return-to-work date, physical capabilities, and work restrictions that may apply
- Working with the employer to determine if modified/alternate work opportunities are available
- Providing direct services and coordination of benefits, such as assistance in obtaining a physician or other

health care provider appointment (and if necessary taking the client to the appointment) and ensuring requests for services are processed in a timely manner

- Working closely with the injured worker and the employer to establish recovery and rehabilitation goals and objectives
- Monitoring the progress of the injured worker in reaching goals as well as any progress or issues once placed in a modified or alternate work program
- Reporting evaluation and monitoring outcomes to the employer and the union, as applicable
- Serving as a liaison with outside professionals, the workers' compensation insurance carrier, and the workers' compensation Board
- Working closely with the injured worker and employer on development of a return-to-work program
- Conducting vocational assessments and then, as applicable, working with vocational counselors on an appropriate training program for the injured worker
- Providing organizational consultation and programs for employers to their employees in attempts to minimize injuries
- Providing expert testimony

Keys to success of disability management include the following:

- Early intervention
- Timely provision of services
- Development and implementation of a timely and safe return-to-work program for injured employees
- Knowledge of the laws and how they apply to or affect the workers' compensation processes
- Ensuring the injured worker maintains a positive approach to the disability and is cooperative with the processes involved

- Ensuring that goals are meaningful and goal-oriented, and that they include work that matches the injured worker's new capabilities
- Ensuring that union jurisdictional issues are addressed and resolved in a timely manner
- Ensuring that the return-to-work program recognizes the worker's diminished capabilities and does not compromise his or her recovery or safety
- Ensuring that the general workplace environment is not compromised by the implementation of the return-to-work program
- Ensuring that the return-to-work program is not used as a disciplinary tool

Many disability management specialists are certified through a program similar to the one used to certify CMs. For more information on certification, see the Disability Management Commission's website at www.cdms.org.

Life Care Planning

Life care planning began in the early 1980s and has its roots in rehabilitation and rehabilitation evaluations for litigation. The initial purpose of a life care plan was to have a tool that could be used to project the impact of catastrophic injury on an individual's future. In 1997, the American Academy of Nurse Life Care Planners defined a life care plan as "a dynamic document based upon comprehensive assessments, data analysis and research which then provides an organized concise plan for current and future needs with associated costs for individuals who have experienced catastrophic injury or have chronic health needs." The academy further states a life care plan may be created as a result of the nursing process and may be developed as an outcome of case management."[9]

Life care planning is the methodology for analyzing medical and medically-related goods and services that will be needed over the lifetime of an individual due to his or her disabling injury or disease. In the planning stages, a systematic logical approach is used to glean information on a variety of sources and trace all needs relating from the disability to the end of life expectancy. All past medical, social, psychologic, vocational, educational, and rehabilitation data are taken into consideration to the extent it is available and applicable. Three methods are commonly used to calculate costs:

1. Analysis of past medical expenditures
2. Determination of local community resources
3. Analysis of costs for optimal care, utilizing model systems and national cost data

The final plan is designed to provide for services that will be needed to prevent or significantly reduce known complications, minimizing potential complications, as well as optimizing quality of life.

Life care planning has emerged as the most consistent and objective methodology for projecting medical and therapeutic services. Life care planning is no more than an advanced professional practice with the life care planner serving as the author of the final document. The actual development of a plan is completed with a team approach, as the final plan requires such breadth of clinical experience and expertise. Due to the depth and breadth of a life care plan, one should encourage the use of a certified life planner. Life care planners usually have a primary educational background in nursing, medicine, vocational counseling, social work, or rehabilitation.

Life care planners must possess a thorough understanding of diagnoses, appropriate medical treatments, cost of treatments, factors affecting outcomes, psychosocial implications, and understanding of the individual's needs. They must also have a thorough knowledge of community resources as well as the creativity to develop alternative plans while incorporating a variety of preventive, curative, and rehabilitative services into a plan.

Completion of life care plans requires comprehensive assessments, data analysis, research, and careful integration of the data. The final document must be consistent with the individual's needs and should reflect risk factors that have the potential to affect available resources. It must also be clear and concise and outline the patient's long-term care needs with appropriate linkage to resources and cost projections. Life care plans contain five basic elements[9]:

1. **Record review**—This includes review of all pertinent medical records, school and military records, specialty evaluations, treatment reports, and reports from various community agencies and services.
2. **Assessment**—This occurs during interviews with the patient and family and includes both documented findings but also those gleaned from direct observation. The assessment covers such areas as medical and health history; complications since the injury or illness; current medical diagnosis; current treatment plan; current status of activities; functional skills and abilities; psychosocial status of both the patient and family; educational and vocational history; financial status; current use of medications, supplies, medical devices, or adaptive devices; environmental assessment and the need for any environmental changes; and other care needs and community services used.
3. **Collaboration**—This includes contact of key treatment professionals and promotion of communication to verify the care regimen and compliance.

4. **Data analysis**—This is critical because it is the driver for accurate recommendations for long-term care and services. The data analysis must be clear, and it must concisely document the patient's needs, necessary care and services, rationale for care and services, and expected outcome of services and variables that may affect costs for care and services, including risk factors. Data analysis covers the following areas: periodic medical care expected as a result of the diagnosis, episodic medical care likely as a result of a risk factor, durable medical equipment needs, disposable medical supplies, medications, vocational services, transportation, counseling, personal care attendants, housing needs, clothing modifications, and community re-entry programs.

5. **Research**—As long-term care needs are identified and costs are assigned to needs, knowledge of actual costs, contracted costs, and geographically specific data is critical. Costs can be researched through direct contact with vendors or via review of actual claims and charges.

The final document produced for life planning must cover areas such as those shown in Box 14-1.

Telemedicine

As lengths of stay decline, patients are leaving inpatient settings more quickly and with more complex care needs (e.g., the average length of stay for a spinal cord injury patient has decreased from 75 days in 1986 to 35 days in 1998). Telemedicine is another mode of monitoring patients. With shorter lengths of stay, patients return home emotionally overwhelmed, socially isolated, or educationally unprepared to participate in their care. Leaving inpatient settings more quickly also affects the abil-

> **BOX 14-1**
> **Life-Planning Document**
>
> Medical history
> Social history
> Family issues
> Vocational/educational history
> Projected medical evaluations
> Projected therapy needs
> Future medical care
> Therapeutic supplies
> Personal items
> Diagnostic testing
> Medical equipment and supplies
> Recreational equipment
> Aids for independent functions
> Home/facility care
> Transportation
> Architectural renovations
> Potential medical complications
> Compromised financial status

ity of patients to integrate preventive behaviors into their lives.

During the past three decades, technologists and clinicians have investigated using telecommunications and information technologies as a way to bridge the gap among people with medical needs and their clinicians. Telemedicine has emerged as a significant component to the health care delivery system. Telemedicine is defined as using telecommunication technology to deliver health care services when the person with medical needs is at a distance.[10]

The goal of most telemedicine programs is to match technology with the medical needs of the patient. Depending on the unit used, images can be captured for the following: evaluating and monitoring patients and their medical condition, facial expressions, gait, and seating posture; preventing and treating pressure ulcers; evaluating home situations for compliance to the plan of care; interacting among patient and family; and providing assistive technology support for home modifications and training.

For telemedicine to work, all equipment runs over telephone lines and makes use of a camera and a monitor. The camera captures the image and displays the activity on a monitor. The image is sent via the videophone to the telemedicine center where the physician or technicians are available to view the image. Treatment can then be rendered according to findings.

The benefits of telemedicine include improved access to quality health care, especially for patients residing in rural areas or urban underserved areas, reduced provider isolation in geographically distant locations, and reduced costs for care. Although barriers exist to the acceptance of telemedicine (e.g., liability, confidentiality, privacy), reimbursement and licensing remain the two biggest barriers.[10]

Workers' Compensation

While workers' compensation is among the oldest of professions for case management, it is important to mention since many carriers have taken on a managed care focus during the last few years as the CM attempts to return the injured employee to work. Many models for today's medical case management have evolved from successes seen with case management under workers' compensation. In contrast, as medical case management for managed care has evolved, workers' compensation has also benefited and many of its processes include managed care techniques. The primary differences between medical case management and workers' compensation are the laws under which each function.

Much of medical case management activity is dependent upon an organization's contractual demands. In contrast, workers' compensation state statutes very heavily dominate workers' compensation case management activity. While statutes vary from state to state, the goals are the same—to provide services to injured workers and assist them in returning to work when possible.

Thus, CMs working with workers' compensation must be very familiar with the laws in their state. Workers' compensation is a social contract by the state government that mandates such areas as the "first dollar" or total coverage of medical bills and a percentage of lost wages for on-the-job injuries or illnesses. Injured workers are precluded from recovering from their employers or coemployees reimbursement for negligence or other claims apart from the workers' compensation claim.[11]

The majority of workers' compensation cases will not require case management. The cases that require case management ideally should start at the time of the first report of injury. The goals of workers' compensation case management are as follows:

- Return the claimant to his or her previous state of health or to a condition of maximum medical improvement (MMI)
- Ensure the treatment plan is appropriate and allows progression
- Ensure compliance with the treatment regimen
- Ensure the claimant is not engaged in activities that would jeopardize his or her recovery

To meet the goals, the workers' compensation CM must have basic medical and surgical skills as well as the following:

- Strong skills and knowledge of the state's workers' compensation laws and how they relate
- Strong assessment skills including job site assessments and return-to-work mechanisms
- Orthopedic, neurologic, and physical medicine and rehabilitation skills (since many injuries are related to fractures, carpal tunnel, head injuries, trauma, and back and neck injuries)

- Common knowledge of medical and behavioral health practitioners and providers in the claimant's immediate area who treat work-related injuries
- Ability to read and evaluate rehabilitation provider records
- Ability to work with attorneys and at times deal with hidden agendas
- Ability to work with employers for an effective return-to-work program

While many states have vocational rehabilitation training and placement structured into their workers' compensation laws, many provisions for vocational rehabilitation have been relaxed by recent law revisions. This is because the vocational component tends to drive up costs and has shown to be of little value especially when the economy is in a depressed cycle. With or without vocational rehabilitation, the general rule of thumb for return to work is as follows: If the worker is not back to work in 6 months, there is a 50% chance of return; if not back to work in 1 year, there is a 25% chance; if not back in 2 years, the chance is near 0%.[11] In addition to relaxation of laws on vocational rehabilitation, many workers' compensation programs have assumed some components of the managed care processes as they attempt to contain the spiraling costs associated with work-related injuries.

Managed Care and Case Management

As indicated in this text's section on managed care and insurance, all types and forms of managed health care dominate the U.S. health care system as attempts are made to reform health care and contain costs. As we all remember, the Clinton administration made attempts at reform in health care and it failed. Despite the failure, health care reform continues with the real drivers the large employers or health care purchasers. It is from employer demands as contracts are generated or renewed that attempts are made at all levels to cut health care costs and reduce spending.

In response to employer demands to contain costs, Congress is aiming many health care reform bills toward encouraging people to join managed care. It is no secret that managed care is the structure that drives costs and spending down. While managed care has been conceptualized in many ways, it is a brokerage of health care services for specific population groups with an emphasis on quality of care and controlled costs. A 1990 study showed that if the entire U.S. population were in an HMO, there would have been a reduction in health care expenditures by 12.2%.[12]

As managed care models increase, case management will be the preferred delivery system if the demands and challenges established by employers continue to reform health care. Another study on managed care identified the following seven major trends that will shape managed care and case management systems[13]:

1. **Capitation**—This evolving system of reimbursement and managed care provides for a more coordinated and efficient team-based approach to care delivery. The major focus is on efficient and effective resource management. With capitation, providers receive a fixed amount of reimbursement per enrollee regardless of whether services were provided. It is through case management that quality of care will be delivered under a capitated system.

2. **Information systems**—These systems will flourish, and the delivery of care will be database-driven. These systems will ensure appropriate management and integration of all care delivery. This is happening to meet the need to move more quickly and efficiently when

dealing with complex, multisystem information. Information systems will fully support the operations of case management models.

3. **Physician control**—These providers must and will provide the degree of leadership necessary to be successful in the world of managed care. They must and will play major roles in the development and implementation of case management models and systems. Although nurses will be the driving force behind case management systems, physician support and leadership are needed to ensure commitment to the model.

4. **Medicare-Medicaid enrollees**—To save money, states are requiring a greater percentage of their Medicaid recipients to be in managed plans and networks. The same is true of the federal government and Medicare recipients. Because each group presents its own unique health care needs, case management systems will be modified and redesigned to address this trend.

5. **Carve-outs**—MCOs will escalate their practice of subcontracting for various health care services. Nurse CMs practicing in case management models will be in great demand as subcontractors of health care delivery. This trend will foster the rapid development of entrepreneurial nurse CMs and move the nursing profession to the forefront of point of service care.

6. **Insurance company ownership**—These entities will own their own networks. They will use case management systems and nurse CMs to drive the efficient and cost-effective delivery of care. Nurse CMs will play significant roles in insurance-owned groups.

7. **Increased decentralization**—MCOs will seek out relationships and models that move them more closely to patients. Case management is the ideal model to realize this goal.

As case management is now offered both internally and externally by a variety of organizations, a close collaborative nonadversarial working relationship between both entities will be paramount. The most effective relationship will be ones in which both parties focus on the health care needs of the patient with the ultimate goal of quality, cost-effective care. To do this requires *accurate* assessments and *excellent* communication. In cases in which the CM is external to the MCO, he or she has essentially the following seven functions:

1. Provide accurate assessments
2. Provide accurate planning of care to be provided
3. Organize staffing
4. Identify and coordinate interdisciplinary and interagency/facility disciplines
5. Identify resource allocations
6. Implement the case management plan
7. Monitor and evaluate the case management plan to ensure standards are met

From the MCO, the internal CM has essentially five functions[14]:

1. Assess eligibility
2. Validate the plan of care against benefit coverage
3. Define payment systems (in the world of managed care and risk arrangements, it is imperative to know who will be authorizing care and who will assume responsibility for payment of bills)
4. Coordinate benefits, if more than one payer is involved
5. Conduct performance evaluations and provider audits to ensure quality providers are available for use

On-Site Versus Telephonic Case Management

Historically, the modality for conducting the majority of case management activity was via on-site visits. Efficient and effective case management organizations allow a combination of both telephonic as well as on-site visits. A combination approach to case management is most useful for cases that are catastrophic in nature and expected to be long-term. While much can be done telephonically (as these cases often require a large quantity and variety of resources and vendors at a high cost), on-site visits allow one to capture realistically what is occurring. They also assist in validating when skilled care is no longer required or the patient or family requires additional teaching to ensure the case management plan remains effective. A primary reason is to solidify a closer working relationship with the patient and family for enhanced compliance to the plan. Additional benefits to on-site case management are as follows:

- An avenue to convey a personal interest and an interest in personal well being
- An avenue for more in-depth exploration of issues so that realistic planning can occur, because the CM can view firsthand issues that affect the case, such as patient-family dynamics, the actual living environment, and the patient's ability to function within his or her environment
- An avenue for more effective assessments, education, exploration of issues, mutual problem solving, and face-to-face negotiation
- If the on-site visit occurs while the patient is in a facility, it will serve as an avenue to conduct a thorough clinical assessment and discuss issues and overall case management plans with the multidisciplinary team

However, to ensure success and the cost-effectiveness of visits, the CM must always examine whether the on-site visit will produce the results desired or if other methods be as useful (such as input from the physician or home health agency or via telephonic conversations with players on the case).

In telephonic case management, phone, mail, fax, e-mail, or other electronic transfer provides services. As a rule, telephonic case management is used in the following cases:

- Cases that are expected to be short-term and noncatastrophic
- When emphasis is on utilization rather than case management
- When rapid decision making is expected to occur
- When there is good rapport with providers or vendors in the area and they are known to report honestly on case findings
- When there are no other CMs in the area and travel would be too costly
- When dollar limits and timeframes are expected to be short-term

Making use of telephonic case management is a way to save considerable time as well as costs. Through telephonic case management, CMs have the ability to handle larger caseloads because there is no down time as with driving to and from an on-site visit. One tremendous downside of especially long-distance telephonic case management is the lack of knowledge and trust of the providers and miscommunications that can occur for a variety of reasons.

Unfortunately, as the Prospective Payment System (PPS) takes effect on all levels of health care, the use of telephonic case management as well as telemedicine will likely increase. These modalities will be necessary because organizations will no longer be paid for every outpatient or home health visit; they will now be paid the same whether they make three calls/visits per week or three calls/visits per day. Also, as lengths of stay grow shorter and patients leave the hospital more quickly, telephonic case management and telemedicine as it relates to case management will take on new meanings.

While telemedicine can be used in many settings, especially those that are remote, if used as part of the case management process it allows the ability to communicate with the patient, assist with patient care, and view the patient and his or her environment. Through the latter part of the process, the CM can often find reasons for noncompliance with treatment regimens or medication administration. Through the use of telemedicine in case management, patients have assistance when it is needed most, along with greater access to a clinician and to information that can produce greater self-directed and controlled care.[10]

Components of Successful Case Management Programs

Overall, the literature supports the broad benefits of successful case management and its multifold processes. To meet goals and thus success, it is paramount for the program to have the following requirements:

- Customized to the individual organization or institution's needs and the population or populations to be served
- Developed in order to allow individual case activity to center on methods to decrease fragmentation, increase timely access to services, streamline care and resource availability, standardize plan of care, improve interdisciplinary collaboration and communication, decrease readmission rates, and improve responses of the patient and family through the use of educational efforts

All of the above can result when there is personal involvement with the patient and family. This personal involvement enhances opportunities for education and consequently compliance and commitment. It also assists in increasing the patient's and family's awareness of financial and quality implications. The ultimate goal of successful case management is to enable the effective measurement of quality and cost outcomes.

Similarities

While there are many models for case management in existence today, all models have similar characteristics that serve as their foundation. The major characteristics are as follows[15]:

- **Nurse driven**—Case management development and its use in health care can be attributed to nursing efforts. Nurses have traditionally been the managers of care. The complexity of the case management system of care requires knowledge and skills of professional registered nurses. While other disciplines and technical nursing personnel can assist in the delivery of health care services, it is the professional nurses, through the nursing processes, that drive the entire care process and retain responsibility for achieving quality outcomes.
- **Patient focused**—The patient must always be the common denominator as the CM uses whatever services are planned, implemented, and provided. This includes staying attuned to all facets of care, levels of care, and resources to provide the care, and knowing where gaps exist so as to prevent fragmentation of the case management plan. A patient-focused system also encompasses one's performance as it does the following:
  - Enforces and ensures patient rights
  - Enforces and ensures assessments are individualized and comprehensive (e.g., physical, psycho-

logic, psychosocial, and socioeconomic)

- Enforces and ensures patient treatment plans are developed using a multidisciplinary and collaborative approach, identifying and operationalizing the resources and services needed throughout the continuum of care
- Enforces and ensures patient and family education is timely, constant, appropriate, and provided in a culturally and linguistically correct venue (e.g., audiovisual, booklets, classes) to enforce understanding and compliance
- Enforces and ensures care plans and processes are monitored and corrective actions are taken when needed

- **Family focus**—Because the family and/or significant others are critical to the patient's recovery, they become a vital focal point in the overall planning for care. Case management is designed to include family in all aspects of care and during the episode of illness. While many patients are alone and get sick in isolation, healing cannot take place in such a setting. Case management systems recognize the position of the patient within his or her family system and use that reality to the maximum benefit of the patient. Case management models incorporate family teaching. Included in this teaching is educating the patient and family so that they have an understanding of the illness process, taking part in self-management, and then compliance. From this, the family can provide the support and at times the resources required by the patient. Case management as a vehicle of care delivery also focuses on care of the family or caregiver, as without them, the case management plan may not succeed.

- **Protocols**—While medical, nursing, or treatment protocols will be the hallmarks of a case management system for quality case management to occur, the importance of using these protocols and guidelines cannot be overemphasized. Protocols are in essence the multidisciplinary teams' written map to achieving the goals of case management as they provide increased efficiency, improve decision making, assist with reduction of costly variations in practice, eliminate inappropriate use of resources, and rationalize and standardize approaches to care.

- **Multidisciplinary**—Case management requires CMs and the other health care team members to function as a multidisciplinary team. As the nature of case management is to provide comprehensive full continuum services to populations, the CM role has become multidisciplinary with all professionals coming together for the common good of the patient. Using a multidisciplinary process is instrumental in breaking down barriers to and fragmentation of health care delivery.

- **Multiservice**—Case management systems provide for a wide variety of health care services. Effective and efficient case management systems bring the multitude of services together to ensure a comprehensive system for care is in place. When services are successfully integrated, quality care and successful outcomes will be superior.

- **Brokerage of services**—As the services needed by case managed cases often require the use of a multiservice approach, the CM serves in a key role as a broker. The ultimate goal is to ensure the patient is referred to all appropriate and applicable services required. The CM may need to serve as an advocate or negotiator of rates or resources to reach the goal.

- **Specialized**—Case management systems continue to be specialized. They are specialized in the sense that they have come into their own right and they are an art and science unto themselves.
- **Continuum of care**—Case management acknowledges that people evolve along a continuum that requires lifelong health care services.
- **Research based**—The development and design of case management systems are based in research.
- **Outcomes and goal driven**—Quality effective case management systems are outcomes and goal-driven. Case management systems must be designed to move the patient through the care delivery processes toward the defined outcomes. Outcomes must be clearly defined and measurable. As outcomes are developed, they must be communicated to and agreed upon by the patient, family, and health care team.

Goal Driven

Whatever the focus, successful case management organizations will ensure their programs and plans established for patients are goal-driven and favorable to both patient and organizational outcomes and that there is satisfaction at all levels. The goals of case management flow from the case management definition. These goals include the following[15]:

- **Quality of care**—Case management has its roots in a strong focus on quality of health care delivery. Services must be therapeutic and beneficial to the population being managed. Quality outcomes must be identified, and interventions must be planned to meet them. Outcomes demonstrate that care delivery through case management has had a therapeutic effect on the client's condition, problems, and needs
- **Length of stay**—A focus on reducing inpatient length of stay is inherent to the concept of case management as a cost-control mechanism for hospitals. The system is designed to move patients rapidly through the care process while maintaining quality of care. Timeliness of the process becomes paramount. This is also achieved by reengineering systems and processes to support the efficiency of the case management model. Studies show that the best-run hospitals have reduced their length of stay to one-half the national average. Thus, length of stay is correlated to systems of efficiency.
- **Resource utilization**—Case management reduces and controls resource utilization. This is achieved by protocols that guide care delivery based on research and the evaluation of patient outcomes. Protocols define a plan of care that is careful to avoid inappropriate resource utilization. This is a hallmark goal of case management.
- **Continuity**—Case management provides continuity of care during each episode of delivery. Models are designed to provide clients with a full range of services by familiar professionals. Continuity evokes client ownership and collaboration of services received. Case management also focuses on the entire episode of illness. This concept of continuity also merges nicely with the collaborative approach inherent in case management systems.

- **Cost control**—A most important goal in this era of capitation, case management achieves reduction of costs and decreased spending through the interface of the previously stated goals. In this way, cost control becomes the primary outcome of the system.

Tools to Improve Case Management Practice

Clinical Information

A key tool for successful case management is for management to ensure staff are kept up-to-date with the clinical knowledge and the tools required for doing their jobs. Managers of case management units must continually ask how this can be accomplished, effectively done, and as cost-effective as possible. Medical practice is data driven. As medical advances are made for better diagnosis and treatment, staff must be clinically astute and the data they need must be readily available.

Clinical information comes from two primary sources: clinical experience and research. This is further divided into two categories: consensus-based and evidence-based. Consensus-based information consists of documents produced that are based on the clinical expertise of a small group of experts. These experts agree that a specific treatment or sequence of treatments will produce optimal outcomes for a particular issue. Evidence-based information is the data generated from clinical trials or the information collected by specific disease registries.

Relationships

A key process in reaching goals and successful positive outcomes is the use of relationships. These relationships can be broken down into four major components: consumer, team members, insurer, and continuum of care providers.

- **For consumers**—Relationship building is important for the patient or family and CM to develop a partnership concept in which mutual goal setting can occur. Consumer relationships might also include consumer groups with like interests or disease processes.
- **For team members**—This relationship involves all members of the multidisciplinary team, starting with the physician. These relationships can be built using either a group setting or an individual one-to-one setting with team members. If a group is involved, the CM often will serve as facilitator to guide the group toward mutually agreed-upon appropriate outcomes. Team member relationships are key to improvements in process as well as resource management.
- **For insurer or payer relationships**—Positive relationship building is important when the CM is external to the insurer or when the CM's organization and insurer are in a shared-risk arrangement. It is imperative to keep the insurer apprised of case actions to ensure timely approval of services and payment.
- **For the continuum of care providers**—The last relationship to build and cultivate is one with the various providers across the continuum of care. Building of such relationships strengthens and builds effective transition of care processes. Openness and honesty are key to effective communication and this relationship.

For most case management programs, nurses make up the majority of staffing. However, a well-functioning case management program also augments the staff with social workers, as they are key players of the multidisciplinary team. As with nurses, social workers are licensed and bound by a Code of Ethics that is produced by the

National Association of Social Workers. These codes embody certain standards of behavior for the social worker and the professional relationships developed with other health care professionals, colleagues, and the community in general. A social worker may be involved with a case singly or in combination with the nurse CM. Social workers usually will be involved in the following types of cases:

- The patient is homeless
- The patient lacks an external support system
- There is known or suspected child or adult abuse or neglect
- The patient is a minor seeking sensitive services often protected by law
- Adoptions
- There is known substance abuse or chemical dependency
- The patient needs assistance with the Medicaid, Social Security, In-Home Supportive Services, Supplemental Security Income (SSI), general welfare assistance, Conservatorship, Durable Power of Attorney, General Power of Attorney, Vocational Rehabilitation, or other public programs
- The patient or family is in a profound family crisis due to the impact of the illness, injury, or death
- The patient or family is highly dysfunctional
- The patient requires psychiatric interventions
- The patient has sustained a catastrophic injury (e.g., gunshot wound, multiple trauma), and the social worker is used for grief and other counseling for the patient, family, or both
- The patient sustained sudden or unexpected death, and the family needs grief counseling
- The new diagnosis (e.g., trauma, cancer, acquired immunodeficiency syndrome [AIDS], congenital anomaly, terminal diagnosis) is life-altering, and the patient or family requires assistance with expected coping issues (e.g., grief, loss, denial)

Communication

One of the most valuable skills and tools an effective CM possesses is the skill of communication. Effective and successful case management depends on the ability to put patients and families at ease while conducting communication sessions at the level, frequency, and type from which issues can be addressed, details can be extracted, and plans can be made.

Effective communication is measured by the extent of information gathered and by the degree of participation and cooperation of the patient, family, and health care team members. Additionally, communication can be enhanced through keen listening skills and the elicitation of suggestions and preferences of the patient and family. Equally as important is honesty. It is important to be honest with the continuum of care providers as the patient moves to the next level of care. It is even more important to be honest with patients and families, letting them ask questions, listening, and then answering. If the answer is unknown, do not guess. Let them know you will research the issue and get back with them. Then do it.

The art of communication also involves the art of listening. This includes what is said as well as what is not and the body language used as one speaks. So, keep your eyes open and aware of how the patient and family are acting. In all cases avoid medical jargon. Keep it simple and ask questions appropriately (e.g., open-ended questions may be appropriate for most patients, but certainly not for Alzheimer's patients; they need questions that limit choices, minimize the use of pronouns, and break down tasks into simple steps, along with repetition).

Just as important as simplicity, honesty, and frequency, communication must be conducted at a level that facilitates understanding by all parties. This is a critical link. Success also involves old-fashioned teamwork in which the CM, regardless of his or her employer, becomes an integral part of the team. A successful CM must act and approach the family or health care team in a proactive manner rather than a reactive one. The power of communication with all parties—patient, family, physician, and health care team—cannot be overstated or underestimated.

Communication with the patient is by far the most critical area. An effective case management plan evolves from an exhaustive knowledge of the patient. This includes the patient's actual care needs versus perceptions, support systems and lifestyle, attitudes, beliefs, values, and the environment in which he or she lives. If the patient is conscious, the patient and CM relationship will be the most important relationship a CM will have. As one speaks with the patient and family, it is of utmost importance to create an atmosphere of trust. Once this occurs, the flow of communication necessary for appropriate treatment decision making can evolve. As one interacts with the patient and family, it is important to capture as much information as possible as it relates to the following:

- One's perception of past medical conditions and treatments
- One's perception of the present illness or injury and treatments
- One's plans for care and the location
- One's financial resources for payment
- One's family and caregiver support systems
- One's attitude toward illness and being sick
- One's beliefs and values from a personal, religious, or cultural perspective
- Foreseen barriers or obstacles

If communication is not kept open and simple with the patient and family, the health care team will find themselves faced with one crisis situation after another. When these situations occur, it is wise to work closely with a social worker or psychologist and conduct as many team or family conferences as possible. For example, while working with alert and oriented ventilator-dependent patients in the ICU, patients and families are often extremely frustrated when their loved one cannot communicate or make wishes known. One of the best ways to assist all involved (personnel, patient, family, physicians, and staff) is to schedule frequent patient or family and team conferences. These conferences can be scheduled at any frequency but in many cases they will be needed weekly. The actual frequency of communication depends on the individual case. In all cases, communication must always be frequent enough with all parties to ensure sharing of information and awareness of the latest details affecting a case.

Regardless of the CM's affiliation, communication with the medical team is just as critical. This requires the development of a mutually agreed-upon course and a balance of authority. You may need to recognize provider or physician authority while you generate authority and respect for yourself.

Communication with the insurer is equally as important in the cycle of communication as case management plans are developed. Each insurer (e.g., private or public) has its own unique requirements if they are to pay the tab. Not providing proper or adequate information to the insurer can cause two serious problems: delay or denial of the request for authorization or delay or denial of payment. When communicating with an insurer, specific information is always needed. This includes the following:

- Patient name, age, and date of birth

- Social security number (patient's or subscriber's)
- Diagnosis and at times prognosis (ICD9 or DSM)
- Requesting provider
- Treating provider (e.g., provider name, address, phone number, and tax ID number if a nonnetwork provider)
- Location of care (e.g., facility name, address, phone number, and tax ID number if a nonnetwork facility)
- Proposed treatments (some require actual CPT code)
- Proposed equipment (some require actual HCPCS codes), duration of need, and medical supply items
- Date proposed treatments will start and frequency and approximate number of treatments planned
- Insurance carrier's name, case tracking number, and name and phone number of internal contact if the patient is insured by a secondary insurer.

In addition, it is wise to send applicable medical records (e.g., history and physical, consultations, latest progress notes, therapy notes) that describe the patient's medical history as well as treatments rendered to date and the responses to such.

Educating Patients and Families on the Importance of Communication

Educating patients and families to communicate with their physician or other providers can be an arduous process if the physician or health care professional does not listen, the patient or family is intimidated or uneducated, or when language or cultural barriers exist. Thus, CMs must continually teach patients to be better prepared for interactions with their physician or provider. This is accomplished through simple strategies they can use before, during, and after their examination or visit. It is through this simple process that CMs can increase the likelihood that patients

will receive satisfactory care and compliance and successful eventual overall medical care results (Box 14-2).

Many patients and families will have a high anxiety level as one teaches them how to communicate effectively with the health care team. It is wise to educate them to read as much as possible about the medical condition and any literature supplied to them (e.g., medication labeling and warnings) and to keep a pad and pencil nearby for questions that come to mind. Also, as they ask questions, they must be educated to write down responses for review at a later time. As they read articles or literature, they should be encouraged to make copies to prove their point when they discuss issues with the health care team member. They can then be prepared

---

BOX 14-2

Checklist for Patient-Physician Communication

Patients need to be prepared to do the following:
- Tell about their medical history
- Tell details of family members and their medical history
- Tell about medications they take (including over-the-counter medications) and their dosages and frequency
- Tell about medications that cause reactions, and list the reactions to each
- Relay current symptoms or those that surfaced since the last visit
- Relay questions they wish to have addressed at each visit

During the examination, patients need to be prepared to do the following:
- Be honest about compliance or issues
- Speak up if treatments or medications are not working as they feel they should
- Not minimize or exaggerate symptoms

After the examination, patients need to be prepared to do the following:
- Repeat the proposed treatment regimen or schedule
- Discuss the cost of proposed treatments
- Ask the questions prepared prior to the visit or ask questions related to what was said during the examination that is unfamiliar[16]

to "scientifically justify" what is said. A process such as this allows patients to stay better informed through active participation in communicating with their health care providers.

Verbal and nonverbal communication is important if one is to ensure psychologic factors or stressors associated with the case are recognized. The patient and family must be allowed to express their feelings, and the CM must listen. Depending on their responses, linkage to peer support or professional counseling may be necessary. Naturally, if threats of violence are made, these need to be reported and acted upon as per any established organizational guidelines.

Written Communication

Effective communication (verbal or written) is an absolute must when helping patients and families deal with the stress of a situation. Whenever possible, the patient and family should be informed of the actual and potential stressors they can expect to encounter as well as the mechanisms to alleviate them. This information allows them to recognize stressors as they occur and make appropriate arrangements to deal effectively with them. The best way to ensure this occurs is to address problems as they arise and, if needed, list the actual resources or mechanisms in the written case management plan.

Collaboration

Just as important as communication, collaboration is critical in working with complex patients and their issues. Unfortunately, this is a process often spoken but not always practiced. Collaboration is time-consuming, but it offers enormous benefits, satisfaction, and effective outcomes when used effectively.

To ensure effective outcomes, collaboration requires excellent communication. This means that all parties must have input with the final objective: achieving a plan

that clarifies differences and focuses on complementary approaches to achieve common goals. Six elements are linked to effective collaboration[17]:

1. Communication
2. Contribution
3. Commitment
4. Consensus
5. Compatibility
6. Credit

Successful collaboration is not always and easy task for some. However, the key elements to becoming a successful collaborator include the following[18]:

- Putting values aside and focusing on the needs and wishes of the patient
- Understanding the value and the contributions others can have on the plan
- Being easy to work with and accessible
- Looking for agreement
- Refraining from acting as if you know more than others
- Keeping your promises to other team members and especially the patient

When building a team, its success depends on the strengths of each team member, their individual expertise, and the ability of the team to work together and tap potential as a whole. A collaborative team requires the following:

- A vision
- Alignment toward common goals and purposes
- Coherence to activities
- Assistance to individuals so that they can put aside differences and work together cooperatively
- Processes that allow and encourage the ability to compliment each other's efforts

A clearly stated vision is the first step in building a collaborative team approach to case management. Collaborative teams don't just happen when people come together for a meeting. They are created through clear communication and up-front agreements about roles and decision making, which builds trust. The agreements the team begins with will enable it to sustain its focus and achieve its outcomes.[19]

An example of a collaborative team is one that was established at a Kaiser Permanente Hospital in Sacramento. A team was assembled to assist the discharge planning and utilization review staff in their efforts with difficult patients. The goals were to decrease prolonged hospitalizations, ensure a timely discharge (decrease days per thousand and the average lengths of stay), and ensure appropriate discharge plans were in place to prevent readmissions). The ultimate goals were to ensure quality of care, appropriate level of care, and patient satisfaction. As the team was assembled, the following had to be considered:

- Purposes for each team member and the team as a whole
- Scope of what the team could do as a whole
- Number and variety of team members that would be necessary to assemble and their roles
- Norms and ground rules for the team to follow (e.g., what information was needed from each team member, the type of information required, and how it would be shared)
- How the information would be relayed for others to see, if not present.

The team is comprised the following:

- Patient's physician or hospital rounding physician
- Patient's floor nurse
- Patient's discharge planner
- Nursing supervisor
- Social worker
- Clinical dietitian
- Physical therapist
- Occupational therapist

- Speech pathologist
- Pharmacist
- Home health liaison
- Skilled nursing facility liaison
- Mental health liaison
- Neurology CM
- Chronic care management representative
- Geriatric clinical nurse
- Nurse educator
- Infection control nurse (patient-specific and as needed)
- Patient's family (as case activities and events dictate)

While patient age and diagnosis played a role in selection, patients were generally selected based on length of stay (more than seven days) and identification by team members as patients with foreseeable discharge problems. Prior to the weekly meeting, a notice was sent out via e-mail to participants of the patients selected for discussion that week (often 15 to 20 patients). The team met weekly at the same time (for one and one-half hours) and the same place, and followed the same agenda. A five-minute time limit was placed on each patient, so team members had to be prepared in order to be concise in their descriptions of issues.

Each patient's attending physician led his or her discussion. Team members then reported on specific issues they were dealing with, issues they saw as a potential barrier, issues in need of a change to the treatment plan (e.g., medication change), and additional referrals or consultations required. If issues were identified for which there were no immediate solutions (e.g., patient still acute; planned length of stay excessive but was based on accepted clinical practice patterns for the diagnosis and patient/family was coping and readied for DC; patient awaiting Conservatorship or Medicaid but was stable and team had completed all actions), the team would collectively agree that the patient does not warrant weekly team reporting and their case discussion would be postponed pending discharge.

Once all team members had presented, the discussion was summarized onto a patient-specific progress note (placed in the patient's chart immediately after the meeting). The information shown in Figure 14-2 was captured using a preprinted or stamped progress note.

This team was highly effective and all team members attended the majority of meetings, with often the physicians arguing over who would present first. Each team member was valued for his or her input and expertise. The team process was evaluated every six months (through both e-mail and an open discussion among team members) to evaluate effectiveness of the team and to identify areas for improvement.

Maintaining Confidentiality

Whether written or spoken, communication is a key element to success. As data are collected or communicated, all team members must ensure that maintaining confidentiality is a top priority. This has always been a key function, but it is now more critical as federal laws now mandate it. Restrictions have been imposed on confidentiality through passage of the Health Insurance Portability and Accounting Act (HIPAA).

Most organizations have historically had detailed policies for maintenance of confidentiality, places where information can be discussed, and processes necessary for dissemination of medical information and health care records and their disposal. However, as the list of persons or organizations asking for medical information seems endless, it is important to keep the following in mind when releasing medical information[2]:

- What needs to be kept private
- Who should have access to the information

A team conference was held on (date) _____ at (time)_____

Facilitator: _____

Team members present: MD ( ) Nursing ( ) Nursing Sup ( ) DCP ( ) SW ( ) Pharmacy ( ) Nutrition ( ) Educator ( ) PT ( ) OT ( ) ST ( ) SNF ( ) HH ( ) MH ( ) Inf. C ( ) Geriatrics ( ) Neuro ( ) CCM ( )

Other:

Problems identified:

Which discipline will handle the issue or is needed to consult on the case:

Other team recommendations:

Figure 14-2   Team conference notes.

- How long the organization maintains records, where are they stored, and if the area is secured;
- If written information is to be discarded, what protections are in place to ensure privacy (e.g., is there a shred box or shredding service for the destruction of the old records?)
- If a third party needs information, how much can be conveyed and how?
- If information goes into a computerized medical record, who will have access to the data, how will it be transmitted, and what requirements does the organization have in place to protect documents while allowing access to those who have been given authority to access specific data

Cultural, Linguistic, and Literacy Sensitivity

The health care environment is changing due to our country's ever-increasing population. The U.S. Department of Commerce's website reveals that by 2000 33% of Americans were members of ethnically diverse cultures and by 2050 the majority of people living in the United States will be from ethnically diverse cultures. These changes will present significant challenges to CMs if they are unfamiliar with different cultures and their practices and beliefs. Consequently, CMs must take stride to constantly be attuned to cultural, linguistic, and literacy sensitivity of their clients.

Ignorance of cultural beliefs and practices can lead to serious problems that compromise efforts to build a solid relationship between the CM and the patient or family. Any CM who works regularly with culturally diverse groups must be extremely familiar with the population's language, customs, folklore, diet, religion, behavior styles, body language, habits, and attitudes as well as the cultural reactions to health and illness. For instance, religious beliefs influence the lifestyles of most cultures. In many cultures, illness, injury, and death are believed to be "punishments" sent by God for sins committed. Therefore, whereas persons of one religion may believe that God is punishing the sick person, others may view sickness as a "test of strength." Providing culturally relevant care is not a simple process. As such, CMs must be aware of differing health practices and beliefs of patients and their families to optimize compliance with care. Efficient and effective case management links culturally specific health patterns with prevailing health resources.[20]

Insensitivity to cultural differences can lead to a potentially dangerous outcome. For case management, this is often failure of the case management plan. In addition, dishonoring or ignorance of cultural beliefs and practices can result in a perception by the patient or family of being harmed or insulted. An attempt by the CM to impose his or her beliefs onto others accomplishes nothing other than failure.

Both verbal and nonverbal communication is learned through culture. The task of observing and interpreting a patient's nonverbal behavior is made more difficult because behavior and verbal cues are often quite subtle and mean different things to different cultures. For example, in some cultures adult patients may show fleeting changes in facial expression and small or quick eye movements, while in others hands or other bodily gestures are used. Subtle communication cues vary from culture to culture but are essential to know if one is to optimize communication. Nonverbal communication also includes space or the physical distance among people to enhance communication. Spatial requirements vary among individuals of different cultures and all communication occurs in the context of space.

Nonverbal communication is an area that can easily be misunderstood when dealing with various cultures. Consequently, CMs must be careful in the content and context of their communication with patients. This often includes the manner and tone used, the space required, as well as the following[21]:

- Dialect (among the same ethnic group there can be a variety of dialects)
- Words—even when the language is the same, words may be used differently
- Language style
- Volume and silence and the meaning of silence
- Touch (often assists communication, while in some cultures it may be forbidden)
- Context of speech or emotional tone (use of small talk or emotions when speaking)
- Body language—stances, gestures, eye contact (eye-to-eye contact may have different meanings), how hands are held (posture and body movements readily convey positive and negative attitudes)

As one deals with cultural issues, it is imperative to also consider such additional cultural factors as the following[21]:

- **Social organization**—This relates to both role and role assignment. In these cases, the CM must look at family structure and its organization as well as the person's religious values and beliefs. Failure to do this can lead to noncompliance to the case management plan. The way the patient and family view the authority of the CM and his or her ability to problem solve also influence compliance. For example, many cultures focus on the past and maintaining tradition, so there will be little motivation to form future goals. Likewise, cultures that focus on the present are unappreciative of the past and may not plan for the future.

- **Time**—In the United States, our culture equates time with money. However, this is not true with many other cultures. Therefore, as the CM plans events in the care plan, it may be necessary to schedule them around social interaction events (e.g., meals, bedtime) rather than real clock time.

- **Environmental control**—This refers to the ability to plan activities that control nature. Unlike Americans who believe they have control of their health and are more likely to seek care before serious illnesses occurs, this is not true in many cultures. In many cultures illness and death are viewed entirely differently, and the patient may not be as receptive to lifestyle changes.

- **Biologic variances**—Here one must look at the biologic differences in people. There is a direct relationship among race and body structure, skin color, enzyme differences, genetic variations, physiologic jaundice, twining, susceptibility to disease, and nutritional deficiencies.

Because the American population is so diverse, CMs must attend workshops and training seminars and make use of printed literature to ensure they are educated and can effectively and competently work with multicultural patients. If one is to provide culturally competent care and optimize care among individuals, families, and communities, there must be an understanding of the differences and similarities among individuals from different cultures.

Language barriers are a readily evident cross-cultural issue, and one of the most difficult aspects of dealing with culturally diverse patients is the need to achieve effective communication. This is one of the most significant challenges. Communication is particularly difficult if not impossible when the patient's primary language is not the primary language of the CM. If an interpreter is used, the CM must be cautious that the communication intended is received as intended as content is often lost during translation.

Thus, every effort should be made to assign CMs who speak the dominant language of the patient and family. If this is not possible, the CM must arrange for the presence of a professional interpreter (e.g., on-site or telephonically) who is familiar with medical terminology and the conveying of accurate medical information. Using professional interpreters is important as they are more objective and information is translated as it was intended. This is important because much information can be lost or misunderstood if not interpreted correctly. This factor can be the primary reason for noncompliance. It is one thing to have access to a general interpreter, but another to know that an interpreter can relay comprehensive medical instructions without losing the context or meaning of the message when it is spoken or written.

In most communities, one can find an interpreter through use of language banks or from community centers designed to handle specific ethnic groups. If local interpreters are not available, phone companies such as American Telephone and Telegraph (AT&T) or other specialized language services can provide a full range of interpreter services for a price.

Cultural and linguistic services are not a convenience or added service an organization affords its clients. It is a *requirement* of several federal acts (e.g., the Civil Rights Act of 1964). Thus, the availability of such services is critical and resources must be readily available for use should key medical information be required. While one can use the services of local interpreters (most now require payment), health care organizations and providers must have arrangements in place that allow access of their staff to telephonic language services.

Another key element to compliance and the case management plan's ultimate success will be the ability of the patient or family to read and use what was read to understand basic directions for medical care. Basic literacy skills help most people follow road signs and read prescription bottles. What happens when a person lacks these skills? If a person misreads directions, the consequences can be serious and sometimes deadly. According to the Center for Health Care Strategy, a nonpartisan health and social policy resource center in Princeton, New Jersey (www.chcs.org), a study among persons with chronic illness showed more than 40% to be functionally illiterate. A 1993 National Adult Literacy Survey revealed that 44% of adults over age 65 are functionally illiterate. Studies are further validating that low functional health literacy leads to more trips to the hospital, inappropriate use of health care services, and inability to understand prescriptions along with higher health care costs and repeated and prolonged hospital stays. The same studies show that individuals who are illiterate or marginally literate are more likely to report physical, mental, and other health disabilities that hinder their participation in work and daily activities. Other studies indicate that patients with low health literacy are less likely to know their discharge diagnosis, reasons for taking their medications, plans for follow-up treatments, implications for filling out forms, and making lifestyle changes for staying healthy.

As a result of these and other studies, many health plans are promoting campaigns to address the issue. The same is true with the primary accrediting bodies such as JCAHO and NCQA. Both agencies have established guidelines that address the readability of patient materials. The Food and Drug Administration is likewise undertaking efforts to promote simpler labels with clearer warnings of prescription drug side effects and drug interactions.[22]

When a CM knows the patient is illiterate or has a limited vocabulary, it is important to maintain a slow steady conversational pace and explain issues or meanings of words (e.g., *diet* doesn't mean the person has to necessarily lose weight as it may pertain to what diet he or she is to follow). Other approaches involve (1) using pictures, models, or actual samples as part of the demonstration process, (2) using short videos that demonstrate what needs to be taught, (3) including a literate friend or relative in the discussion or demonstration, and (4) encouraging the patient to call if he or she cannot remember or understand the directions.

Other Key Components

Caseloads

Balancing caseloads with other responsibilities is a constant concern of case management departments and staff. However, without appropriate caseload assignments, case management is doomed for success. If caseloads are too high, the department only puts out fires and runs from one crisis to another. If too low, the department will not be cost effective or will not reach productivity goals. Unfortunately, if senior management does not have a positive role or does not support the concept, requests for additional staff are often ignored.

Assigning caseloads and determining what factors to consider is dependent upon multiple factors such as the following:

- CM's level of expertise
- Senior management's commitment to case management and the resources available for staffing, including availability of administrative assistance support
- The type of clients or populations served (e.g., Medicaid and Medicare populations may require a different level of case management than a younger and more healthy insured population in an HMO)
- Insurer or payer demands
- Type of case management services (telephonic or on-site) allowed or offered by the organization
- Geographic distances covered by the CM's organization
- Role of the CM—either the dual role of utilization reviewer and CM or the single role of CM
- Age of the patients and the intensity and severity of their condition (e.g., ventilator-dependent patients and children with special needs)
- Intensity and complexity of care required as well as availability of resources necessary to meet these needs

Caseloads must be adjusted according to details of the cases. Factors such as family dynamics, psychosocial factors, and socioeconomic issues all play heavily on the final determination for caseload assignments.

As management sets out to determine caseloads, it must consider the time for the CM to gather, analyze, and report patient care data. This is necessary if one is to develop utilization management, case management, and quality improvement strategies for cases handled. While a CM might have a caseload of 20 to 30 cases, one high-acuity case can destroy the ability to manage all details of the other cases (see Figure 14-2).

In December 2000, American Healthcare Consultants (AHC) and the Case Management Society of America (CMSA) conducted a national survey on CMs to clarify issues surrounding the caseload debate. More than 520 CMs working in a variety of settings responded. While caseloads vary with the organization, finding the appropriate caseload depends upon multiple factors such as the organization's definition of case management, the type of case management offered, and how the organization structures its case management department. While the study cannot serve as a benchmark, it is the first national effort to clarify the issue. If more information is needed, it can be obtained through the AHC website at www.ahcpub. com. The study revealed the following[23]:

- 12.3% reported managing 1 to 15 active cases each month
- 23.9% reported managing 16 to 30 active cases per month

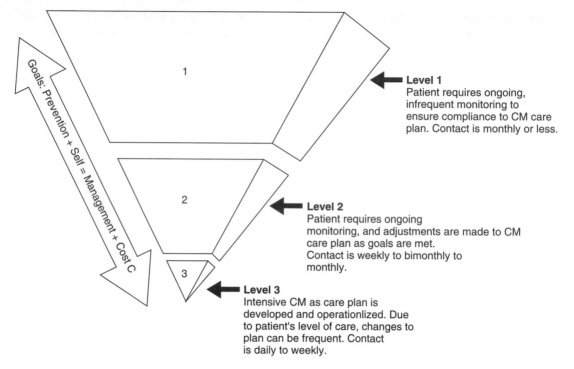

Figure 14-3   Level of case management: a three-tiered program.

- 14.8% reported managing 31 to 50 active cases per month
- 21.6% reported managing 51 to 75 active cases per month
- 10.5% reported managing 76 to 100 active cases per month
- 16.9% reported managing more than 100 active cases per month

Diane B. Williams in her editorial for *Nursing Case Management* indicates the average caseload of hospital-based CMs is among 15 to 20, and that MCO CMs have similar caseloads if they are reviewing patients in a hospital setting and higher caseloads if they conduct telephonic case management.[24]

Some issues that affect caseloads are as follows:

- High acuity of cases
- Other work responsibilities
- Lack of adequate administrative or clerical support
- Lack of tools, such as practice guidelines, clinical pathways, general versus detailed policies and procedures, computer access or incapability among programs, cell phones, community directories, inability to access resource information (e.g., manuals or Internet access)
- Travel distances and yet imposed daily or weekly productivity standards
- Lack of organization or redundancy of paper or workflow (e.g., diagnosis or disease-specific assignment versus unit assignment)
- Insurer/payer requirements for prior authorization (e.g., amount of information or details required for a coverage determination)

Caseloads are further affected by various other conditions such as the following:

- Patient age and sex
- Principal diagnosis and the severity of illness or injury
- Principal diagnosis and the intensity of services required

- Extent and severity of comorbidities and the intensities of services required
- Physical functional status
- Psychologic and cognitive status, factors, and behaviors (past and present)
- Socioeconomic status
- Prior health status and compliance
- Patient preferences and attitudes toward health, wellness, and compliance
- Patient support systems and functioning of the support system

Managing caseloads and individual case management plans within the financial constraints placed by an insurer's reimbursement is no longer a task only associated with managed care. It affects all organizations that provide health care to individuals. As case management has evolved, so has the list of responsibilities. These responsibilities must likewise be taken into consideration as caseloads are determined.

Increased responsibilities are the result of increased documentation requirements, reporting requirements, and complex financial calculations in an ever-growing paper-intensive and cost-containment environment. Consequently, the CM's responsibilities now include the following:

- Performing readmission reviews and preadmission costing and coding
- Performing initial patient-specific clinical and other assessments
- Verifying benefits and eligibility
- Coordinating benefits with other known insurers or payers to ensure that the appropriate one assumes responsibility for claims
- Referring patients to other public or entitlement programs when patients meet the criteria
- Educating patients, families, and professionals as educational opportunities are identified

- Reviewing and approving or seeking approval for services
- Reviewing questionable cases, referrals, or requests with a medical director and having access to other physician advisors in various specialties when special circumstances arise
- Having knowledge of the Internet and how to obtain scientific evidence when it is needed for review and a determination of approval or denial, especially when the request appears experimental in nature or is not usual and customary for the diagnosis
- Reviewing utilization limits and outliers to ensure coverage is allowed for such events
- Coordinating with the multidisciplinary team
- Identifying preferred providers and vendors and alternate choices
- Ensuring drug costs and other high-cost items are covered and/or approved
- Managing contract inclusions and if exclusions exist, the location of alternatives and negotiations for coverage
- Managing care plans to ensure favorable outcomes
- Determining appropriate care settings and planning as the patient is readied for differing levels of care as they progress or regress
- Reviewing claims or other data for validating or trending outcomes or capturing events for reporting purposes
- Documenting final results for measuring outcomes

Failure to manage any one of the foregoing has the potential to lead to loss of revenue for an organization. This is not to mention the toll such actions have on unnecessary out-of-pocket expenses, the stress of the situation, and the hassle of appealing an unnecessary denial by the patient or family. Such inefficiency also leads to the inability to demonstrate effective outcomes. To effectively analyze referrals and case actions, CMs must be well-trained, financially astute, capable of using complex forms, and knowledgeable about laws that affect health care, reimbursement methodologies, and tools associated with the reimbursement.

If case management practices are inefficient or poorly executed, severe financial consequences can result for an organization. Unfortunately, the tools needed to effectively manage activities have not always been available or able to keep pace with an organization's growth. While it may seem costly on the surface, effective information technology support and the necessary coding and other manuals are a must.

However, it is anticipated that the HIPAA of 1996 will positively affect case management and the standardization of electronic transmission of data. Hopefully, the information technology of a CM's world will be expanded and updated as attempts are made to meet the demands of HIPAA. The three pillars of HIPAA-defined standards are as follows:

1. Privacy
2. Security
3. Administrative simplification through the development of a uniform set of electronic formats (transaction sets, identifiers, and code sets) for use by organizations

When looking for a case management system, an organization must consider several essential criteria that will meet these new HIPAA standards. First and foremost, the system must integrate both clinical and financial data. It also must at a minimum track the following functions[25]:

- Eligibility
- Referrals
- Authorizations
- Utilization
- Contracts

- Claims, if the case management organization is affiliated with a payer

To implement the mandates of HIPAA, the Department of Health and Human Services (DHHS) has been given the authority to mandate the use and implementation of the standards. HIPAA compliance is expected to affect all health care organizations and include operational, legal, regulatory, process, security, and technology divisions if it is implemented. Each HIPAA rule must be carefully monitored and audited before an organization can deem itself fully compliant with HIPAA.

Thus, every time a CM discusses patients, requests health information, and coordinates a referral and processes, he or she must be fully cognizant of the need to comply with HIPAA privacy requirements. HIPAA standards include mandates for the following:

- Electronic exchange of health care data.
- Specification of medical and administrative code sets that should be used within those standards for an organization.
- Requirement to use national identification systems for health care patients, providers, payer, plans, and employers.
- Specifications for the types of measures required to protect security and privacy of personally identifiable health care information.

To be compliant with HIPAA case management, organizations must do the following[26]:

- Incorporate HIPAA regulations into their practices
- Assess operations from receipt of referral to case closure
- Develop HIPAA compliance strategies
- Ensure updated and current understanding of security and privacy regulations are in place

- Advocate for protection of patient health information
- Establish a concentric role for providers and patients through use of HIPAA-compliant CMs

Following are some guidelines to help a case management organization ensure HIPAA compliance[27]:

- Understand and adhere to written privacy procedures.
- Ensure training is obtained.
- Work with the compliance officer of the organization to clarify and interpret policies.
- Ensure and monitor procedural compliance.
- Ensure information of personal health information is de-identified, especially if it will be used for quality or research issues.
- Communicate and implement a grievance process that offers a means for patients to make inquiries or complaints regarding privacy of their records.
- Obtain consent for case management services, including release of information before the information is released.
- Provide patients a copy of the signed consent.
- Ensure the consent is not coerced.
- Ensure patients have access to written information on their privacy rights and how the information may be used.
- Ensure patients have access to their medical records, including the ability to copy, inspect and understand their right to make amendments.
- Maintain logs of all health care information disclosures, which is also accessible to patients.
- Release only minimal information necessary for the intent and purpose of disclosure.
- Do not disclose personal health information to employers or financial institutions without the patient's explicit authorization.
- Maintain an audit trail of those who received information for purposes other than for treatment, payment, or health care operations.
- Educate patients, families, providers, peers, and the community about HIPAA requirements as needed.
- Disclose only personal health information necessary for treatment, payment, and operations.

The HIPAA website for additional information is www.cms.hhs.gov/hipaa/.

Technology Support

In today's world of increased confidentiality awareness, managed care, and the integrated health care delivery system, CMs often assume ownership in the role as a health care guardian. It is through this guardian role that patients are led through a complex health care delivery system and appropriate care can be coordinated.

CMs have the responsibility and perspective to weave thoughtful and consistent care into the fabric of an integrated health care delivery system. No caregiver within the multidisciplinary health care team has a more comprehensive role. Without proactive patient observation, intervention, and documentation of variances from the individual care path, measurable data for useful outcome analysis fall far below an acceptable standard. These functions cannot be performed independently. Performing them effectively requires the assistance of a software program that can support case management.

Case management systems that offer strong support for clinical judgment and decision making foster the advocacy role of the CM. Instant accessibility to information and standards enhances the effectiveness of the case management process, grounding it firmly within the dynamic care delivery environment. Finally, the ability to capture analytically useful information (not simply free-form notes) ensures the delivery of better health care worldwide.[28]

When looking for a case management software vendor, in addition to ensuring the system will support and generate the reports and other data required, managers must also evaluate the following components[29]:

- What operating system does the software program require?
- What is the minimum software configuration needed to operate the program (processor speed)?
- What is the recommended computer configuration to run the program satisfactorily?
- What is the license fee of a nonnetwork single-user version?
- What product services are included in the license fee?
- How much free technology support is included in the license fee?
- What is the price of a network version and how many users are allowed?
- For which network program is the software certified (Windows, Novell)?
- Is there a sunset date?
- Is a training manual available, how detailed is it, and is it understandable by the average user?
- Can the license be transferred to another person in the company?
- What is the warranty on the software?
- Is there a money-back guarantee?
- Can someone demonstrate the program?
- Is there a promo demonstration program?
- If the computer business fails, who will support the product purchased?
- Can export information from the software program be transferred to another software program?
- What export methods are available?
- Can information be imported from the current software into the new program or does the information need manual data entry?
- Can the company assist with the importing of data from the old system?
- Is there a monthly or yearly maintenance fee?
- What is covered in the maintenance agreement?
- Are on-site installation and training recommended or required with the purchase of a site license?
- Is any on-site training and installation technical support included in the license fee?
- What is the cost of on-site training?
- Are training programs offered at regional locations?

Problem Solving

Ongoing changes in the health care arena continue to present CMs and others in health care management with new challenges and problems. Added to the complexity of care required by patients are factors such as the following:

- Increased insurer/payer constraints
- Increased nursing shortage at all levels of care and thus the need for increased patient and family education related to accepting alternatives when options for ongoing care are limited (e.g., SNF level of care is unacceptable and home care must be arranged or vice versa).

Thus, CMs in today's health care arena are finding they cannot address patient problems in ways that were previously effective.

To meet the new and old challenges effectively, individual CMs, case management companies, health insurance companies, and other health care organizations and providers are changing how they address and solve everyday business challenges and problems.[30] Traditionally, problems are classified in many ways, for example by their size (large problems versus small problems), degree of complexity (simple versus complex) and type (medical, social, economic, rehabilitative). Case management problems require creative problem solvers as well as the use of productive and reproductive thinking skills.

Productive thinking generates a new solution for each new problem. In contrast, reproductive thinking reuses an old solution to solve a new problem. The CM approaches a new problem by drawing on past solution experiences and simply reproduces one for the problem at hand. Experienced CMs use both productive and reproductive thinking, breaking with old problem-solving habits and solutions when new problem situations occur.[30] Regardless of the type used, there are three main ingredients and components that the problem solver must address:

- **Problem givens** an initial state that includes conditions, objects, and informational processes that are present before the problem solver begins to work on the problem
- **Problem goals**—the desired, terminal, or goal state
- **Problem obstacles**—impediments to reaching the goal state

Taking the foregoing ingredients, problems are then broken down into the following components[30]:

- **Problem solver**—the person who makes decisions, for example the CM
- **Controllable variables**—aspects of the solution the problem solver can influence or control (decision variables of the CM)
- **Uncontrolled variables**—aspects of the problem situation the problem solver cannot influence (in case management the insurer or insurer representatives often dictate uncontrollable variables)

- **Constraints**—limitations imposed on the possible values of the controlled or uncontrolled variables as constraints can take several forms that further impose limits and boundaries on such things as benefit levels, costs, network provider usage, medical technology, and experimental procedures
- **Possible outcomes**—outcomes produced by the problem solvers' choices of the variables they control (controllable) and those variables controlled by others (uncontrolled)

How a CM goes about defining and solving problems is the driver for the number, nature, and quality of proposed solutions as well as the one finally selected. The art of problem solving involves gathering facts and then making assumptions about the problem components, especially those that influence constraints or problem boundaries. The boundaries are then used to determine how information is organized and processed, how research is conducted, and how the CM finally attacks the issue or problem at hand. To find the optimal solution, the CM must always (1) keep an open mind about exactly what the problem is; (2) know and never lose sight of the goal to be attained; and (3) refrain from discarding reasonable solutions early in the process.[30]

The key to becoming a better problem solver is the ability to generate innovative ways to achieve the optimal solution. The best way to do this is to discard old habits and ways of defining problems, avoid insurer and physician lock-ins, and reject quick-fix solutions. This requires "thinking outside the box" (at which CMs are often the best). The best way to achieve beyond the boundary or box thinking is by aggressively challenging the givens, constraints, and uncontrolled variables. New rules for creative problem solving are listed in Box 14-3.

Isabel Briggs Myers describes an ideal win-win problem solving method that

BOX 14-3
New Rules for Creative Problem Solving

- Define the problem as broadly as possible
- Reject the status quo
- Look for solutions in new places
- Look for solutions outside your area of expertise
- Break away from your practical side once in a while
- Generate as many ideas and solutions as possible
- Be a nonconformist
- Use errors as a learning experience
- Solve the problem without constraints
- Have fun solving the problems[30]

minimizes failure, increases success, and allows everyone involved to maximize his or her potential and satisfaction. Good decision making and problem solving involves four basic components[31]:

1. Gathering facts and details of the problem at hand
2. Brainstorming possibilities to help develop possible causes of and solutions to the problem
3. Analyzing objectively by considering the cause and effect of each solution to the problem
4. Weighing the impact by considering how the problem will be affected by each solution

Due to a multitude of issues as well as coping abilities to address problems, CMs must also possess the ability to serve in an advocate role when needed.

Advocacy

The common thread that brings CMs together despite varying practice settings or professional disciplines is the fact that case management, when practiced in its truest sense, is serving an advocate role. While the CM assumes many roles, one of the greatest challenges will be that of being a patient advocate. This is especially difficult when the CM is assigned to an organiza-

tion and ends up in a dual-advocate role. Here one must serve as both patient advocate and organization advocate. CMs may feel as if they are performing a balancing act on a tightrope. In contrast, an independent CM serving in the CM role without link to an insurer, payer, or provider may feels in a less precarious position. This type of case management can at times be a more impartial advocate for a patient. This is especially true in situations in which the CM must lobby for client needs when these needs are not in line with the fiscal priorities of the insurer or organization. When caught in the crossfire of the insurer, payer, physician, hospital, and patient, the CM must serve as the patient advocate.

Thus, how CMs fulfill their role varies and depends on the employer and contractual requirements the employer may have with health care purchasers. Regardless of the setting, being a patient advocate takes on different characteristics. The important element throughout is to ensure the patient remains at the center of the process.

Literature supports the fact that less than 20% of the population uses 80% of the health care resources. The key is to identify these patients and triage them into a case management system. Sadly, even with the multitude of sophisticated systems available in the health care industry, many patients are vulnerable (e.g., financial, health, functional, developmental status, communication, race, educational circumstances) and fall through the cracks of a health care system that is not user-friendly. Thus, early assessments using available data to capture patients and then using a telephonic as well as an on-site approach to case management is essential. CMs then have a better opportunity to work with patients and advocate for their needs while teaching them how to advocate for themselves so that they can make it through the health care maze.

In addition to advocating for the patient, CMs must also support physicians in the processes of accessing services and resources. This is necessary as most treating physicians and providers are being forced to see more patients in their daily routine or take on multiple other tasks. They often do not have the time or energy to serve as the old fashioned "doc" of yesteryear. Efficient CMs can often make up for lost time by following up with patients, making sure they understand the treatment plan, educating them, helping them advocate as needed, and ensuring any new treatments are working.

By ensuring patients needs are met and the patient or family can advocate for themselves, patient advocacy can ease a patient's or family's physical, emotional, and mental burden. This is needed as patients and families are often over whelmed by the emotions of the disease and by their care-giving role. As such, they are unable to focus on more than one issue at a time. Serving as a patient advocate allows them a voice when they are least able to help themselves. To serve in an advocate role one must have the following[32]:

- Knowledge of the patient's situation, benefit packet, clinical needs, and health care resources
- A trusting relationship with the patient and family
- Persuasion skills and the ability to temper persistency with realism
- Ability to clearly and concisely communicate
- Understanding of risk tolerance and power brokering
- Ability to mobilize resources and build coalitions
- Ability to deal with role conflicts
- Bureaucratic know-how
- Time and energy to serve as the advocate (heavy caseloads or playing various roles can dilute advocacy efforts)

- Ability to conduct cost-benefit analysis

Unfortunately, there are times when the CM is forced to choose among the best interests of his or her employer, the insurer or payer, and the patient. Almost all CMs at one time or another will face this potential conflict of interest while trying to accommodate the patient's differing needs and wants and preserving and protecting the financial interests of the insurer. This is when the CM will walk the finest of lines, hoping to find a middle ground that allows them to fulfill both roles. A key element to advocacy is education of the patient and the ability for them to be empowered. CMs must educate patients on their medical condition, how to better handle their care, what they need to know about the workings and benefits of their health plan, how to locate community resources, and what to expect with denials and appeals. Education such as this helps develop patient empowerment skills and the ability to advocate for themselves when the CM is no longer around.

Advocacy Competencies

As stated by Schielke,[33] there are a variety of skill sets that are required for competency. Some of these changes are as follows:

- Supporting autonomy
  - Determining and documenting the patient's decision-making capacity; ensuring that agency or institutional policies specify how this is to be done, and identifying responsible parties
  - Protecting the right of patients with decision-making capacity to be self-determining through facilitation of communication and documentation of patient preferences; anticipating the types of treatment decisions that likely will need to be made; and assisting with the preparation of advanced directives

- Promoting authentic autonomy since authentic decisions reflect the individual's identity, decisional history, and norms
- Identifying a morally and legally valid surrogate decision maker for patients who lack decision-making capacity
- Supporting the surrogate decision maker and clarifying his or her role
- Identifying limits to patient, surrogate, and caregiver autonomy
- Developing agency or institution policies that identify the caregivers and procedures to be used to identify and support appropriate decision makers
- Promoting patient well-being
  - Determining medical effectiveness of therapy
  - Weighing the benefits and burdens of therapy
  - Ensuring that all interventions are consistent with the overall goal of therapy
  - Ensuring that all of the patient's priority needs are addressed (biologic, psychosocial, and spiritual needs)
  - Ensuring continuity of care as the patient is transferred among services within and without the institution
  - Weighing the moral relevance of third-party interests (family, caregiver, institution, society)
  - Identifying and addressing forces within society and the health care system that compromise patient well-being
- Preventing and resolving ethical conflict
  - Establishing that preventing and resolving ethical conflict falls within the authority of all health care professionals engaged in the care of a patient

- Developing an awareness of and sensitivity to both the conscious and unconscious sources of conflict
- Facilitating timely communication among those involved in one-on-one decision-making meetings and periodic patient, family, and interdisciplinary team meetings to clarify goals and plan of care
- Documenting pertinent information on the patient record
- Referring unresolved ethical issues to the ethics consult team or the institutional ethics committee
- Identifying and addressing system variables that contribute to recurrent ethical problems

This author has had firsthand experience in advocating for two family members, my sister and daughter. In both cases, each had had a craniotomy for an aneurysm repair and both had a history of drug sensitivities. Postoperatively both developed adverse effects of the drugs they were taking. Despite my facts (drug fact sheets and information from my pharmacist with whom I supervise), it was almost impossible to make the physicians and nurses understand the postoperative symptoms being dealt with, and in the case of my daughter her aggravated stroke symptoms were the result of today's strong medications and patient sensitivity to such. I was labeled "hysterical" (which I was not), "an overprotective mother" (which I had to be). The list goes on. It was not until another physician entered both pictures and confirmed that I was right that the issue changed. However, I was prepared to fight and had already made arrangements for a second opinion and if necessary a change in physicians. So, as CMs if we do nothing else, we must teach our patients how to advocate and advocate effectively and not only complain.

Networking

As one advocates for clients, the power of networking can never be underestimated. This is true whether it is in one's professional or personal life. Networking abilities are individual-specific. However, if one is not intimidated, networking opens unending opportunities. From a professional stance, this includes asking or seeking help from peers, looking for new customers, negotiating for services or rates, or advancing one's career. The following list of recommendations can serve as a guide to learn the dynamics of networking[34]:

- Set specific and realistic networking objectives.
- Create a positive first impression with new contacts.
- Find common ground for discussion to develop mutual respect and trust.
- Carry plenty of business cards.
- Write identifying informational notes on the back of the business cards received.
- Tell people what you do, not just who you are.
- Ask people what they do and how you can help them.
- Be willing to connect people with mutual areas of interest.
- Follow up on leads and information gained, as well as commitments made.
- Don't hard sell or monopolize people's time.
- Take advantage of chance encounters to network.
- Assume that everyone you meet possesses valuable networking information.
- Ask yourself the following: Do I know the right people? Do the right people know me?
- Practice making networking come naturally: Don't force yourself on others.
- Think of yourself as being useful to others.
- Ask carefully selected, open-ended questions, and then listen.
- Show your sense of humor.
- Smile frequently. Be at ease, composed, and engaged.
- Say, "thank-you" often, both verbally and in correspondence.
- Be willing to give information freely, as long as it is not proprietary.
- Never repeat or perpetuate rumors.
- Be positive, enthusiastic, and confident.
- Develop true enjoyment in meeting new people.
- Ask for a personal introduction to a friend of a networking contact.
- Avoid offensive jokes and emotion-laden topics when networking.
- Look for opportunity in every conversation.
- Make sure your handshake is firm and brief.
- Don't interrupt when someone is talking.
- Become an artist in small talk.
- Develop an "information needed" list before networking.
- Think about how you can create value with every conversation.
- Project positive body language.
- Prepare a "30-second commercial" to explain your occupation. "Mirror image" (but don't mimic) your conversation partners.
- Visualize the skills you'll use in your networking experience.
- Visualize anticipated outcomes for each networking experience.
- Remember that some people are not receptive to networking.
- Develop "reciprocal relationships."
- Remember that each person you meet knows an average of 250 people you do not know.
- Avoid mention of racial, sexist, or ethnic bias when networking.

- Look for opportunities to make yourself visible in a variety of social settings.
- Get involved in organizations that will enhance your personal development.
- When attending a conference:
  - Plan ahead to identify and prioritize people you want to meet.
  - Arrive early to circulate and network.
  - Wear your nametag on the right, where people tend to look when shaking hands.
  - Act like a host rather than a guest and introduce yourself.
  - Position yourself in high-traffic areas near food tables, bars, or doors.
  - Willingly introduce peers and associates to new contacts.
  - Mingle or sit with people you do not know.
  - Ask yourself how you can turn today's contacts into tomorrow's opportunities

Negotiations

Just as communication, advocacy, and networking are skills necessary for successful case management, CMs assume a unique role in the health care environment and their skills of negotiation plays an equally crucial part in their role. Successful negotiating to meet the patient's identified needs requires special considerations including exemplary communication. While one automatically assumes negotiations are used for monetary purposes, this is not always true. In case management there are times one has to negotiate an agreement on the arrangements necessary to implement the case management plan (e.g., the patient wants to go home and it is unrealistic or the patient is a narcotics user and a contract is required to help with compliance).

Successful negotiation requires creating an atmosphere in which negotiations can be a win-win situation for all parties. It also requires open lines of communication. Open lines of communication create the framework from which the desired goal can be reached. Creating an atmosphere for winning negotiations can be compared to cooking a meal. If you accidentally forget one ingredient, the finished product will be lacking the perfect result. Selecting the right recipe for effective negotiations mandate the correct proportion of basic ingredients. These ingredients are fundamental to building successful relationships.[35]

Requirements of successful negotiations include the following:

- Focus on issues that are negotiable.
- Ensure that both parties are interested in taking and giving.
- Develop mutual respect for others as individuals and their opinions and positions.
- Develop a shared goal.
- Develop a trusting environment or atmosphere.
- Learn to use empathy because it helps promote desired decision making.
- Listen actively and concentrate on the message.
- Glean the facts and then organize the details.
- Collaborate as needed with others.
- Make every effort to enhance communication by keeping lines of communication open and two-way.
- Use "I" rather than "we."
- Do not make assumptions.
- Verify information through continual feedback.
- Finalize negotiations in writing, when applicable.

Criteria to evaluate the success of negotiations are listed in Box 14-4.

Patient Contracting

Along with provider negotiations for payment discounts, one must continually

BOX 14-4

Criteria to Evaluate the Success of Negotiations

- Was the process worthwhile for both parties?
- Did both parties feel self-respect was maintained?
- Did both parties leave with a positive impression?
- Were both parties sensitive to the needs of the other during the process?
- Did both parties achieve most of their objectives?
- Would either party be willing to negotiate again with the other?[36]

strive to negotiate with patients for their buy-in to a case management plan and assume the role as their own CM. Demonstrating the value of case management is often accomplished by capturing details on cost-saving reports, utilizing management activities, or via reports used in the return on investment reports generated. However, the real value of case management is demonstrated in one's ability to manage all patients (including difficult ones) and ensure compliance to treatment plans. Therefore, as one goes about capturing details from which a case management plan can be developed, CMs need to focus on the process of setting mutually compatible goals (e.g., patient, CM, and physician) and establishing a final contract.

Contract development starts with an informal introductory interview. This is the first step in developing a relationship. CMs should liken this to a job interview for a patient mentor or coach.[6] During the introductory interview, it is important to outline and clarify one's background and experience, the services expected, time frames and fees, client expectations, motivations of involved parties, and limits upon each one's expectations.

If patients are difficult, the plan is not working due to noncompliance, or there seems to be one crisis after another due to many factors, it may be wise to develop a written contract in addition to any case management plan. Keep in mind that your plan is ineffective if misunderstandings exist, therapy or services are ineffective, or the patient is noncompliant with treatments. It is important to realize that ineffective therapy or services may by definition be deemed inappropriate as they do not produce the progress expected by insurers. Consequently, they can end up being a noncovered service by many insurers.

As the case management plan is developed, the patient must be given a clear understanding of his or her role in the process and what realistic options will be. In an article by Newell, he reports that the goal must be the growth of the patient as a human being, employing not the curative aspect of the medical treatment so much as the healing component of the nursing intervention. He further states, "health is, after all, our relative ability to cope with our external and internal environments; Optimum health is our coming to terms with impairments resulting from disease or injury, our appraisal of our place in the world and our quest for the meaning in our lives. Our mental attitudes, belief systems, values and life expectations all impact our ability to cope with the slings and arrows of outrageous fortune."[6]

As the case management plan is further developed, it is wise to set goals that are personalized to the patient as these then become "real" goals. In developing the case management plan, one may find that a treatment may not be any better than the next. If this occurs, one must query the patient and ask, "What course of action feels better to you?" Once personalized goals are set, they can be used to assist the CM in keeping on target and for the activities necessary to reach the goals. Goal statements must be written and shared with the patient, family, and members of the health care team.

When dealing with the foregoing issues, formalizing contracts into written agreements can have several advantages such as the following:

- It gives the patient a greater sense of personal power and self-worth.
- It gives caregivers and providers the ability to focus on the more important issues of the case.
- It enhances the moral voice of the CM.[6]

Dealing and Negotiating with Noncompliant and Difficult Patients

Noncompliance is a reality. So is dealing with difficult patients. So is the use of multiple medications (polypharmacy). While many patients will make the right choices and agree to take an active part in their health care, many will not. Making bad choices is a patient's right, even though health care professionals do not support them. If the CM identifies a patient at risk for noncompliance or as one who is using multiple medications, it is wise to conduct further assessments and take the following steps:

- Identify the areas at risk.
- Identify the risk level.
- Develop a case management plan or strategy that attempts to enhance compliance.
- Continue to monitor and scrutinize the patient's encounters with the health care system (e.g., patients who overuse the health care system and resources, especially those who frequent the ED for drug-seeking behavior or go from one provider to another in their quest for a cure).

CMs who are involved with patient education and managing patients across time can significantly improve patient adherence by being catalysts of change rather than commanders of change. CMs must learn to be catalysts if patients are to be directed toward self-care. A key component to adherence is ensuring the patient and family know who their treatment team members are, their role, the reason they are involved, when to work with them, and how to reach them if issues arise. Adherence also involves a positive relationship between the patient and the treatment team.

CMs must also learn to pay close attention to details, especially when the patient has symptoms, the diagnosis is not clear yet, and the patient is a high consumer of health care resources including drugs. Although sometimes difficult, "tough love" is an approach that is helpful with this type of patient. This often involves making frequent contact with the patient to help build rapport, validate symptoms, and offer empathy while not enabling the sense of disability (even when you as CM feel that their symptoms are not as severe as they indicate). This further involves treating them with respect, not being cynical, offering encouragement to undertake small accomplishments even when symptoms are "disabling," or offering advice on learning to identify their limits so that they can have some activity. The main idea is to work closely with the patient, physician, and other providers to ensure a consistent message and theme is given (e.g., "we believe what you are saying is real, we are here to help you as you recover, and it takes us all working together to make it work"). It is important to keep the following in mind as one works with patients on adherence[37]:

- Recognize the predictors of nonadherence.
- Openly discuss adherence importance with patients and incorporate adherence strategies into their daily care and routine.
- Intervene as needed to foster patient adherence.
- Use the right tools at the right time.
- Use websites and other technology to enhance adherence, but not to replace a personal relationship with patients.

- Be ready and willing to learn from patients.
- Constantly work on helping patients build a network of support beside yourself.
- Never promise more than you can give.

It has been found that there are a handful of truths regarding adherence[38]:

- Adherence is highly personal because illness has particular meaning to each patient.
- Adherence requires readiness and stamina on the part of the patient and usually on the part of the family.
- Real changes take time and consistent behavior changes take even longer.
- Change toward adherence involves perceived gains and losses for the patient, and the overall benefits must outweigh the costs (real and imagined).

For the general clients served, adherence is more likely when the following apply[38]:

- Treatments are derived from a high trust, responsive, concerned, sympathetic, collaborative provider-patient relationship
- Treatments are short term and related to an acute medical condition
- Treatments are supervised (direct observed therapy)
- Treatments are simple
- Long-acting drugs are used
- Drugs with few side effects are used
- Focusing on a painful condition that responds to treatment
- Centering on a patient with a positive attitude
- Benefits outweigh costs
- Visits to the health care provider are satisfactory

When working with the elderly effective adherence strategies include the following[38]:

- Use of predeveloped medication schedules
- Use of medication reminder cards
- Use of pharmacist-led educational programs
- Visual as well as verbal cues
- Comprehensive geriatric assessments, including functional assessments
- Telephone follow-up after the teaching session
- Personal health planning and counseling
- Provision of large print, specific, easily readable information

When working with persons identified as polypharmacy users, adherence strategies include the following:

- Comprehensive assessment and identification of causes for multiple medications
- Identification of all medications and pharmacies used as well as prescribing clinicians
- Identification of primary clinician who will assume responsibility for coordination and signing of all prescriptions
- Identification that all drugs are necessary and if others will be as effective
- Identification of treatment alternatives
- Development of a contract and case management plan for which the patient and treating clinicians have buy-in

Adherence poses special problems with the elderly and with patients who have conditions such as mental illness, tuberculosis, human immunodeficiency virus (HIV), and other chronic medical conditions. Poor adherence is often attributed to the following:

- An inexperienced CM
- Lack of insight and awareness or denial
- Lack of insight and awareness of behaviors and medication effects

- Treatment dropout or missed appointments
- Homelessness
- Substance abuse
- History of poor compliance or noncompliance
- Emotional distress
- Lack of transportation or difficulties in consistency of transportation resources
- Behavioral issues
- Dissatisfaction with health care in general
- Lack of understanding of managed care (many people are now covered by managed care because it means lower out-of-pocket expenses; however, they continue with an attitude that health care is a right or they still want indemnity-type rules to follow)
- Misdirection from their physician or establishing the right of expectation (e.g., reporting to the ED if not feeling better; offering services of a tertiary provider or specialist without obtaining prior approval)
- Lack of family or social support
- Migrant status
- Low literacy
- Lack of education
- Cultural/personal/racial stigma
- Unemployment
- Low income or other economic hardship reasons (e.g., Medicare patient without drug coverage on several medications, but also on a limited income)
- Minority status
- Complexity and duration of treatment
- Medication or treatment interferes with lifestyle
- Medication or treatment requires attention to a myriad of details
- Lack of knowledge about the disease (many patients do not even have a basic understanding of their disease process, nor do they understand the effect of taking prescribed medications or following a correct diet)
- Skepticism exists about the treatment effectiveness
- Caregiver is absent
- Stigma and uncertainty of the illness
- Conflicting forces in everyday life
- Poor health care provider communication
- Lack of trust in the physician or health care providers in general

When dealing with a difficult or noncompliant patient, it may be necessary to hold a case conference with at least the patient, CM, and primary attending physician in attendance. The realities of the behavior can be broached and hopefully a realistic case management plan developed. In dealing with difficult patients and helping them reach their goals, a CM can expect to assume any number of roles—advocate, parent, friend, coach, or advisor. Unfortunately, there will be times when the CM must play the role of a "bad cop." This type of role is used when individuals respond only to strong boundary-setting behavior. While the bad-cop role is distasteful to most CMs, it may be a necessary response to the limited options such patients present due to their unrealistic expectations of the system.[6]

A patient who has been declared competent has the right to make choices, whether bad or good. As good CMs, we can only guide them to their choices—we cannot force our likes, dislikes, views, or values on them.

While the following statistics are related to transplant patients and were presented at the First International Symposium on Transplant Recipient Compliance, they validate many of the effects of noncompliance[39]:

- Patients with chronic conditions with few or no symptoms are most likely to be noncompliant.
- Noncompliant transplant patients were readmitted to the hospital 5.9

times compared to 2.5 times for compliant patients.

- Between 15% and 18% of kidney transplant patients are noncompliant, and 91% of noncompliant patients lose their grafts or die from medical complications.
- About 50% of all prescriptions written in the United States are taken improperly.

Many of the following predictors of noncompliance can be addressed and overcome given enough time. The reasons for noncompliance are often linked to such factors as the following[39]:

- Required length of prescribed treatment
- Complexity of treatment
- Lifestyle restrictions
- Cost of treatment
- Severity of symptoms
- Beliefs about severity of the disease
- Failure to fully understand the regimen
- Effects of disease on activities of daily living
- Frequency or difficulty of getting to follow-up appointments
- Past behavior
- Inadequate social support
- History of substance abuse
- Personality disorders (may not be easily overcome)

Compliance is in the eye of the beholder. Compliance is defined in the American Heritage Dictionary as "the act of complying with a wish, request or demand." In health care most often it refers to the client's ability to make, keep, and follow-up with medical care and appointments. Other applications may include adherence to medications, diet, therapy, nutrition, and exercise regimens.[40] The following strategies can be used when dealing with difficult patients (especially those with alcohol, drug, and mental health issues):

- **Communication**—It must be persistent and consistent either by phone, mail, or by home or office visits. Documentation plays a just as important part so that the entire team is given the same message.
- **Engaging clients**—Constant attention must be paid to keep the client and medical/social services systems engaged. Keep in mind that traditional health care services are not designed for difficult patients and as a CM you may need to serve as the "middle man" to help negotiate the system.
- **Negotiation**—Negotiating with the client for compliance to medical care involves more than arranging an appointment. This may include a variety of activities that allow the appointment to be kept.
- **Follow-up**—This must be prompt. This involves paperwork, patient education, appointment scheduling, referrals, and obtaining necessary services.
- **Documentation**—This is critical. Do not allow others to duplicate what has been done, undo what has been accomplished, or do nothing to address the client's needs.
- **Expectations**—Lower expectations and success levels. Take small steps or set short-term goals that allow client participation.

Past behavioral patterns, anger, cognitive impairments, and many other factors can lead to maladaptive behavior, the label of a difficult patient or one of noncompliance. When dealing with difficult patients, CMs must be creative so that they can assess the nature, scope, and depth of the problem as well as the patient's ability to cope or respond appropriately. It is from this base that additional creativity can be used to work with the patient and treatment team to map out the actions needed to allow the patient to obtain the services and goods required. By assisting clients in this way, CMs can open doors to compliance. It also helps to create a caring and sensitive environment that promotes trust. When dealing with patients labeled as noncompliant, one must think creatively while digging deeply to uncover the underlying motives and issues.[40]

Another strategy many case management organizations use when dealing with patients with maladaptive behaviors as they attempt to guide the patient to compliance is as follows[40]:

- Come to agreement with the patient that a problem exists.
- Define the nature of the problem from both the patient's perception as well as that of the health care team.
- Mutually discuss treatment alternatives.
- Mutually agree upon an action plan.
- Follow up to ensure the plan is being carried out.
- Recognize achievements as they occur.

For example, several years ago while reviewing drug utilization, it appeared on the surface we had a noncompliant drug-seeking patient. As we did our research, we discovered that the patient was using the ED frequently and using various physicians and pharmacies on almost a daily basis. It was found the patient was receiving in excess of 50 pain pills per day. When we called the patient to interview him about what was happening and to ask if we could help, the man broke down and started to cry as he gave the following information:

- He was 32 years old and had an old back injury with resultant multiple spinal surgeries, all without relief. He reported that he was actually worse and now wracked with chronic incapacitating pain.
- He had lost his job due to the amount of time off work, and his family's lifestyle was drastically altered because his wife now had to be the breadwinner.

- He had lost his bid for Social Security Disability Income (SSDI) and was now in the appeal process, but he was panicky because his state disability would end soon.
- He had two small children with whom he could not play.
- He spent most of his day crawling around on his stomach and had difficulty conducting his own activities of daily living because standing and moving were too painful.
- He and his wife were fighting continually due to financial issues, lack of sex, and the strain that the pain's effect was having on their life.
- He had gone from one physician to another, and none would treat his pain other than to prescribe pain medications.

After taking the information and with his agreement, a case conference was planned. To do this we called one of the physicians with whom he felt he had the most confidence and explained the situation. The physician agreed to participate in the case and take the lead. We then called a local university pain management program and spoke with the coordinator who also agreed to participate in the case conference. From the conference it was found that the patient had been horribly undertreated and was viewed as a narcotics addict. However, a detailed case management plan was developed that included the following:

- The young man's physician would cooperate with the pain management's requirements, and the pain management center would serve as the primary prescribing entity.
- The patient would receive assistance to allow him to appeal his SSDI determination.
- The patient would be enrolled in the pain management program on an outpatient basis.
- Transportation was arranged from the local paratransit authority.

- The patient was linked to a vocational rehabilitation counselor.
- In addition to the emotional/psychologic support the patient was to receive in the pain program, he and his wife agreed to enroll in marriage and family counseling sessions.

Although this case had a happy ending, many do not. This is true when the patient, family, or practitioners are not willing to cooperate. Despite any plan or contract, if the patient continues in a noncompliance mode, there often is no alternative other than to close the case.

Undertreatment of pain is a reality. However, with the recent $1.5 million award to a California family from a physician (hospital paid out-of-court), this may change. The reasons for the undertreatment of pain are complex and derive from both patient and physician attitudes, as well as from a social focus. The undertreatment of pain is not caused by a lack of safe or effective medications. For example, barriers to good pain management include the following[41]:

- Health system barriers
  - Pain is "invisible" because pain assessment historically has not been integrated into patient charts or made a part of a nursing care plan.
  - Regulatory barriers on the federal and state level cause prescription renewal problems for persons with chronic pain and make health care professionals wary about prescribing opioids for fear that misguided oversight will jeopardize their medical license.
  - There is a mistaken belief that pain management is expensive and must be saved until the end-of-life issues.
- Provider-based barriers
  - Health care providers fail to ask about and systematically assess pain.
  - Health care providers distrust indirect subjective measures of pain and fail to display a willingness to believe patient reports of pain as essential to good pain management.
  - There is an unfounded fear that patients will become addicted to strong opioids.
  - Medical board oversight of prescribing practices often has the unintended effect of inhibiting the prescription of opioids.
- Patient-based barriers:
  - Patients may be reluctant to tell health care professionals when they are in pain, fearing it will distract physicians from further treating their illness or injury.
  - Patients mistakenly believe pain is an inevitable and untreatable aspect of some disease. In fact, pain can lead to depression, other bodily functions, and in some cases rejection of standard treatments due to their despondence.
  - Patients confuse illegal use and medically supervised use of drugs and believe they should say no.
  - Patients fear opioids will compromise their alertness and don't realize this can be avoided by good dosage adjustment, use of combinations of appropriate medications, and/or changing from one opioid to another.

Recently JCAHO introduced new pain management standards as the fifth vital sign. This has been applied to all ages across the continuum. In the standards, all patients have the right to initial pain assessment, routine reassessment, and ongoing adjustments of treatment plans. Unfortunately, many people continue to experience pain unnecessarily. CMs are in an ideal position to help patients by discussing the plan, improving assessment, and designing and coordinating a plan of care that includes appropriate pain management. As the CM develops a plan to address adequate pain control, the plan should contain the following elements[42]:

- The plan should be individualized and specific for the patient and the management of his or her pain.
- Each individual should be assessed for pain first at the initial contact and then routinely screened for pain during other evaluations or contacts. To do this, assessments should be conducted using a thorough history, physical examination, and workup with the outcomes of pain interventions tried recorded along with the responses (e.g., description of the pain using possibly a pain rating scale of 1 to 10, with 10 being the worst; individual responses to the treatments; medication side effects; and any personal concerns about the pain or its treatment). This assessment must also cover such issues as side effects and bowel regimen management.
- The plan should be communicated to all team members.
- Individual goals and outcomes should be documented.
- Pain medications should be prescribed appropriately. This may mean development of round-the-clock dosing and elimination of PRN dosing.
- Pain medications should be dosed systematically and based on individual client responses.
- The plan should be monitored for the dosages of nonopioid analgesics (e.g., do not exceed maximum dose limits per day as prescribed by the physician).
- Laboratory values should be monitored to detect complications or impaired bodily functions.
- A prophylactic bowel management program should be developed and ordered when opioid therapy begins.
- Other interventions such as no-drug therapy (physical therapy, yoga, applications of heat and cold) should be used as appropriate.
- The patient should be educated to increase knowledge of what to report and to whom.
- Lack of knowledge or any outdated attitudes and beliefs should be identified.

Comprehensive management of pain and pain-related disability requires an integrated process that treats the physical, psychologic, social, and emotional aspects of people with chronic pain.[43] In their attempts to alleviate pain, many patients have been to multiple physicians, clinics, and other entities with the same result—unsuccessful outcomes in diagnosis and cure. The focus of their pain management must shift from physician shopping, overuse of health care providers and resources, and at times hospitalizations for pain control to a coordinated plan that addresses all aspects of their pain-related dysfunction. The following goals must be included in the coordinated plan[44]:

- Measures that will decrease suffering (e.g., depression, psychologic distress, anxiety, sleep problems)
- Measures that will restore function (e.g., maximize functional capacity, facilitate vocational rehabilitation)
- Measures to control pain

To measure the outcomes for a pain management program, the team uses reliable tools that are multifaceted and easy to administer. The current tools used are the Sickness Impact Profile (SIP), the Multidimensional Pain Inventory (MPI), and the Medical Outcomes Study Short-form General Health Survey (SF-36). The SF-36 includes measurement of limitations in physical, social, role performance, vitality, health perception, bodily pain, and general mental health.[45] As part of the team, CMs are in an ideal spot and play an integral role in facilitating effective functioning of the team through communication. Their role to ensure that each area of life dysfunction is addressed by the appropriate discipline. They must also do the following:

- Ensure communication of pertinent medical history and prior treatment information is relayed to the other team members as well as communication of ongoing reports as to the progress and any post discharge follow-up plans
- Ensure communication occurs among the patient, family, and team
- Keep the insurance reviewer appraised of case actions and of the reasoning for the use of independent pain management strategies to replace costly, passive previous interventions (e.g., ED visits, prolonged manipulation, injections, massages) to ensure coverage for the multiple disciplines and the duration of the pain program

The ultimate goal of a pain management program is to alter the pain experience through self-management and active participation in one's own care. To accomplish this, an accurate diagnosis should be made (physical and psychologic) and education should be used, as it will play a key role in recovery, as will interventions that are acceptable to the patient. According to the recommendations of the International Association for the Study of Pain (IASP) at their website (www.halcyon.com/iasp) the descriptions of chronic pain syndrome should not be used as a diagnosis because it eludes the requirement for accurate physical and psychiatric diagnoses.[46]

Other Competencies

To function as a CM, one must possess not only clinical expertise but also a variety of other competencies. Basically, competency is the demonstration of one or more skills and is based on a person's education and expertise. Competency can be broken down into components that are departmental, job-specific, or age-specific. Through the use of competencies and the development of a competent staff, case management organizations can expect results such as the following:

- Improvement in quality of the staff's ability to perform
- Economic efficiency
- An atmosphere that will improve the reputation of the department
- Enhanced departmental functioning
- Enhanced patient care

The core competencies of a CM are very basic, but in reality the expertise and knowledge must be extensive. Skills include the following:

- Clinical expertise of disease processes
- Assessment skills
- Leadership skills in order to manage and facilitate a patient's care planning
- Decision-making, critical-thinking, and problem-solving skills
- Communication skills (the foundation of a CM's role)
- Knowledge of financial matters, insurance, managed care, coordination of benefits, managed care plans, benefit plans, capitation, prospective payment systems, and public entitlement programs
- Knowledge of community resources, whether local, regional, or national

Integrity and Moral Competency

As with all novices, new CMs must learn through experience to make appropriate professional judgments over time. The root of case management is professional integrity—acting consistently to advance the good of patient care, the organization, the practice of case management, and society in general. Along with integrity comes moral competency to which all CMs should be held accountable. In short, professional integrity and moral competency are traits that distinguish a good CM from a bad one. Integrity and moral competency come into play on a daily basis.[47]

In most simple cases rarely is professional judgment, integrity, or moral competency an issue. However, they do surface when a CM approaches a case and finds there is conflict that could compromise the processes to be proposed or implemented. Unfortunately, some cases will be more complicated and there will be conflict from the start. At that time, one must back off and ask if he or she is the right person to handle the case. In an article by Meaney on professional integrity, he states six steps to follow[47]:

1. Consider whether self interest may interfere with care management when facing a conflicted case.
2. Discern whether a person is a relevant decision maker based on whether he or she has any intention of doing the right thing.
3. As a decision maker, define and agree on a definition of the ethical conflicts in the case.
4. List the alternative that will address the conflicts identified in step 3 and try to predict each alternative's effects on the relevant stakeholders.
5. Evaluate the alternatives only after performing a thorough ethical analysis of the case.
6. Implement the decision, communicate it to relevant stakeholders, and follow up on it to address the remaining negative consequences.

Age-Specific Competencies

Erik Erikson, a neo-Freudian, is best known for his work in the field of identifying characteristics of the healthy personality. The major thesis of Erikson's work was the concept of achieving "ego identity." Erikson described a dialectical process as a conflict between two opposing forces with each developmental stage resulting in an ego strength or failure, depending on how well the stage was negotiated. Age-specific competencies are broken down into eight stages and it is imperative for health care professionals, especially those who work in the medical case management field, to have a knowledge of these competencies and how they affect reactions to health care environments and other stressors. Also, age-specific competencies are now a factor evaluated by JCAHO during their accreditation processes. As such, most hospitals use age-specific testing as part of their annual evaluation of staff. The eight stages of personality are as follows:

Stage 1: Infancy—Age 0 to 1 Years

Crisis: Trust versus mistrust

Description: In the first year of life, infants depend on others for food, warmth, and affection, and therefore must be able to blindly trust parents (or caregivers) for providing these basics.

Positive outcome: If parents consistently and responsively meet the infant's needs, the infant will develop a secure attachment with the parents and learn to trust his or her environment in general as well.

Negative outcome: If not, infants will develop mistrust toward people and things in their environment and even toward themselves.

Stage 2: Toddler—Age 1 to 2 Years

Crisis: Autonomy (independence) versus doubt (or shame)

Description: Toddlers learn to walk, talk, use toilets, and do things for themselves. Their self-control and self-confidence begin to develop at this stage.

Positive outcome: If parents encourage children's use of initiative and reassure them when they make mistakes, children will develop the confidence needed to cope with future situations that require choice, control, and independence.

Negative outcome: If parents are overprotective or disapproving of children's acts of independence, they may feel ashamed of their behavior or doubt their abilities.

Stage 3: Early Childhood—Age 2 to 6 Years

Crisis: Initiative versus guilt

Description: Children have newfound power at this stage as they have developed motor skills and become more and more engaged in social interaction with people around them. They now must learn to achieve a balance between eagerness for more adventure and responsibility and learning to control impulses and childish fantasies.

Positive outcome: If parents are encouraging but consistent in discipline, children will learn to accept without guilt that certain things are not allowed, without feeling shame when using their imagination and engaging in make-believe role plays.

Negative outcome: If not, children may develop a sense of guilt and may come to believe that it is wrong to be independent.

Stage 4: Elementary and Middle School Years—Age 6 to 12 Years

Crisis: Competence (industry) versus inferiority

Description: School is the important event at this stage. Children learn to make things, use tools, and acquire the skills to be a worker and a potential provider. They do all these while making the transition from the world of home into the world of peers.

Positive outcome: If children can discover pleasure in intellectual stimulation, being productive, and seeking success, they will develop a sense of competence.

Negative outcome: If not, they will develop a sense of inferiority.

Stage 5: Adolescence—Age 12 to 18 Years

Crisis: Identity versus role confusion

Description: This is the time when we ask the question "Who am I?" To successfully answer this question, Erikson suggests the adolescent must integrate the healthy resolution of all earlier conflicts. Did we develop the basic sense of trust? Do we have a strong sense of independence and competence and feel in control of our lives? Adolescents who have successfully dealt with earlier conflicts are ready for the "Identity Crisis," which Erikson considers the single most significant conflict a person must face.

Positive outcome: If adolescents solve this conflict successfully, they will come out of this stage with a strong identity and ready to plan for the future.

Negative outcome: If not, adolescents will sink into confusion and be unable to make decisions and choices, especially about vocation, sexual orientation, and their role in life in general.

Stage 6: Young Adulthood—Age 19 to 40 Years

Crisis: Intimacy versus isolation

Description: In this stage, the most important events are love relationships. No matter how successful you are with your work, said Erikson, you are not developmentally complete until you are capable of intimacy. An individual who has not developed a sense of identity usually will fear a committed relationship and may retreat into isolation.

Positive outcome: Adult individuals can form close relationships and share with others if they have achieved a sense of identity.

Negative outcome: If not, they will fear commitment and feel isolated and unable to depend on anybody in the world.

Stage 7: Middle Adulthood—Age 40 to 65 Years

Crisis: Generativity versus stagnation

Description: By "generativity," Erikson refers to the adult's ability to look outside oneself and care for others, for instance, through parenting. Erikson suggested that adults need children as much as children need adults and that this stage reflects the need to create a living legacy.

Positive outcome: People can resolve this crisis by having and nurturing children or helping the next generation in other ways.

Negative outcome: If this crisis is not successfully resolved, the person will remain self-centered and experience stagnation later in life.

Stage 8: Late Adulthood—Age 65 Years to Death

Crisis: Integrity versus despair

Description: Old age is a time for reflecting upon one's life and its role in the big scheme of things and seeing it filled with pleasure and satisfaction or disappointments and failures.

Positive outcome: If adults achieve a sense of fulfillment about life and a sense of unity within self and others, they will accept death with a sense of integrity. Just as the healthy child will not fear life, said Erikson, the healthy adult will not fear death.

Negative outcome: If not, the individual will despair and fear death.[48]

It is from these eight stages that organizations must develop specific competency requirements for their staff. As such the competencies developed must be reflective of the type of care provided by the organization and the environment in which the client will receive care. For example, for the competencies one might find in the vari-ous acute care hospital settings, the educational department must develop expected competency standards for all ages. In contrast, for skilled nursing facility staff, the primary emphasis will be related to competencies as they apply to the older age groups and the environment in which the patient resides. Also, competencies for a hospital setting may be different from those used by a home health agency or an MCO that supplies case management services to enrollees.

Training

As managers develop training programs and ongoing educational sessions, one must develop the programs to cover any topics applicable to the clients served as well as case actions and outcomes expected. If case management is to be successful, training programs must, at a minimum, cover the following to ensure skills are kept current:

- Clinical data and information as well as the resources needed and any changes to clinical care guidelines or processes
- Legal, legislative, financial, and contractual changes that affect the type of care and how it is provided
- Clinical knowledge of home medical equipment, transportation requirements, and community resources, and the processes required or recent changes to processes
- Current clinical knowledge of drug therapies, treatment modalities, and other drug or pharmaceutical issues that affect cases, costs, and outcomes

As case management firms vary, so will training and orientation programs. However, to meet the demands placed on CMs, a structured comprehensive orientation and training program is critical. In establishing the initial training, management must allow a minimum of four to six weeks of training for all newly hired CMs.

Based on the skills of newly hired staff, training and preceptorship/mentoring can then be customized according to individualized personnel needs. For new CMs, training programs must include the following:

- Let the person become acclimated to the new company and role— this will include introductions to personnel as well as a tour of the organization.
- Use a combination of individual sessions with classroom-style instruction to cover key elements or policies and procedures.
- Use self-directed study by reading policies and procedures.
- Use videos on various topics.
- Use one-on-one experienced persons to serve as a mentor; this allows the new CM to sit side by side with the experienced person and learn.
- Schedule new CMs with other key departments that interface with the CMs.
- Schedule weekly meetings during the initial orientation process to ensure the new employees have their questions answered.

Elements for education of newly hired CMs might also include the following:

- Overview of the concepts and evolution of case management within the organization
- Overview of job description and expectations
- Concepts and principles for use of the multidisciplinary team
- Use of clinical pathways or other care map processes
- CM organizational goals
- Roles, responsibilities, and relationships internally and externally
- Organizational tools available for CM
- Patient educational tools
- Role of discharge planning
- Time management

- Variance reporting and monitoring

As education is a continuous process, ongoing educational sessions may cover the following:

- Schedule weekly or more frequent meetings to discuss case-specific issues; this is an invaluable educational tool.
- Meet regularly with CMs to staff cases and provide information and suggestions as to what works and what does not.
- Review cases and files on a regular basis (using peer review and a pre-developed checklist based on performance standards) to ensure cases are being worked properly and that reporting and recommendations are appropriate; this helps to identify both strengths and areas of weakness.
- Review documentation on a regular basis (again using peer review for this process is an excellent educational tool) to ensure whoever reads the documented notes can decipher what is being done and actions are clear.

If weaknesses or deficits are found from the foregoing, they can serve as the guide for future educational topics. In addition, it is wise to schedule in-services on a regular basis to cover such topics as the following:

- Overview of new laws and their effect on processes
- Overview of changes to the health care system such as new technology, processes, or techniques
- Overview of changes in community resources and processes
- Overview of home medical equipment requirements
- Overview of changes in drug or other therapies and modalities for care
- Overview in technology and the changes in chronicity as patients survive and live longer

In addition to any internal training programs, staff must be given the time and opportunity to attend local, regional, and national educational sessions. This process alone allows for additional training as well as for the global approach needed by CMs to effectively manage cases (e.g., firsthand view of how others handle similar situations).

Another tool to assist in establishing training programs is to conduct individual audits of case files. This can be done either by a supervisor or developed as a peer audit process. The simplest tool to use for this type of an audit will be a checklist covering the elements the organization expects as cases are worked. Use of a checklist also helps in the final tally and capturing of topics for future educational sessions. When developing a checklist for auditing files or charts, some critical elements for quality controls as well for identifying training issues include those listed in Box 14-5.

As one audits charts for opened and closed cases, the following elements should also be evaluated[49]:

- Have realistic objectives been established? Are they described in terms of who, what, where, when, why, and how much?
- Do objectives and recommendations appear cost-effective?
- Have alternatives been thoroughly explored to identify and compare options to maintain quality of care?
- Have the client's assets and limitations been clearly identified?
- Are there areas of concern that need further evaluation or does it appear there are extraneous conditions that are impeding progress?
- Have cost savings issued been identified and have price negotiations taken place, if applicable?
- Does case activity correspond to case notes and claims payment?
- Are services being delivered in a timely manner?

- Are there any ethical issues that need to be addressed?
- Is the CM maintaining professional objectivity?
- Is the file well-organized? Is anything missing?
- Is the case actively being managed or is the CM performing passive monitoring activities?
- Is case closure warranted?

In addition to ensuring training programs are in place and effective, departmental managers need to ensure there are sufficient policies and procedures to cover the specific functions and processes as they relate to the type and scope of case management services provided by the organization. In addition, policies and procedure manuals must also cover topics such as the following:

- Confidentiality and the importance of using the necessary form when release of information is required;
- Regulations, rules, restrictions, and responsibilities as required by laws or various insurers, and contractual requirements
- Handling conflict of interests and when, to whom, and how reporting must be done
- Detecting fraud and abuse and when, to whom, and how the reporting must be done
- Detecting and reporting patient abuse, when, how, and to whom the reporting must be done, and within what timeframe; this is necessary as law mandates that health care professionals report suspected or real abuse.
- Reporting incidents and what needs to be reported, to whom, and when
- Reporting and handling exposure to communicable diseases of the CM as well as expectations for reporting it, as well as how to ensure universal precautions are carried out

BOX 14-5
Checklist for Auditing Case File

Case Opening
___Is screening tool available that validates the rational for case opening?
___Is basic patient demographic information present (e.g., face sheet or data sheet that shows name, address, phone numbers, date of birth, family identifying information)?
___Are initial assessments completed and present?
___If medical records were needed to support requests or case activity, are they present?
___If initial approval was required, is it present? If ongoing approval was required, was it obtained and is it present?

Consent Form
___If a patient consent form is part of the process for case opening, is one present?
___If medical records or information are to be obtained from or shared with other providers, is a signed consent form present?

Case Notes
___Are case notes in order, and are they clear, concise, and descriptive enough so that case activity and plans are apparent without the need to review the entire chart?
___If recommendations have been made, are they completed, or what actions have been taken and what actions are outstanding?
___If notes are linked to authorization requests, is there sufficient information contained from which claims can be paid, reports generated, or actions taken? If the authorization is linked to a nonnetwork provider or other entity for which an authorization letter must be generated, is the appropriate letter present? Is it accurate and free from any typos or errors?
___If the patient is participating in a clinical trial, are all required documents and forms present? Has a physician and/or attorney reviewed the case and case actions? If an authorization was issued, was the applicable letter generated? Is it accurate and free from typos or errors?
___If billable hours are part of the case management activity, are billable activities documented as required in the case notes? Do the notes match the billing?

Denials
___If a denial was generated or a case issue was in dispute, is there documentation that a physician advisor reviewed the request or case issue, and the final coverage determination issued by him or her?
___If a denial was issued, was the appropriate letter generated and the appropriate physician denial language used? Is it free of any typos or errors? Is appeal language present?
___If a denial was issued, was the denial and letter issued within the time constraints established for the type of request (urgent or routine prior authorization, concurrent review, or retrospective review)?

Reports
___Are reports being written at appropriate intervals or as requested?
___Are data being entered into a database as required so that system-generated reports can be produced in a timely manner and according to any contractual requirements or specific contractual requests?
___Are the data entered correctly and accurately?
___Are data current and relevant? Or are data repetitious or duplicative?

Cost Savings
___If case rate negotiations were part of cost savings, are they documented and reported according to organizational policy so that claims can be paid without delay?
___If cost savings is part of the CM's activity, are savings tabulated accurately and does the documentation support the activity that generated the cost savings?
___Are cost savings reports being generated as contractually required?

Billable Hours
___If reimbursement is based on billable hours, does the file reflect time recordings that should be appropriate for the activity undertaken?

- Reporting of violent situations or potentially dangerous encounters and how to handle it, the rights and responsibilities of the CM, and when and how the reporting must be done
- Handling and charting of sensitive issues
- Handling of potential suicide and when, how, and to whom reporting must be done

As CM training is undertaken, it is important to include classes to teach staff how to deal with stress. Stress is a reality for CMs as they continually try to "fix" things when, often they cannot. This is further complicated by the fact many cases are sad and emotionally draining. It is also important as CMs are like most caregivers; they are much better at taking care of others than themselves. CMs have strong intuitive abilities to heal or care for others. However, they must also learn to make use of the same healing, nurturing, and intuitive senses for themselves.[50] To do this, one must first recognize the signs of stress and then exercise techniques such as breathing exercises or mindfulness exercise in which one focuses on the present moment and lets go of distractions. Additionally, one can use any number of books for dealing with stress and its reduction as well as learning to cope with change.[50]

Office Efficiency

The importance of the knowledge and competency base of CMs cannot be understated for success of case management, but the department and staff's efficiency and effectiveness depends on having a department that is well-organized. This includes making use of technology and having simple items at one's fingertips. While these will be organization-specific, they often include the following:

- A phone system with phone mail capability or a phone tree that routes callers to appropriate personnel
- A computer system that can electronically capture all case specific activity into an electronic medical record format and generate such final reports as the case management plan, cost analysis summaries, letters, and other electronic data historically completed on paper and stored as a hard copy
- A computer system with electronic calendar and interdepartmental communication capability as well as eligibility, claims, and payer information; if a computer system does not exist, preprinted communication sheets to capture all such activities and efforts
- A fax machine dedicated to the case management department with capability to record confirmation data and enough memory to capture the volume of faxes in any given period of time
- A fax machine at the CM's individual workstation to expeditiously submit information electronically to vendors and other outside resources as well as to send and receive referrals, and prior authorization requests, and other electronic chart or medical information
- If case management is within a medical group or MCO, electronic or hard copy benefit matrixes or other guides, including limitations and exclusions for all payer sources and policyholders
- If not electronic, preprinted patient referral and other sheets used to consistently document and capture activity
- Colored folders to prioritize case functions, specific case types, or specific policyholders
- If not electronic, quality referral sheets to document quality issues as

they are discovered or for the data needed for Health Plan Employer Data and Information Set (HEDIS) reporting.

■ If not electronic, forms for patient complaints or appeals to forward to applicable staff for handling issues to ensure timeframes and other functions are performed as required

■ Card file or electronic database with all contracted vendors, facilities, and community agencies used, along with main contact names, phone numbers, addresses, and other pertinent information

■ If not electronic, drug-pricing manual that shows average wholesale prices (AWP) of drugs

■ Other manuals or electronic databases to support case activities and functions (e.g., Interqual, Milliman and Robertson, St. Anthony's, Length of Stay Manuals, Current Medicare Handbooks, Hayes Inc. Medical Manuals and Journals, Medical Dictionary, and other texts that can be used for reference)

■ Lists of community, state, and federal referral sources and a brief description of what is required for referrals, along with names of contacts/departments, phone numbers, and addresses

■ Electronic or hard copy of all letters required in the course of business

While the foregoing section has briefly covered the elements necessary for a competent and fully functioning case management unit and staff, of key importance will be the actual processes used as one conducts the functions necessary for case management to work and reach successful outcomes.

Case Management Processes

Most organizations that offer case management use the same basic processes, although many players may be involved and referral criteria may be different and dependant upon the population served. To avoid crises, a key element is to ensure the true planners, the patient, and the family, are informed and involved in every step of planning. Another critical element as the final case management plan is developed is to ensure it focuses on the individual family or caregiver's needs as well as patient needs. Case management plans developed without patient and family input are likely to fail.

Also critical to the development of any case management plan is the involvement of the patient's physician and the interdisciplinary health care team. CMs must realize their case management plans are nothing other than extensions of the treatment plans ordered by the physician. The eventual case management plan when executed will serve as the guide to ensure goals established by the health care team are reached, resources required by the patient to meet goals and needs are identified, and linkage with resources is made in a timely manner (Figure 14-4).

While many of the following steps can occur at any given time and some will be simultaneous, the processes common to case management are as follows:

■ **Screening**—Gathering information from which one can make a decision if the case will benefit from case opening.

■ **Assessment**—Gathering as much in-depth information about the patient, family, and resources as necessary as this will serve as the base of the case management plan finally developed. This process requires the clinical expertise of the CM as the patient is assessed for the appropriate level of care. Assessments must include patient demographics, medical history and current health status, financial assessment, functional assessment, environmental assessment (home);

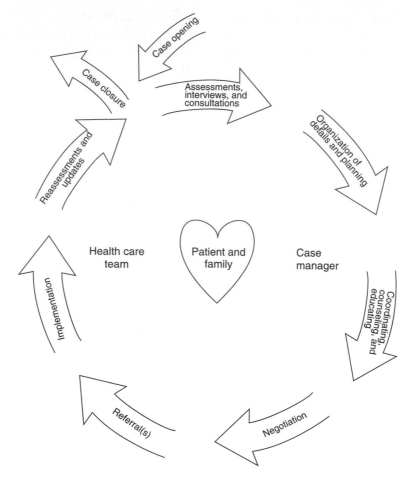

Figure 14-4   Cycles of case management processes.

activities of daily living (ADLs), assessment and psychosocial assessment (mental status or cognitive abilities, cultural and religious values and beliefs, language, formal and informal support systems, hobbies, work and education history).

■ **Planning**—Developing a plan of care that involves input from the patient, family, health care team, and community resources. Challenging situations arise as health care resources are stretched to meet the demands, and there is greater cultural diversity as well as financial stressors placed on patients and families. Thus, a constant challenge

for CMs is the identification of real or potential barriers that will affect the plan of care as well as outcomes. The first step in planning involves the setting of goals and what must be accomplished and within what timeframe. Additionally, goals must be prioritized. Once goals are established, the resources necessary to meet the goals must be explored.

■ **Documentation**—Keeping records on actions taken and used as a form of communication among all parties.

■ **Approval**—Getting the case management plan approved prior to implementation; this could be buy-in from the patient and family and health care team as well as the entity that will be paying for the services.

- **Implementation**—Decision-making and critical-thinking actions needed to coordinate, establish, and activate the approved plan.
- **Follow-up**—Monitoring the plan once implemented and taking the necessary actions to ensure it continues as planned, or actions are taken when alternatives or changes are required.
- **Evaluation**—Measuring outcomes and the effectiveness of the plan; this will be either ongoing or after case closure and data is studied.

During any part of the referral or assessment phase, solicitation of facts and input from the patient, family, physicians, and other health care team members are vital elements for the success of the eventual case management plan. To ensure all data elements are collected and recorded properly, a questionnaire specifically developed for interviewing the various parties is an excellent method for recording data. As with all forms, questionnaires will be specific to the organization, the clientele to be interviewed, the type of case management offered, and the populations served. However, questionnaires serve as an excellent way to document answers to specific questions as later these answers might be useful as the case management plan is developed.

While the planning and processes of case management will in most cases focus on the patient, family and health care team, it is important to remember in today's world of litigation and multiple CMs, there will be times when these entities will also be involved. Thus, as plans and interviews are scheduled, it will be important to recognize their presence and when possible their inclusion to the process.

Dealing with Attorneys

Because case management often involves patients who have survived severe or catastrophic injuries and litigation is pending, it is common to encounter attorneys. Their presence may not be known at the time of referral. If an attorney is involved, many organizations require staff to review the case with the organization's legal counsel before proceeding.

In many cases, the presence of an attorney poses its own set of issues and challenges. For example, if the case has proceeded to litigation and the patient is represented by an attorney, all contact with the patient may have to be approved by the patient's attorney as they have the right to deny a CM's involvement with the case. If an attorney is involved it is also common for case handling directions to come from the organization's legal counsel, and it will be common for this direction to override any of the usual case management procedures.

CMs should not be intimidated by the presence of an attorney. Many attorneys may be skeptical of the CM's intent, but the CM should merely state his or her reasons for involvement in the case. A CM's purpose is to assist the patient and the family to gain access to care while ensuring quality of care is maintained. However, like physicians, most attorneys are a delight to work with once you get to know them.

Attorneys should be contacted in the same manner used to contact others on the case. If an interview is planned, the CM should have questions prepared as they would for any other interview.

It is often during the interview that the attorney will set his or her expectations or stipulations. Although the following scenarios are case-specific, it is common for attorneys to do the following:

- Allow involvement and services to proceed without stipulation.
- Set specific stipulations.

- Allow involvement in the case but no access to the patient unless the attorney is present during every contact with the patient.
- Require approval for any phone or personal contact with the patient and family.
- Tape all conversations among the CM, patient, or family.

Some attorneys allow the CM to work with the patient and family once the attorney understands the CM's role and purpose. However, if the attorney poses too many stumbling blocks or denies the CM access to the case, the organization's best decision may be to close the case. If case closure does occur, the CM must carefully document the reasons for the closure in the event questions arise at a later date.

Outside CMs

If the CM is not part of the internal multidisciplinary team but will continue to work with the patient upon discharge, there are some suggestions that will be key to promotion of positive and effective relationships. The following factors should be considered throughout the comanagement process:

- Clearly define your role and the scope of your involvement up front to avoid conflict and misunderstanding later.
- Clarify what responsibilities are yours on a case-by-case basis, as this will avoid duplication and fragmentation and maximize the time and skills for all parties.
- If you represent an insurer, be aware the team may perceive your interests to be focused solely on the financial aspects of care and not on the patient's best interests. Take every opportunity to alleviate these fears and take into consideration their perspective, including incentives, scope of responsibility, and ability to impact.

- Identify ways that you can be of added value to the team. Utilize ideas to make everyone's jobs easier while simultaneously achieving goals and establishing, building, and gaining mutual respect.
- Recognize that your on-site presence may initially add tension until the team fully understands how you can work collaboratively with them. Alleviate the tension by taking the first step and asking what the concerns are.
- Recognize that you will not always agree with each other. This does not necessarily determine whether you can enjoy a good working relationship.
- Initiate communication when necessary and minimize communication barriers by being concise and consistent and by answering questions if you know the answer. If you don't know the answer, indicate that you will locate the answer and get back with them; then do it.
- Provide them with any information you learn that is relevant to the case or discharge planning process.
- Educate them of the importance of your help with the process.
- Facilitate communication regarding request for services and authorizations in a timely manner.
- Follow through with activities, and provide timely responses to build trust.

In today's world of health care, it is common to find "CMs" within every agency used. While each will have a place in their organization's scheme of things, having too many CMs on a case is very frustrating for all. If not careful, confusion, gaps, fragmentation, or duplication can occur. When there are multiple CMs, those primarily affected will be the physician, patient, and family; in most cases, those affected will be frustrated and confused when it comes to who to call and when, or having to repeat what was already communicated. Therefore, if there is more than one CM involved, it is important to establish guidelines for the patient, family, and physician directed as to who will be their primary contact. In addition to other duties, the primary CM's duty will be to serve as the contact for the flow of communication to all parties. Guidelines for effective dual management of a case include the following:

- Selecting one person to serve as the primary CM
- Maintaining regular and consistent communication with the primary CM
- Working with the primary CM, proactively identifying treatment gaps or fragmentation or duplication of care to prevent complications or increased costs
- Working with the primary CM, ensuring specific contingency plans have been discussed with all members of the team in the event the implemented plan is not as effective as anticipated and modifications are required
- As directed by the primary CM, conducting any follow-up with aftercare providers to ensure the timely delivery and provision of services, equipment, or supplies has occurred; if you represent the payer ensuring claims are paid as agreed upon
- Working with the primary CM, ensuring the provision of comprehensive patient and family teaching by appropriate members of the patient's care team is occurring as needs are identified
- Working with the primary CM, ensuring the provision of quality of care in coordination with cost-effectiveness
- Working with the primary CM and ensuring the case management plan is focused on prevention of complications and there are no gaps or fragmentation

If you represent the insurer or payer, do the following:

- Inform all disciplines of the scope of the insurer's liability, including benefits and policy provisions of the patient's individual health care coverage.
- Investigate the clinical feasibility based on availability and accessibility of benefit coverage and contractual agreements for resources.
- Get the facts before you offer any alternatives or coverage.
- Never promise services without knowing they will be covered—once you set up the right of expectation, the insurer may be obligated to pay for care.
- Ensure safety of the plan through appropriate selection and use of vendors.
- To ensure quality and appropriateness, know options and know levels of care as well as policy coverage for the various levels of care.

Referrals

Case management is not required on every case nor does every organization use the same red flags for referral purposes. Some cases neither require nor benefit from case management. Therefore, while a diagnosis may be one on an organization's referral listing, it does not necessarily mean it will be opened once screened. This does not mean if it is not accepted initially it will never qualify. Events change. If they do, the case should be re-referred and re-screened for potential case management. Most organizations will produce a listing of the top "red flags" likely to warrant case management. For most organizations, many of the referrals will be internal; however for others they are accepted from a variety of sources.

While referral criteria may be extensive or specific to the type of case management offered (disease management), any medical condition that necessitates a major lifestyle or quality of life change must be assessed for case management. The same is true for patients for which the medical condition negatively affects physical, sexual, or self-image or self-care functions, or when there are unrealistic expectations about the prognosis or proposed treatment plan or discharge plan. Other indicators that commonly trigger referral include the following:

- Insurer or payer source (some may contractually require some form of a case management process)
- Hospitalizations beyond 5 or 7 days
- Cases with the potential to have charges in excess of a set amount (e.g., $25,000 for a large medical group; $75,000 for a hospitalization)
- Readmissions within or less than 7 days
- Lives alone or lives with a disabled significant other; for the frail elderly, lives with an elderly spouse
- Age over 65 years (all should be screened despite the fact the actual age range is often greater than 75 years)
- Specific diagnoses, diagnosis-related groups, or procedure codes
- Substance abuse, including overdoses
- Chronic mental illness
- Chronic pain
- Dementia or Alzheimer's disease
- Noncompliance
- Persons with a factitious disorder
- Uncooperative or manipulative behaviors
- Frequent use of ED services
- Other disorders as indicated by the organization or at times the reinsurer

Other high-risk indicators generally termed *socioeconomic issues* include the following:

- Adult or child abuse
- Dysfunctional family situations
- Lack of family or other support systems
- No health insurance or inadequate amounts, or care needed is limited or excluded
- Limited or no financial resources
- Incompetency and the need for Conservatorship
- Homelessness
- Poor home environment (inadequate housing, sanitation, lack of water or electricity, multiple structural barriers; if in an apartment, the restrictions imposed by the landlord and at times the fire marshal)
- Out-of-state or out-of-country patients
- Persons with illegal or questionable alien status
- Persons residing in rural communities with limited or nonexistent resources or where physician care is not available or not willing to assume responsibility for overseeing the care plan
- Single parents
- Needs upon discharge may include a move to a skilled nursing facility or other sheltered living facility
- Persons in need of skilled home health services
- Persons in need of assistance in coordinating custodial care services upon discharge
- Admission from a skilled nursing facility or other sheltered living facility and plans for a return upon stabilization of the medical condition

When evaluating targeted groups for case management, it is wise to first evaluate the volumes of patients within a specific diagnosis or population. For example, one might look at how many patients are in specific ICD9 codes or populations that can be classified as "at risk"; what are the top costs for resource consumption; what is an average number of encounters with the health care system for patients within a specific category of medical conditions studied; if days or visits are reported, what are the variances for these patients from any known standards; and, is there a potential for control of resource consumption or an opportunity to improve the quality of care for these patients.

Once diagnoses or the specific population is targeted, as with all aspects of case management, diagnoses or situations not on a list are not exempt—any diagnosis or known situations that pose a risk should be evaluated for possible inclusion. Similarly, although a diagnosis may be listed as one causing automatic referral, it may be evident the patient does not require case management once all the data in a particular case has been collected and assessed. Typical high-risk diagnoses include the following:

- Cardiovascular and thoracic disorders such as the following:
  - Cardiac arrest
  - Cardiac tamponade
  - Cardiomyopathy
  - Congenital anomalies of the cardiac or thoracic system
  - Congestive heart failure (severe)
  - Endocarditis
  - Gangrene
  - Heart failure
  - Heart transplantation, heart-lung transplantation, or rejection
  - Malignant hypertension
  - Mesenteric infarction
  - Myocardial infarction or complications
  - Myocarditis
  - Neoplasms of the cardiovascular or thoracic system
  - Pericarditis
  - Pulmonary hypertension (severe)
  - Stasis ulcers (severe, complicated)
  - Thrombophlebitis, phlebitis
  - Vascular disease (severe)
- Connective tissue disorders such as the following:

- Progressive systemic sclerosis (scleroderma)
- Rheumatoid arthritis
- Severe osteoarthritis (multiple sites or complications)
- Spondylitis and ankylosing spondylitis or spondylolisthesis
- Systemic lupus erythematosus
- Alimentary tract, hepatic, and biliary system disorders such as the following:
  - Biliary atresia
  - Cirrhosis
  - Congenital cystic disease of liver
  - Esophageal varices
  - Gallbladder cancer
  - Hepatic coma, encephalopathy
  - Hepatic decompensation (severe)
  - Hepatic or portal vein thrombosis
  - Hepatitis (primarily B and C)
  - Hepatomegaly
  - LeVeen peritoneal shunt
  - Liver abscess
  - Liver cancer
  - Liver laceration (major)
  - Liver transplants or rejection
  - Pancreatic abscess
  - Pancreatic cancer
  - Pancreatitis
  - Portal hypertension
- Disorders associated with high-risk pregnancy such as the following:
  - Age under 15 years or over 35 years
  - HIV, AIDS
  - Early, threatened labor
  - Excessive vomiting
  - Fetal abnormality (known or suspected) affecting management of mother or unborn fetus
  - Hemorrhage in early pregnancy
  - History of or antepartum hemorrhage, abruptio placentae, placenta previa, fetal deaths, or previous neonatal history of sudden infant death
  - Hypertension complicating pregnancy

- Infectious disease during pregnancy
- Multiple gestation (known)
- Maternal diabetes
- Other placental or fetal problems affecting management of mother
- Pulmonary or other emboli
- Toxemia
- Venous complications
- Musculoskeletal system disorders such as the following:
  - Complicated fractures (traction, spica casts)
  - Complications of reattached limbs
  - Congenital muscular or skeletal anomalies
  - Crushing injuries
  - Multiple fractures
  - Muscular dystrophy
  - Osteomyelitis (complicated or with repeated admissions)
  - Severe decubitus, gangrene
  - Spinal cord injuries
  - Traumatic amputation
- Metabolic and endocrine disorders such as the following:
  - Congenital anomalies of metabolic or endocrine system
  - Diabetes insipidus
  - Diabetes mellitus (with complications or frequent admissions)
  - Hyperthyroidism (toxic)
  - Neoplasms of endocrine system
  - Pancreas transplant
  - Parathyroid disorders with complications or tumors
- Neonatal disorders or congenital anomalies such as the following:
  - HIV, AIDS
  - Amyotonia congenita (Oppenheim's, Werdnig-Hoffman)
  - Atresia of bladder, esophagus, duodenum, liver, rectum, or anus
  - Birth trauma
  - Bronchopulmonary dysplasia (BPD or RDS)
  - Cerebral palsy

- Chromosomal disorders
- Cleft palate, cleft lip
- Conjoined twins
- Cystic fibrosis
- Exstrophy of abdominal organs
- Hirschsprung's disease
- Intrauterine hypoxia or birth asphyxia
- Malformation of central nervous system
- Malformation of heart or vascular system
- Malformation of urinary system
- Malformation of respiratory system
- Microcephaly
- Myelomeningocele
- Multiple anomalies
- Prematurity (severe complications)
- Neurologic disorders such as:
- Abscess (intracranial or intraspinal)
- AIDS with neurologic complications
- Amyotrophic lateral sclerosis (ALS)
- Anoxic brain damage
- Brain or other central nervous system (CNS) neoplasms
- Cerebral palsy
- Cerebrovascular accidents
- Congenital neurologic anomalies (common)
- Convulsive disorders (severe)
- Guillain-Barré syndrome
- Head or intracranial injuries
- Subarachnoid hemorrhage, or other cranial bleeding
- Spinal cord injuries or tumors
- Tuberculosis of neurologic system
- Paralysis, quadriplegia, or paresis
- Hereditary and other degenerative or neurologic disorders such as the following:
  - Friedreich's ataxia
  - Huntington's chorea

- Myasthenia gravis
- Tay-Sachs disease
- Wilson's disease
- Multiple sclerosis
- Parkinson's disease (severe)
- Poliomyelitis
- Respiratory disorders such as the following:
  - AIDS (fungal pneumonia, *Pneumocystis carinii, Candida*, and cytomegalovirus infections)
  - Apnea
  - Asphyxia with complications
  - Asthma (severe)
  - Bronchopulmonary dysplasia
  - Chest trauma or flail chest
  - Chronic tracheostomy with complications
  - Congenital anomalies of respiratory system
  - Chronic obstructive pulmonary disease (primarily end-stage or frequent admissions)
  - Crushing injuries to chest
  - Cystic fibrosis
  - Pneumonia, staphylococcal
  - Pulmonary emboli
  - Pulmonary fibrosis
  - Respiratory failure (RDS)
  - Systemic fungal infections (coccidiomycosis)
  - Tracheostomy (complications or new)
  - Tuberculosis with complications
  - Ventilator dependency
  - Emphysema
  - Laryngectomy
  - Legionnaires' disease
  - Lung abscess
  - Lung injury
  - Lung transplants or rejections
  - Major neurologic disease with respiratory complications
  - Neoplasms of respiratory system
- Renal or urinary system disorders such as the following:
  - Complications of implants, grafts, or external stoma
- Glomerulonephritis (acute or chronic)
- Renal abscess
- Renal artery sclerosis
- Renal artery thrombosis and fistulas
- Renal failure (acute or chronic)
- Renal or bladder neoplasms
- Renal or bladder rupture or trauma
- Renal hypertension
- Renal transplants or rejections
- Stricture or trauma to ureters or urethra
- Other high-risk disorders such as the following:
  - Blood disorders (severe with complications):
  - Anemia (severe with complications)
  - Hemophilia
  - Leukemia
  - Sickle cell anemia
  - HIV, AIDS
  - Amputation with complications
  - Anorexia nervosa
  - Bone marrow transplants
  - Burns
  - Crush injuries
  - End-stage malignancies
  - Esophageal trauma, tumors
  - Failure to thrive
  - Fistulas (with complications)
  - Flail chest
  - Gangrene
  - Gunshot wounds
  - Intestinal malabsorption disorders
  - Lye or poison ingestion
  - Multiple trauma
  - Nutritional or vitamin deficiencies (severe intractable nausea, vomiting, or intractable diarrhea)
  - Obesity with complications, including those patients who undergo gastric bypass
  - Peritonitis
  - Radical neck dissection for malignancy

- Septicemia
- Short bowel syndrome
- Stab wounds (if complications)
- Ulcerative colitis (if complications)
- Wound infections (multiple sites or complications)

Assessments

To be effective, assessments must be thorough and systematic. Assessment is defined as a process by which one collects and analyzes data about the client. Data collection includes gathering information from physical, psychosocial, spiritual, cognitive, and functional abilities, and developmental, economic, and environmental dimensions. The Commission for Case Management Certification (CCMC) defines assessment as "the process of collecting in-depth information about a person's situation and function to identify individual needs in order to develop a comprehensive case management plan that will address those needs. In addition to direct client contact, information should be gathered from other relevant sources (patient or client, professional or nonprofessional caregivers, employers, health records, and educational or military records."

According to these definitions, the clinical assessment of the patient and the assessment of the family must be comprehensive enough to reflect their total needs. These assessments must capture details pertinent to the social, financial, cultural, religious, physical, and psychologic functioning of both the patient and the family. For instance, the initial and ongoing clinical assessments are used to determine the patient's physical care needs, psychologic factors, and functional limits and abilities. Assessments also emphasize the family's and caregiver's physical, mental, and emotional ability to cope with these immediate care needs as well as the stresses and emotional demands of caring for a patient who

may have complex or lifelong needs. During the initial assessment, the interview processes and subsequent conversations with the family, the CM must always strive to obtain and maintain a clear picture of how the family functioned prior to the illness as well as during the present acute phase.

Assessments, while organization-specific, are best accomplished by on-site visits using such techniques as chart reviews, visual observation of the patient and family, interviews with the patient and family, case conferences, and consultations with the health care team members and the patient's physicians. A CM who is based in a facility or is a clinical nurse specialist has an advantage because he or she may be able to conduct an actual physical examination of the patient, which can be a bonus for actual case planning.

On-site visits allow the CM an opportunity to see and communicate directly with the patient and family, visualize the personal dynamics operating in the case, and bond with the patient and establish a level of trust. More importantly, on-site assessments allow the CM to view the actual facts of the case without third-party interpretations. Unfortunately, because of budgetary constraints, senior management directives, or remote geographic territories covered by the case management organization, on-site assessments and reassessments are not always possible.

Using Assessment Tools

Measurements of functional health status have long been used in medical rehabilitation to justify the care rendered. While they have not yet reached wide acceptance, they are slowly making their way into the assessment processes used by medical CMs. As with all tools used to conduct business, assessment tools will be organization-specific. As in the past, most measurement tools focus on evaluating the degree of assistance patients require to perform ADLs and must be age-specific. The following are examples of the most commonly used assessment tools in the health care industry:

- The Expanded Disability Status Screen as it focuses on mobility;
- Two tools used to focus on the effectiveness of the rehabilitation program are:
  - The Level of Rehabilitation Scale (LORS) used for communication
  - The Patient Evaluation Conference System (PECS) used for interpersonal skills
- The Functional Independent Measures (FIM)
  - Self-care
  - Sphincter control
  - Transfers
  - Locomotion
  - Cognitive
  - Communication/Comprehension
    - Expression
  - Social cognition
    - Social interaction
    - Problem solving
    - Memory
- The WeeFim (used for children ages 6 months to 7 years)
- Medical Outcomes Study Short Form 36 (SF36) is a widely used measure of health-related quality of life. It is completed by the patient, is composed of 36 items, and measures the following eight health concepts:
  - Physical functioning
  - Role limitations due to physical health problems
  - Social functioning
  - Bodily pain
  - General mental health
  - Role limitations due to emotional problems
  - Vitality (energy/fatigue)
  - General health perceptions

The Functional Independent Measures or FIM and the Wee Functional Independent Measures or Wee FIM are based on the World Health Organization's definitions of impairment, disability, and handicap. These definitions are as follows[51]:

- **Impairment**—Abnormalities or disturbances of structure or function. Disturbances at organ level include anatomic, physiologic, and psychologic.
- **Disability**—Restriction or lack of ability to function normally as a consequence of impairment. Disturbances at the level of a person; concerned with restriction of compound integrated activities (tasks, skills, and behavior).
- **Handicap**—Disadvantage resulting from an impairment or disability limiting or preventing an individual from fulfilling a role that is normal for that individual. Handicap reflects the cultural, social, and economic consequences of the impairment or disability. Handicap is shaped by values and attitudes.

The FIM is an 18-item, 7-level ordinal scale. It was originally a four-level scale with three sublevels, and it later became seven levels. The FIM emerged from a thorough developmental process overseen by a national task force of rehabilitation research, clinical, and administrative experts and was sponsored by the American Academy of Physical Medicine and Rehabilitation. The FIM incorporates concepts and items from multiple other functional assessment instruments. The FIM was designed to do the following:

- Assess areas of dysfunction in activities at the person level that commonly occur in patients with progressive, reversible, or fixed neurologic, musculoskeletal, and other disorders and disabilities;
- Represent a minimum dataset of items likely to reflect cost of disability in terms of consumption of social and economic resources

- Be discipline free, reliable, easy to use, and completed by clinicians within a short period of time
- Be consistent with terminology used by clinicians to describe disability
- Be sensitive to change over the course of a comprehensive medical rehabilitation program
- Be a meaningful element within the broader context of measurement of health status and quality of life

As brain injury rehabilitation has surfaced as a modality of care, the functional assessment measure (FAM) was developed for use with the brain-injured individuals. It consists of 12 items that emphasize the cognitive and psychosocial aspects of disability. These items do not stand alone and are used in conjunction with the 18 items of the FIM. The total 30-item scale is referred to as the FIM+FAM. The 30 items of a Functional Independence Measure (FIM) and Functional Assessment Measure (FAM) are as follows:

- Motor items
  - Self-care
    - Eating
    - Grooming
    - Bathing
    - Dressing upper body
    - Dressing lower body
    - Toileting
    - Swallowing*
  - Sphincter control
    - Bladder management
    - Bowel management
  - Mobility
    - Bed, chair, wheelchair transfer
    - Toilet transfer
    - Tub, shower transfer
    - Car transfer*
    - Walking, wheelchair locomotion
    - Stairs
    - Community mobility*
- Cognitive items
  - Communication
    - Comprehension

- Expression
- Reading*
- Writing*
- Speech intelligibility*
- Psychosocial adjustment
  - Social interaction
  - Emotional status*
  - Adjustment limitations*
  - Employability
- Cognitive function
  - Problem solving
  - Memory
  - Orientation*
  - Attention*
  - Safety judgment*[51]

Other assessment tools commonly include the following:

- Karnofsky Performance Status Scale (this rates a person's ability to carry on normal activities)
- For cardiac patients – the New York Heart Association (HYHA) Functional Classifications
- Functional Assessment Staging (FAST)
- Burden assessments (for use with caregivers)
- Mini-mental assessment

In addition to any of the foregoing tools used by the treating team, assessments by the CM of the patient and family will be just as critical. For successful planning, the foundation of the final case management plan must be solid. For this to be solid, assessments must be performed on all facets affecting a case once screening is completed thoroughly. Equally as important is solid knowledge and understanding by the CM of community resources (local, state, regional, or federal) and a patient's entitlement to such as well as to health insurance benefits and those offered by public funding programs. To start a case management plan, a thorough assessment must be conducted of the following areas:

---

*FAM items.

- Physical condition and needs of the patient:
  - Current physical and medical condition and responses to treatments for all body systems
  - Laboratory, radiologic, and diagnostic results and plans for ongoing care, if results are negative
  - Planned interventions and ongoing care needs—skilled or custodial
  - Future plans for care and level of care required for each (e.g., high-dose chemotherapy only provided as an inpatient; participation in a clinical trial in a center of excellence; eventual transfer from SNF to acute rehabilitation)
  - Patient endurance and prognosis
- Psychosocial needs of both the patient and family or caregiver:
  - Personal relationships and dynamics among patient and family members and significant others
  - Competency of patient
  - Cultural influences (values and beliefs)
  - Linguistic abilities and level of communication and understanding both orally and written
  - Spiritual (values and beliefs)
  - Coping abilities of patient and family
  - Emotional status of patient and family
  - Perceptions and attitudes of patient and family toward illness or sick role
  - Priority of illness or sickness within life's context
  - Level of involvement of family, friends, and community
- Socioeconomic needs of both patient and family or caregiver:
  - Effect of wage loss as well as other family members affected by the potential wage loss and monthly income
  - Financial ability to pay for basic living (food, shelter, and clothing) in addition to needed health care services (limited income directly influences a patient's compliance and adherence to the case management plan)
  - Eligibility for public funding or entitlement programs
  - If the spouse or primary caregiver works, what will be the effect on their abilities—emotionally, financially, and physically, as well as the ability to continue to work while still serving as caregiver
  - Eligibility for community programs and resources
- Environmental issues that will affect the case.
  - Location of care, such as home, outpatient, or facility (local versus out-of-area)
  - Home environment and setup (safety issues, ease of mobility, or barriers)
  - Home environment and access to phone, water, heat/air conditioning, and electricity
  - Access to transportation resources
  - Resources (local or regional to meet the patient's level of care as well as access, availability, cost, and requirements for acceptance.
- Health behavior and views that will affect the case:
  - Patient and family awareness and basic understanding of the disease or injury
  - Perception of both patient and family regarding the illness or injury
  - Commitment to treatment compliance not only to proposed methodologies for care but for wellness in general
  - Expectations of both patient and family for plans and prognosis

- Self-care abilities:
  - Patient's ability to performing activities of daily living both mentally and physically
  - Patient's or family's ability (both mentally and physically) to perform any skilled care
  - Patient's mental status, willingness, and commitment to self-care
- Teaching needs of patient or family or caregiver or at times professionals:
  - Level, type, and frequency of training needed
  - Level of education of both the patient and family or caregiver and ability to understand, read, and write; interpretation of the facts in the patient's primary language may be necessary
  - Willingness to be trained
  - Sex of patient and dominant caregiver and their relationship and ability or inhibitions to render care to the opposite sex
  - Resources necessary to accomplish training

It is important to note that the distinction between screening and assessment is often misunderstood. Screening involves the collection of data from which potentially high-risk patients can be identified. Assessments require the detailed collection of data from which the CM can determine whether the high-risk patient actually requires case management intervention, and what deficits or needs must be acted upon if they do.

Thus, once screening is completed, assessments, development, and revision of the case management plan continue throughout the duration of the case. Accurate and comprehensive assessments of all details of the case are absolutely critical to the development of an effective case management plan. Assessments this comprehensive are not developed in a vacuum.

They require input not only from the patient's chart but also through interviews and conversations with the patient, family, and the various multidisciplinary team members involved in the patient's care.

Assessments for case management planning focus on the medical needs of the patient and also on the entire picture—family, psychologic, socioeconomic, and cultural factors—with all pertinent facts used in the final plan. Although the referral and preliminary screening assessment data can be gathered by phone, the actual clinical assessment is best accomplished during an on-site visit.

On-site visits and assessments allow actual review of the medical records and also an opportunity to meet the patient and visualize his or her care needs. The formal evaluation of the case starts with the patient's clinical assessment and an assessment of the family. These are the most crucial steps in developing a case management plan. These assessment phases involve the accumulation of pertinent and accurate data from all parties. These data elements give the CM an opportunity to identify alternatives and resources.

To collect the data, one of the best mechanisms is to capture the data on an assessment form. As one interviews the patient, family, and professionals, there is nothing wrong with telling those involved at the beginning that you will be taking written notes. For hospitalized patients, it is important to collect as much information as possible as in most cases phone calls for linkage of resources may not occur with the patient's chart readily available. A data-collection tool also allows the capturing of all critical data components.

Assessment Components

Assessments involve a continuous process of gathering information to ensure the patient's needs are being met. They also include a monitoring process to ensure, at a minimum, the patient's health care benefits are not exhausted, the patient is always at the appropriate level of care, and the caregiver is following the techniques as required and is not becoming worn out by the demands of the tasks. Monitoring is defined by the Commission for Case Management Certification as "the ongoing process of gathering sufficient information from all relevant sources about the case management plan and its activities or services to enable the CM to determine the plan's effectiveness." Consequently, the assessment phases of case management are never completed.

The initial assessment process should cover at least the following components:

- Demographic information on the patient and family
- Patient's past and current physical health
- Patient's current functional status
- Patient's mental health status, memory, and behavior
- Patient's psychosocial function and perception of the illness or injury
- Financial data
- Caregiver capabilities
- Home environment
- Nutritional needs and abilities and resources
- Resources and providers
- Actual physical assessment of the patient and his or her physical care needs, medications, and feedings

Most case management organizations have established standards requiring CMs to complete the clinical assessment phase within a specified period of time after referral. For instance, although a facility-based or community-based case management program may start the assessment process within 24 hours of admission, an insurer's or independent case management program may allow a seven-to ten-day time frame after referral in which the initial assessment can be completed. The time frame must be realistic enough to allow the

CM to capture as much relevant data as possible. The primary purpose of the initial assessment phase is to determine a baseline of abilities prior to the illness or injury and the subsequent needs and corresponding resources to meet the needs.

If the patient is hospitalized, the initial family assessment is best accomplished in the home environment. CMs have a big advantage over discharge planners in that the latter never see firsthand the actual home environment and the family's interactions. Thus, final case management plans developed using this process can be far more detail-oriented than is possible with discharge planning. If on-site visits are allowed, the CM has a dual advantage—he or she can assess the family and the home simultaneously. Home interviews allow the CM an opportunity to see the following:

- Actual environmental risks and barriers
- True living situation
- Environment in which activities of daily living occur (bathroom, bedroom, kitchen)
- Interactions among all parties
- Cognitive abilities of the patient and, at times, the identified caregiver

Regardless of where they are conducted, family assessments should determine at a minimum the following elements:

- Names, addresses, and phone numbers (including work phone numbers)
- Work history of spouse
- Family health problems and limitations
- Perception of the patient's illness or injury
- Emotional status of family
- Transportation availability and mode
- Identification of potential barriers within the home, if the home is to be the discharge destination

- Identification of the person who will be the caregiver
- Caregiver's physical, emotional, and mental capabilities and availability
- Cultural, ethnic, and religious beliefs

As one interviews the patient and family or conducts assessments, the following questions might be helpful for capturing additional information for case planning:

- What are the patient's clinical or medical needs with consideration to limitations and potential for improvement and recovery?
- In what setting or location and in what projected time frame can the care be met?
- Does the treatment plan include aftercare services or can the patient safely be discharged to a lower-level, less-intensive setting in lieu of acute hospitalization?
- What are the patient's and family's goals?
- Are their goals realistic?
- Are the patient's and family's goals consistent with the physician's and health care team's goals?
- If so, what are the options for discharge?
- If not, what is needed to achieve consensus?

Case Management Plan

Once the initial clinical assessment process is completed, all information elements captured must be documented in some written form. The data gathered during interviews and assessments serve as the basis for the written case management plan. Although actual formats vary from organization to organization, the final summary must include and identify the following minimum information elements:

- Date of assessment
- Date of referral
- Patient's name and identification number

- Name of primary physician
- Diagnosis and prognosis
- Summary of medical procedures carried out
- Current level of care and specialty unit, if applicable
- Summary of pertinent past and present medical history
- Summary of special needs (e.g., intravenous therapy, oxygen, suctioning, wound care)
- Medications (frequency and dose)
- Allergies
- Summary of mental status and memory deficits
- Summary of neurologic status and functional deficits
- Summary of problems related to skin integrity
- Summary of mobility status and deficits
- Pain and pain control, route, frequency, and type
- Elimination or bowel and bladder status and deficits
- Feeding and nutrition status (type and mode)
- Communication abilities and deficits
- Behavioral characteristics
- Sensory, visual, and auditory status and deficits
- Safety concerns
- Summary of capabilities in activities of daily living
- Amount and type of teaching required and appropriate teacher (caregiver, patient, professional)
- Planned date of discharge, if applicable
- Level of care anticipated
- Agencies thought to be needed
- Equipment anticipated
- Type of facility anticipated for placement, if patient is not to be discharged home
- Person who is to assume financial responsibility for costs or if assistance is needed from another fund-

ing source; who will assume the application process and, if already started, the status of the application and eligibility of the patient

■ Other (e.g., known barriers)

Goal Setting

Short- and long-term goals are a necessary component to the plan. Although as the case progresses the goals and case management plan may need to be modified, developing realistic and measurable goals allows for the most successful outcomes both qualitatively and quantitatively. Goals must be written so that they are observable, measurable, and time-limited. One way to make a goal measurable is to use terms that have few interpretations. This helps to ensure consistency in understanding. Avoid terms that can mean different things to different people. Establishing goals is the initial step in the planning process and sets the direction for the activities to follow. The nature of the goal will depend on the type of outcome one is trying to achieve, but it is common for goals to be in the following categories:

■ **Educational**—These goals express the desired learning outcomes.

■ **Behavioral**—These goals are related to achieving a desired level of behavior.

■ **Health restoration**—These goals are aimed at restoring a designated level of health.

Once assessments are completed, goals are established, and the resources are identified to meet the needs of the patient and family, the plan must be implemented. Key to ultimate success is to have plans readied for implementation as discharge approaches or as the patient moves to the next level of care.

Implementation, Monitoring, and Changing the Case Management Plan

The development, implementation, frequency of monitoring, and changes in the actual case management plan vary with the individual case. In most cases, referrals are generated early enough to allow time for planning the case and educating the patient and family so as to avoid a crisis atmosphere of discharge or an unexpected move to another level of car. Unfortunately, when referrals are untimely, a crisis atmosphere surrounding the discharge or move is common.

In such cases, the discharge and implementation of service often occur almost simultaneously with the referral. In these cases, there is inadequate time to plan for appropriate linkage of patient and family to necessary resources or to teach the patient and family. Equally as important, communication with the patient and family is not always pleasant.

Early referrals provide the benefit of adequate planning for locating appropriate resources and for smoothly implementing the plan. By all means, if a last-minute referral reveals the discharge is not safe, the CM must be prepared to substantiate opposition to the discharge either through documentation or discussion with the attending physician, utilization reviewer, or other members of the health care team.

In all cases, the intensity and complexity of care required affects the frequency of monitoring as well as the type of monitoring technique used (by telephone versus on-site visits) and varies patient by patient. However, the importance of performing reassessments on a regular basis cannot be overstated. The frequency of reassessments depends on such factors as the following:

■ Medical or physical changes in the status of the patient (improvement, deterioration, or failure to change) or in his or her level of function

■ Changes in the psychosocial status of the patient (e.g., loss of income, marital discord and separation, other crisis or stressors)

■ Evolving educational needs (e.g., changes in the treatment plan that necessitate a new teaching plan and then a new regimen of teaching or monitoring)

Reassessments must be performed at regular intervals throughout the case. These are necessary for monitoring purposes as well as making adjustments to the case management plan as the patient's condition progresses, slides backward, or stays the same. Reassessments evaluate the patient's progress, give the patient and family the reassurance they need that all is going well, and ensure they have the information they need. The frequency and type of reassessments made and whether they are accomplished by telephone or on-site depends on many factors. Among these are the intensity and severity of the patient's condition; the quantity, quality, and complexity of the resources necessary to manage the patient's required level of care; and the patient's and family's emotional and coping abilities.

As the case management plan is monitored and the patient assessed, the following are general questions that may be asked either by the CM as he or she reviews case events or as a supervisor evaluates a CM's actions on a case:

- At the time of case opening and assessment, were all needs identified and addressed? If not, what was missed and what bearing did it have on the success of the plan?
- Was the patient linked to the appropriate resources? Do the resources remain applicable? If not, what needs to occur. Is a decrease or increase in frequency, amount, or duration of services needed, or should care be shifted to another provider?
- Were the interventions taken effective and efficient? If not, what must be changed to ensure effectiveness and efficiency? Is it too late to change?
- Are the goals of the plan being met? If not, were they too stringent or

aggressive given the facts of the case and the patient's or family's ability or coping patterns? If changes have occurred, what new goals must be set?

- Were all services delivered as planned? If not, why not? What needs to be done to correct the situation?
- Is this a quality issue and if so, due to whose role (CM, physician, patient or family, or agency)?
- Have new needs surfaced? If so, what are they and are they serious enough to destabilize the plan? What is needed to ensure stability of the plan?
- Were all phone calls and communications handled in a timely manner? Were the actions summarized supportive of good communication?

If the patient had a change of condition (improvement or deterioration in mental, physical, or functional condition or mobility), were actions taken in a timely and aggressive manner to ensure the patient was receiving the right care at the right price and at the appropriate level? If not, what was the reason for the delay?

- Were the issues addressed with the attending physician and what were the orders? What was the final outcome?
- If the patient had a change in social stability (e.g., loss of a job, housing, pet, family member is ill or died), did the added stress of such factors affect the case? If they did have an impact on the case, was prompt attention given to these needs? Were modifications made to the plan? Were appropriate resources implemented (e.g., counseling, referrals to public funding programs)?
- If an accident or oversight was detected, was it acted upon immediately? Did the CM take the necessary

steps to prevent or impede further adverse outcomes?

- If teaching is identified (initially or ongoing), was a teaching plan developed? Was it timely? Was it adequate (scope, duration) to meet the goals of the teaching plan? Did it cover the needs? If not, why not and who dropped the ball?

- Has a contingency plan been established in the event that an unforeseen situation occurs? Are the patient and family comfortable with the plan and know what is needed to implement the plan, who to call, or where to go?

- After reality has set in, have the patient's or family's expectations changed? If so, were proper steps taken to activate a contingency plan?

- If the patient has a caregiver, is the caregiver able to continue in the role? If so, are the support systems in place and capable of supporting the caregiver long-term? If not, what referrals need to be made? What is the anticipated timeframe for a contingency plan for caregiver support?

If the patient or family is not satisfied with care or services, the case management plan is not going as planned, there are unnecessary re-admissions, or the patient deteriorates, the following questions might be helpful as analysis of the case is conducted:

- When the patient and family originally consented to the plan, were they willing participants or were they pressured or coerced into agreement? In some cases did they agree, as there was a lack of understanding or informed consent obtained?

- Was the patient or family in denial or unrealistic about their options?

- Was there a change in the patient's medical condition that occurred without revisions to the case management plan?

- Was there poor, inadequate, or no plans made for ongoing care?

- Did the plan not go as intended due to inadequate financial resources or because the patient refused available options or was prone to making bad choices?

- Did the agency or provider used not handle the case as was agreed upon? In some cases, did they not pull a staff member or agree to transfer the case to another vendor when it was known there was friction between the patient or family and staff member or agency?

- Were phone calls and other communication with the patient and family timely and as needed in response to their needs?

Case Closure

In case closure, the decision to close a particular case must be based on specific, identifiable, tangible, and potentially measurable factors. Once a care plan's goals have been met, case closure should be considered. However, factors to consider before closing a case include the following:

- Is the patient at risk for re-admission due such factors as comorbid diagnoses or complications?

- Have services been provided in a consistent and reliable manner?

- Can the patient (or caregiver) administer the care and verbalize appropriately how to perform the care?

- Has the necessary patient teaching been completed?

- Will the patient's health care benefits continue to be available and able to support continuity of care needs?

- Is the patient's caregiver support system reliable?

- Does the patient or family have a backup plan for specific situations?

For example, do they know what to do if (1) a home care agency does not deliver necessary supplies; (2) a nurse or therapist does not show up to provide necessary care; or (3) treatment or transportation needed for outpatient services does not arrive.

- Is the patient receiving ongoing treatments that might cause future re-admissions?
- Does the patient know whom to contact if he or she needs services again?

In addition to goals being reached, cases may be closed for the following reasons:

- Treatment or services is discontinued
- Treatment plan is not covered or in lieu of a covered service
- Treatment or services requested is no longer medically necessary
- Benefits are terminated
- Another insurer or payer provides financial risk
- Patient or family refused services
- Patient is noncompliant with the treatment plan
- Physician refuses to participate in discharge planning process
- Patient died

Capturing Cost Savings

Although cost savings is the ultimate goal, this is not the only or even the most important factor for quality case management services. Not every case has a cost savings that can be shown in black and white. Also, every patient does not need universal case management. Many high-cost diagnoses may trigger the need for case management activity, but a person's diagnosis is a poor indicator of how much money will be spent or saved on the case over the course of the patient's disease or injury. Thus, dollar thresholds are not good predictors of the usefulness of case management because at times the treatment course is

planned and the resources needed are pre-determined as they will be needed to treat the disease. In case such as these, the CM can do little if anything to influence the course of care and costs.

For many cases, a cost savings will not be evident. However, if all activity prior to and after case management is reported and analyzed, often cases will show a decline in costs that is generally attributable to less encounters with the health care system. Sometimes the key to a decrease in costs will be due to such actions as early assessments to identify patients at risk, education, and linkage with appropriate resources and the implementation of lifestyle changes.

The direct impact of case management can equate to such outcome measures as the CM being effective in performing the four key case management functions: assessor, planner, facilitator and advocate. These four functions positively affect the overall outcomes: improved knowledge and adherence, improved coordination of care, enhancement of patient empowerment, and involvement in self-care. However, the major outcomes include the following[52]:

- High-quality care
- Decreased or appropriate costs
- Improved health care status

In addition to the positive effect case management can have with patients, policyholders, subscribers, insurers, payers, and providers, cost savings that are captured or reported *must* be valid, accurate, defensible, and reflective on the reality of the case, case activity, and the true efforts of case management. Maintenance of quality is a cost-savings mechanism as it eliminates or reduces complications and other costly factors.

Outcomes and Other Reporting

In an uncertain health care industry, two things are fact when it comes to outcomes: (1) Regardless of the decision makers (government, managed care, businesses, others), cost constraints will continue to tighten. (2) As data become more available and reliable, it will be used increasingly in decisions related to quality. The driver of competition strategies will come from this data. Health care organizations that can show data verifying that they provide the best quality outcomes at the lowest cost will be in the best position to compete for their share of the market. Management has the ultimate responsibility to be accountable for quality outcomes. In collaboration with staff, management is responsible for developing processes and systems for delivery of care and services to the patients served. If the processes are sound and the staff follows them, targeted results will be achieved. If the processes are designed to use resources most efficiently, the targeted results will be achieved at the lowest possible cost.[53]

In the broadest sense, case management is a reflection of the phases in the nursing process. Very simply put, it represents the nursing process in action. Through the integration of case management techniques and activities as well as use of the nursing processes, nursing can effectively manage all facets of patient care and have a tremendous impact on outcomes and costs. In addition to any cost savings, there are general goals and outcomes that one can expect from any well-organized, efficient, and effective case management model.

Whether goals are client-oriented or system-oriented, outcomes are further enhanced when the case management model is supported by a common vision of what case management is and can do as well as the commitment of senior management and the health care team members at all levels. As clinical processes are streamlined and integrated and as desired outcomes are projected, it is important to evaluate such factors as the following:

- What population will be served?
- What outcomes are to be achieved?
- What processes will achieve the outcomes most cost-efficiently?
- What resources are required?
- How will the processes flow—ideally and realistically?

Despite the variability in type, model, and setting, certain commonalities are always present in successful case management outcomes. These include the following:

- Effective and efficient use of all resources whether related to medical, psychologic, or financial needs
- Improved health status including physical and emotional health and well-being
- Social responsiveness of community agencies and professionals
- Better educated patients who are knowledgeable about their disease or condition and able to accept it, while assuming self-management skills such as activation of the strategies and interventions to maintain health and prevent relapse
- Patients who emerge from case management with a sense of responsibility for their overall health and lifestyle and a greater sense of the need to incorporate preventative health care practices into their daily living
- Professional collaboration and mutual respect
- For patients with life-threatening illnesses, the ability of the patient and family to receive multidisciplinary support that allows death with dignity

Other critical elements to successful outcomes are as follows:

- To have an adequate informational system in place that can capture the data required for reporting purposes
- To have adequate resources available for use by the staff (e.g., code books, Internet access, other disease-specific reference books)

including technologic capabilities (e.g., cell phones, laptop computers, preprogrammed forms, automated health plan benefit information, other automated databases specific for the region or populations served)

- To have a management team that ensures and advocates concurrently for a solid organizational structure for case management as well as for the clarification of team member roles and responsibilities and adequacy of staffing
- To ensure the department is staffed with highly educated and skilled professionals
- To ensure education of the staff is ongoing and supportive of the needs of the case management team and the clients served
- To ensure policies and procedures and the standards and protocols are adequate to serve the department as well as for contractual requirements and the client populations served
- To ensure that outcomes and time frames established are realistic for the populations and clients served as well as for the staffing level of the department

Variance Reporting

As case activity occurs and cost savings are calculated, it is important to capture the variables that impede care as these often impact quality as well as the total costs. Capturing and reporting of such activity is a key process if management is to be kept apprised and can act on issues affecting not only case success but also the organization's bottom line. Variance data are of two types. The first variance kind is when patient care activity is not performed as ordered and is cancelled, omitted, or delayed. The second variance type involves expected outcomes to not be met for whatever reason. In addition to negative (unde-

sired outcome) and positive (patient progresses faster than anticipated) variations, variances can be divided into six broader categories or causes:

1. Clinical
   - Delays related to clinical issues include the following:
     - Patient's severity of illness and intensity of services do not meet criteria for acute care admission
     - Patient comorbidity, secondary diagnosis, or allergy
     - Appropriate acute care bed (e.g., center of excellence, rehabilitation center) is not available
     - Unscheduled return to surgery
     - Postoperative complication
     - Readmission within seven days of discharge
2. Community or alternate level of care
   - Delays related to SNF or subacute placement include the following:
     - Ventilator dependency
     - Tracheostomy care or suctioning requirements greater than every four hours of suctioning
     - Skilled care that is required more than every four hours
     - Complexity of care is greater than facility or agency can accommodate or is in excess of the hours for their RN to patient acuity ratio
     - Chronic infection (MRSA/VRE) and infection requires private room
     - Behavior problems (e.g., restraints or locked unit)
     - Awaiting Medicaid or other financial reasons for delays
     - Awaiting Conservatorship
     - Care is custodial, and appropriate bed or funding is not available
     - Bed is not available for the applicable sex

- Admission refused by facility or agency staff due to weekend or holiday
- SNFs or home health agencies refuse, as patient is known to them
- Home health agency or skilled nursing facility does not have adequate staffing or the training required to manage the level of care required

3. Patient or family
   - Delays related to patient or family issues include the following:
     - Family is indecisive, nonaccepting, uncooperative, or refuses suggestions
     - Family changes their minds about day of discharge or implementation of plan
     - Family is fighting and unable to reach a decision
     - Family is slow to select a facility
     - Family is unavailable (e.g., for planning, teaching, consultation, transporting, or decision making)
     - Family is unwilling to be trained
     - Family is slow or noncompliant, or refuses to complete any required paperwork (e.g., admission papers, application for Medicaid or Conservatorship)
     - Patient is homeless, and care is beyond what a shelter can provide
     - Issues related to placement of patients into a board and care (B&C) or Assisted Living (AL)
     - Legal delays (e.g., abusive situation and APS or CPS involved, attorney, or awaiting Conservatorship proceedings)
   - Patient-specific issues include the following:

- Patient refuses treatment or plan of care
- Change in condition
- Allergic reaction
- Signed out against medical advice

4. Practitioner or physician
   - Delays related to practitioner or physicians include the following:
     - Unwilling to accept plan of care
     - Medication error
     - Refuses to discharge patient
     - Untimely ordering of applicable services or consults
     - Ordering unnecessary tests or procedure
     - Omission of test or procedure
     - No consent obtained
     - Patient is stable, but physician does not write transfer orders in a timely fashion and bed availability is placed in jeopardy
     - Physician infighting or conflicts regarding appropriate care

5. Service or treatment delays
   - Service or treatment delays include such activities as the following:
     - Patient's treatments do not meet criteria
     - Delays in consults (e.g., cardiology or other specialty service, therapy, social services, discharge planning, nutrition)
     - Surgery scheduling or availability of room or anesthesia
     - Appropriate physician is not available
     - Prep is not done
     - Orders are not carried out
     - Nursing treatments are not done or timely
     - Nursing medication error
     - Diagnostic delays (e.g., radiology, treadmill, nuclear medicine, cardiac lab)

- Timely ancillary services (e.g., therapy, nutrition)
- Teaching is not done (e.g., availability of educator or family)

6. System or operational delays
   - System or operational delays often include the following:
     - Services are not available on weekends or holidays
     - Machine is not operational
     - Lost requisition slip, request, or specimen
     - Hospital technician or personnel not available due to weekend, holiday or after-hours
     - Untimely delivery of equipment or wrong equipment delivered
     - Transportation issues
     - Home health agency or SNF not available or staffing inadequate to handle patient
     - Infusion agency not available or staffing inadequate to handle patient
     - Hospice agency not available or staffing inadequate to handle new admission
     - Costs are beyond contracted amount (e.g., medications or equipment)

Evaluations of the effectiveness of the case management plan and the final reporting of outcomes are as important as the development and implementation. One of the best ways to conduct such evaluations is through the use of data collection and analysis whether this is done manually or via automation. To do this, one critical task of case management is a daily review of the case management plan, capturing any expected outcomes whether anticipated and achieved as well as any cause for delay. If a delay or problem is encountered, the CM must determine why such arose and then take whatever steps are needed to correct the situation.

SECTION II—DISCHARGE PLANNING

Medicare Conditions of Participation are designed to ensure the quality of hospital care. Equally as important, they reinforce the fact that effective discharge planning is vital to continuity of care. Discharge planning has been around as a profession since the mid-1960s and the passage of Title XVIII or Medicare of the Social Security Act. For details of the legislation on discharge planning, see Section 1861(ee) of the Social Security Act. This legislation requires the following:

- All patients who are likely to be at risk must be identified early.
- Discharge planning evaluation must be provided for patients who are identified as likely to be at risk and for patients referred by his or her representative or physician.
- Discharge planning evaluation must be timely to ensure appropriate arrangements for discharge and to avoid unnecessary delays.
- Discharge planning evaluation must include the patient's likely needs and availability of appropriate post-acute resources.
- Discharge planning evaluation must be part of the patient's medical record, and the results must be discussed with the patient and his or her representative.
- Upon request by the patient's physician, the hospital must arrange for the development and initial implementation of a discharge plan for the patient.
- A registered professional nurse, social worker, or other appropriately trained staff must develop or supervise the discharge planning evaluation or plan as required by the Act.

The goal of most organizations is to ensure discharge planning is integrated into overall patient care plans. While 80% of patients can be effectively handled using standardized care plans, critical pathways, and other tools that facilitate the discharge process with a primary care nurse, the other 20% cannot.[54]

Unfortunately, as hospitals downsize and reorganize, duties are often shifted. In many cases, discharge planning is eliminated and shifted to the duties of the primary care nurse or combined with other functions such as utilization review. If discharge planners assume dual roles, both processes are diluted. Discharge planning then takes a back seat to other duties, and there is not enough time to adequately assist and coordinate the needs of the 20% who truly require devoted time upon discharge.

The Conditions of Participation can bring attention to the complexity of the discharge planning process and the need for specially designated staff to conduct only discharge planning and thus meet legislative standards. Discharge planning programs require professionals dedicated to carry out at least the following functions:

- Provision of direct care coordination to achieve a timely and safe transition to post-acute care for patients who are likely to suffer adverse health consequences if discharged without adequate discharge planning
- Development of listings of alternate care programs and services that can be used as a resource tool for all staff providing discharge planning
- Provision of expert consultation to other staff members assuming the discharge planning is part of the overall plan of care for all hospitalized patients
- Education of other discharge planners about clinical and social factors as they affect functional status for discharge
- Assurance that policies and procedures are written and correctly implemented

- Participation in research that identifies clinical outcomes and projects designed to improve the continuity of care process[54]

The continuum of care is generally defined as the patient's entire sequence of interactions with the health care system.[6] As a rule, references to continuum of care come into play as the patient is readied for discharge and then moved through the various levels of care as he or she either progresses or regresses. Readiness for discharge varies with diagnoses, the patient's response to treatment, the treatment course's progression, and a multiplicity of factors. Readiness is generally considered when the following occur:

- The outpatient treatment or alternate level of care is financially feasible and more cost-effective than continued inpatient care.
- The patient is clinically stable.
- The patient is taking a drug that is appropriate for home use.
- The patient has tolerated the initial course of treatment or chemotherapeutic agent without problems.
- The patient and family accept home care or the alternate level of care.
- If the plan is for home care, the patient and family or caregiver is taught all techniques required.
- For patients with anticipated need for long-term infusion, there is an appropriate venous access line in place.
- In the case of home care, the patient's home has an adequate physical layout and a clean environment.
- The necessary medical resources and services required for ongoing care, further diagnosis, and treatments required are available.

As indicated earlier in this chapter, in today's health care environment there are CMs within almost every health care entity. Thus, when CMs are external to a hospital and need information for concurrent review or for continuum of care planning, the following questions may be useful to capture the details needed:

Discharge readiness in general:

- When is discharge or transfer to another level of care anticipated?
- What treatments are currently being rendered (intensity of services), and are treatments currently at a level that can be managed outside the hospital?
- What is the level of assistance required upon discharge?
- If there is pain, is it under control and what is the plan for ongoing pain management?
- Have side effects resolved or been stabilized?
- If on a high-dose medication, is it approved for use outside the acute hospital?
- Has the cost of care been explored with the patient and family? If not covered by insurance, are they prepared to assume the cost? If not, has a referral for Medicaid been started?
- Do the patient and family have an understanding of what will be needed upon discharge?
- How is the patient and family coping with illness and impending discharge?
- Have the patient and family completed any or all training if the plan is for home care?
- If teaching is required, have the patient and family been adequately trained in the aspects of care required?
- If the plan is for home care and the patient requires more care than provided through intermittent visits of a home health agency, has the patient and family explored caregiver needs? Are these arrangements in place?
- If emergency situations are anticipated, has a plan been developed for

how the patient and family is to handle it, whom to contact, or what process to use?

- Has the patient been instructed in medications and treatment protocols?
- How motivated are the patient and family about compliance to the proposed treatment and discharge plans?
- What referrals to care or services are anticipated upon discharge?
- Have all referrals been generated, and has the patient been accepted at the next level of care?
- What are the timeframes or dates for return appointments or examinations?

In analyzing readiness for discharge, the following questions may be helpful:

For the Physician

- What is your treatment plan for the patient?
- What are your short-term and long-term goals for the patient?
- What is your perception of the patient's support system and the proposed discharge plan?
- Is the patient realistic regarding discharge plans, treatment goals, and diagnosis? Is the family?
- Does the patient have any unmet needs?
- Is the current support system consistent and reliable?
- What do you estimate as the time frame for recovery?
- What aftercare services do you perceive the patient to have beyond this hospitalization?
- If the patient's discharge needs are proactively addressed with patient teaching and the family or caregiver's commitment to assist the patient, what specific services would need to be in place to achieve a timely discharge?
- What is your assessment of the patient's clinical status?

For the Social Worker, Discharge Planner, or Primary Nurse

- What is the proposed discharge plan for the patient?
- What is your perception of the patient's support system?
- Is the patient realistic regarding discharge plans, treatment goals and diagnosis? Is the family?
- What is your assessment of the patient's discharge needs?
- What is your perception of the patient's coping ability?
- What is your perception of the patient's motivation for self-care or participation in treatment?
- What do you think will be needed upon discharge?

Discharge delays are a reality. When they occur, they must be captured and the reasons clearly stated. Delays are frequently broken down into two categories: variance days and avoidable days. Variance days occur when the patient remains acute but operational issues are encountered, such as scheduling delays, staffing, or broken equipment. Avoidable days occur when the patient is medically stable for discharge but barriers are encountered, such as no beds or resources for transfer to a lower level of care, no financing for long-term care, the patient is awaiting Conservatorship, or delay in accessing equipment or medical supplies. When a variable or avoidable delay occurs, one may ask the following questions:

- What are the reasons for the delay?
- What actions have been taken to correct or overcome the variance situation?
- How soon will the issue be corrected?
- What is the expected time frame for bed procurement, nursing agency, DME or medial supply items, issuance of Medicaid or a temporary Conservatorship, and other such issues?

- If corrected, what is the anticipated length of stay or discharge date?

While variances will account for some delays in discharge, the biggest delays will be those termed avoidable, because barriers must be cleared before discharge can occur.

Common Barriers to Discharge

Historically, most treatments have been administered in the clinical setting of acute care hospitals. With the advent of shorter lengths of stays and the proliferation of outpatient services, many treatments are now available in the home or in various outpatient settings. However, caution must be exercised when patients are discharged. Caution is needed to ensure any postacute care the patient requires can be administered safely and efficiently in an outpatient setting or at home. This is necessary because some treatments, according to the standards of care for the condition or treatment modality, can only be given safely in an acute care setting.

Developing a case management plan for the discharge of a patient requiring complex care or depending on technologic equipment requires considerable lead-time (several days to weeks). This time frame is necessary for the patient and family to gain full acceptance of the plan, for training to occur, and for all resources to be in place and ready to assume responsibility for the patient's care. For patients discharged to the home, the patient, family, or caregiver must be fully trained and the home environment must be readied for the discharge. This can be the reason for delay, but it is not the only one. Costly delays can be encountered for any number of reasons. Although some of these are case-specific, the following factors are often primary culprits in the delays.

For Home Planning

- Inadequate home environment or in some cases, no home

- No family or caregiver
- Family in-fighting, family resistance to the plan, or noncompliance with the plan
- Local physician unable or unwilling to accept responsibility for care
- Local resources or agencies not available or able to assume the required level of care
- Transportation for follow-up appointments or services not available
- Financial reserves are inadequate and patient is ineligible for alternate funding
- Multiple psychologic factors present in either the patient or the family
- Patient, family or caregiver nontrainable (e.g., language and cultural barriers, care is perceived to be too repulsive, or dexterity problems are encountered)
- Care too complex or beyond the standard of care for home care
- Conservatorship has not been started or completed
- Care is custodial and patient and family do not have financial resources, and referral to alternate funding has not been made or the family is resistant to applying as they feel their "insurance will pay for services"

For Out-of-Home Placement

- Facilities are not available or inadequate to manage the level of care required (this is especially true for patients who are children or who require total care or complex skilled care).
- Staffing is inadequate in number, type, or skill level (e.g., depending on state licensing laws, in many skilled nursing facilities a registered nurse [RN] is present on the day shift and a licensed vocational or practical nurse [LVN or LPN] is present on evening and night shifts; or the staff may not have the skill level and training to manage the patient.).
- Facility available is out of area, but this is unacceptable to family.

- Facility administrator is unwilling to hire additional staff or to train existing staff.
- Financial resources of patient or family are limited and they cannot afford the ongoing care if the patient's care needs shift from skilled to custodial.
- Patient requires custodial care (often the patient requires total care and skilled care is not needed), health care insurance will not pay for this level of care, and the family does not have the financial resources to pay privately for help.
- Total care is required and the facilities have a waiting list.
- Patient has an infectious disease, and the facility has no private room or cannot accept a patient with an infection.
- Patient's weight is a problem (Many facilities will not accept patients who weigh more than 200 to 250 pounds because this factor increases the probability of staff back injuries and increases workers' compensation claims).
- Intravenous therapy is required and staff is not certified to provide it or the toxicity or complexity of the solutions is approved only for acute level use.
- Delays in application for alternate funding are encountered.
- Delays in Conservatorship are encountered.
- Rates are unacceptable to health care insurer or payer, or rates must be negotiated prior to a transfer.
- Care needs are of such intensity and complexity or frequency that skilled nursing facility cannot manage the level of care (e.g., complex wound care).
- Cost of the care is prohibitive and beyond contractual rates for the post-acute facility, and the facility will be inadequately reimbursed for the type and level of care required.
- Patient is confused, noisy, or combative.
- Facility is full and there is a waiting list.
- Patient is a child or young adult, and the staff is unfamiliar with the care needed for this age group.

It is a well-known fact that health care professionals have an automatic tendency to blame barriers to discharge on the health care system in general. However, patient and family barriers are often encountered as well. These include such experiences and emotions as the following:

- Fear (e.g., fear of the unknown)
- Unrealistic priorities
- Insufficient motivation
- Lack of buy-in
- Previous unhappy experience with providers or resources
- Lack of knowledge of resources
- Lack of understanding of the problem (e.g., denial, emotions, language)
- Poor self-image
- Cultural or language factors
- Financial limitations
- Pride (too proud to apply for Medicaid because it is "welfare")

Rural Areas

Another barrier or problem encountered is the difficulty of providing care to persons who live in rural areas. These cases are often the most challenging for CMs. Although many rural communities have advantages for most residents, residents needing medical care may experience major difficulties in obtaining access to care or services. Also, when managing rural patients, the CM must often deal with lack of good roads, flash flooding, blackouts from electric failures, and homes without running water, indoor plumbing, electricity, or adequate heating or cooling systems.

These barriers and many other factors place a burden on the CM, patient, and family. For example, for the CM establishing the required services, this may entail making a multitude of phone calls before needs are linked to the appropriate services. In many cases, resources and services are not available. For the patient and family, getting home help especially when care is custodial is often a challenge. Worse yet,

if the patient is not homebound but continues to require services that can only be provided by an outpatient facility, the benefits of the treatment are often eroded due to travel distance or getting in and out of a car.

When patients reside in rural areas and care can be provided at home, there are times when ordering medial supplies in bulk or for several months at a time will be appropriate. If blackouts are a reality, one must consider a generator as part of the equipment.

For rural patients, often the key will be locating a physician willing to accept the patient and provide the care as dictated by the treatment plan. If the local physician is willing and the treatment plan complex, one of the best plans is to have the actual treatment plan and updates generated by the tertiary care physician but actually implemented and monitored by the local physician.

Urban Underserved Areas and Alien Status

For CMs serving some urban and underserved areas, their skills are equally as challenged as the nurse working in a rural community. CMs serving urban and underserved areas often find multiple challenges and additional barriers such as homelessness or lack of services as agencies refuse to provide services in the area due to known violence. In dealing with patients in urban or underserved areas, there will be cultural, educational, and linguistic challenges. These factors can be further complicated by the fact that attempts to locate resources or funding to pay for such resources cannot be done as the patient is an illegal alien or alien status must be determined before Medicaid can be obtained.

The latter recently happened in a hospital in Sacramento. A patient was admitted, and during the Medicaid eligibility application process it was discovered that

Medicaid eligibility could not be determined and it would not be a financial resource for arranging the discharge needs. All research by the Medicaid worker was pointing to the fact the patient was possibly an illegal alien. Fortunately, as arrangement for financing was proactively started shortly after admission, these extra weeks required for the patient's condition to stabilize allowed the patient to progress to a point where a home plan could be arranged. Although there were postacute needs for DME and outpatient therapy, a local loan closet provided the equipment and the hospital's outpatient rehabilitation department provided the follow-up therapy. Long after discharge, it was finally determined the patient was indeed an illegal alien. This case ended successfully for the hospital, as they were able to discharge the patient. However, many hospitals are not so lucky. As a result of unknown residency or when illegal alien status is known, the social services staff, discharge planners, and other health care professionals spend countless manpower hours attempting to locate resources to manage postacute needs. Unfortunately, many such patients tie up needed acute beds, as the patient cannot be moved.

Durable Medical Equipment

While DME will be discussed in more detail later in this chapter, it is important to recognize it as there will be times when the actual barrier to discharge will be lack of equipment. This delay can be due to a variety of issues such as the need for specialized or customized equipment or, in the case of an obese patient, locating bariatric equipment that can accommodate the patient's weight. There will be other times when it will be difficult to find DME companies to provide the needed services especially when the patient is technology-dependent. Many DME companies require patients to live within a 1-hour driving distance from their place of busi-

ness. The travel distances make it unproductive for the agency to serve such patients. More importantly, if the patient requires immediate assistance, the distance places the patient and equipment vendor at risk. By accepting the patient as a client, they have indicated they can meet the needs when, in essence, if distance is an issue they cannot. DME companies find this restriction necessary if they are to successfully manage the care required.

An example of the travel distance occurred many years ago when the author was case managing a ventilator child. The child resided in a small community several miles from the nearest large town. Finding an agency that could provide the skilled services needed took months as traditionally none of the agencies served this region. It was soon found that the closest agency that would consider taking the case had never serviced a child. Thus, they had no pediatric nurses much less ones who had provided care or been around the equipment necessary to manage a ventilator-dependent child. Once the agency agreed to take the case, they had to advertise for nurses. Between the agency and hospital, a training program was established to train these nurses prior to discharge. For the same child, finding a DME company that could serve the child was equally as challenging. While the DME companies in Sacramento were familiar with ventilators for children, the patient lived more than an hour commute, and winter fog and flooding to the area precluded the company from accepting the child. After many months of research and calling, a company was located as they were relocating one of their offices to the immediate area. The discharge took many months, but the child was finally discharged safely to home.

Although barriers vary with each case, the CM frequently must make many daily calls to various local or regional facilities to locate a suitable facility that can accept and render the care required or to ascertain the patient's status on the waiting list. Case management has inherent pitfalls, and it is very important to recognize that barriers can occur both internally and externally. Many of the foregoing barriers are considered external, and it is important to ensure contingency plans are devised expeditiously and efficiently to handle various situations. However, internal barriers are just as common and can cause delays as well. Unfortunately, not all internal barriers are fixable if there is no senior management buy-in. However, it is important to recognize internal barriers. If they are present, one must be willing to bring these to the attention of senior management and support the need for change. Internal departmental barriers often include the following:

- Expectations set too high by management
- Lack of support from senior management
- Lack of departmental leadership
- Inefficient reporting relationships or leadership support for decision making
- Misplaced accountability
- Inadequate support of the case management process by management, physicians, or team members
- Lack of policies and procedures
- Unrealistic timeframe or outcome expectations
- Inadequate staffing
- Inadequate technical support (e.g., computers or lack of automation in the office)
- Lack of ongoing education of the case management staff
- Turf issues

Services Required for Discharge

As discharge approaches, plans will be underway to arrange the services required. Unfortunately, there is no formula that states what and how much should be ordered. The final orders vary with the patient's actual diagnosis and medical need, with the treating physician ordering any the following in any combination:

- For homebound patients, orders can include any combination of home health agency services for intermittent or private duty (hourly) skilled nursing care or skilled rehabilitation therapy services
- For patients who are not homebound, services provided by an outpatient facility or center
- Social worker services
- Infusion services
- DME and medical supplies
- Laboratory or radiologic services that are portable and serve the homebound (if patient is not homebound, linkage to an outpatient provider)
- For both homebound patients those who are not homebound, transportation to follow-up appointments or outpatient services
- Detailed medication regimen and a pharmaceutical provider

Preventable Admissions

As CMs work with patients and they are readied for discharge, it is imperative to ensure the case management plan addresses the resources and techniques to avoid unnecessary hospitalizations. If it appears the discharge is not safe or resources are not in place, the discharge planner must inform the treating team of the reasons. There will be times when an aggressive approach is needed. For example, a physician wanted to discharge a patient in reverse isolation with a very low blood count. This placed the patient at risk of an opportunistic infection. The patient was receiving daily blood products. Due to the need for beds, the physician presented the discharge to an unsuspecting family indicating the patient would be "better off at home." However, home was not an option for many reasons. One reason was that the patient continued to require daily blood products after discharge. The home health agency could not do it, so the patient had to come to an outpatient infusion setting every day. In the end, the patient was maintained at the acute level until safe for discharge. The case went all the way to the chief of staff, as it was simply not a safe discharge. Consequently, while readmissions are costly for the health care system in general, the emotional and physical toll they take on patient and family is immeasurable.

CMs must continually ensure safe and unplanned rehospitalizations do not occur. Preventable hospitalizations are generally linked to the following:

- Diagnoses for which timely and effective care can help reduce or eliminate the risks of hospitalizations
- Adequacy of or inappropriate use of outpatient services
- Prevalence of diseases
- Physician practice patterns
- Demographics, education and literacy, or cultural factors
- Lifestyle factors

The diagnoses most frequently included under preventable hospital conditions are as follows:

- Asthma
- Congestive heart failure
- Diabetes
- Hypertension
- Pneumonia[55]

Services That May Be Needed at Discharge for Various Diagnoses (Not Limited to the Following)

- Cardiovascular and thoracic disorders
  - ADLs (retraining)
  - Antiembolic stockings
  - Cardiac rehabilitation
  - Counseling (role reversal, lifestyle changes, depression)
  - Energy conservation and mobility techniques
  - Job retraining
  - Nutritional counseling for weight control or reduction or fluid retention
  - Pain management
  - Wound care
- Alimentary tract, hepatic, and biliary system disorders
  - ADLs (retraining)
  - Counseling (body image, sexual function, lifestyle, depression)
  - Energy conservation and mobility techniques
  - Nutritional counseling for dietary and fluid restoration
  - Edema monitoring
  - Total parenteral nutrition
  - Gastric suctioning
  - Ostomy care and supplies
- Connective tissue disorders
  - ADLs (retraining)
  - Counseling (body image, sexual function, lifestyle, depression)
  - Energy conservation and mobility techniques
  - Gold therapy
  - High-dose steroids
  - Interarticular joint injections
  - Job retraining
  - Pain control
  - Pool or water therapy
  - Nutritional counseling for weight control or reduction
- High-risk pregnancy
  - Antiembolic stockings
  - Bed rest
  - Blood pressure monitoring
  - Counseling (frustration, lifestyle changes, altered sex life, depression)
  - Edema monitoring
  - Fetal monitoring
  - Nutritional counseling for weight control
  - Terbutaline therapy
- Musculoskeletal disorders
  - Antiembolic stockings

- Energy conservation and mobility techniques
- Counseling (frustration, lifestyle changes, altered sex life, depression)
- Hyperbaric oxygen
- Muscle or nerve stimulation
- Nutritional counseling for weight control or reduction
- Pain control
- Pool or water therapy
- Wound care
- Metabolic and endocrine disorders
  - Vitamin B_{12} injections
  - Growth hormones
  - Diabetic education
  - Glucose monitoring
  - Insulin regimen
  - Nutritional counseling for dietary planning and weight control
  - Pain management
  - Wound care
- Neonatal problems or congenital anomalies
  - Specific to the diagnosis or anomalies
- Renal or urinary system disorders
  - Blood pressure monitoring
  - Counseling (lifestyle changes, role reversal, sexuality)
  - Nutritional counseling for dietary and fluid restrictions
  - Pain management
  - Ostomy care and supplies
- End-stage renal disease
  - Blood pressure monitoring
  - Counseling for coping, role reversal
  - Dialysis shunt care
  - Energy conservation
  - Nutritional counseling
  - Possible self-dialysis
- Neurologic disorders
  - Antiembolic stockings
  - ADLs (retraining)
  - Cognitive retraining
  - Counseling (coping, frustration, lifestyle changes, altered sex life, depression)
  - Job retraining

- Mobility training and energy conservation
- Pain management
- Rehabilitation
- Wound care
- Respiratory disease
  - Antiembolic stockings
  - ADLs (retraining)
  - Counseling (role reversal, coping)
  - Energy conservation and mobility techniques
  - Job retraining
  - Nebulizer treatments
  - Respiratory rehabilitation

Typical Equipment Needs upon Discharge (Not Limited to the Following)

- Cardiovascular and thoracic disorders
  - Antiembolic stockings
  - Adaptive clothing
  - Blood pressure cuff and stethoscope
  - Electric carts
  - Electrocardiogram supplies
  - Feeding pumps (portable and stationary) and supplies
  - Respiratory monitor and supplies
  - Infusion therapy, equipment, and all medications and supplies
  - Oxygen (stationary and portable) and supplies
  - Prosthetic devices
  - Ramps
  - Self-help devices (for feeding, dressing)
  - Suction equipment (portable and stationary) and supplies
  - Wedge pillow and other pillows or devices for positioning and support
  - Weight scale
  - Wound care supplies
- High-risk pregnancy
  - Blood pressure cuff and stethoscope
  - Glucose monitor
  - Infusion pump, solutions, supplies, and medications
  - Home uterine monitor and supplies (not always allowed as a covered benefit)

- Alimentary tract, hepatic, and biliary system disorders
    - Blood pressure cuff and stethoscope
    - Dressings, irrigation solution, and supplies
    - 50-cc syringes (rectal neomycin)
    - Gastric suction or similar devices and supplies
    - Glucose monitor and supplies
    - Humidifier or cold mist
    - Infusion therapy equipment and all supplies (portable and stationary), medications, formulas, and solutions
    - Ostomy supplies
    - Oxygen (portable and stationary) and
    - supplies
    - Scales (weight)
    - Tape measure
    - Wound care supplies, when applicable
- Connective tissue disorders
    - Adaptive clothing
    - Adaptive eating, cooking, and writing utensils
    - Other ADL and self-help devices
    - Ramps
    - Rails for shower, commode, or hallways
    - Splints and other orthotics
- Metabolic and endocrine disorders
    - Assistive and self-care devices
    - Button infusor if insulin is required more than four times per day
    - Glucose monitor
    - Infusion pump and supplies (portable and stationary)
    - Regular or blind insulin syringes and supplies
- Neonatal problems or congenital anomalies
    - Stationary units and battery-operated backup units or monitors for all electronic equipment
    - Feeding pumps and supplies
    - Oxygen and supplies
    - Tracheostomy suctioning equipment and supplies

- Infusion therapy supplies, solutions, and equipment
- Ostomy supplies (common with neonates)
- Suction equipment (stationary and portable)
- Musculoskeletal disorders
    - Adaptive clothing
    - Alternating air mattress and pump
    - Antiembolic stockings
    - Bedpan (regular or fracture) or toilet and bars and elevated toilet seats
    - Call system if confined to bed
    - Infusion pumps (stationary and portable), supplies, solutions, and medications
    - Pillows for patient lift, body support, and positioning
    - Ramps
    - Slide board
    - Traction unit (Bucks, pin, pelvic)
    - Wedge pillow and other pillows or devices for positioning and support
    - Trapeze (freestanding or bed)
    - Wheelchair (regular with removable armrests, elevating leg rests, or reclining)
    - Wound care
- Renal or urinary system disorders
    - Blood pressure cuff, stethoscope
    - Hemodialysis or ambulatory dialysis equipment and sterile supplies and solutions
    - Infusion pumps, solutions, supplies, and medications
    - Ostomy supplies
    - Weight scale
- Neurologic disorders
    - Adaptive clothing
    - Adaptive feeding equipment
    - Adaptive ADL devices
    - Alternating or special mattress
    - Antiembolic stockings
    - Call system
    - Catheter supplies (if self-catheterizing, mirror)
    - Communication devices
    - Decubitus supplies

- Electric mobility carts
- Elevated toilet seat or toilet rails
- Feeding equipment and supplies (stationary and portable)
- Foot board
- Grab bars for toilet, shower, or hallway
- Incontinent pads
- Infusion equipment, solutions, supplies, and medications
- Orthotics
- Patient lift
- Patient restraints
- Prism glasses
- Protective head gear
- Ramps
- Seating systems and supports (customized)
- Slide board
- Special cushions (often customized)
- Splints, braces
- Suction equipment and supplies (stationary and portable)
- Trapeze (free-standing or bed)
- Trunk supports
- Walker (platform or regular)
- Wedge pillow and other pillows or devices for positioning and support
- Wheelchair (regular, reclining, specially made, removable armrests and leg rests)
- Respiratory disease
  - Antiembolic stockings
  - Alternating air mattress or pump
  - Communication aids or call system
  - Dressing and supplies
  - Electric mobility carts
  - Feeding pump and supplies
  - Grab bars for toilet or shower or hallway
  - Humidifier or vaporizer
  - Infusion pump (for antibiotics or pain; stationary and portable), solutions, supplies, and medications
  - In-home respiratory (apnea) monitor
  - Oxygen equipment (stationary and portable) and supplies

- Percussors
- Pump-driven or handheld ultrasonic or intermittent positive pressure (IPPB) nebulizer
- Sterile tracheostomy tube (extra) and other tracheostomy supplies
- Suction equipment and supplies (stationary and portable)
- Wedge pillow and other pillows or devices for positioning and support
- Ventilator and all supplies
- Other high-risk diagnoses
  - Dressings, solutions, other supplies for wound care (on occasion, continuous intermittent suction machine)
  - Feeding equipment (stationary and portable) and supplies
  - Infusion therapy (stationary and portable) equipment and supplies

SECTION III—SHIFTS OF CARE

Technology

Technologic advances are often the biggest challenge for discharge planners and CMs. The next challenge is keeping current and knowing what and where treatment alternatives are available to patients. According to research by the Health Insurance Associate of America (HIAA) and the BlueCross and BlueShield Association of America (BCBSA), the cost of medical technology may account for up to one-third of projected increases in U.S. health care spending over the next 5 years. The fundamental issue raised by BCBSA's CEO is that "at a time of significant across-the board cost increases in our health care system and with finite resources to pay for everything, consideration must be given as to how best to use new technology available to patients and then work with patients and providers to ensure appropriate information is available from which wise choices can be made." *The Impact of Medical Technology on Future Health Care Costs* examined how medical technology affects the cost of health care and gives these three conclusions:

1. Technologies that may save costs for some people often increase overall spending.
2. In addition to price, volume is also a only determining factor behind overall technology costs.
3. Incentives of the health care financing system play a critical role in how new technology affects costs. In the absence of clinical guidelines (which happens when new technology is introduced), the reimbursement structure influences how a physician makes use of new technology.[56]

In addition to investigating appropriate treatment settings, CMs may need to be aggressive in helping patients seek appropriate treatment options and providing to patients information regarding appropriate new therapies available. One key role of CMs is to educate the patient in using experimental treatments. If the patient does not respond to traditional therapies or treatments (and these have been exhausted), one may help the patient pursue more high-tech or invasive procedures that often fall into the experimental or clinical trial arena. If the patient wants an experimental treatment and it is covered (which is often not the case, except with new Medicare guidelines), the CM must help the patient make the necessary arrangements. If not covered (which is often the case), the CM will need to assist the patient in the facilitation and location of funding or appropriate clinical trials. The key is to focus on how the patient perceives his or her condition and the latitude allowed by the CM's organization for advocacy. For example, if the CM is only to fit patients into existing benefit structures (and these do not cover such treatments), it is fruitless to foster false hope. However, if the CM is allowed to advocate for the patient, he or she can help the patient

locate the alternate ways to have the treatment covered.[57]

Chronicity

Historically, acute illnesses have dominated the health care payer scene due to their resource consumption and the attention they have gotten from insurers. However, advances in technology, newer more effective medications, and other treatment modalities have shifted the emphasis for care from acute to chronic. As a result, the health care system in general deals with an older population, many with chronic illnesses. The system also deals with persons with injuries and long-term disabilities or medical conditions, all of which have a high propensity for utilization of health care resources. While chronic conditions traditionally have been associated with prematurity, birth defects, diabetes mellitus, cardiovascular disease, pulmonary diseases, renal failure, arthritis, many neurologic disorders, cancer, and AIDS, this is no longer true.

As case management is critical for the growing population of chronically ill persons, CMs must continue to increase their knowledge of acute and chronic care processes. They must stay abreast with the most current treatment modalities, know target outcomes, and understand common complications of disorders. They must also maintain current and accurate listings of common providers, support groups, and community resources for any disease that shifts from acute to chronic. Additionally, as the cultural, religious, racial, and age environment changes, a CM's knowledge of cultural, religious, racial, and aging dynamics and how they affect cases must also be current.

Chronic illness is not immune to any age. However, with each age, cohort trajectories and resulting consequences occur. Typically, consequences relate to psychologic, physical, and socioeconomic realities of sustained illness. Chronic illnesses are slow, insidious, characterized by periods of exacerbations and remissions, and have irreversible pathologic changes. These illnesses require vigilance by the chronically ill person, significant others, and key health care providers; they also require resources to confront the long-term impact on health care and emotional, functional, and financial needs. Lifelong treatment and behavior changes are required for the management of such illnesses. To be successful, the patient must be active in self-care management and be supported by key health care providers (e.g., nurse CMs). While a community-based model is ideal for chronic conditions, insurers usually do not cover this type of care.[2]

Case management is evolving in complexity and effectiveness. In many parts of the country, contemporary health care systems continue to struggle as they deal with chronic illness as a series of events rather than a trajectory of illness requiring systematic support of self-management skills and care coordination across the continuum. Nurse case management as a strategy supports the ability of chronically ill persons to maintain self-management skills while increasing coordination of care, decreasing fragmentation of care, and decreasing consumption of health care dollars. Through the addition of a nurse CM to the current set of primary care providers and relationships, the nurse CM has the ability to influence self-management capabilities as well as interaction of the primary provider and health care organization with the chronically ill person. The resulting alteration in relationships leads to changes in the amount and type of health care resources consumed. The ongoing continuum-based relationship between the chronically ill person and the nurse CM is critical if trajectories of chronic care are to be altered and hence health care consumption.[58] As care is shifted from acute to chronic, one might ask the following questions:

- What is the specific diagnosis?
- What does the treatment plan look like, and is it appropriate?
- Will this be a high-dollar case despite the fact that it may be chronic?
- Will hospitalizations be required? If so, how many should one expect and for how long should each be?
- Will other encounters with the health care system be needed? If so, how many should one expect, for how long, and for what providers or services?
- What tasks must be taught to the patient and/or family to enable them?
- What are the expected functional outcomes?
- Will other financial resources be needed to manage the shift from acute to chronic?
- While shifting from acute to chronic, are advanced directives in place if the condition shifts to acute? Who can make decisions for continuation of life verses end-of-life care?
- Where and at what level can care be rendered to keep the patient in the most appropriate but least restrictive environment while promoting the highest functional level and quality of care?
- What nonprofessional assistance will be needed (e.g., activities necessary to allow personal care or attention to ADLs)?
- What bargaining with insurers must occur to allow additional services (e.g., therapy) that improve the patient's quality of life and functional ability since this is often denied once the patient is deemed custodial, chronic, or long-term care?
- If pain is an issue, what pain management activity must continue to ensure pain is effectively addressed and measures remain in place?

In working with the chronically ill, one must take the foregoing into consideration as well as the primary diagnosis, severity of illness, and the number of secondary diagnoses. These antecedents are necessary to create a continuum-based relationship. Once established, the relationship ultimately and significantly influences self-management capabilities as well as the family's ability to support and influence the effectiveness of what the chronically ill can do as it relates to self-management. While working with patients, a critical junction that makes a significant impact is the relationship between severity of illness and self-management skills. In a study done by Lamb and Stempel in 1994, the relationships among nurse CMs and patients were studied. It was found that growing together as insider-experts developed through a process of affective, cognitive, and behavioral changes and that the following three interpersonal phases emerged: bonding, working, and changing.[58]

The patient's ability to improve self-management skills and develop a therapeutic relationship of trust and mutual respect with the CM is paramount to reaching case management outcomes. The final outcome related to chronically ill patients is often multidimensional (maximal quality, managed costs, and enhanced accessibility due to appropriate use of resources). However, outcome measurements for chronically ill patients and their families include a cross-sectional examination of resources consumed. These are typically expressed as emergency and acute-care service consumption, cost per patient day, and use of community services. They are further expressed through reporting of well-being as measured in terms of functionality, stabilization of physical symptoms, extent of self-management ability, knowledge of the illness and the health care system, and satisfaction.[58]

To effectively measure self-management and effectiveness of services as they pertain to outcomes and chronicity, one must evaluate the patient's medical history and the number of encounters with providers from the start of illness to the present. It is equally important to measure the patient's satisfaction with treatments and responses to date. As one evaluates the health care record using a then-and-now approach, one might evaluate the following:

- Consumption of emergency services
- Consumption of health care resources (costs and encounters with the health care system)
- Consumption of acute care services (costs and days)
- Consumption of community resources (costs and visits)
- Comparison data for pre- and post-screening of functionality
- Increased knowledge of the disease and how to access resources
- Periodic patient satisfaction surveys

As one works with patients with chronic illnesses or injuries, the following statistics shed light on the magnitude of problems faced by this population. They also point out major deficiencies in care and where the case management plan may need to focus attention. According to a Harris Interactive survey released by the Partnership for Solutions (led by Johns Hopkins University and the Robert Wood Johnson Foundation), the following statistics raised awareness of challenges faced by children and adults with chronic conditions:

- 72% of Americans said it is difficult for people living with a chronic condition to get the necessary care from health care providers
- 74% said it is difficult to obtain prescription drug medications
- 89% said it is difficult to find adequate health insurance
- 78% said it is difficult to get help from their family

Additionally, this survey showed:

- 10% reported that in the past year they were unable to see a primary care physician
- 11% reported that in the past year they were unable to see a specialist
- 22% of those who had insurance reported that it does not cover all types of care needed
- 45% reported that costs of their care are a financial burden
- 14% reported that in the past year different doctors diagnosed them with various medical problems for the same set of symptoms
- 17% reported that they had received contradictory information from health care professionals
- 16% reported that they had been warned by a pharmacist about possible harmful interactions among medications prescribed by one or more physicians[59]

Alternative Medicine

As well as chronic illness, it is important to mention the need to address alternative medicine. While traditional health care techniques include surgery, medicine, or radiation, about one-third of Americans use alternative medicine at some time, and many with complex illnesses or injuries turn to nontraditional medicine in their quest for a cure.

Alternative medicine is a blanket term used to describe several interventions not taught widely in American medical schools or used in American hospitals. Some alternatives come to America from foreign countries.[60] Alternative therapies might include but are not limited to the following:

- Aroma therapy
- Folk remedies
- Mega-vitamin therapy
- Relaxation therapy
- Hypnotism
- Reflexology
- Herb therapy
- Spiritual therapy
- Magnetic therapy
- Homeopathy

Alternative medicine comprises nonallopathic interventions that are noninvasive. Many arise from cultural or religious traditions and are generally not reimbursable by insurers. Treatments such as naturopathy, massage techniques, chiropractic, acupuncture, midwifery, celation, diets, herbs, and laying of hands all come under the heading of alternative medicine. Alternative treatments are generally nontoxic and do not interfere with allopathic treatment. For this reason, they are sometimes called complementary treatments. There is no social sanction given by insurers and no listing in the physician-controlled current procedural terminology (CPT) book, so these therapies are generally paid for out-of-pocket.

However, due to consumer demands, many large employer or health care purchasers allow reimbursement for some alternative medicine treatments. If alternative treatments are allowed, they should be guided by the following conditions:

- They are initiated by the patient or family request.
- Other treatment modalities have failed, and there are a few other viable therapy choices or the therapy is part of a cultural tradition.
- The alternative or complementary treatment will not interfere with the ongoing course of treatment or otherwise harm the patient.
- Outcome expectations are clearly stated, and how intensive the treatments are is clearly prescribed and preapproved.[60]

Shifting from Inpatient to Outpatient Care Providers

Fortunately, many chronic and long-term care patients can now have the majority of care provided through outpatient or ambulatory care providers. This shift to outpatient care is not surprising. It is due to the decline in inpatient hospitalization rate and shorter lengths of stay during the past decade. This decline is attributed to the increase in post-acute care setting changes, ambulatory care, and same-day surgery. All have been made possible in the past 20 years through advances in treatment modalities, new surgical techniques, and less invasive procedures.

According to the National Hospital Discharge survey conducted by the Centers for Disease Control and Prevention's (CDC's) National Center for Health Statistics, the average length of stay for hospital inpatients was 5 days in 1999 down from 7.3 days in 1990. The hospital rate varied by region. It was 93 days per 1000 in the west and 133 days per 1000 in the northeast. Six diagnostic categories: heart disease, delivery, pneumonia, cancer, psychosis, and fractures accounted for 13 million of the 32 million hospitalizations in 1991. Heart disease was the most frequent cause with 4.5 million patients discharged. In 1999, over 41 million inpatient procedures were performed with almost three-fourths falling into four categories: diagnostic and therapeutic procedures, obstetrical procedures, operations on the cardiovascular system, and operations of the digestive system. Men accounted for the majority of patients requiring cardiovascular procedures, while women had the higher rate in digestive disorders.[61]

SECTION IV—ETHICAL ISSUES
Change and Loss

The need to adjust to change and loss is one of the most important and difficult tasks an individual must face. While especially apparent in later years when change and loss occur at an increasing frequency, this problem can be seen as patients in all age brackets face chronic and long-term care.[62]

Although some changes may be positive, many are viewed negatively. The change process and subsequent feelings of loss are normal behaviors and occur in a variety of situations. Loss occurs when a spouse, friend, or relative dies; one is separated from a place, home, or role in the family; or one is no longer independent and must rely on others for the basic necessities of life. These are activities the average person takes for granted while conducting his or her life (ADLs).

It is human nature to respond to loss in ways that allow us to cope. Loss of function, body image, comfort, job, self-esteem, self-concept, freedom, control, and quality of life can be devastating to patients and families. People handle loss differently, and some react negatively. For others, loss will have a positive effect. It often brings families closer and reminds them of what is most important in life. Change and loss frequently interfere with consistency in human contact and intimacy and therefore result in loneliness.

Change in relation to performance of daily living increases with age. The number of persons needing help with ADLs falls in the age 85 years or older bracket. This population is increasing more rapidly than younger old age groups and represents approximately 4.2 million persons in the United States. Also, it is estimated that the number of persons older than 85 years will increase to 19 million in the next two decades. Additionally, stressors that accompany old age often appear to precipitate feelings of loneliness as well as other factors contributing to the onset and persistence of loneliness, powerlessness, and grief. Powerlessness is evident as a person ages and loses the ability to function due to physical, mobility, or mental handicaps or sensory deficits or as society relegates power to the young and withdraws it from the old. Feelings of grief are frequently connected to change and loss.[63] Interventions that can assist in helping patients of all ages to adjust to change and loss are listed in Box 14-6.

End-of-Life Issues

Unfortunately, while end-of-life issues are real and affect all health care professionals who handle terminal patients, the majority of professionals have very little if any training in end-of-life issues. This is further affected by the fact that many professionals do not know how to talk realistically and comfortably to patients about end-of-life issues, nor do patients wish to engage in advanced end-of-life discussions or planning. While the Institute of Medicine issued seven recommendations for dealing with end-of-life issues in 1997, very little training exists. Despite the push for Advanced Directives and the advances made in pain control, many patients die without their wishes carried out. Worse yet, many die a painful and horrific death.

According to an editorial by Gary S. Wolfe, "While we have made significant advances in medical care and the critically ill as a result of new treatments, procedures and medications, recent studies showed that 40–80% of the patients with terminal illnesses were *inadequately* treated for pain—even though pain is treatable." He also says that health care professionals are often frustrated at not having the resources or skills to effectively and efficiently manage end-of-life issues. "Consequently, reimbursement for end-of-life care ranges from over-utilization, under-utilization or no-utilization."[64] Wolfe further states that as CMs are in a pivotal position to influence quality of care and quality of life for terminally ill patients, they must do following:

- Acknowledge that problems exist with end-of-life care
- Commit to improving end-of-life care
- Effectively ensure the patient's pain including accompanying symptoms is prevented or relieved
- Prevent or manage physical and psychologic symptoms that present during the advanced illness
- Advocate for system changes when needed
- Conduct research on end-of-life care
- Measure quality of life and other outcomes of care for dying patients
- Participate in or lead public discussions about end-of-life care
- Know all available provider resources for end-of-life care
- Identify one's feelings or issues surrounding end-of-life care[64]

To manage patients with terminal illnesses, it is important to educate them about their rights, encourage them to have an advanced directive in place that specifies their last wishes, and ensure they have the care and support that they require.

Ethics

Ethical issues shift as health care practices change. For example, much has changed during the past several years as technology has advanced and health care in general is seeing a much older more technologically dependent population. We have also seen societal changes as well. Many years ago, patients believed that the things their doctor said were gospel. Now patients question and make demands to the point that health care has become a perceived right.

Ethics in health care is about choices and morals. Ethical issues are influenced

---

BOX 14-6
Change and Loss Interventions

- Assess clients for ability to cope with change and loss
- Assess clients for suicidal risk
- Facilitate verbalization about change and loss
- Assist clients to develop and utilize coping strategies
- Promote positive relationships with others
- Use positive reminiscing to promote a positive outlook
- Discuss the future with hope
- Give the elderly control where possible[62]

by free choice as well as our professional and personal values and morals. Ethical dilemmas are more difficult as one must often select a course of action that may result in an undesirable outcome.

Facing an ethical dilemma is an inevitable and almost daily function with health care professionals. This is true as in making the best decision, there is not always a clear choice between what is right or wrong. The best choice may seem right to one but not another, or may often result in an undesirable outcome such as death.

CMs continually balance the needs, wants, and concerns of all parties—the patient, family, physician, payer, CM's organization—with varying goals and expectations. For example, these can run the gamut from individual patients to families and from generic to case-specific issues. Dilemmas occur for all ages. Although there is a finite number of ethical challenges, each case can present a new twist to a problem. Examples of ethical dilemmas often include the following:

- A patient and family will not consent to a do not resuscitate (DNR) when the patient is faced with a life-threatening illness or injury and health care professionals know that if a code occurs and the patient survives the outcome, the costs of care will be horrific.
- A baby is born with multiple anomalies that are almost incompatible with life, yet the family wants everything done.
- A patient is borderline incompetent and refuses nursing home placement despite all indications of need for a nursing home.
- A battered spouse or elderly person elects to return to a known abusive situation.
- A patient without a signed advanced directive does not wish treatments, but family members are insistent.

- Family members want one approach and argue with other family members who want another approach.
- A pregnant mother refuses an abortion when it is known there will be adverse birth defects.
- A pregnant mother refuses an abortion when she has a medical condition that is incompatible for a pregnancy and the end result will probably be death to both or a premature birth for the fetus with unknown outcomes for survival or care.
- A family wants a loved one removed from life support but meets resistance from the medical team as a clearly defined advanced directive was not in place (this scenario often happens with young children).
- A patient and family cling to hope and go from one treatment center to another in hope for a cure.
- A medical professional places false hope on a hopeless situation.
- Balancing what is right for one patient and not considering it for another.
- Balancing personal wants with the possibility of accepting kickbacks (e.g., wanting to attend a seminar knowing there is no reimbursement from the employer or enough personal money to cover the cost, yet vendor sales staff propose payment in full in exchange for kickbacks, such as referrals).
- Balancing what is best for the patient while operating within financial constraints or limits of what the CM's organization or the payer wants in return.
- Balancing what to include in a report versus what not to include (a huge dilemma for nurses working in the workers' compensation arena).

- Rationing health care resources as costs continue to spiral and insurers and payers attempt to maintain their bottom line (e.g., Medicare does not cover drugs, and many insurers only cover generic drugs). If a patient needs a brand-name drug, the patient pays out-of-pocket or does without it. If they do without the drug, it often leads to a disastrous outcome. Also, there are times when the payer is on a different course other than what the physician or CM feels is necessary for good patient care.
- Becoming emotionally invested and taking a personal stance that interferes with professional judgment.
- As a patient advocate, wanting to offer the patient more than the payer or the organization allows.

Nurse CMs are in a perfect role to educate patients and families to articulate their wants and views on an issue and hopefully keep cases from going to court. Unfortunately, some ethical issues will go to court, and the court's decision doesn't always solve the issue. Many cases in the court records validate this issue. The most famous case is that of Nancy Cruzan. Her case is the impetuous for the Patient Self-Determination Act of 1990. Today, every patient entering a hospital is affected by this Act, as they must be aware that they have the right to sign an advanced directive.

It is imperative for those involved in case management to be cognizant of the importance ethical competency has on case activities and decision making. This need is enforced by the 1991 professional standards published by the American Nurses Association (ANA). These standards hold all nurses accountable for ethical practice, regardless of their role and affiliation. For more information on the standards, see the ANA website at www.nursingworld.org/.

Today, nurses are legally liable if their practice is ethically deficient.[65] Ethical conflict is inherent to health care. Among the forces contributing to this conflict are factors such as the following:

- The multiple therapeutic options available for most health problems and the lack of consensus about their medical effectiveness, benefits, and burdens
- The raging debate about who should get how much of our scarce health care resources and the increasing tendency to dismiss certain patients as poor investment risks or simply unworthy of indicated medical care
- The condition of moral pluralism; the fact that we seem to grow more heterogeneous daily in our religious and cultural beliefs and values[65]

What then are the components of ethical competence? Taylor indicates that ethically competent nurses are able to do the following:

- Be trusted to act in ways that advance the best interests of the patient entrusted to their care
- Hold themselves and colleagues accountable for their practice
- Act as effective patient advocates
- Mediate ethical conflict among the patient, significant others, health care team, and other interested parties
- Recognize the ethical dimensions of practice and identify and respond to ethical problems
- Critique new health care technologies and changes in the way we define, administer, deliver, and finance health care in light of their potential to influence human well-being[65]

To meet the challenges of ethical competency the following characteristics are necessary:

- Commitment to patient well-being—The nurse's first challenge and core responsibility is to be committed to the patient and to keep the entire system of care and the caregiving team focused on meeting the needs of the patients it purports to serve.
- Responsibility and accountability—As systems for delivering health care are fragmented, it is not unusual for patients to flounder through the system not having their needs addressed or met. CMs are in the perfect role to assume responsibility for monitoring the effectiveness of the plan and ensure all disciplines are held accountable.
- Ability to act as an effective advocate—CMs are in the perfect position to ensure the system works and the patient's needs are met in all levels and settings for care.
- Ability to mediate ethical conflict—CMs need to be skilled in identifying patients, families, and caregiving teams that are at risk of ethical conflict and in addressing the issues contributing to the conflict.
- Ability to recognize ethical dimensions of practice—CMs must be able to recognize such ethical dimensions and know when and how to intervene.
- Ability to critique the potential to influence human well-being—CMs must be able to critique new technology and the chances they require (e.g., administration, delivery, financial impact).[65]

Not every organization has an ethics committee. Those organizations that do are at an advantage because this type of committee often takes the burden of the final decision making off a specific individual—often the attending physician. The core membership of an ethics committee includes physicians, nurses, clergy, an attorney, and at least one layperson. The ethics committee is given a chance to review both the patient's medical records as well as an update of the patient's present status and a realistic prognosis. All possible treatment options are discussed, and various ethical tools are applied before a decision is made.

Despite the fact a CM may not have a case that is presented to the ethics committee, it is wise to attend one. A CM can learn to be better equipped to handle ethical issues from this experience. If a committee is not available, attend educational sessions to learn how to handle issues. Better yet, network with seasoned colleagues to discuss ethical issues and potential ways to resolve them.

SECTION V—SPECIAL COMPLEXITIES

As one can see by the listing of diagnoses appropriate for referral and possibly case management, CMs often deal with the sickest of sick, many with multiple comorbid diagnoses, one equally as complicated to deal with as another. There are no rules for the management of patients because every patient, family, and situation is unique. In addition, each case is affected by the patient's or family's coping ability or emotional stability, the intensity and severity of the illness or injury, the intensity and complexity of the care required, and the resources available or required to prevent rehospitalization or deterioration of the patient's condition. These variables affect all decisions made as well as the patient teaching required, the barriers to discharge, the overall case management plan, and the outcome. As stated earlier, the CM's own organization and its policies, procedures, and criteria dictate the type and level of case management offered and the scope and depth of care planning. However, the final medical case management plan is often based on the following components:

- The treating physician's orders
- The standards of care for the illness or injury outside the acute care facility
- The patient's actual physical and psychologic needs
- The family's or caregiver's physical and psychologic needs
- The financial means or resources available to pay for the care
- The availability of resources to meet the patient's level of care

In all cases, the orders or services requested must be based on the patient's individual needs and must be specific to the patient or ordering physician. Standards of care for the community, region, or facility affect the success of any case that requires continuity of care. Because of the importance of standards of care, CMs must be familiar with the standards that affect health care providers and the health care delivery system. This familiarity must encompass local, regional, and national standards. Recent legislation has also changed how health care payers must act on experimental issues or clinical trials. Without this knowledge, case management of all patients, especially technologically dependent patients, is likely to be unsuccessful. CMs must remember that what might have been done for one patient may not be necessary or appropriate for another. The same is true for hospital versus home care. What can be done in an acute care facility may not be possible in the post-acute health care arena. The case management plan, if developed and employed correctly, serves as a guide to obtaining access to care and linking patients to the necessary resources in a time-efficient manner as well as ensuring that resources are used effectively as the patient moves through the continuum of care.

Because many case management clients have multiple diagnoses and multiple needs, referrals are necessary to all resources specific for each diagnosis or issue. For example, if a patient with severe diabetes has an amputation that is further complicated by a stroke and cancer, referrals to community agencies for all three diagnoses are in order. In this case, the American Diabetes Association, the American Heart Association, and the American Cancer Society may be among the agencies utilized. Services from these agencies can range from information, education, and support groups to volunteers. In most cases, the services obtained from these agencies will augment or enhance the patient's health care benefit coverage and the services reimbursed by the health care payer.

Head injuries may result in dual diagnoses (e.g., medical needs and psychiatric needs). When this occurs, the medical CM and the mental health CM must confer and determine which diagnosis is paramount. Likewise, they must decide which discipline, mental health or medical case management, is to assume responsibility for coordinating the resources necessary to manage the patient's care appropriately. Regardless of which CM assumes the primary role, mental health and medical benefits, resources, and services must be coordinated if both problems are to be treated.

Far too often, roles overlap or role conflicts occur in patients with dual diagnoses. Likewise, there is potential for fragmentation and gaps in the care provided and the establishment of resources available to aid the patient. These gaps and fragmentation of care can be avoided through close collaboration and excellent communication among all CMs involved. These two keys are essential if the patient is to meet the goals established by the health care team.

Unlike psychiatric diagnoses, managing patients with a medical and psychiatric diagnosis, a medical and addictive diagnosis, or a combination of all three presents a real challenge. These dual diagnoses often complicate the recovery process and at times the success of the case management plan. Dealing with dual diagnoses takes careful coordination of the patient's health benefit package and use of medical and mental health benefits. When CMs find they are managing a patient with dual diagnoses, it is wise to ensure a mental health CM or social worker is also assigned to the case. Therefore a joint case management plan can be developed that ensures both conditions are treated adequately and linkage to applicable resources and services occurs in a timely manner. Also, the CMs must ensure their individual medical directors or applicable physicians, psychiatrists, or other mental and medial health care providers are involved with case planning.

As stated in the postacute care section of this text, health care professionals repeatedly hear that home is the best place for patients because they do better in their own surroundings. However, this is not always true in today's era of patients being discharged when they require very complex care. Home care can be very expensive and worse yet, it is not always appropriate for every patient. Therefore, when home care is contemplated, some basic factors must be considered. The following four factors can serve as guidelines in determining whether the patient can benefit from home care, whether the cost is reasonable and acceptable to the health care insurer, and whether out-of-pocket expenses for the patient and family are manageable:

1. The patient is ambulatory and can seek care provided by specific outpatient services, programs, or providers; if this is not true, it must be determined whether the patient meets the criteria for homebound care and whether the level of care can be adequately provided by home health care providers.
2. The patient's medical, psychologic, or psychosocial needs require continued care or supervision that can be provided in a home setting.

3. The home environment is conducive to the treatment plan and to achieving the desired goals.
4. The costs of the home care plan are comparable to or less than inpatient alternatives (e.g., continued hospitalization in an acute care facility, skilled nursing facility, subacute care facility, or rehabilitation unit), but the quality of the care is essentially the same.

For many patients, the costs of basic nursing care and equipment necessary for home care may exceed thousands of dollars per month. Not included in the costs are other charges (e.g., physician home visits, outpatient laboratory or radiologic services, pharmacy charges) for services that are necessary to meet the patient's needs. Thus, when evaluating all costs, home care can be far more expensive than placement. In other cases, numerous daily visits by professionals (e.g., nursing, physical therapy, speech therapy, occupational therapy, laboratory, radiologic services) requiring out-of-pocket patient copayments can make home care financially impossible for many patients. Consequently, out-of-home placement until the patient's condition is medically stable and can be managed more easily at home is usually the best plan.

Children with Special Needs

Children with disabilities differ from adults with disabilities in a variety of ways. With this comes a myriad of ethical issues and dilemmas. Working with chronically ill or technology-dependent children presents its own special challenges. Not only are there differences in patient care management techniques, but CMs must deal with the needs of the pediatric family and their own emotions as they relate to children with special needs in general. In addition, children with special needs and their parents, especially if technologically dependent, consume large amounts of case management time and resources. Also, there are three major differences in dealing with children versus adults:

1. The changing dynamics of child development affect the needs of children at different developmental stages and alter their expected outcomes. Illness and disability can delay a child's normal development (sometimes irreversibly).
2. The epidemiology and prevalence of childhood disabilities with many rare or low-incidence conditions and few common ones differs markedly from that of adults in which there are few rare conditions and several common ones.
3. Because of children's need for adult protection and guidance, their health and development depend greatly on their families' health and socioeconomic status.

Nationwide the number of children with chronic and special needs currently receiving Supplemental Security Income (SSI) is approximately 1 million. Of this number, the following are estimated:

- Approximately 50% have mental or nervous system disorders (about 90% of these with a primary diagnosis of mental retardation and 10% with behavioral disorders)
- Approximately 30% have respiratory diseases
- Approximately 10% have musculoskeletal disorders (e.g., cerebral palsy)
- Approximately 10% have other disabilities

In general, most programs consider children with special needs as individuals age 22 or younger who are disabled, receiving SSI, and their chronic physical developmental, behavioral, or emotional conditions require services of a type or amount beyond that of other children.[66]

It is important to note that the Personal Responsibility and Work Opport-unity Reconciliation Act of 1996 changed the definition of disability for children under the Supplemental Security Income (SSI) program. The definition of disability for children now includes the following:

- The child must have a physical or mental condition or conditions that can be medically proven and which result in marked and severe functional limitations.
- The medically proven physical or mental condition or conditions must last or be expected to last at least 12 months or be expected to result in death.
- A child may not be considered disabled if he or she is working at a job that is considered to be substantial work. However, the law did not change the rules that allow certain children already on the rolls to continue to receive SSI even though they are working.

The law also changed the way certain behavioral problems caused by a child's condition or conditions are considered. The law requires that the child undergo continuing disability review (CDR) to determine whether or not the child remains disabled. As such, the CDR must be done as follows:

- At least every 3 years for recipients under age 18 years whose conditions are likely to improve
- Not later than 12 months after birth for babies whose disability is based on their low birth weight

Any individual who was eligible as a child in the month before he or she reached 18 years of age must have his or her eligibility redetermined. The redetermination will be done during the 1-year period beginning on the individual's 18th birthday.

With these statistics in mind, it is critical that as case management models are designed to assist children with special needs, the model must integrate both acute and chronic services while allowing for a family-centered and community-based system that focuses on the child and family. The family must be an equal partner in all health care decisions particularly when it comes to choosing the child's primary care physician and in the development and implementation of the treatment plan and case management plans and the care processes.

As plans are developed, they must be designed using a multidisciplinary team approach. The team should include the child, family, primary care physician, specialty physicians, CM, and other health care professionals as needs are identified. The team must develop an individualized and comprehensive plan that will serve as the foundation for the delivery of health care services. Included within the plan must be components that will be supported through public programs such as the school district, the state Title V/Children's Medical Services programs, and the Department of Mental Retardation or Developmental Disabilities. As SSI or Medicaid may cover many of these children, it is important to include services traditionally mandated by Medicaid for Early, Periodic, Screening, Diagnosis and Treatment (EPSDT) in the treatment and case management plans. As such, the plans must include routine treatments and services needed to support the physical or medical needs of the child as well as services such as immunizations, vision and hearing screening, and preventative well-child visits. Once developed, the plans must be updated at least every 6 months or sooner if there are significant changes in medical condition or further needs that are reflective of EPSDT services and any entitlement to other funding programs.

This update is necessary as many children will have private health care insurance as well as eligibility for many public programs that include the following:

- Public health clinics

- Title V/Maternal and Child Health block grants
- Title X/Family Planning programs
- Public schools, particularly those receiving services as a result of the Education for All Handicapped and Individuals with Disabilities Education Act (IDEA) Amendments of 1991 (including Part H—Early Intervention for Infants and Toddlers with Disabilities)
- Women, Infants, and Children (WIC) nutrition program
- Head Start
- Pediatric Vaccine Programs[66]

When working with children and their families, it is very important to evaluate all funding programs to which they might be eligible. This is important as many programs have age limits but if referred by a specific age, services can be provided long-term. Using strategies such as this helps optimize child health outcomes and assists parents with care and other services traditionally excluded or limited by benefit provisions of the private health care insurance.

Although children with relatively minor special health care needs may require double or triple the expenditures made on average healthy children, an estimated 5% of children with special health care needs account for slightly more than 35% of the health care costs of all children and adolescents. These children have more complicated disabilities (e.g., multiple, lifelong and/or technology-dependent) that compound their needs. These children often require such services as subspecialized and inpatient care, often at tertiary facilities; ongoing complex outpatient management; community-based services; home nursing services; and a multitude of medical supplies and DME (often requiring customization).[67]

In 1988, the Task Force on Long-term Health Care determined that "...all technology dependent children should have the opportunity for family centered, coordinated and community-based care." Home care shifts responsibility from the team of medical caregivers to the family. Before a child is sent home, the family needs to be made aware that no matter how stable their child, there is always the possibility an emergency situation or death is a potential outcome. With home care, it is imperative that families be trained to ensure they are capable of caring for their child in the event a nurse is not present. It is also imperative that someone be trained as a backup caregiver, especially when round-the-clock nursing is not provided or available.[68]

As with all complex cases, early discharge planning, preparation, and training of the family for events is critical. Moves or referrals made without planning will almost always have disastrous consequences. When a high-technology dependent patient is discharged, especially to home, a multitude of services must be put in place. However, although home care is desirable for many reasons, it is not always applicable or the best choice for every child, family, or medical condition. Families who do not wish to establish a home plan must be supported in this decision. If a child is to be discharged to a facility, it is critical that parents be allowed an opportunity to familiarize themselves with the facility and staff prior to the transfer. As discharge approaches to home or a facility, it is essential to involve the parents in the transitional phase so that they can become familiar with the specifics of care (e.g., suctioning, feeding, medication management, equipment use, and troubleshooting). As the CM works with the family, he or she will have the ability to view the family and their responses to providing the care. This will also allow the opportunity to assess potential options for alternative care if needed.[68]

As most families will desire to take their child home, CMs must be very familiar with any state Medicaid waivers as services to children were expanded with passage of the Omnibus Reconciliation Act of 1981. The Omnibus Act enables children to be cared for at home as part of Model Waiver programs. These waivers are separate programs from traditional Medicaid.

It is necessary to be familiar with the waiver programs as the application process is arduous and it is common to encounter long waiting lists. More importantly, there will be times when the hours allocated under the waiver may not be sufficient to meet the needs of the child. In cases in which traditional Medicaid covers the child, the child will qualify for inpatient services but not home care services. This is generally due to the fact that care needs are greater than can be provided by a home care agency and, as the hours allocated are insufficient, the child is not eligible for a waiver.

Children with disabilities and other chronic conditions often require the services of pediatric subspecialists in addition to primary care pediatricians. Access and availability of pediatric subspecialty services must not be significantly impeded. Despite the fact that it is contrary to managed care thinking, CMs may need to advocate for a complex pediatric patient to ensure the child has a pediatric subspecialist as a primary care physician. This is especially true when the child's health insurance is linked to a managed care plan. It is ideal for the primary care physician to manage and coordinate the care for most children they serve. However, the complexity or rare nature of a particular child's condition frequently makes it difficult for the primary care physician to meet all needs of the child and family adequately without additional expertise.

In addition to any medical care, all children regardless of their illness or injury are entitled to a free and public education. However, to assist parents in locating educational resources that can meet their child's needs, an excellent website primarily designed for TRICARE beneficiaries (military) is at www.odedodea.edu/communities/. TRICARE's websites are an excellent resource when educating families of children with special needs about other types of resources available.

The Aging Disabled

With technology and the advances in science and medicine, people are living longer. Aging takes on a special significance when combined with chronic disability. When superimposed on physical disabilities, normal changes of aging may lead to functional changes at an earlier age than that encountered in the nondisabled population. Without effective case management services, there is often decreased access to medical and therapeutic services after school-age years. For example, adults with cerebral palsy often present with chronic back pain from poor trunk control or posture; scoliosis; cervical spine pain; sequelae of hip dislocation and spastic deformities of the feet and toes; and a high incidence of bowel, skin, cognitive, and dystonic problems. In the nonambulatory group, musculoskeletal wasting increases the risk of osteoporosis and renal calculi with pulmonary and vascular complications further intensified. Consideration must then be given to the physiologic changes associated with aging and the increased reliance upon medical services and personal care needs.[9]

With aging and disabilities come a variety of problems. Unfortunately, many of the aging disabled do not qualify for Medicaid. As a result, the elderly person is caught between whether to pay for food and shelter or medicines. This age category is further hit with the ever-decreasing availability of affordable housing for low-income families and the elderly. When the aging disabled have special housing needs, there is often not enough money to cover the costs of home modifications or copayments needed for simple equipment. There is often not enough money to cover equipment that allows independence if it is deemed as a convenience and not medically necessary. This factor alone forces many elderly into board and care homes or other assisted living facilities. Thus, as CMs work with these patients, it is very important to ensure an individualized plan so that appropriate linkage to resources to meet patient needs will occur.

Patients with Factitious Disorders

Factitious disorders are defined by DSM-IV as the "intentional creation or feigning of physical or psychologic signs and symptoms in absence of external incentives for such behavior." A CM using observation, history taking, and review of medical records and claims are often the first ones to suspect a factitious disorder. Fortunately, most CMs will rarely encounter patients with factitious disorders. However, it is important to realize the need to be cognizant of the facts surrounding detection of this disorder. Factitious disorders are commonly discovered when one finds a patient who is a poor historian, yet has a medical history of frequent hospitalizations, surgeries, and other invasive procedures and there are marked discrepancies in comparisons with physician reports, current medical data, and the patient's perception of their medical history. While there are many elements of factitious disorders, patients predictably will do the following:

- Deny self-harm refusing to be unmasked
- Be skillful at eluding detection
- Be legally competent and able to make health care decisions
- Like to be the center of attention
- Seek help but then often refuse it
- Not be motivated to be involved in sustained treatments
- Have a long history of procedures or hospital admissions
- Often be aggressive

- Often have disruptive tendencies yet be very believable
- Often not be good historians
- Often express competence in coping with typical life stressors, but may minimize or smooth over shortcomings or faults
- Threaten malpractice
- Often flee the care of an attending physician or hospital when exposed

Further characteristics include the following:

- Growing up in a family of somatizers
- Being raised by parents who were demanding and unrewarding when they were well but caring and loving when they were ill
- Experiencing an environment in which one or more coping mechanisms for dealing with psychosocial crisis are unavailable
- Developing a repertoire of actions used to withdraw from usual life activities or to engage or punish others
- Consciously feigning illness to attain something to avoid punishment or responsibility or to avoid required duties
- Being raised by parents who were excluding or rejecting or in broken homes that lead to foster home placement or adoption[69]

There are five specific motivations for individuals to maintain the ruse:

1. Manipulation of interpersonal relationships
2. Privilege of the sick role including sanctioned dependency (one may conclude then that this disorder is quite cultural)
3. Financial gain
4. Communication of ideas or feelings that are somehow blocked from verbal expression
5. Influence of intrapsychic defense mechanisms[69]

An essential element in factitious disorders is to get one's psychologic needs met through the assumption of a sick role.[70] Factitious disorders, somatoform disorders, and malingering represent various degrees of illness behavior characterized by the process of somatization. Somatization is a process by which an individual consciously uses the body or bodily symptoms for psychologic purposes or personal gain.[69]

As CMs work with this category of patients, they must understand that factitious disorder patients often will not respond as hoped and they will continue to feign or induce illness despite all interventions. This reflects the challenges inherent in the treatment of such patients. It is critical while working with these patients that CMs build rapport and continue at every avenue to reinforce positive health behaviors while encouraging the patient to maintain a consistent treatment plan with the attending physician and encourage a multidisciplinary treatment and evaluation approach.[70]

Malnutrition

CMs have a unique opportunity to easily incorporate nutritional screening into routine or socioeconomic and medical assessments. One of the first steps a CM can take in this area is to assess all patients for risk factors that contribute to malnutrition. The greater the number of occurrences or characteristics and the longer they persist, the greater likelihood that poor nutritional status will ensue. When assessing patients, the risk factors to assess for are as follows:

- Inappropriate food intake (assess meal or snack frequency, quantity and quality of food groups, self-imposed modifications or compliance impact, or substance abuse)
- Poverty (access to and choice of food and ability to pay for food after housing, utilities, medications, and other expenses are paid)

- Social isolation (primarily the elderly, but any person who experiences loss of family, friends, or support systems; income; independence; self-esteem; and situations where loneliness and possibly depression has set in). Assess support systems, living arrangements, cooking and preparing food, and how shopping is done.
- Weight loss or gain (a recent change of 10 pounds in body weight). Assess meal or snack frequency; quantity and quality of food groups; new or increased medication usage, including over-the-counter medications; and change in mental status.
- Dependence or disability. Assess functional status including ADLs and instrumental ADLs, inactivity and immobility as physical decline can impede mobility and the ability to perform self-care activities, including shopping, meal preparation, and eating
- Acute or chronic diseases or conditions (recent hospitalizations, surgery, trauma, and infections have the ability to affect weight). Assess over and under body weight, alcohol use, cognitive and emotional impairment such as dementia and depression, poor oral care, pressure sores, and sensory impairments
- Chronic medication usage (this increases the potential for adverse effects of drug-nutrition interactions, metabolism, and drug absorption due to malnutrition). Assess use of all drugs whether prescribed or over-the-counter, poly-pharmacy, vitamins and mineral supplements.
- Advanced age (chronologic age and functional capacity do not always equate). Evaluate the individual's circumstances and ability to function)[71]

Using screening assessments to identify appropriate patients, CMs have six referral sources to assist in implementing planned interventions when nutritional deficiencies are uncovered:

1. Social services
2. Oral health
3. Mental health
4. Physician or pharmacist
5. Nutritional education and counseling
6. Nutrition support

As organizations implement nutritional screenings and implementations, most will not be required to "re-invent the wheel." Successful nutritional screening programs are built on existing health plan systems of care. Some of the possible ways to screen patients for nutritional deficiencies and malnutrition include the following:

- Telephoning as part of welcome-aboard calls or periodic check-in calls
- Mailing as a stand-alone a nutritional screening form referred to as a Short Form 36
- Inserting screening forms in new member or client packets
- Printing screening forms in existing plan newsletters
- Having screening forms available in physicians' office waiting areas
- Offering screening forms at wellness programs or through employer-sponsored events
- Handing out screening forms after group tours of a health plan[71]

The processes for incorporating nutrition screening and interventions into routine care are essentially the same used to diagnose and treat a patient with any health problem. Therefore, organizations should consider the following:

- Much of the data regarding risk factors for malnutrition have already been collected (e.g., persons already have their height and weight, alcohol and medication usage, and functional status recorded, which can be used as a tool to identify risk for nutrition-related health problems).

- Most of the professionals who need to implement nutritional interventions are already involved with the patient's care.
- Knowing a patient's nutritional risk identifies where there is a greater need for early intervention or utilization of services. For example, in some cases a patient may need a referral to a dietitian or social worker or to be enrolled in a disease management program; therefore interventions such as these bring early involvement of the team members into the case.
- Nutritional screening and interventions ensure more effective and appropriate use of staff time and services before health problems are exacerbated by poor nutritional health.
- Because most patients will have only a few risk factors or indicators of poor nutritional status, interventions may be simple and few.
- Benefits to the patient and to the health care provider far outweigh the temporary adjustments of adding new nutritional screening and intervention programs.[6]

Patients and their families must be aware of and able to respond to the warning signs of malnutrition and to ensure the patient receives a proper diet that is healthy, balanced, and offers variety. Caregivers can learn these warning signs of malnutrition: unplanned weight gain or loss of 2 to 3 pounds over a 7- to 10-day period; dry skin; noticeable daily hair loss; loss of grip strength or inability to use an eating utensil; decrease in urine output; concentrated urine; constipation; lethargy or fatigue; or the slow healing of wounds.[72] As one educates the caregiver and develops and monitors the case management plan, it is imperative to link any patient identified as at risk for malnutrition to a dietitian. Here the dietitian can help develop a nutritional plan that is individualized for the patient and his or her disability (e.g., dysphagia, special diets, living alone) (Table 14-1).

Difficult Wounds

Many cases followed by CMs will have compromised outcomes due to difficult-to-heal wounds. Difficult-to-heal wounds can result from a variety of conditions such as burns, punctures, and cuts (inflicted by accidental trauma or induced passively or intentionally); traumatic injury; diabetes; peripheral vascular disease; complications following surgery; rheumatoid arthritis; congestive heart failure; arterial or venous ulcers; lymphedema; and many other conditions or activities in which circulation is compromised. Additionally, it is a known fact that infection is very common in patients with diabetic ulcers, and this often is the leading cause of tissue necrosis, sepsis, gangrene, and added costs to the overall health care bill.

CMs can play a critical role as providers struggle to provide quality cost-effective care for wound care management. This can only be done through the reduction of hospitalized timeframes, achieving faster recovery, accomplishing a higher rate of limb salvage, and preventing prolonged or permanent disability. To ensure optimal outcomes, CMs must assume a leadership role in educating patients and managing the utilization of services and supportive devices, medical supplies, or other related items needed for wound care management. At the same time, it is critical they keep informed of the latest technology, approved treatments, dressings, and clinical protocols. Candidates for wound care management include patients with pressure ulcers, venous stasis ulcers, ulcers on ischemic limbs, and neuropathic ulcers. Motta indicates that diabetes and its complications have increased sixfold since 1958, mostly due to overweight Americans.

TABLE 14-1
Diagnoses or Conditions That Are Considered High Risk for Nutritional Deficiencies

Adult	Pediatric
Aging	Bronchopulmonary disease
Burns	Burns
Cancer	Cancer
COPD	Congenital disorders
Diabetes	Cystic Fibrosis
GI and pancreatic disorders	Developmental delay
Heart disorders	Failure to thrive
Hepatic failure	GI disorders
HIV/AIDS	Hepatic disorders
Impaired wound healing	HIV/AIDS
Inflammatory bowel disease	Inborn errors of metabolism
Metabolic stress	Obesity/Pickwickian syndrome
Obesity	Solid organ or bone marrow transplant
Renal failure	Type I diabetes
Short bowel syndrome	Ventilator dependency[73]
Solid organ or bone marrow transplant	
Ventilator dependency	

HIV, Human immunodeficiency virus; *AIDS*, acquired immunodeficiency syndrome.

Yet 6% of the population (the number with diabetes) accounts for 15% of total health care costs—$119 billion spent annually. Consequently, these patients should be a CM's primary focus.[18]

Over the past 5 years, many advances have been made in wound care. This includes products now available due to advanced technology and due to the fact that we now have many professionals who specialize in wound care. It is through this combination of expertise and new techniques that wounds can aggressively be managed. As a CM, it is critical to ensure wound patients are linked to appropriate professionals as early as possible in their diagnosis and treatments. This will help to ensure simple wounds do not turn into chronic complicated ones.

Unfortunately, what often happens is patients stay with their primary care physicians and family practitioners too long or insurers want the cheapest treatment modality available or delay making a coverage determination on an expense treatment modality. So it ends up costing more.

This includes total wound care costs and patient suffering in terms of pain and infections, at a minimum. Often by the time the patient is referred, limbs are lost and wounds that might have been healed earlier are now chronic. This means healing and treatments will be long-term.

In addition to the use of new wound care techniques, another key will be timely referrals to specialists, aggressive and early interventions, and patient education. Some of the new wound care techniques include any one or more of these techniques at a given time:

- Regranex, a platelet-derived growth factor that stimulates healing and has proven to be tremendously beneficial for wound care in appropriate patients
- WoundVAC (a vacuum-assisted device that applies negative pressure to the wound to facilitate closure)
- Hyperbaric oxygen therapy (HBOT), which is also the primary therapeutic modality for patients with carbon monoxide poisoning and those

with air or gas embolism; it has proven to be an important adjunctive therapy for many other conditions including gas gangrene, radiation tissue damage, compromised skin grafts, crush injury, acute traumatic ischemias, necrotizing soft-tissue infection, and chronic refractory osteomyelitis

- Deep, sharp debridement to remove necrotic tissue from the wound helps minimize the risk of infection
- Wet-to-dry dressings
- Gel dressings (sheets, granules, or liquids)
- Warm-up therapy
- Moist wound healing, which is currently the most advanced wound-care technique; these dressings fall into six categories: thin films that are transparent but waterproof; hydrocolloids; alginates that are absorbent; polyurethane foams; hydrogels; and collagens
- Silver dressings
- Many new wound care dressings that make it possible to have wounds cared for on an outpatient basis thus avoiding costly inpatient care

As wound care is incorporated into the overall case management plan, the CM must ensure the resources and frequency of care necessary for reassessments are identified. The assessments most often needed on a regular basis include the following:

- **The wound**—This must be assessed at least weekly or sooner if deterioration of the ulcer is noted
- **The patient's medical condition**— This must be assessed to watch for other complications such as amyloidosis, endocarditis, maggot infestation, meningitis, peptic arthritis, systemic complications of topical treatment, and signs of infection. Preventing infection in wounds is

the key to rapid and successful healing. New dressings are providing health care workers with an edge in the fight against wound infection, and careful monitoring in the early stages of healing can dramatically reduce the probability that complications will develop if infection occurs, treatments will be implemented earlier, and the overall costs of care reduced.

- **The patient's nutritional status**—A nutritional assessment should be performed at least every 3 months for patients at risk for malnutrition.
- **Pain**—This must be assessed at regular intervals to ensure the causes of pain are identified and ensure pain medications are effective and adjusted as necessary.
- **The patient's psychosocial or socioeconomic status**—This must be reassessed at regular intervals to ensure the environment and financial resources are adequate to ensure adherence to the treatment plan.

As more surgery and wound-care patients are discharged earlier and cared for at home, patients and their families will be increasingly responsible for participation in the care of the wounds. Thus, education will play a key role if risks are to be minimized and compliance to treatment is to occur.

The many changes brought about by the Balanced Budget Act of 1997 (BBA) have significantly affected case management and at times impeded a successful transition of care. As changes brought about by the Act are implemented onto different health care providers (skilled nursing facilities, home health agencies, and outpatient clinics), the Act is also bringing changes in reimbursement for wound care patients. The Act now places a new reimbursement method, the prospective payment system (PPS), onto home health agencies as well as skilled nursing facilities; thus, their ability to effectively manage some wounds is impeded.[74]

For example, under PPS for a skilled nursing facility, payment is not based on the level of care provided but on what level has been documented. Medicare now pays a fixed amount each day based on a person's documented specific care. Separate billing for supplies is now a thing of the past. In addition to other services, the new PPS amount also includes all therapy services performed (physical, occupational, and speech).

The basis of the payment is derived from what is termed the Resident Assessment Instrument. Within this rests assessment and screening elements referred to as minimum data set (MDS) that are used to evaluate each resident. MDS is a tool used to assess the skin condition of all Medicare residents in long-term care facilities and requires providers to assess pressure and stasis ulcers using a I to IV staging system. The evaluation continues and includes service blocks known as Resource Utilization Groups (RUGS) that categorize anticipated treatments per diagnosis. Wound care falls under the following two RUGS:

1. Residents receiving treatment for pressure or stasis ulcers on two or more body sites or who have a surgical wound or open lesions
2. Residents with clinically complex wounds (e.g., burns, septicemia, or foot wounds).

Staff documenting on the MDS play a critical role in the final reimbursement for the facility. Failure to include all needs or follow timeliness standards established by Medicare can have severe financial consequences.[74]

In late 2000, Medicare implemented its new home health prospective payment system (PPS) and made changes to its Part B surgical dressing policy. The main goal of this new payment system is twofold:

1. To control runaway costs

2. To consolidate payment for all Medicare Part A home health benefits into a single payment the agency receives for each 60-day episode of home health care.

This new payment methodology requires home health agencies to operate under a very different wound care philosophy—an enormous task for agencies that have not trained their staff and physicians to provide state-of-the-art wound care and have not tracked their clinical and economic wound management outcomes.

For payments under PPS and most insurance rules (if medical necessity guidelines are met), the following services are covered:

- Both primary and secondary dressings are covered when either of the following criteria are met: they are medically necessary for the treatment of a wound caused by or treated by a surgical procedure; or they are medically necessary when debridement of a wound is medically necessary.
- If a surgical procedure or debridement is necessary, it must be performed by a physician or other trained health care professional and to the extent permissible under State law. Debridement of a wound may be mechanical, surgical, autolytic, or chemical. Dressings used for mechanical debridement are also considered a covered benefit.
- Surgical dressings must be ordered by a physician, nurse practitioner, clinical nurse specialist, certified nurse-midwife, or physician's assistant acting within the scope of his or her legal authority as defined by state law or regulation.

The documentation needed for Medicare or insurance reimbursement for wound care and supplies includes the following:

- History, previous treatment regimens if applicable, and current wound management

- Dressing types and frequency of change
- Changes in wound conditions, including precise measurements, quantity of exudate, and presence of granulation and necrotic tissue
- Concurrent measures being addressed relevant to wound therapy (e.g., debridement, nutritional concerns, support surfaces, positioning, and incontinence control)
- Documentation that supports regular evaluation and treatment of patient's wounds
- Monthly documentation of quantitative measurements of wound characteristics including wound length and width (surface area) and depth and amount of wound exudate (drainage) indicating progress of healing
- A signed order by the physician or other health care provider legally allowed to sign such orders must be present, and this includes the following:
  - Type (category) of dressing
  - Size of dressing
  - Number or amount of dressings to be used at one time (if more than one)
  - Frequency of dressing changes
  - Expected duration of need
  - A new order is needed when a new dressing is added, the quantity of an existing dressing increases, and at least every 3 months even when the quantity remains the same

While most skin and wound care professionals are familiar with Medicare's requirements for reimbursement of dressings and supplies, CMs must be equally as familiar. This is necessary because most insurers follow Medicare guidelines and criteria.

Medicare's DMERC

In 1993, the Health Care Financing Administration (HCFA; now the Centers for Medicare & Medicaid Services [CMS]) and the Department of Health and Human Services (DHHS) entered into contracts with four carriers to perform all duties associated with processing claims for DME, prosthetics, orthotics, and medical supplies (DMEPOS) under Part B of the Medicare program. These four carriers were designated as Durable Medical Equipment Regional Carriers (DMERCs), and they include the following:

- **Region A DMERC**—BlueCross and BlueShield of Western New York, operating as HealthNow NY. Region A covers Connecticut, Delaware, Maine, Massachusetts, New Hampshire, New Jersey, New York, Pennsylvania, Rhode Island, and Vermont.
- **Region B DMERC**—AdminaStar Federal. Region B covers Washington DC, Illinois, Indiana, Maryland, Michigan, Minnesota, Ohio, Virginia, West Virginia, and Wisconsin.
- **Region C DMERC**—Palmetto Government Benefits Administrators. Region C covers Alabama, Arkansas, Colorado, Florida, Georgia, Kentucky, Louisiana, Mississippi, North Carolina, New Mexico, Oklahoma, South Carolina, Tennessee, Texas, Puerto Rico, and the Virgin Islands.
- **Region D DMERC**—CIGNA Health Care Medicare Administration. Region D covers Alaska, American Samoa, Arizona, California, Guam, Hawaii, Idaho, Iowa, Kansas, Mariana Islands, Missouri, Montana, North Dakota, Nevada, Nebraska, Oregon, South Dakota, Utah, Washington, and Wyoming.

If a CM has questions about wound care supplies or other Part B coverage of services, these carriers are often the most valuable for resources and are willing to send applicable information about Medicare's stance on an issue.

SECTION VI—CAREGIVERS, TRAINING, AND OTHER POINTERS

Caregiver Statistics

While caregiving can be needed at any age, a survey conducted by the National Alliance for Caregiving (NAC) and the American Association of Retired Persons (AARP) revealed that 22.4 million U.S. households, accounting for about one-fourth of the population, are involved in caring for an elderly relative. The Census Bureau estimates that more than 4 million Americans are older than age 85 years and forecasts this same age population will grow to about 18 million in the next 30 years. CMs will play an increasing role in helping adults develop plans for older parents as they carry on their own personal responsibilities.[75] Unfortunately, it is estimated that only 6% of employee benefit plans offer in-depth programs for family or bereavement leave or for programs to help employees cope with a terminal illness or a terminally ill family member. According to the Department of Labor, approximately 30% of employees have caregiving responsibilities for an elderly relative, but 54% expect to assume a caregiver role within the next 10 years. According to MetLife, aggregate expenses of caregiving costs American business approximately $11.4 billion annually in lost productivity.[76]

As professionals know, the core of any team starts with the patient and family. Professionals can plan, and the plan can be ideal. However, if input and agreement from patient and family is not sought, plans, while good in intent, are doomed for failure. Thus, if plans for care are to be successful, the patient's and family's buy-in and acceptance are critical. Also, if case management is to likewise be successful and caseloads kept within reason to allow for new cases, the CM must continually strive to maximize the patient and family's ability to assume the role of the CM so that they can advocate for their own needs.

While working the case, the CM must set up appropriate resources, ensure the patient is at the right level of care at the right time, and also teach the patient and family how to assume the role as soon as possible.

Where does one start when teaching the patient and family to be a CM? A CM needs to start on day one of involvement with the patient. While there are many factors to be taught, a key element will be empowerment. To ensure the continuity of care, six basic requirements must be satisfied in the process of training the family to manage their own case. These requirements are as follows:

1. Identification and early referral to case management must take place, and all CMs must be introduced early to the patient, family, and health care team. Early referral allows time to build trust, rapport, and confidence. Also, the patient and family must have someone to guide them through difficult situations in which they can learn first-hand how to manage their case.

2. Planning any case requires open, frequent, honest, and personal communication with all involved. As stated repeatedly in this manual, good communication is critical to prevent misinterpretation, duplication, fragmentation, omissions, and discrepancies in care. Good communication ensures that the plan meets the patient's needs and that it is implemented in a timely and effective manner when the patient exhibits readiness for discharge. It also allows the patient and family to express their ideas and input, strengthens their confidence, and helps them to build communication skills in preparation for their assumption of the CM role. Good communication also

allows the ability to promote self-responsibility. To avoid miscommunication and unrealistic expectations of patients and families, the CM must take every opportunity to engage the patient in open and honest conversations, always seeking the patient's perceptions.

3. Crisis intervention mechanisms should be included in the plan to ensure that crisis atmospheres (which are common with case-managed patients) are alleviated. The use of a social worker or clinical psychologist is an excellent resource that can assist in this area. Personal experience validates that some of the best discharges and case management plans are those in which the social worker and CM work hand in hand with the patient and family. In situations such as this, the CM assists the patient and family in establishing ties with community resources, and the social worker helps them with coping skills. Provision of these mechanisms reassures the family and patient that they will not be abandoned in a crisis. More importantly, if a written guide or a list of resource personnel can also be given, these tools can be used for assistance when they are on their own and working through the crisis themselves.

4. A keen awareness on the part of the CM to all available community, regional, and national resources and the patient's entitlement to their use builds the trust and confidence of the patient and family. This awareness is the pivotal element in case management and determines the success or failure of the plan. This often occurs when referrals are not limited to individual health care providers but frequently encompass a broad array of medical health care resources as well as social, financial, or other supportive formal and informal services or resources. Referrals may be made for direct care skills, counseling, meals, attendant care, respite care, support groups, transportation, or out-of-area placement. If the patient and family are involved in the decision-making and provider selection process and are given tips on how to access resources, they gain the confidence they need when they must do it on their own.

5. Teaching the patient and family the physical care techniques and how to access resources and exercise their appeal rights is required. Patients and family must know how to refuse to take a simple no from community resources or a denial from their insurer and how to insist on receiving all denials formally in writing. This allows them to file a formal appeal and exercise their rights to services to which the patient may be entitled. If the request is related to reimbursement, referral, or provision of services and is denied, the patient and family must be educated as to their appeal rights and the levels of appeal available to them. If the request for services or denial relates to an acute condition, the CM must educate the patient and family as to the requirements and processes related to an expedited review or appeal. Expedited reviews and appeals are available to patients when they involve the following: preadmission requests (acute, SNF, rehabilitation, or psychiatric); continued stay denial (acute, SNF, rehabilitation, or psychiatric); a reduction in home health services

(nursing or therapy); preservice arrangements for ambulance transportation services a physician deems urgent; out-of-plan urgent service requests; and requests related to a medical condition considered terminal or the patient's life, health or ability to regain maximum function may be jeopardized using the standard appeals and review process. While the standard appeal process is limited to 30 days, the expedited appeal determination must be rendered within 72 hours of the filing of the appeal. For an expedited preservice referral, the request likewise must have the final determination made within 72 hours of the referral.

6. Patients and families must know when and how to obtain access to a professional CM or other support system if their own attempts at case management or gaining access to care and resources fail.

Empowerment

Key to the success of a person becoming his or her own CM is the ability to assume the responsibility to become one's own advocate and obtain successful outcomes. This is necessary as a professional CM or a medical professional may not be available long-term to "advocate" for the patient or their family when it is needed the most.

As chronic illness or injury frequently results in lifelong care needs, services needed to maintain quality to one's life are not episodic. Bartering and obtaining authorizations for necessary services whether the person is a professional or a layperson requires skill and finesse and will be an ongoing process during the patient's lifetime. Appropriate advocacy does not occur when frustration or anger prevail. It does not occur when one is intimidated with the "system," afraid to speak out or ask pertinent questions, and

seek a higher authority for an answer. Therefore, it is important that patients and families must be taught as soon as possible the power or ability to act as their own spokesperson if they are going to be CM.

Empowerment to be a CM must start immediately or as soon as the reality has set in that long-term care will be needed. Empowerment is important as access to a professional CM may be in the early stages of the illness or injury. However, this luxury does not last long. In today's medical health care arena, lengths of stays are shorter and in most cases funding for specific services such as case management is limited to short-term episodic "skilled-care events." When long-term care is needed, it is frequently classified as "custodial," and the patient and family are frequently left to fend for themselves. Thus, other than a public payer such as Medicaid, the payer sources and the services provided are no longer existent.

As the patient or family starts the process to be CM, one often encounters fear and lack of assuredness of how to tackle the necessary tasks. Thus, they need a guide from whom to take direction and learn. One key element as one teaches is to stress the need for them to take notes and ask questions no matter how simple or "stupid" they may feel the questions are. They also need to observe what and how the professional does the bartering or negotiation for services and care. The professional CM needs to help them and serve as the mentor until they feel comfortable in speaking up and assuming the role as their own advocate.

How does empowerment occur? It is very simple. The patient and family must learn all they can about the medical condition. They must know their rights to health care. They must know what coverage they have and what is covered versus what is excluded. How is this done? By researching the medical libraries, the Internet, or the literature that is available from national and local community agencies. Additionally, their member handbook from the insurer must become their "Bible"; they must be familiar with their insurer's appeal and grievance processes as well as what their state regulatory agency allows. Equally as important is to know their state's rules and regulations related to specific health care issues. For example, in most states this will be the Department of Insurance or, if the patient is a member of a Health Maintenance Organization, the Department of Managed Health Care. By all means, they need to be encouraged to not be afraid to take actions such as the following:

- Writing questions down prior to any visit to the doctor or encounter with the health care workers; it is key to ensure they ask the questions and get an answer.
- Asking about their rights of appeal or due process should they get a "no" answer; it is key to inform them that they must request a written denial.
- Asking for clarification or written directions to what has been said when the reasoning for an action is unclear; they have problems understanding the language as they are frustrated, tired, or angry; or they do not understand; it is key to obtain written directions or bring another person to appointments.
- Seeking a second opinion when they are unsure of their treatment and they desire an option prior to consenting to the proposed treatment or they are unhappy with their current treatment plan; it is key to know their health care rights, how the insurer views second opinions, and if they are protected by laws that allow second opinions.
- Learning to proactively speak up for what they feel is right or needed. The patient may have to change doctors if they are unhappy or dissatisfied with the care or approaches taken. The patient may initially have to deal with supervisors or leaders of the organization for answers prior to making changes. In some instances, the patient may have to write letters to state their case or file a complaint, grievance, or appeal about their dissatisfaction. As a final resort, the patient may have to propose litigation.

There are several keys to becoming one's own CM. Three keys will be honesty, ability to communicate effectively, and ability to not be intimidated while seeking help or attempting to access services or resources. Other keys include the following:

- Knowing their rights as "informed" health care consumers and having available concrete information that supports their views (e.g., drug literature, literature from scientific-based studies, their appeal rights)
- Learning all they can about the medical condition and what treatments are available ("standards of care" treatments as well as those classified as "experimental" or "investigational")
- If the treatment is experimental or investigational, knowing where they can seek help (e.g., from national agencies such as the American Cancer Society and the National Institutes of Health) so that they have as much information as possible about the following:
  - Knowing what treatment and processes will be involved
  - Locating centers of excellence that participate in the studies and then calling them and speaking with the clinical nursing staff or doctors about their case, options, costs, and other requirements of participation in the study (if not a

candidate, what other options might be available)

- Reading and knowing what insurance benefits they have, the limitations or exclusions, and their out-of-pocket costs; this means reading their health insurance benefits handbook (if they do not have one, CMs must educate them of the importance of calling for a copy and of always having a current copy readily available
- Knowing their appeal rights should they encounter a "no" or denial and knowing the importance of requesting all denials in writing
- Keeping accurate records, notes, and copies of their medical records
- Being honest and open with their physician and other health care professionals involved with their care
- Learning to be proactive versus reactive
- Researching local community, regional, and national resources and learning what community or national resources are available to help with either direct services, information, or literature
- Learning definitions and the "lingo" of health care

Knowing their rights as a consumer involves reading their insurance handbook and reading information supplied by their state's Department of Insurance or other regulatory body for health care insurance (e.g., Department of Corporations or Department of Managed Health Care). It also entails seeking advice from local support groups and from persons who have been in similar situations as they are encountering. It also includes researching their rights by reading laws and regulations, many of which are on the Internet and can be found by typing in *Patient Bill of Rights*. Other key websites for patient rights include the following:

- www.cms.hhs.gov/media/press/release.asp?Counter=40

- www.cms.hhs.gov/media/press/release.asp?Counter=7
- www.nami.org/update/unitedbill.html
- www.cc.nih.gov/ccc/aboutcc/partners/billrights.html

Information can also be found by visiting a local library, medical library, or local state law library. All states have what are called administrative codes for how they will enforce federal laws as they pertain to health care provided under such Acts but not limited to the following:

- Social Security Act and Title 18 and 19 (Medicare Title 18 and Medicaid Title 19), Children's' Medical Services (Title V of the Social Security Act), and the many amendments to the Social Security Act
- Americans with Disabilities Act of 1990
- Privacy Act of 1974
- Individuals with Disabilities Education Act of 1991
- HMO Act of 1972

Patient and Family Chart

Taking notes and keeping accurate records in some form of a chart is vital to the patient's or family's success as a CM. This action equates to a professional CM documenting findings. Therefore, patients and families must be shown how to start and maintain their own chart.

To do this, they must be encouraged to keep copies of all pertinent medical records, especially history, physicals, consultations, and discharge reports generated by their physicians and other health care professionals.

In addition, they must be encouraged to keep records that validate the dates and times they called their physician, agency, or other health care provider for support or services. Also, if they actually filed a hard copy of an application with an agency for a service, they must be encouraged to keep copies of all on file in their chart.

It does not matter how information is filed in their chart, as long as it is filed and available when they need it most. As we know, the best way to maintain a chart is by keeping all documents in chronologic order by dates of service and separated by type in separate labeled folders or sections of a binder or expandable file (e.g., receipts, medical records, notes made of calls, and letters in different sections).

Addressing Needs

As CMs work with families, it is important to ensure their needs are addressed as well as the patient's. This is especially important if they are to be given the information they need as well as an opportunity to cope with the realities of the situation. By sharing accurate information, the patient or family become empowered and are able to make informed decisions and gain the ability to gain understanding and a feeling of control. Some key needs that require astuteness and attention by the CM (this may mean delegating the task to another nurse if the patient is hospitalized) are as follows[77]:

- Families cling to hope, which can create a delicate balance between giving too much or too little
- Families want their questions answered honestly
- Families want to know the prognosis
- Families want specific facts about the patient's progress; if hospitalized, this would be on a daily basis
- If hospitalized, families want to see the patient frequently
- Families want to know what is being done and why
- Families want an opportunity to speak with the physician; if hospitalized, this would be on a daily basis
- If hospitalized, families want to be called when the patient has a change of condition

- If hospitalized and the family cannot make it to the hospital, families want a designated nurse with whom they can speak to for updates
- If hospitalized, families want to be told about transfer plans
- Families want to feel accepted by the staff
- If hospitalized, families want to know what they can do at the bedside
- Families want to talk about the possibility of death

To fully assess caregivers and their abilities, some organizations use a battery of testing tools developed by a variety of universities and organizations. The tools used often include the following:

- Caregiver questionnaire as the one offered by theSilberstein Aging and Dementia Research Center (ADRC) at New York University
- Caregiver Physical Health Questionnaire
- Patient Physical Health Questionnaire
- Social Network List and Satisfaction Scoring
- Family Adaptability and Cohesion Evaluation Scale
- Short Psychiatric Evaluation Scale
- Affective Rating Scale
- The Burden Interview
- Memory and Behavior Problems Checklist
- Caregiver Home Evaluation (ADRC)
- NEO Personality Inventory

Care of the Caregiver

Long-term care is the most common reason for caregiver stress and burnout. Often this is not a life-and-death issue but is just from the day-to-day routine of needs of the total care patient. While long-term care is one of the most common reasons for caregiver burnout, additional reasons include:

- Lack of help to provide the care required

- Lack of sleep, rest, or respite for the caregiver
- Lack of socialization for both the patient and caregiver

If CMs or other nursing personnel are involved with the care, they are often in the best position to detect signs of stress. As such, they can serve as a safety net before families reach the breaking point. Expressions regarding the illness and its resultant care, feelings of isolation, and signs of exhaustion are often the three warning signs of caregiver stress and the ones nurses should heed. Other common signs are depression, hyper-responsiveness, lashing out, a sense of hopelessness, anxiety, and argumentativeness.[78] Therefore, as CMs work with caregivers they must make every attempt to ensure linkages to support groups, respite services, and financial resources including any resource appeal rights and processes are included. They must also work with the health care team to ensure the caregiver is using proper body mechanics as care is rendered.

There are times when a CM may have to give the caregiver permission that it is okay to take a break. Keep in mind that the best way to help patients and their caregivers is to tailor the case management plan and its interventions to all individuals (patient and caregiver) involved. As stated earlier, although some families are resilient and are able to cope, others are not. Many family structures may be stressed to the point of abandonment, frequent arguments, abuse, or divorce. For these reasons and others, care of the caregiver and family is as important as care of the patient. If the caregiver system fails, the consequences may be deterioration in the patient's condition or costly rehospitalization.

Serving as a caregiver frequently places a heavy burden on the family mentally, physically, and at times financially. If the caregiver system fails, often the case management plan fails. Therefore, the overall plan must address appropriate training of the caregiver or caregivers and the necessary resources they will need to perform the caregiving role. Caregiver burnout is possibly the number-one reason for unnecessary anger and frustration for all parties, and the result is costly and unnecessary readmissions or neglect of the patient.

The ability to cope with stressors is affected by many factors, some of which are related to past experiences in dealing with crisis situations. It is also dependent upon the emotional well-being of the patient and family, their ability to cope in general, and the actual situation or circumstance causing the stress or crisis. Although stressors are not limited to the following situations, CMs commonly encounter the following factors and emotions:

- Feelings of frustration are present because the patient and family believe they are receiving conflicting answers or are not receiving the "true story" (e.g., they may have difficulty in communicating with or in obtaining access to the medical staff or absorbing what is said).
- Tempers are on edge and denial is the primary coping pattern.
- Feelings of hostility emerge owing to the unfairness of the situation or because the patient and family cannot accept the changes that have occurred in bodily functions or in body image (e.g., loss of the ideal or "normal" image of self or loved one).
- Emotions are so high that they only hear what they want to hear.
- Exhaustion results from countless sleepless nights, worry, improper nutrition, and hurried hygiene; thus, personal needs are forgotten.
- Feelings of disbelief are present, and they cannot believe the situation is happening to them or the condition might not improve.

- Feelings of overwhelming guilt occur and the effect of the responsibility they must face may or may not have set in.
- Fears of the unknown are always present and the effect of finances, bills, and care responsibilities may or may not have set in; although it is often not spoken, the fact that death is a real possibility is in the background.
- Feelings of frustration and anger with the "system" are common when denials are issued and resources or services are unavailable, limited, or not affordable.
- As chronicity sets in, other stressors arise such as those related to lack of help, respite, financial assistance, loneliness, isolation, and exhaustion.

As the patient's condition changes or becomes chronic, it is common to see many or all of the foregoing reactions. To assist in identifying any stressors and to prevent social isolation or escalation of the situation, it is imperative to link the patient and family with disease-specific support groups or agencies, professionally trained counselors, or social workers and document it in the case management plan. From these resources and peer support systems, the patient and family can learn how to cope and more importantly, how to navigate the health care system.

Social Isolation

Social isolation is a reality for many technologically dependent patients and their families. It must also be addressed and solutions given for prevention in the case management plan. As a result of social isolation, patient and caregiver are forced to be with each other twenty-four hours a day. Situations such as this frequently result in extreme stress for all parties. In addition, family structures are often stressed to the point of abandonment, neglect, or abuse of the patient, frequent arguments, or divorce. CMs must continually stress the need of the caregiver to take care of themselves. They must be encouraged to research their community for sources for socialization for both themselves as well as their patient. Social isolation is frequently due to situations such as the following:

- The patient and family live apart.
- The burden of care is overwhelming, the family or caregiver is physically and emotionally exhausted, and an outing "is not worth the effort."
- Moving all the equipment and supplies for an outing is too tiresome and overwhelming.
- The family's car or mode of transportation is inadequate to accommodate the patient and all the equipment. In some cases, there is no car because the patient and family rely on public transportation.
- Family members and friends may react negatively or be repulsed by the physical condition of the patient and some of the care that is required.
- Families and patients are embarrassed about the patient's disabilities or appearance.
- After paying for medical expenses that are not covered by the health care insurer, the patient and family cannot afford other expenditures even if they are for fun and offer a means to "get away."

The foregoing list is by no means all-inclusive, but it gives some idea of why social isolation and caregiver burnout can occur if arrangements for socialization and respite are not included in the case management plan. To encourage socialization, the CM should at a minimum urge patients and families to join disease-specific support groups when they are available. Disease-specific organizations and support groups are an invaluable resource for patients. In these groups, the patient and family can learn firsthand how to solve problems and can share ideas. The power and ability these groups have with peer support are immeasurable.

The power of community disease or injury-specific support groups cannot be underestimated. Patients and families can be with persons in similar situations or with similar feelings. In most cases, many of the same supporters have already encountered similar situations or feelings and can help the new patient and family work through issues. In these groups, both caregiver and patient can learn by sharing firsthand how to solve problems or traverse the health care resource or health payer maze. Also, groups such as these often have the power in numbers that are needed to make changes.

Whether disease-specific, church, or ethnic, support groups are an invaluable resource and an economical way to get the support and guidance the patient or family will need. These groups offer the support needed to "cope," and they offer an excellent outlet for socialization.

Consumer Information and Teaching

Historically, the consumer's voice has been silent as the patient's physician or other health care professional spoke for them. However, this is changing and consumers are more aware and educated than ever before. There is a wealth of information now available to consumers. Consumers can now rely their physician as well as the Internet, radio, magazines, television, newspapers, lectures, and seminars as they attempt to become informed. Unfortunately, some of the information is misleading as it is haphazardly obtained, there is no uniformity or consistency in how it is supplied, and often it is only in English.

As CMs work with patients and educate them on how to make wise informed choices, patients must be given good, clear, understandable information that describes the following:

- What they need to know about their disease and care
- What their benefits, exclusions, and limitations include
- What the cost of care will be
- How the health care delivery system works
- How to locate and use resources
- How to appeal a health care decision
- How to resolve a complaint
- How, why, and when they should contact their health plan directly or an ombudsman or state agency

When consumer information is developed and then used, it should do the following:

- Provide information that will empower all consumers to make informed decisions about their health care. Empowerment must be for all levels of ability to understand, in various languages, and from a variety of sources. From the information, patients must be knowledgeable enough to make informed decisions about their choices regarding medications, treatments, physicians, facilities, or the right to refuse care.
- Provide as much information as is required by the patient to address his or her individual needs including alternative choices.
- Improve communication among consumers and health care professionals. The communication must also be enhanced among those who administer health care plans and expect consumers to understand and use the plans effectively.
- Be provided in a manner so that it can be received and acted upon by all potential users (it must be tested for understanding by all levels of users; as a result, many organizations use a fifth grade reading level for publications).
- Aid and encourage effective use of the health care system.[79]

Teaching

In all cases, teaching of the patient and family is of critical importance. Teaching and a means of monitoring the teaching-learning process throughout the duration of the case must be incorporated into the case management plan. While a great deal of teaching will be started while the patient is still hospitalized, in many cases it will continue after discharge. During training, the family and patient must have a professional to oversee its effectiveness. More importantly, the professional must remain involved until the patient or family or both are proficient in all aspects of care.

In planning an educational program for teaching patients, it is important to keep in mind the learning barriers that affect how materials are received. These six barriers are as follows:

1. Literacy level (it is best to assume most patients will have a low reading level)
2. Resistance to instructions (remember many people are in denial)
3. Cross-cultural differences (language as well as other cultural barriers)
4. Professional and layperson differences (health care professionals have their own spoken and written language, lingo, abbreviations, and symbols)
5. State-dependent learning (an educational theory concept of a person's receptiveness to learn under various conditions; studies show that a person recovering from anesthesia has a learning level no higher than someone who is drunk)
6. Budget constraints[80]

The CM may not be involved in the development of the training materials used. However, it is very important that the CM, at a minimum, has knowledge of what is presented to his or her patients. This also means going over the material with the patient to ensure learning indeed did occur.

If the patient is hospitalized, teaching is not an option; the Joint Commission on Accreditation of Healthcare Organizations (JCAHO) mandates it. Despite the setting, any teaching undertaken must take into account the physical and psychologic influences and their impact on a patient or family's readiness to learn. If the patient is the one to be taught, many of the following examples must be taken into consideration as the teaching plan is developed: pain, weakness, nausea, drowsiness, manual dexterity, cognitive abilities, shock of the illness, depression, denial, and refusal to participate.

Some patients and families simply refuse to participate in any teaching. Learning cannot be forced. For learning to occur, the patient or family must be willing and cooperative with the plan. Otherwise the information will not be accepted or absorbed. Patient and family education must do the following:

- Facilitate and enhance a patient or family's understanding of the health care status, options, and consequences of options selected
- Encourage patient or family participation in decision making about health care options and their rights to making an informed decision
- Increase the patient or family's abilities to follow the proposed health care plan
- Maximize the skills necessary to render actual care
- Increase the patient or family's abilities to cope with the illness, health status, and prognosis
- Facilitate and enhance the patient or family's role in continuum of care
- Promote a healthy lifestyle as well as maximize functional abilities and the ability to remain in the least restrictive environment

Due to the complexity of care required by most case-managed patients, teaching and mastery of all care techniques, troubleshooting of problems, and correction of problems are the most vital of all the processes needed in planning for a move to an alternate level of care. Teaching is even more vital if the alternate level of care is to be the patient's home. Occasionally, patients being discharged to a postacute care facility will require care that is so complex that the facility staff may require training in the specific details of the patient's care before the transfer is allowed.

Although training the family concentrates on direct hands-on care, it is not limited to this type of training. Sometimes teaching in the early stages of an illness may center on issues such as gaining an understanding of the specific diagnosis, performing common techniques such as ADLs, and proper body mechanics as care is rendered. It may also include such issues as gaining access to and use of resources, making lifestyle changes, planning the diet, and making decisions.

Studies show that patients retain only 10% of the information given to them in teaching sessions. To augment teaching, it is important to use visual demonstrations, books, audiovisuals, and handouts as often as possible. As the patient's and family's readiness and receptivity increase, they can review the material as needed. Studies show that informational material is best understood if it is written in large print at a sixth grade level and contains several illustrations.

CMs and all health care professionals must keep in mind that patients and caregivers must become as familiar with care techniques (skilled and nonskilled) as health care professionals. Unlike professionals who may be in the home for a relatively short period of time during the day or week, the family or caregiver often assumes responsibility for care for the greater part of a 24-hour day, 7 days a week. More importantly, patients and families are expected to learn in a relatively short period of time what it may have taken the health care professional weeks or

years to master. So, as the training program is developed, keep this fact in mind.

Naturally the substance of teaching varies in each case, but for all patients it must be started as soon as possible. Every patient who is capable of self-care must be taught this care or allowed the opportunity to learn it. With all patients, active participation in their own care must not be limited merely to their physical ability to perform the actual tasks. Self-care must encompass physical care as well as the chance to contribute actively to the choices and decisions necessary for care. Physical self-care for many patients is not always possible. However, the ability to contribute and make informed decisions helps patients do the following:

- Reduce their fears and anxieties about the unknown
- Alleviate passive dependence on others
- Encourage motivation and compliance

If self-care is to be effective, it must be a collaborative effort between patient and teacher. The teacher must allow ample time for performance of tasks and be patient if they cannot be completed in a reasonable time frame. Likewise, the creativity involved in performing a task must not be thwarted if the patient's method accomplishes the same result. Choices about how to accomplish the care are individual. Such choices are not the teacher's decision but the patient's because the patient must live with the consequences.

The key to teaching is that *every* body system must be assessed thoroughly and all physical needs must be identified. From this needs assessment checklist, a plan for teaching can be developed. Possibly one of the best means of assessing each body system is to use a predeveloped questionnaire or checklist that can be modified to meet individual teaching needs. In the course of asking questions, if other issues surface that may have an impact on the final plan, notes must be added to the checklist to ensure that these issues are captured and addressed in the plan. Because proper teaching is so critical for home care, many case management organizations have developed assessment forms for their staffs. If such a form is not available, one can be developed using the guidelines listed below. When properly developed, this assessment checklist serves as the database for the teaching program. Assessments for teaching must be inclusive and all needs identified addressed. Teaching for all patients must encompass at least the following areas:

- Understanding of the disease
- Knowledge of the drug (action, side effects or toxic reactions, dose)
- Care of intravenous catheter and venous access site, if applicable
- Safe handling and storage of the drug and disposal of waste products
- Signs and symptoms of complications or problems
- Nutritional needs, hydration and antiemetic use, pain control, and bowel elimination regimen
- Procurement of DME and other medical and nonmedical supplies
- Troubleshooting of equipment, infusion therapy, tubes, etc.
- How to use community resources and agencies and how to ascertain availability
- Techniques, strategies, and resources to use for coping with the illness, psychosocial changes and limitations, physical changes, and, at times, death

Keep in mind that the list of issues to be covered when one teaches can be extensive just for the basics of care. Add to this any other teaching the family may require (such as care of the patient with diabetes or a transplant or wound care), and the list becomes even more extensive. Not only must the family or caregiver be trained in all aspects of the care required, they must

also know basic information about body mechanics, infection control, how to protect themselves when lifting or moving the patient or handling waste, soiled linens or dressings, and how to manage all equipment. Teaching of such information is necessary because in many cases the caregiver will be alone and if injuries or infections are to be prevented, training in basic care and preventative techniques is imperative.

Once the teaching needs have been identified, the teachers of each task must be assigned and an actual teaching schedule agreed on by the caregiver, patient, and teacher. Because not all teaching can be done on the day shift, teachers must be found on all shifts. This ensures that the teaching schedule is maintained and kept within the time parameters established, thus minimizing delays in discharge.

One of the best ways to identify who will be responsible for teaching each task is to have a predischarge conference with as many team members as possible present. At this time, teaching duties can be assigned and one team member can also be given the responsibility of serving as the primary teaching coordinator. The patient, family, and all health care team members who have the day-to-day responsibility for care should attend team conferences such as this. These conferences must also include all postacute care health care professionals who will be responsible for continued teaching, monitoring of the teaching-learning cycle, and the ongoing care for discharge.

Teaching Tools

Teaching tools vary but in most cases training consists of basic hands-on care. In some cases, teaching can be accomplished by using audiovisual materials and written literature. Depending on the facility, teaching can be further augmented by a home care manual. This manual enforces teaching accomplished and, more importantly, serves as a reference tool once caregivers are on their own.

Both patients and families benefit greatly when teaching is started long before discharge. Early teaching and actual practice of the physical care techniques required alleviate some of their concerns. The benefits are further enhanced if the family is allowed to troubleshoot problems and issues with professionals nearby. For technology-dependent patients with long-term hospitalizations, one of the best ways to validate the fact that teaching has been successful is to allow the patient a trial weekend pass (or several) before the actual discharge occurs.

Trial Passes

Although allowances for trial passes are health plan and facility specific, a trial pass (generally 48 hours) is critically important in the care of any technologically dependent patient because it allows an opportunity to identify areas that may require additional teaching. For a trial pass to work as intended, it must be remembered that all equipment, supplies, and staffing must be in place just as they would be if the patient were actually being discharged.

Depending on the patient and the rules and regulations of the facility or health care insurer, one mechanism that may be used when a pass is allowed is to simulate and actually plan for a real discharge (all dependent upon the approval of the attending physician). In this case, prior to the transfer home for the trial pass, the family makes all arrangements with the business office as if a discharge were to occur. A team member on each shift is identified who will assume responsibility for communication with the family during the pass. The family is given instructions in how and who to report to during the pass. If the pass is successful, this information is relayed to the business office and the official discharge occurs at the end of the trial pass. The patient is readmitted only if

problems arise or when additional training needs are identified. Use of such a plan can potentially save hundreds of dollars in unnecessary ambulance fees not to mention the stress and anxiety of readmission. Why readmit the patient only to discharge him or her home again, especially if success was the outcome the first time?

Postdischarge Planning Teaching

In many cases teaching continues even after discharge. In all cases, a mechanism for evaluating the teaching plan must be developed to ensure that monitoring of the plan continues throughout the duration of the care. It is important to identify a person who can assume a position after discharge similar to that of the inpatient teaching team coordinator. Someone must be responsible for performing ongoing assessments of teaching-learning needs and for identifying areas that require further teaching.

A postdischarge teaching plan is essential to ensure that what was taught prior to discharge was relevant and that the family is not encountering problems or not reporting them. It is common for the team not to hear from a patient or family if things are going smoothly. In other cases, families do not call at all because they feel their questions may be judged wrongly. Fortunately, others do call when unexpected problems arise or when they need reassurance.

On the proactive side, if case management continues after discharge by the same CM and a good relationship and trust has been established between both parties, the patient or family often confides in the CM realistically about the problems or limitations they encounter. In these cases, issues can be dealt with and the educational plans revised immediately. Such communication allows an excellent opportunity for continual monitoring of the teaching-learning process.

For some patients (e.g., respiratory or infusion therapy patients) much of the postdischarge teaching is continued by the respiratory therapist or the nurses affiliated with either the DME company or the infusion therapy company. As a rule, this teaching and any patient assessments, adjust ments to equipment or therapy, and report ing of responses to treatment to the physician are done at no additional cost. These professional disciplines are used because these services are included in the cost of the equipment or the overall nursing program established for use of the equipment.

Fortunately, for many case-managed patients, a home health agency is involved after discharge owing to the patient's need for skilled care. Such agencies and their staffs are in a perfect position to serve as the person responsible for monitoring the teaching-learning process on an ongoing basis. If a home health agency is not involved and case management ceases at the time of discharge, one excellent means of monitoring the teaching-learning process is to establish a callback system. Either a discharge planning team member, the facility-based CM, or the MCO's CM can be assigned this duty. Such a system allows an informal evaluation of the situation by a health care professional and offers a way to identify problems and find solutions before the problem leads to disastrous consequences. More importantly, it covers all patients and nothing is left to chance.

In all cases, ongoing teaching-learning assessments are necessary to ensure that additional teaching occurs when issues are identified. Additional teaching is necessary when new caregivers are found, new equipment is required, changes in procedures occur, and new skills are required or there are changes in the level of care or condition.

Assessing Caregivers for Their Equipment Needs

The equipment ordered for each patient depends on the diagnosis and the patient's specific medical needs and functional abilities. However, as the CM prepares the patient and caregiver for home care, an evaluation of the equipment needed by the caregiver in order to render care must be undertaken and is a critical element in overall planning.

While the equipment used by the caregiver is critical for ease of care of the patient, it rarely will be covered by the patient's health plan, as it will be deemed not medically necessary. As it will not be covered, the family must be educated of this fact. The most frequently ordered equipment that caregivers need includes the following:

- Hydraulic lift devices
- Hospital beds—where the caregiver can elevate the patient to an adequate height for the provisions of care
- Overbed tables—for convenience of the caregiver and ease of reach for items needed for care
- Commodes or shower benches

In all cases, decisions about selection of equipment must be based on its suitability for the patient's home care needs, lifestyle, and home environment. Early identification of equipment needs well in advance of discharge is critically important.

Physicians

There are going to be times when the patient or family is not satisfied with their physician or they wish a second opinion. When it comes to selecting another physician, if the patient is linked to an MCO they will be required to select another physician from the MCO's network and work with the MCO's member services staff. If not linked to an MCO, the patient should be encouraged to call the local medical society for physicians in the immediate area. If changes are made, they will be assigned their new physician at the first of the following month. While the MCO will discourage requests for middle of the month enrollment, this process is possible and they can accommodate the change as they have policies in place relating as to how to handle such requests. Such requests are "prorated" with each physician paid accordingly his or her fees for the month in question.

Patients and families must be educated when getting a reference from a person who is familiar with the physician. They must inquire as to the physician's capabilities and personality traits as well as their availability and promptness to appointments and telephone calls. Once a physician has been located, it is important to encourage the patient or family to make a "get-acquainted appointment" and draft some questions to ask during the appointment. Also, when they call to make the appointment, it is important that they listen to the receptionist's tone of voice to see if it seems friendly, and note whether questions are answered. They also need to make note of how long it took for the person to answer the telephone and how he or she handled interruptions. Examples of questions that patients and families may wish to ask include the following:

- Does the provider take the patient's particular insurance?
- What are their fees for routine office visits and do they expect only cash or payment at time of visit?
- What are the fees should the patient require assistance with any additional paperwork completed (e.g., insurance or other forms or applications)?
- What are their office hours and if important do they see patients after 5 P.M. and on Saturdays?
- How is coverage handled after the office closes?
- What hospitals do they use and have admitting privileges?
- What laboratories do they use for testing and are they reasonably accessible to the patient?

- What are the provisions for emergency or urgent care situations, including situations that occur during office hours?
- How are medication refills accommodated (must the patient see the physician before the prescription is refilled or can one be called in)?
- When an appointment is made, what is the length of time allowed for each patient with the physician?
- If they employ nurse practitioners or physician's assistants and the patient wishes to only see the physician, will these wishes be honored?
- Do they employ a CM or other personnel to assist them with teaching or accessing additional services or care should it be warranted?
- If the patient requires special provisions to access the office or use the bathroom, can he or she be accommodated?
- If the patient must take public transportation or rely on volunteers, can the schedule be flexible enough to accommodate the patient's arrival or departure?
- If the patient does not speak English or has poor understanding, what are the provisions for an interpreter?
- If the patient has specific cultural or religious preferences, is the physician willing to honor them?

Possibly the biggest barrier to good care or a lack of understanding is the lack of communication among physicians and patients. Traditionally, many people without question have accepted what a physician said as gospel. The feeling was whatever the doctor says must be true, so why ask questions? However, as health care has evolved and become more complex and families are now often geographically separated, this type of one-sided communication no longer serves anyone.

If a second opinion is requested, most MCOs allow this process. However, the actual process and authorizing body will be state-specific, and MCO-specific when the person is linked to an MCO. For example, in California, second opinions are legislatively allowed by the passage of AB 12, but in most cases the MCO is the one that serves as the approval body for such requests. For Medicare, there are no established standards for second opinions.

While the reasons for a second opinion will be varied, for complex cases with complex care needs, a second opinion is truly often what is needed if the patient is to be compliant with the treatment plan or accept what the attending physician is recommending.

Consumer Rights

Health care consumers in the United States have many health care rights. While some are not officially mandated, many large employer groups mandate that health plans offer certain rights. Among these include the following:

- The right to participate in candid discussions about medically necessary treatment options and decisions; this must be done in such a way that if the patient has difficulty in understanding or speaking the language or hearing what is said, an interpreter or person must be present during the conversations
- The right to refuse treatments or express preferences about future treatment decisions
- The right to change doctors or providers should the patient be dissatisfied with the current one; this includes the right to expect their medical information will be forwarded immediately to the new provider
- The right to have their medical information kept confidential, and if information must be shared with other doctors or providers it is only released if the patient grants approval

- The right not to be discriminated against regardless of age, sex, national origin, race, ethnicity, mental or physical disabilities, sexual orientation, genetic makeup, or source of payment for health care
- The right to treatments with specialists despite the fact the specialist may not be a provider in the patient's insurance company's network of providers
- If the patient has a complex or serious medical condition and requires frequent specialty care, the right to continue treatments with the specialist and have direct access to the specialist by virtue of an extended authorization; in some cases this may include issuing an authorization for up to a year at a time if the medical necessity of such an authorization can be justified
- If the patient is a woman, the right to have direct access, without prior authorization or direction from a primary care physician, to a gynecologist for her yearly examination
- If the patient, as a prudent layperson, feels his or her life is in serious jeopardy due to serious illness or injury, the right to access emergency services without prior authorization or direction from a primary care physician or a representative from his or her insurance company, regardless of whether he or she uses the insurer's emergency department or whether the event was emergent

In exchange for these rights, patients must also do the following:

- Take responsibility for themselves, maximizing health habits such as exercising, not smoking, eating a healthy diet, and having regularly scheduled checkups (not just seeing the doctor when they are sick)
- Become involved in their own health care and the decision-making

processes and carry out agreed-upon treatments and instructions from their physicians or providers. This includes asking questions about their diagnosis, treatments recommended, cost of treatments, side effects, and amount of time it may take. Questions they may ask include the following:

- If they have symptoms—"What do the symptoms mean and what can be done for them?"
- If the doctor prescribes a new medicine—"How often do they take the medicine?" or "Are there things they can or cannot eat, drink, or do when taking the medicine?" or "What side effects should they look for?"
- If a test is ordered—"What is the test for?" or "Will it make them sick?" or "Are there things they should or shouldn't do before the test?"
- If a treatment is ordered—"What is the risk of such a treatment?" or "What are the other options?" or "Can they get a second opinion before proceeding?" or "How do the benefits of the treatment compare with the risks?" or "What symptoms should they be worried about enough to call their physician?"
- If a treatment requires a hospital stay—"How long will they be hospitalized?" or "Will they need help after discharge?"
- Other questions may include— "Must they limit activities" or "What emotional reactions should they expect?"
- Inform their physician when a reaction to a treatment or medicine occurs or when their symptoms worsen
- Inform their physician when they cannot follow a treatment plan and the reasons why

- Take responsibility to provide, to the extent possible, accurate information about their health and medical history; this includes information about all medicines taken (those prescribed as well as over-the-counter), allergies, the number and types of surgeries, admissions to a hospital, or accidents
- Have reasonable expectations of their physician or other providers (e.g., don't expect to see the physician any time of the day or night) and know where to seek care in the event of an emergency when they cannot reach their physician
- Keep appointments and if they are going to be late or need to cancel them notify the physician or provider at least 24 hours in advance when possible
- Keep appointments within their allotted time frame by having questions or other information written in advance of the visit

Dealing with Death

While none of us like to deal with the topic, at one time or another death touches all our lives. While discussion of death may go unspoken, the reality is in the backs of the minds of many patients with chronic or long-term illnesses. We in the medical profession can certainly attest to the countless number of persons with chronic conditions who die without having the briefest of discussions with their loved ones about their wishes.

Therefore, as CMs work with patients and families and help them plan for death, patients and families must be encouraged to make arrangements as early as possible and avoid making decisions during a crisis event, where they may not be the same as decisions made in a noncrisis atmosphere. Also, the CM must be encouraged to locate, label, and store valuable documents in a logical place for loved ones to easily access. More importantly, documents should be current. What are some of the key documents and minimum information necessary? First and foremost, survivors must have a Social Security number and death certificate to activate many of the deceased's accounts and insurance policies or conduct business. Also, it is important to establish Advanced Directives that list the patient's desires for resuscitation, life support, and organ donation. Patients and families will also need to know the following:

- If the patient does not desire organ donation, whether there is a wish for the body to be donated to science
- If there is a will, the name, address, and phone number of the attorney who drew up the will
- Life insurance policies, including the following:
  - Policy numbers
  - Amount of coverage
  - Company names and phone numbers
- Burial arrangements, including the following:
  - Mortuary
  - Cemetery
  - Desires for cremation or burial
  - Where burial is desired (e.g., crypt, plot, private mausoleum) or if cremated what is to be done with the remains
  - Desires for the actual ceremony— a memorial versus no ceremony
- If the patient is retired and drawing benefits other than or in addition to Social Security:
  - Retirement papers that designate who provides the pension and/or retirement income
  - Addresses and phone numbers of who to contact for pension income
  - If the spouse survives, papers that validate what percentage of their

pension income designated as a "widow's allowance"
  - If the patient has an employer, union, or individual burial policy, the amount and how and where a claim can be filed
- If there are bank accounts:
  - Names of each bank, address, and phone number
  - Passbooks with the account numbers
- If there are stock or certificates:
  - Names of all accounts, addresses, phone numbers, and/or name, address, and phone number of all stockbrokers
  - If certificates, actual certificates
- If there is real estate property:
  - Addresses of all real estate properties
  - Names of all mortgage companies, addresses, and phone numbers
  - Next loan payment coupons
  - Deeds to all properties
  - Name of homeowners insurance company, address, and phone number
  - Tax records that show record of last taxes paid
- If the patient owns a car:
  - Pink slip, if paid for; if not, names, addresses, and phone numbers of loan company
  - Automobile insurance company name, address, phone number, and policy number
  - If license tags are soon due, if paid or not
  - Next loan payment coupon

SECTION VII—TRANSPORTATION, TRAVEL, AND OTHER ACTIVITIES

As CMs work with patients and families, it is important to add to the list of educational and training opportunities the importance of understanding the various modalities for travel and the importance of including recreational activities into their lives as soon as possible.

Recreational Activities

As a result of our society's emphasis on wellness, many communities now have a full array of recreational activities available to healthy as well as disabled individuals. Information about the recreational activities in one's region can often be located by calling the following:

- Local city parks and recreation department
- National Park Service
- Chamber of Commerce
- Centers that offer service to the disabled or offer training in independent skills
- Disease-specific or other community service agencies
- Easter Seals Society
- Services available from the local school districts
- Services available from local colleges
- Organizations such as Special Olympics

The recreational activities offered are designed to allow and encourage a physically or mentally challenged person to continue as active a life as possible since such activities are essential to one's physical and mental well-being. Recreational activities are no longer merely designed for the "normal, healthy" person. Programs for the physically or mentally challenged often include activities such as the following:

- Hiking
- Mountain climbing
- Camping
- Dancing
- Rafting/boating
- Basketball/softball
- Football
- Bowling
- Skiing
- Swimming
- Tennis
- Track and field
- Weight lifting

Unfortunately, for a variety of reasons some patients are not interested in participating in such activities and they may wish to take a more sedentary approach. While day care may not be the answer for many, for some it will be. Here the patient can play cards, get involved with crafts, or socialize by visiting with other patients. In some cases, low self-esteem will be present and the patient may require peer group support or professional counseling before acceptance of recreational activities is granted. In other cases, nothing will change the patient's mind about participation, and pressure will only create frustration and anger.

Transportation and Travel

CMs must also educate patients and families about transportation modalities that may be available. This will include any variety of modalities. Education about transportation options often include what may be needed if they:

- Desire information on an adaptive driving program or equipment
- Rely on public buses for transportation
- Want to take a trip or rent a car
- Rely on volunteers
- Use ambulance services (air, emergent or nonemergent, or life flight)

Adaptive Driving Programs

If the patient's previous driving record is good and they are capable of passing a road test, even severely physically challenged persons can drive legally. To obtain a license to drive, the person must take the test that is performed by a licensed occupational therapist. A training program that is certified to offer an adaptive driving program must employ the therapist. For information about current training programs in the patient's immediate area, they can contact their local Department of Motor Vehicles, state Department of Rehabilitation, a hospital that offers acute rehabilitation, or local agencies that serve the disabled (e.g., Centers for Independent Living). However, as a rule most adaptive driving programs are located at regional spinal cord rehabilitation facilities.

The adaptive driving test takes approximately 5 hours, and the cost ranges from $75 to $100/hour. Costs for such services will not be paid by private health insurance. However, if the injury is a result of workers' compensation and the person has vocational goals and is capable of returning to gainful employment, a state's Department of Rehabilitation may consider paying the fee. In most cases, the patient or family assumes the cost.

The driving test consists of two sessions. The first session consists of a physical assessment, and the second session is spent behind the wheel. To be considered for an adaptive driving program, the patient must have the following:

- A doctor's prescription specifying that the patient is stable mentally and physically to participate in an adaptive driving program
- A valid driver license or permit
- A prearranged appointment with the program

The patient is tested for their ability to drive, and they are assessed for the following:

- Proper positioning behind the wheel.
- Proper transfers into and out of the vehicle.
- Necessary modifications or driving equipment that will be required for their van or car.

General Information About Automobiles

If the patient is disabled, he or she can apply to the local Department of Motor Vehicles for a handicapped placard or a disabled person's license plate. To obtain the placard or license plate, the patient's physician must complete the necessary paperwork that specifies the extent of the disability and length of time the disability will last. While there is a slight fee for the placard, it is often the most favored as it can be transferred from vehicle to vehicle; a license plate is most often free and in many cases is favored by those who will use it long term or for those classified with a permanent disability. As one educates patients and families, it is important to cover the following rights for the disabled:

- Car insurance rates cannot be increased, the policy canceled, or insurance denied because a person is considered disabled.
- At gas stations, state health and safety codes allow the disabled the right to full service at self-service islands for self-service prices. The patient is encouraged to carry a copy of the law in the glove compartment of the car should problems occur. If an attendant refuses to honor the law, the patient and family can contact the local consumer affairs office of the District Attorney's office to initiate court action.

Modified Vehicles

The cost of modifying a car or van varies from person to person and depends upon the person's physical challenges. As with testing, the cost of vehicle modification is not covered by private health insurance and in most cases the cost must be assumed privately. It is possible to get coverage through the state Department of Vocational Rehabilitation. If the disabling injury was a result of a work injury, modifications are possible through the workers' compensation carrier. Also, the patient may be covered by the Veterans Administration (VA) for a service-related disability. The cost for modifications and equipment vary with the following examples:

- Hand controls range $500 or less
- Actual modifications to a van range from $7000 to $15,000 or greater excluding the cost of the vehicle

Bus Services

Local Handicapped Bus Services

Many cities and their transit authorities offer handicapped bus services for the disabled, elderly, or mentally challenged at a nominal cost. As each city varies with schedules and costs, the local regional transit authorities should be contacted for full information in one's area. As a rule, the process from application to actual services takes 3 to 4 weeks. Should transportation be required in the interim, other arrangements must be made.

Once accepted as a client, the patient must call several days in advance of needing transportation services and reserve a date and time for pickup as well as other round-trip arrangements. Because delays are common, it is wise to alert the physician's or other provider's office of the approximate time for arrival and departure. Most providers are willing to adjust their schedules to accommodate someone who uses public transit modes.

To assist in determining eligibility, functional and therapeutic classifications as well as a medical statement from the physician must be included with the application. As a rule, conditions indicative of a disability are divided into three categories: physical, mental, and developmental. Examples of each category are as follows:

- Physical
  - Ambulatory or coordination disabilities
  - Uses mobility aides such as a walker or cane
  - Arthritis
  - Amputation
  - Stroke or other neurologic disorder with deficits that limit endurance or mobility
    - Pulmonary or cardiac problems where endurance can be an issue
    - Dialysis
    - Sight difficulties
    - Hearing difficulties
- Mental
  - Mental disorders recognized by the American Psychiatric Association
  - Persons residing in a board and care home or group home
  - Persons who participate in sheltered workshops or other training programs
- Developmental
  - Mental retardation
  - Cerebral palsy
  - Epilepsy
  - Autism
  - Neurologic handicap

Local School Bus Services

If the patient is a child, the Individuals with Disabilities Education Act ensures access to a free education for all children. This includes children with disabilities and limitations regardless of their severity. This also means the school district is responsible for transporting the child free of charge from home to the classroom and back. To use this benefit, parents must contact the local school administration and make sure this need is included in the Individualized Education Program (IEP) developed for their child. If the child has special needs, the school district is required to develop an education plan that must be individualized to the child's needs and updated at least annually. Until the IEP is developed and the plan is in place, the parents may be required to offer alternative transportation.

Commercial Bus Service

Travel by commercial bus lines is by far the most economical mode of transportation. However, it is also the most restrictive and often the least favored mode of travel for the disabled. Traveling by bus is very restrictive when it comes to accommodations and accessibility in boarding, unboarding, seating arrangements, and using the restroom should one be on board.

Airlines

Many commercial airlines can accommodate minimal to moderate handicaps. However, the accommodations vary from airline to airline and are regulated by the Federal Aviation Administration (FAA). If the disabled person must travel by commercial airlines, it is wise to contact the airline's medical department (located at the airline's central headquarters) well in advance of any scheduled travel to discuss accommodations, requirements, or restrictions.

While most airlines will offer wheelchair or escort service to board and unboard the plane, there are oxygen and other requirements that must be met when a person requires anything other than assistance with walking. In reality, few commercial airlines can accommodate the severely disabled or those who require oxygen in route.

Trains

As with bus services, train services for the disabled are equally as limited. The disabled encounter difficulties with boarding and unboarding, and cramped isles and bathroom facilities. If travel by train is desired, contact the national headquarters of Amtrak by calling 800-872-7245 for information about availability and accessibility of travel, or visit their website at www.amtrak.com/plan/accessibility.html. If the travel exceeds a certain amount, Amtrak offers the elderly and disabled a discounted fare.

Ships and Cruise Lines

As with commercial bus and train travel, travel by ship is very limited. Most ships will not allow motorized wheelchairs. If equipment is needed, the disabled person is required to use the ship's equipment. Few ships can accommodate the disabled due to lack of accessibility to most areas as halls and doorways are narrow, steps are frequent, and bathrooms are small, cramped, and often have a step. If travel by ship is desired, one should call the ship's headquarters and discuss the feasibility of accommodating the person and his or her disabilities.

Rental Cars

When a car is rented in a major city from a major car rental agency, a person who must drive using hand controls can be accommodated at no additional cost. In most cases, a 2-week notice is required to install the controls.

Volunteer Pilots

If a patient needs a transplant or specific "urgent" service from a large medical center (often referred to as a tertiary center), does not require the services of an air ambulance, and cannot afford a commercial airline ticket, the patient or family may wish to contact a group of volunteer pilots who operate a service called "Air Life Line." AirLifeLine is based in Sacramento, California, and has been offering such services for more than 20 years to the entire continental United States, Canada, and Alaska. Unfortunately, this group does not offer services to Hawaii or the Virgin Islands nor do they fly internationally. To reach them call 916-641-7800 or 800-446-1231.

Volunteer Drivers

Despite the fact that the frail elderly or disabled may use a walker or cane; experience problems with sight, balance, endurance, or hearing; or have other medical problems that limit their driving abilities, finding transportation for this category of persons is often a community's greatest challenge. If the caregiver cannot transport the patient by a private car or make use of public transportation, they may want to explore community agencies to ascertain if such services are available from volunteer drivers. If volunteer services are available from a church or other community agency, there are often no charges associated with the service. Local agencies or groups that might offer such services can be found in the Yellow Pages of the local telephone book and may be listed under such categories as the following:

- Churches
- Community services
- Disease-specific agencies (e.g., Children's Medical Services, American Cancer Society, United Cerebral Palsy Association or American Lung Association)
- Fraternal organizations

When volunteer transportation is needed, keep in mind that due to insurance regulations the volunteer will not offer to help the person get into or out of the car. Also, if transportation is needed between one county to another, the volunteer agency may have restrictions against transporting persons from one county to another (e.g., going from Sacramento County to Yolo County or Nevada County to Sacramento County).

For some disease-specific agencies, funds for reimbursement of mileage costs might be available. For example, if a child is eligible for services from the local or state Children's Medical Services agency or the person is a dependent of an active duty military person and is covered by the military's Program for Persons with Disabilities (PFPWD) and transportation is required to obtain medical services, reimbursement of some costs associated with the transportation may be possible. If reimbursement is made, it often is at a reduced amount. If money is paid, it will be for gas but calculated and limited to the number of miles actually driven.

Travel and Other Pointers

If the patient or family cannot locate a volunteer driver from an agency or other organization and transportation is not available, it may be necessary to call upon friends and relatives for such assistance.

Regardless of the type of volunteers used for transportation, if frequent trips are necessary it is wise to educate patients and families of the need to use a calendar so that they can write in dates, times, and places for pickup and delivery and who will transport the patient.

Many of the major chain fast-food restaurants offer some services for the visually impaired as they have menus printed in Braille. The menus are available upon request.

Air Ambulance or Military Aero Medical Evacuation System

If the commercial airlines are unable or unwilling to accommodate a person who is disabled and air transportation is still required, it may be necessary to arrange for a commercial air ambulance. Most commercial air ambulances fly both domestic as well as internationally. If the patient has a serious medical condition and is a military retiree or a dependent of a military retiree or active duty sponsor, arrangements can often be made with the military's aero medical evacuation unit, which is dispatched from Scott Air Force Base in Illinois.

Details for using the aero evacuation system can be obtained by calling Scott Air Force Base or by speaking with personnel such as a health benefits advisor or a beneficiary representative in a TRICARE office at the nearest military base. The intent of the military's aero medical unit is for use by active duty personnel. However, if not in use or scheduled for use, it can be used at no cost to military dependents, retirees, or their dependents. Civilians can use it, but there is a charge and approval must be obtained from the Department of Defense in Washington, DC.

When a commercial air ambulance or the aero evacuation system is used, it is often necessary to make arrangements for land ambulance or "life-flight" helicopter services or transfers to and from the point of departure for the air ambulance. Arrangements for such ambulances most often are included and coordinated by the air ambulance personnel. However, to avoid confusion or delays, patients and families must ascertain who will retain responsibility for such arrangements. If "life-flight" helicopter use is necessary, such units are as a rule based at large medical centers. Such transportation is needed when the airstrip is located some distance from the patient and the patient cannot tolerate long-distance land travel.

Commercial air ambulances are expensive, often costing several thousand dollars per trip. If the health care insurance company is to pay for the service, the transportation must be "medically necessary" and not considered a family or patient "convenience." If the air ambulance travel is denied, the patient or family must assume the costs and charter their own air transportation.

If the move is for "convenience" (e.g., having the patient closer to family and friends) and the receiving hospital offers services no different than the one currently treating the patient, one alternative is to contact private plane owners or the local airport and discuss the feasibility of chartering a private aircraft and pilot for the travel. If medical equipment or medical personnel are needed to handle the patient's needs, finding and equipping the plane as well as the arrangements for staffing can take several days to weeks. Again, costs any of the foregoing arrangements remain the family's responsibility.

Regular Ambulances Versus Nonmedical Transportation

Transportation is often a key barrier to establishing outpatient and ongoing services the patient requires. While many patients need only an automobile for their use, others will need some form of non-emergent medical transportation, whether from a wheelchair car or gurney van or even an ambulance that offers basic life support (BLS). To meet Medicare's and most insurers' requirements for medical transportation, the following must occur:

- Any vehicle used as an ambulance must be designed and equipped to respond to medical emergencies and, in nonemergent situations, be capable of transporting patients with acute medical conditions.
- In all cases, the vehicle must comply with state and local laws governing the licensing and certification of any emergency medical transportation vehicles.
- BLS vehicles must be staffed by at least two persons, one of whom must be certified as an emergency medical technician (EMT). The state or local authorities where the services will be furnished must issue the certification. The vehicle must be furnished with and the persons in attendance must be legally authorized to operate all lifesaving and life-sustaining equipment on board.
- To serve as an advanced life support (ALS) vehicle, it must be staffed with at least two persons. One of the two must be certified as a paramedic or an EMT who is trained and certified by the state or local authority to perform one or more ALS services.

Historically, patients needing nonemergent transportation home via ambulance have often been limited to persons who need life support modalities readily available. This eliminated consideration for coverage for patients who were bed-confined. Medicare's new rulings on what defines bed-confined as it applies to use of transportation has thus changed the way insurers view nonemergent transport services. However, bed-confined is not meant to be the sole criterion used when making a medical necessity determination. Other criterion may include medial supervision for a medical condition or to ensure proper positioning, airway monitoring, ventilator dependency, cardiac monitoring or restraints to ensure patient safety, IV treatment, or oxygenation. To meet Medicare's requirements, the following must be met:

- The treating physician or other qualified practitioner treating the patient must certify through a written and signed order that all criteria for bed-confined (this is not synonymous with bed rest or nonambulatory) status are met, and these include the following:
  - Patient is unable to get up from bed without assistance
  - Patient is unable to ambulate
  - Patient is unable to sit in a chair or wheelchair for transport
- The origin and destination must meet Medicare guidelines
- The information to support the criteria is clearly supported via documentation in the patient's medical record

Under Medicare rules, the physician's certification cannot be dated more than 60 days prior to the date the services are needed. For patients who are under the direct care and supervision (this generally applies to persons in a nursing facility) and the patients require nonemergent, unscheduled transportation, the physician's certification can be obtained within 48 hours after the transportation occurred. However, for persons who are not under the direct care and supervision of a physician and there is a need for nonemergent, unscheduled transportation, a physician's certification is not required in order for payment to occur.

The area of transportation is possibly the most critical as the CM educates the patient and family of postacute care resources. This is key as health insurance companies often deny payment for the use of ambulances, as the use of the ambulance is deemed not to be medically or emergently necessary. Far too often an ambulance is used, as it is the most convenient way to transport a patient or is thought to be a "covered benefit." Historically, use of ambulances required prior authorization. With the advent of the prudent layperson language now used for emergency department care, prior authorization is not required, but most ambulance bills are reviewed prior to payment by the health care insurance claims unit. If the patient is found to be possibly abusing ambulance usage, the health care insurer may use "pay and educate letters" warning the patient that future use for nonemergent transport could be denied.

Ambulances are a very expensive mode of travel. Consequently, this is the reason most health care insurance companies review ambulance claims on a case-by-case basis before a decision is made to pay the claim or not. In some cases, coverage may be allowed when the patient is unable to be transported by a private vehicle, as the patient is bed-confined. In addition to being bed-confined, other examples for approved ambulance use include the following:

- The person requires oxygen in route
- The person needs suctioning or other medical care and procedures in route
- Stairs pose a risk or barrier
- Physical activity poses a risk
- The person is unable to tolerate sitting
- Restraints are needed

Costs for an ambulance vary, but all charges start with a base rate. Additional charges include a rate for every mile traveled, medical supplies and dressings, and oxygen. If medical personnel are needed over and above those supplied by the ambulance company, there is a separate charge for each person in attendance. Arrangements for additional personnel are made through a nursing staffing agency, and the needs of the patient are matched to the skills of the nursing personnel. If additional nursing staffing is required due to medical necessity, the health care insurer assumes this fee.

For military dependents or veterans whose health care needs are covered by TRICARE (the military's insurance) or for veterans, the VA, every effort must be made to use the military or veteran ambulance or transportation systems and seek approval when required. Otherwise, the cost of the transportation will be denied and must be paid by the patient or family.

Life Flight Services

Life flight services of a helicopter or other air ambulance transfers are available in most major cities and offered by large tertiary, trauma, or specialty medical centers. As a rule, life flight services are used to transport the patient as quickly as possible to the nearest facility that can render the care required. Additionally, during the flight the patient often requires highly specialized care similar to that found in an intensive care unit of a hospital. Trauma victims most commonly use "life flight" services. This mode of transportation is used for transporting critically ill persons or babies that require neonatal or other specialized care that is only offered by a select few hospitals in a given state or region. As most of the cases transported by life flight are of an emergent basis, insurance companies do not require prior authorization.

SECTION VIII—OTHER PLANNING NEEDS

Home Care Is Not Always the Answer

One of the first considerations for ongoing care will be where care will be provided and at what cost. While health care professionals hear it said repeatedly that home is the best place for patients because patients do better in their own surroundings and environment, this is not always true. As patients are being discharged sicker and sooner and requiring more complex and technologically driven care, home care can be very expensive and more importantly, it is not always appropriate for every patient. Therefore, when home care is contemplated, four basic factors must be considered. These factors can serve as guidelines in determining whether the patient can benefit from home care, whether the cost for such care is reasonable and acceptable to the health care payer, and whether out-of-pocket expenses for the patient and family are manageable. The four factors are as follows:

1. The patient is ambulatory and can seek care provided by specific outpatient services, programs, or providers; if this is not true, it must be determined whether the patient meets the criteria for homebound care and whether the level of care can be adequately provided by home health care providers.
2. The patient's medical, psychologic, or psychosocial needs require continued care or supervision that can be provided in a home setting.
3. The home environment is conducive to the treatment plan, and there are adequate caregivers available for achieving the desired goals.
4. The costs of the home care plan are comparable to or less than inpatient alternatives (e.g., continued hospitalization in an acute care facility, skilled nursing facility, subacute care facility, or rehabilitation unit), but despite the reduced costs the quality of the care is essentially the same.

The reality of the situation for home care is that the cost of "basic" care (not even nursing care) and equipment necessary for home care can cost several thousands of dollars per month. It is not uncommon for 24-hour live-in nurse aide care to cost in excess of $10,000/month, while an assisted living facility costs approximately $3700/month. Neither of these costs includes the costs for other charges necessary to meet the patient's needs, which often include physician home visits, outpatient laboratory or radiologic services, pharmacy charges or incontinent pads, gloves, and other personal care items. If the person requires an SNF, the cost is approximately between $4000 and $5000/month and is often all-inclusive. Thus, when evaluating all costs, home care can be far more expensive than placement. In other cases, numerous daily skilled visits by professionals (e.g., nursing, physical therapy, speech therapy, occupational therapy, laboratory, radiologic services) requiring out-of-pocket copayments by the patient can make home care financially impossible for many patients. Consequently, out-of-home placement, until the patient's condition is medically stable and can be managed more easily at home, is usually the best plan.

Dual Home and Out-of-Home Planning

There are going to be cases in which health care professionals know the home plan will not work. Despite any failure that results from the patient's or family's decision to try it at home, many families simply must prove to themselves that they tried. Keep in mind that if the patient has not been declared mentally incompetent or in the case of incompetence, the family member has durable power over health care matters and insists on a home plan, the team often have their hands tied. When discharges surround such issues and the team has major concerns about the safety of the patient and the realism of the discharge plan, accurate documentation of case events and discussions by the various team members with the patient and family is vital. As the case is prepared for discharge, it is critical that such cases are reported to the local protective agencies for follow through. Dual home and out-of-home planning cases often center around the following:

- The patient insists the family never place him or her in a nursing home, and the family is overridden with guilt about possible placement
- Money is an issue (often this covers patients in the gray area, with too much to qualify for Medicaid but not enough to pay privately, or the patient has the funds, but is "saving it for a rainy day")
- Abusive situations where the patient is demanding and the spouse is too intimidated to say no
- Financial gain by the family or friends
- The patient is borderline incompetent and no matter how many times a competency hearing has been held, the court rules the patient competent

If a discharge such as this is allowed, cases such as these must be closely supervised and at times the local protective agencies notified prior to discharge of all details of the issue at hand. More importantly, a contingency plan must be developed and ready to activate as quickly as possible.

Hiring Help in the Home

If the patient is appropriate for discharge to home and as the family prepares for home care, it is wise to also teach the patient or family about the skills they will need should they be required to hire a caregiver or help. Hiring help is often needed when the family lives at a distance, they are physically or mentally unable to provide care, or they have no desire to participate in providing the care required. Most help hired for home care will be for custodial care. This level of care is not reimbursed by the health care insurer and will be a cost that must be assumed by the patient or family.

Because of the high charges associated with hiring help from a home health agency or nursing registry, many patients and families often prefer to recruit their own help. However, this has pitfalls and in many instances can result in higher costs than if the family had elected to use an agency. Unfortunately, if they do their own recruiting they are often not aware of some of the pitfalls of such actions. Fortunately, with education they are able to make an informed decision about how and where help should be hired and what is entailed to be the "employer."

Employer Responsibilities

As a potential employer, the patient and family must become familiar with their new responsibilities as an employer. For example, if they are unfamiliar with paying wages, they must be educated of the need to contact the Internal Revenue Service to discuss the IRS requirements for employers. They must also be educated of other responsibilities such as the following:

- Contacting the Social Security office to obtain Social Security reporting forms and the amount of wages they must report each quarter
- Reporting any wages greater than the quarterly amount specified for Social Security to the state agency responsible for unemployment benefits
- Keeping detailed records on each employee including:
  - Name
  - Address
  - Social Security number
  - Hours worked
  - Amount of wages paid
- Distributing W-2 forms
- Maintaining workers' compensation insurance coverage in case the employee is injured

The patient and family must be educated of the advantages and disadvantages of hiring help directly rather than using an agency. A major disadvantage is the lack of appropriate supervision of the employee. Also, despite the fact the patient may require only custodial care, their new "employee" may not have a clear understanding of the physician's orders, which can lead to confusion and inappropriate care. More importantly, when help is hired directly by the patient or family, there are no provisions for backup help if the person quits, becomes ill, or takes time off.

Recruitment Methods

If the patient or family are insistent upon hiring their own help, and while the following lists of suggestions for recruiting attendants appears lengthy, the actual time needed to elicit a response to an advertisement and hire the attendant varies from a few days to months. Patients and families must be educated of these factors. Consequently, it is advisable for families to advertise in several sources at once. Such sources include the following:

- Newspapers
- Social service agencies
- Vocational schools or other work-training programs
- Church-sponsored or ethnic agencies
- Bulletin boards (e.g., at churches, hospitals [both skilled nursing facilities and acute care facilities] and senior centers)
- Employment agencies
- Friends and other word-of-mouth discussions
- Centers that serve the disabled and offer independent living skills and referral services
- College placement centers

As families are taught the techniques of hiring staff, one must also teach them the importance of how best to do their advertising. Suggestions for this include use a post office box instead of placing their phone number or address in the ad. Doing this allows the patient and family to screen the resumes and references before they make any actual contact with the applicant. The advertisement should include the following information:

- Type of services or specific duties required
- Number of hours required per day, week, or month
- Rate of pay
- Statement requiring resume and references
- Post office box number to which applicant should reply

Hiring Interviews

The patient or family should be advised to prepare a list of questions or issues they desire to cover during the interview. This list should be prepared in advance. The questions serve as a guide during the interview and prevent the interviewer from forgetting to raise important questions or issues. Interview questions must be broad enough to cover specific job requirements as well as give some insight into the applicant's personal characteristics. Due to the Privacy Act, certain questions of prospective employees are illegal, and patients and families must be advised of this fact. Questions must be phrased in such a way that maximum information about the person can be gained without violating this act. However, questions should be directed to the following areas:

- Job qualifications, training, and certification
- Recent work history, work history gaps, length of employment, reason for leaving, and specific tasks performed
- Medical problems that limit the employee's ability to perform any tasks that require strength or physical labor
- Criminal record, including arrests or convictions

- Personal habits such as smoking that may be annoying
- Transportation mode and dependability
- Personal likes and dislikes that the employee would like to share or have known

It is advisable for a second person to be present during the interview to validate the family's impressions and to ask additional questions. The patient and family should keep in mind that the person they hire will be coming into their home, and they must feel comfortable with him or her. Key personal characteristics to look for during the interview include the following:

- Compatibility
- Reliability
- Promptness
- Honesty
- Willingness to learn
- Good listening skills
- Ability to grasp details
- Neat, clean appearance

Other key points the patient or family may wish to consider during the interview are (1) proposal of a 2-week trial for training purposes and (2) agreement by the applicant to accept payment by check to verify that the person was paid if questions arise. To avoid any misunderstanding, families should be encouraged to draw up a contract for the new employee that outlines the duties, rate of pay, pay dates, and time off. In addition, families should maintain a list of nursing registries and agencies that can render the required care if problems arise and help is needed immediately.

Verifying a Candidate's References

References must always be checked! Remind families that when checking references they should look for the following details:

- Length of previous employment
- Reliability
- Dependability

- Specific tasks performed and competence with which they were performed
- Employee's reaction to suggestions and criticism
- Other problems or situations the previous employer would like to share

Common Problems with Hired Help

Although problems among employees can be many and varied, families must be aware that when hiring help they must be alert to signs of the following common problems:

- Thievery
- Abuse
- Sudden termination without notice
- Substitute help during periods of illness or absence of the employee
- Alcohol or drug use
- Criminal record

Hiring Help Using a Nursing Agency

If continuous private-duty nursing is necessary and an agency is used, the patient and family must be educated about the following before the final selection is made:

- What are the capabilities and availability of the agency staff to manage the care required?
- Will necessary staff training be done at no extra charge?
- How do the rates of the chosen agency compare to the rates of other agencies in the area?
- Is the agency willing to discount services and work with the family for possible reimbursement by the health care payer?
- Is the agency certified or accredited and licensed appropriately?
- What is the contingency plan for backup staffing if problems occur?

Even when the health care insurer is paying for the cost of private-duty nursing, the patient and family must understand that they are often the ones to assume final responsibility for the hiring of the individual. Also, they must be informed that the actual contract is between them and the agency, not the health care insurer.

This section highlights the basic information that must be taught and shared with patients or families who are considering the possibility of hiring attendants or home health care workers on their own. Although the rates charged by a nursing or home health care agency appear high, the disadvantages of being the employer often outweigh the advantages. The patient and family must be aware of these issues prior to their decision for help in the home.

SECTION IX—PROVIDERS OF CARE

Health care has changed significantly over the past several years. This is due to many factors such as a shift from inpatient to outpatient care, risk from one entity to another, changes in reimbursement modalities, reduction of reimbursement payments, downsizing, mergers, and even closure. These factors and others have touched every aspect and level of care, and these changes have tremendously affected both health care consumers as well as the health care delivery system.

One positive change that has occurred is the ability to move patients from the acute care facility to other levels of care at a higher acuity care need. For example, stroke patients historically stayed as an inpatient for approximately four weeks and then in rehabilitation another four. This is in contrast to one to two days acute and a week or so in rehabilitation. Therefore, a key step in the planning process is to identify the unique needs of the patients and then locate the resources and vendors that can meet the needs.

In a managed care world, vendor selection is frequently linked to the MCO's contracted network. However, as the contracts are designed to serve the 80% of the insured who often require episodic, noncomplicated, routine care upon discharge and not the 20% who consume enormous resources, CMs must be savvy as to patient needs and the ability of providers to meet the needs. For patients with or without inadequate insurance, the challenge will be to locate the resources that can meet the needs. At times like these, one must be very creative. The importance of appropriate provider selection cannot be underestimated because it plays an essential role in creating a successful plan.

Ideally, selection of the provider should be started as early as possible. Early selection has the following advantages.

- If the organization's network is inadequate and is unable to accommodate the level of care required, there is enough time to locate another provider.
- The provider's staff (those who will actually provide the care) have time to build a relationship with the patient and family, and any necessary staff training can be accomplished before the patient is discharged.
- The equipment can be delivered early and the patient or family can practice with it and become familiar with the actual equipment that will be used on discharge.

Provider Selection

While it is easy to use one provider or organization over others, it is not always wise. First and foremost, patients have the right to be informed of their providers and expectations for care. As one keeps patients informed, CMs must leave nothing unturned as they search for an appropriate provider for the best service possible for the patient. As one evaluates providers, it is important to evaluate all the services they provide and the quality each brings forth to patients. National or large vendors are not always better. Therefore, keep in mind the dos and don'ts listed in Box 14–7 as provider searches are underway.

Centers of Excellence

Owing to the complexities of new treatment modalities (e.g., experimental procedures and clinical trials), many patients now receive their care in centers of excellence or tertiary care centers. Any patient who is hospitalized in a tertiary care center must be evaluated for the feasibility of case management. This is necessary because these patients are sicker and because their medical costs (as well as their out-of-pocket costs) at a tertiary center can be exorbitant. The increase in cost results

---

BOX 14-7
The Dos and Don'ts of Quality Service

Dos
- Do look at data that supports the fact that the companies validate appropriate patient outcomes regardless of the size of the organization.
- Do evaluate the management structure and determine if there is an on-site manager who is willing to work with CMs.
- Do seek companies that are flexible in terms of products, hours, services, and a desire to alter what is routine.
- Do look at getting the best impact for the dollar; look at quality as well as consistency in what is offered.
- Do look for companies that allow access to information in a timely manner.
- Do look for companies that are easy to do business with. Look for businesses that have employees who return phone calls in a timely manner or treat customers as if that customer is the only one they are dealing with.

Don'ts
- Do not be misled by glossy brochures or exteriors; too much time and money is spent to make some companies look better than others.
- Do not be impressed simply by the number of locations; instead look at what is happening internally at each location. One of the best ways to do this is to review state agency reports. Any company can make things look idealistic on paper. Keep in mind that neither small nor large organizations have a monopoly on any one market or business practices.
- Do not be deceived by sales approaches or marketing gimmicks.[81]

from the types and frequency of the care given and the fact that many such centers often will not have nor will they contract with health care insurers. Many centers are also not willing to negotiate discounts or consider other forms of reduced rates for reimbursement. Thus, the full costs of the services must be paid. Out-of-pocket expenses, in addition to copayments and deductibles, can be high because many patients must drive long distances or even relocate temporarily to be near the treating facility.

In tertiary centers, costs can average several thousand dollars per day because charges are based on the full fee-for-service rate. If services and costs are not monitored closely, the patient's health care benefits, if not linked to an HMO, can be quickly eroded. Although cost is a concern, the actual treatment program is a matter of concern also. This is due to the fact that many tertiary care centers are teaching centers, and complex cases make excellent subjects for teaching. Medical students, however, are not attuned to the business world of medical finances. Consequently, lengths of stay must be closely monitored to ensure the patient is moved to a lower level of care or back to the local community as soon as it is medically possible to do so. Such monitoring saves health care costs and, more importantly, ensures the patient's health care benefits are preserved for use at a later time.

Alternate Level of Care Providers

Many levels of post-acute care services are now available for use by case-managed patients. Unfortunately, not all communities offer all levels of care, and it is common to encounter waiting lists for persons in need of complex skilled care. Consequently, out-of-area placement is necessary in many situations. Regardless of the setting of the alternate post-acute care used, the patient's progress must be closely monitored as he or she moves from one level of care to another. Monitoring is necessary to ensure the patient is making progress toward the established goals, is receiving the care required to meet his or her needs, and is moving appropriately through the continuum of care. The following alternate levels of care are those most commonly used by the majority of patients:

- Subacute care facilities
- Acute rehabilitation care facilities
- Skilled nursing care facilities
- Home health agency care for intermittent or hourly private-duty skilled nursing care

Other facilities that may be required, depending on the diagnosis include the following:

- Cardiac or respiratory rehabilitation units
- Inpatient or outpatient pain management units
- Outpatient therapy (physical, occupational, or speech therapy) facilities
- Post-acute care rehabilitation facilities for patients with a brain injury
- Intermediate care facilities for patients with either less intense medical needs or developmental delay
- Mental health facilities including psychiatric outpatient treatment facilities, residential treatment centers, substance abuse programs, and in extreme cases state hospitals

For frail elderly people, patients with a psychiatric disorder, or patients with a mild or moderate developmental delay, explore the following types of facilities before using the more restrictive ones:

- Adult day care centers
- Residential or board-and-care facilities
- Community care homes

Although a subacute care facility, rehabilitation facility, or skilled nursing facility may be appropriate for a child with special needs, these facilities may not be readily available. Consequently, many children are discharged home with any combination of complex needs and requirements for care and resources. This is necessary as the facilities for geriatric patients often lack opportunities that promote activities geared toward a younger population. Fortunately, some communities offer facilities that specialize in pediatric skilled care, and some have day care centers that specialize in providing services to children with special needs. In addition, many communities have specialized care homes that are licensed to provide varying levels of care. For some of the most severely disabled children, the only option for placement may be a state facility that provides long-term care.

Facilities designed to treat children and adolescents with a mental illness are likewise not available in all communities. Although many children and adolescents can benefit from outpatient programs, many require placement in a residential treatment center, community care home, or sometimes a state school or state hospital. If the child requires placement in any of these facilities, close coordination with the CM from the agency responsible for mental health, the Department of Mental Retardation, or the Department of Education is vital to ensure the child is placed appropriately. In most cases, these levels of care are not reimbursed by health care insurance.

SECTION X—DURABLE MEDICAL EQUIPMENT, SUPPLIES, AND DEVICES
Durable Medical Equipment
Durable medical equipment (DME), sometimes referred to as home medical equipment (HME), is the fastest growing area in the Medicare program. Most health insurers cover DME and medical supplies in a variety of settings. The only exception is when the patient does not have DME

included in his or her health benefit package. If this happens, one must rely on loan closets, or the patient and family must pay privately for the cost of the items. If provided by a facility, most DME items are generally included in the facility's reimbursement rates. The only exceptions are very specialized equipment (e.g., pressurized bed). When DME and medical supplies are reimbursed, they are often reimbursed in four different instances:

1. Supplies furnished as a necessary part of the physician's treatments
2. Prosthetic and orthotic devices furnished in the home or facility, if specific criteria are met
3. DME furnished to patients for use in the home, and when specialty equipment is required, for use in a facility (normally, the facility is required to provide equipment needed for the care of the patient)
4. Surgical dressings provided in the home or facility

Historically, DME has been reimbursed according to a fee schedule. However, this has changed since the enactment of the Balanced Budget Act of 1997 and the various modalities now used to reimburse for DME, medical supply items, orthotics, or prosthetics. DME reimbursement is divided into six categories. CMs must be familiar with these categories, their coverage criteria, policies that underlie coverage decisions, and basic payment rules. There are six categories for DME:

1. Inexpensive or routinely used DME. This is equipment with a price that does not exceed $150. It can be purchased or rented based on the fee schedule amount.
2. DME requiring frequent and substantial servicing. This is equipment such as continuous passive motion machines and ventilators. Medicare does not pay to purchase these items but pays to rent them on a monthly basis.

3. General prosthetics or orthotic devices and supplies. These can only be purchased. Prosthetics must replace all or part of an internal body organ or replace all or part of a permanently functioning organ (e.g., arm, leg, or eye).

4. Capped-rental items. These products cost more than $150, are not routinely purchased, are not customized, and are not service-intensive. Examples include hospital beds and wheelchairs.

5. Oxygen and oxygen equipment. This includes stationary and portable gaseous liquid systems, oxygen, and concentrators.

6. Customized equipment, which is uniquely constructed or substantially modified to meet the specific needs of the individual patient.[82]

Although the actual equipment and supplies ordered vary with the patient, disease or injury, and level of impairment, many case-managed patients require an inordinate amount of expensive equipment and supplies. Factors affecting the amount of supplies and types of equipment ordered include frequency of the patient's physical need for the item; patient's mobility status; distance between the patient and the supplier; and presence of inclement weather conditions. Although most case-managed patients require voluminous amounts of supplies and duplicate items, many patients will also require battery chargers and backup batteries or battery-operated equipment. In areas where power outages are frequent, a portable generator will be mandatory.

In addition to requiring expensive equipment, case-managed patients also consume voluminous amounts of disposable supplies. In most cases, supplies should be ordered in 30- to 60-day increments. However, if the patient resides in a remote or rural area or in an area where accessibility is an issue, supplies can be ordered for a greater period of time, such as quarterly or semiannually. In all cases, proper storage (e.g., site, temperature) of all items must be considered when the plan is developed and the actual orders are placed.

For patients with respiratory disease, the same consideration must go into the selection of airways and accessories as for the ventilatory device. This decision alone requires close communication with the health care team throughout the case but especially as the time for discharge approaches. Communication is necessary to ensure that the proper respiratory equipment and supplies are available and have been approved prior to the actual day of discharge and the patient and family or caregiver has had adequate training in their use. Like other technologically dependent patients, many respiratory patients require huge amounts of supplies. Additionally, much of their equipment must be ordered in duplicate because they require both a stationary model as well as a portable battery-operated version.

The portability of equipment for all patients is vital if the patient is to be mobile and is to resume some kind of normal life. This duplicate equipment, however, can pose a problem if the health care insurer will reimburse the provider for only one piece of like or similar equipment within a specified period of time. When this situation occurs, loan closets must be explored to find the alternate equipment, or the patient or family must make the arrangements to pay privately.

In all cases, decisions about selection of equipment must be based on its suitability for the patient's home care needs, lifestyle, and home environment. Early identification of equipment needs well in advance of discharge is critically important to ensure a successful outcome because some equipment may have to be specifically made or adapted for the patient or the home modified to accommodate the weight of the equipment. This requires time. If there is not enough time allowed, costly delays can ensue because the patient cannot be discharged until the equipment is available or the modifications made. In other cases, the discharge may occur but loaned equipment may have to be supplemented in the interim. This latter method is the least desirable, as it may not be appropriate for the patient and thus, may hinder the patient's functional abilities.

The equipment ordered for each patient depends on the diagnosis and the patient's specific medical needs and functional abilities. The most frequently ordered equipment items for most patients include the following:

- Hospital beds, bedrails, and trapezes
- Commodes or bedpans
- Shower and bathroom devices
- Mobility devices

Requirements to Meet Insurer Coverage Guidelines

In addition to requiring patients to use their network of providers to obtain medical equipment, most health care insurers allow reimbursement only for DME that has been approved by the FDA. In addition, they require that the equipment be used within the realm for which the FDA granted its approval. As equipment is ordered, keep in mind that it is not always considered a benefit or medical necessity because a physician orders it. Also, a letter does not necessarily justify the equipment unless the letter and the medical information supporting it testify to the medical necessity of the item.

Most insurers use a DME formulary much as they would a pharmacy formulary. A DME formulary is a compilation of clinical and operational guidelines that have been developed to help clarify benefit coverage rules while providing clinical guidelines that help determine the appropriate and most cost-effective item that

will meet the medical needs of the patient. Most DME guidelines specify the following:

- Type of equipment
- Requirements for its use
- Applicable professional discipline's evaluation that might be necessary for inclusion as the request is reviewed
- Number of units approved in any given period of time
- Suggested frequency of replacement
- As applicable, the recommended rates for usage of associated medical supplies
- References as to who can authorize the request (e.g., nurse, medical director, specific clinical specialist, reviewer)

In order to have the DME covered, insurers require the following basic information.

- Order date
- Diagnosis
- Description and name of the item (add HCPC code; if the item is oxygen, the liter flow, type of unit, and last blood gas level is necessary)
- Duration the equipment will be needed
- Additional supplies needed
- Physician signature

Any additional documentation that can medically justify the request should be submitted along with the prescription. Once the prescription is received, it is then verified against DME formulary guidelines (many organizations use Medicare's criteria). If the DME meets criteria, it is approved; if it does not, it is denied.

A variety of DME items are often excluded or denied, and if so, they generally fall into the following categories:

- Convenience items—duplicate pieces of equipment, bedpans, overbed tables, shower chairs, and chair lifts.
- Environmental equipment—heating devices, air conditioners, electronic sensory devices for turning

lights and appliances on or off, and air filters and air cleaners

- Exercise equipment—exercise bikes, weights, and treadmills
- Nontherapeutic items—fully electric beds (which are convenient rather than medically necessary), hand controls in automobiles, and van lifts
- Comfort items—spas, water mattresses and pads, and hydromassage bath devices
- Hygienic equipment—shampoo trays and other bathing devices
- Education devices—Braille teaching texts and certain computers or electronic equipment used for speech or communication

Ordering Equipment for Various Conditions

The following is an example of a list of the DME and orthotic devices used for a person with quadriplegia. These items are recognized as medically necessary for this condition and compose the standard of care for such patients. As can be seen, many of the items are considered deluxe or convenience or would be so considered for other patients. The items required by a person with quadriplegia may include the following:

- Fully electric wheelchair with tongue, chin, breath, or mouth stick control (customized)
- Custom wheelchair pads (this item is required for patients with all levels of spinal injuries with paralysis)
- Wheelchair trunk supports or seating systems (customized)
- Slide boards
- Lumbar sacral orthotics
- Lapboards
- Arm supports
- Wrist and hand supports
- Adapted grooming and feeding equipment
- Semielectric hospital bed

- Bed rails
- Patient lift and sling
- Standing frame

Of the foregoing, the only items that are truly not medically necessary are the lapboards and adapted grooming and feeding equipment. All the others are medically necessary if the patient is to have proper support and mobility. Certainly, the list is not limited to these items. In all cases, the final list of equipment ordered depends on the level of spinal cord injury in the particular patient.

In other patients, again depending on the diagnosis, DME items ordered may include the following:

- Semielectric hospital beds, bed rails, and trapezes
- Bedside commodes, toilet rails, shower or tub benches
- Standard wheelchairs with removable arm and leg rests
- Transfer benches or slide boards
- Specialty beds (e.g., air beds, fluidized beds; these are generally used for persons with multiple and severe decubitus ulcers and persons confined to bed)
- Continuous passive motion (CPM) devices
- Glucometers (for insulin-dependent diabetics)
- Canes, walkers, and crutches
- Apnea and cardiac monitors
- Oxygen systems (varying from combinations of oxygen concentrators, liquid oxygen, and oxygen cylinders to air compressors) and their related supplies
- Ventilators and all related supplies
- Feeding pumps, stationary poles, and all feeding supplies
- Infusion equipment and all related supplies
- Continuous positive airway pressure (CPAP) devices and supplies
- Suction devices and related supplies
- Urinals and bedpans

Believe it or not, health care insurers or individual health benefit packages exclude most bathroom items, adaptive feeding and dressing devices, and some special items, as they are considered not medically necessary! The most common excluded devices are toilet rails and shower or tub benches. Additional bathroom and sleeping devices often not covered include the following:

- Raised toilet seats
- Grab bars for shower or tub
- Bath lifts
- Whirlpool equipment
- Special pillows (cervical or wedge)
- Air or gel mattresses or pads
- Handheld shower heads
- Compression garments

In all cases where the patient will be wheelchair-bound, consideration must be given to an appropriate seating system. Due to inappropriate seating, many patients are limited as to what they can do. Worse yet, this makes them prone to costly pressure sores. As patients become older and more chronic and dependent upon a wheelchair or prolonged sitting, addressing seating and mobility needs will take on greater importance. The goal in all cases must be to maximize patient function and comfort, prevent or decrease the progression of pressure sores or musculoskeletal deformities, and increase independence and quality of life. When evaluating a patient for seating, a team approach often works best. Here the patient, caregiver, occupational and physical therapists, and the medical supplier, at a minimum, should be included. Once the team is assembled, goals can be established and the evaluations and recommendations for the actual prescription can be made and presented to the insurer.

One of the greatest challenges in procurement of the appropriate seating system often is reimbursement, as without the proper diagnosis or documentation and medical information to support the request, the request may be denied and considered "a convenience" or "not medically necessary."[83]

DME Supplies and Monthly Purchases

Even when a DME item is purchased, it may also require the purchase of monthly supplies to operate the basic equipment. If this is the case, the case management plan must include provisions for this occurrence. Fortunately, some of these related supplies required monthly and sold as "sterile" supplies can be homemade. Therefore, whenever possible the CM must evaluate which supplies can safely be made at home or eliminated merely by using "clean" instead of sterile techniques. However, the final decision for conversion to clean technique rests with the ordering physician. If the patient's supplies can be homemade or used with clean techniques, significant cost savings will result.

Patients who require even the most sophisticated equipment can be discharged. In cases such as these, the homes of the patients are often converted to resemble mini-hospital units. However, to obtain reimbursement, several factors must be considered before any equipment is rented or purchased. Among these factors are the following:

- Is the equipment available from a network provider?
- Have the specific needs and medical justification for the equipment request been documented?
- What is the policy for buy-back, trade-ins, or loan of other equipment during periods of routine maintenance or repair?
- How long will the equipment be necessary? (This answer will assist in deciding whether it is more cost-effective to rent or purchase the item.)
- Is there a need for backup equipment (e.g., if the equipment malfunctions, to allow the patient some independence, or during periods of routine maintenance)?

- Are alternative suppliers available in the area for purposes of cost comparison or in case the equipment or supplies are not available from the first supplier?
- Can the supplier schedule prompt same-day service or delivery with no extra charges for delivery or setup?
- Is the provider willing to provide the equipment or training to the patient, family, caregiver, or professional before the patient is discharged at no additional cost?
- What is the rental versus purchase costs of the equipment (including its maintenance)? If the equipment is rented, can the rental price be applied to the purchase price?

Rental Versus Purchase

Decisions about purchase of equipment vary from health plan to health plan and must be made on a case-by-case basis. In some cases, it is appropriate to rent the equipment for a brief period before an actual purchase is made. This allows enough time to ensure that the patient can be managed safely at home or that the equipment requested is appropriate. In other cases, the actual overall cost of the equipment may be the driving factor for rental versus purchase.

When considering rental versus purchase (there will be times when it is cheaper to purchase equipment), several factors must be considered before the final decision is made. These factors demand answers to the following questions:

- How long will the patient require the equipment?
- Is the patient stable on the present model or are adjustments still being made that could indicate the need for another model?
- Is a service contract necessary? If so, who will cover the monthly service cost?

- If the patient or family cannot afford the cost of a service contract, will the patient be at risk of a costly outcome if the equipment fails and a backup unit is not readily available?

Although the long-range treatment plan may indicate the equipment will be used for the long term, it is sometimes best to rent the equipment for the first 30 to 90 days or longer. This time frame allows changes and adjustments to be made to the equipment. More importantly, if the patient cannot tolerate a postacute level of care, money has not been spent needlessly on equipment. Likewise, if the equipment thought to be the most desirable item at discharge turns out to be inadequate or less desirable and another item is required at a later date, money will not have been wasted. This scenario is especially true for patients requiring ventilators several of which must be tried before the correct one is found. Also, sometimes the family finds that once the patient is home they cannot manage, and placement becomes necessary.

Because for some equipment long-term rental costs can easily exceed the purchase price, this factor must be considered when deciding whether to rent or buy. Ventilators are a good example. The purchase price of a ventilator, even with the cost of a service contract included, is far more advantageous than the rental cost. Most ventilators can be purchased for under $10,000 (the service contract is an additional $300/month) whereas the monthly rental charges average $700 to $1000.

Service Contracts

If the equipment is serviced regularly, it can generally last for years. If it is purchased, routine maintenance will not be included in the purchase price. Thus, the prime drawback of purchase is that someone must assume the responsibility of paying for the routine maintenance and repairs such equipment requires. In contrast, when equipment is rented the item continues to be the "property" of the equipment company, and thus they retain responsibility for caring for it. When the item is purchased, these costs are shifted to the new "owner. " The only alternatives are to pay for the maintenance privately or arrange for it to be provided through a service contract.

A service contract covers the same services as those provided while the equipment was rented. Although a service contract can average several hundred dollars per month, these costs are cheaper than the cost of replacement or of deterioration of the patient's condition if the equipment fails. Unfortunately, this type of service is not routinely allowed by health care payers. Therefore, all factors must be taken into account before purchase of equipment is considered.

Generally, when an item is rented the rental price includes the routine maintenance required by the manufacturer and routine monitoring of treatment responses by the equipment company's professional nursing or respiratory therapy staff. Consequently, payment of a separate service contract is not required. Thus, before a ventilator is purchased the CM must be aware of the health care payer's policies for rental versus purchase. As stated earlier, if the ventilator is purchased, a monthly service contract must be considered or arrangements must be in place for a backup ventilator. This is necessary should the equipment fail or need routine maintenance by the manufacturer and be sent away for a period of time.

Equipment service contracts are almost a necessity for ventilators because the ventilator must be totally overhauled according to the manufacturer's specifications. As a rule, this is required for every 5000 to 8000 hours of use. During these times the primary ventilator is sent out to be serviced and another is supplied in the interim. If a service contract is not maintained, the health care payer must assume the rental cost during the interim.

Most DME companies provide free delivery setup and teaching. Sometimes teaching is required while the patient is still an inpatient and discharge is imminent. In these situations, the company supplying the equipment to the patient should bring the equipment to the hospital so that the patient or family can receive the actual teaching required there. In this way, the patient and family can be taught the procedures in the hospital and become familiar with the equipment. When this type of service is required, most health care payers do not reimburse the equipment company for this service; reimbursement will only start at the time of discharge.

Equipment that must be customized (e.g., wheelchairs, seating pads, or trunk supports) requires outright purchase. However, until the special equipment arrives, similar equipment may have to be rented. This situation is always less than desirable because the interim equipment can cause unnecessary pressure sores or other problems that can be costly if procurement of the customized version is delayed for some reason. For this reason, the patient must be measured and the equipment ordered as soon as the need for this equipment is identified.

Some equipment requires modifications of the home and ramps. These modifications are rarely allowed by health care payers (the prime exception is workers' compensation). Consequently, the cost must be borne by the patient or family. When the family is unable to pay these costs, it may be wise to refer them to a fraternal organization. Volunteers from these organizations may be able to supply the labor, and the organization may assist with covering the costs of any supplies used. Likewise, van lifts and modifications to vans or automobiles are not covered by health care payers (again, this is not true of workers' compensation). Costs then become the responsibility of the patient and family. However, depending on the patient and his or her motivation (and physical and mental abilities) to obtain gainful employment, the state department of rehabilitation or vocational rehabilitation may be a source of reimbursement.

DME and related supplies are commonly billed by using the CMS (formerly the Health Care Financing Administration) common procedural coding system (HCPCS). This is a set of codes used by Medicare and health care organizations for billing purposes because the codes are specific for DME and some other services (e.g., ambulance services).

As mentioned earlier, equipment it is not always a benefit or medical necessity just because a physician orders it. The CM must know which items are medically necessary and which ones are appropriate for either the patient or caregiver's convenience. Depending on the diagnosis, the medical necessity of the equipment and its importance in preventing complications, some items that do not meet the medically necessary criterion may require payment by the patient or family. In some instances, the patient may have to do without the equipment if it is not available through loan closets or other community service agencies. Due to the many limitations and exclusions pertinent to DME, it behooves CMs to be familiar with alternative resources.

Children and Their Equipment Needs

In dealing with children with special needs, their equipment needs most often will not vary from those used by adults. However, as equipment is ordered, care must be exercised to ensure some items will "grow" with the child. This ensures the child's needs are met but costs are kept in line. No matter how careful one is to attempt to maximize the life expectancy of equipment (e.g., for a child's wheelchair, the life expectancy is three to five years),

children sometimes grow faster than anticipated. As a rule, in most cases the equipment will be too small one to two years after the initial wheelchair or device was purchased. While the child's wheelchair or device may be modified, modifications may not be possible and the equipment will not be "growable" if it is not the right type.[84] Thus, when working with parents and their child to order the equipment, CMs must always work in concert with a DME organization that employs pediatric equipment specialists.

Using Loan Closets

Many communities have disease-specific organizations and other organizations that maintain DME "closets." These closets are useful for patients with no insurance or limited income, or for patients who require duplicate insurance but the health care payer denied it. CMs should be familiar with the availability of such closets within the community.

Self-Help Devices, Clean Technique, or Homemade Alternatives

Self-help devices and other factors related to the use of DME and home modifications are very important to the overall success of the case management plan. Because they may be excluded from the patient's health care coverage (workers' compensation is one exception), the patient or family may be required to assume a cost that is unplanned or for which there is "no money."

Key resources that can be used for information or assistance in planning or designing self-help devices or methods used for clean technique can be found by using the knowledge of the therapy team members (physical, occupational, and speech therapy) and the professional nursing or rehabilitation staffs of the local home health agency.

Clean technique and homemade supplies are cost-effective alternatives to the high cost of sterile supplies, once the patient is home and no longer requires the sterile technique and supplies used in the hospital. Many of the following "recipes" are those used by home health agency and public health nurses when the family cannot afford the out-of-pocket costs for "sterile solutions" and the patient can tolerate "clean technique." However, *CMs must always check with the physician first before implementing or suggesting this alternative to the family.*

Most homemade supplies cost less than 10 cents per item, whereas the same item, if purchased, can cost more than $1 to $2. For example, the savings achieved for a tracheostomy patient using clean technique for suctioning and care of the suction catheters versus sterile suction catheters can exceed $300/month. The following sections highlight some examples of cost-effective homemade supplies or tips that are commonly taught by home health agency nurses and can be used in place of costly sterile ones if the attending physician agrees.

Sterilization of Water and Supplies

For disinfecting toilets and bedpans the Centers for Disease Control and Prevention (CDC) suggests using household bleach. Use a ratio of one part bleach to ten parts water. When making any solution, use the following tips:

- The water, storage jars, and jar tops (metal screw type) can be sterilized by boiling the item or solution for 15 minutes.
- Metal or glass containers or instruments should be used whenever possible (e.g., glass syringes and baby food, mayonnaise, or peanut butter jars).
- Two large "boiling pots" are necessary—one for water and one for receptacles or containers.
- Once solutions have been sterilized, they should be stored in sterilized

jars while other items can be stored in self-sealing plastic bags.

Frequent hand washing and the use of hot soapy water and household bleach are two of the most commonly used disinfectants and are recommended by the CDC for disinfecting most items.

Homemade Solutions

In the following recipes the salt, sugar, and soda dissolve better if the water is hot. All mixing and measuring must be done using sterilized containers or utensils.

- Normal saline solution
1 teaspoon salt
1 quart boiling water (sterilized water)
Mix well, store in a sterilized closed container, and replace every 24 hours.
- Dakin's solution
To make a 25% Dakin's solution use:
25 ml chlorine bleach in 1000 ml H_2O or normal saline solution
To make a 50% Dakin's solution use:
50 ml chlorine bleach in 1000 ml H_2O or normal saline solution
Mix well, store in a sterilized closed container, and replace every 24 hours.
- Soda solution
$1/2$ cup baking soda
4 cups sterilized water
Mix well, store in a sterilized closed container in the refrigerator, and replace every 24 hours.
- Acetic acid solution
$1/2$ cup distilled clear vinegar
1 quart sterilized water
Mix well, store in a sterilized closed container in the refrigerator, and replace every 24 hours.

The vinegar solution is used to dissolve mineral deposits from urine that often plug catheters, leg bags, and inlets and valves of equipment. Leg and drainage bags should be soaked approximately 8 hours in the solution. Respiratory equipment should be soaked for a few minutes, rinsed with clear water, then drained and allowed to dry.

Other Tips on Home Care Items

Egg Crate Mattress Care

If the patient has an egg crate mattress, it can be washed in a bathtub with water and detergent, rinsed thoroughly, and hung to dry. Old egg crates can be cut into various sizes and used as protectors for pressure points.

Brace Care

The leather lining of braces should be cleaned with saddle soap or leather cleaner once a month. This increases the longevity of the brace and helps to prevent the leather from cracking.

Incontinent Pads

If the family cannot afford to buy hospital sheeting (it comes by the yard at fabric stores) incontinent pads can be made by using the following:

- Several pillow cases
- One to two sheets of plastic cut to the size of the pillow case
- Several stacks of newspapers folded in half

Place a plastic sheet in the pillowcase and add about ¼-inch thickness of newspapers. When using, place the plastic nearest the mattress. When soiled, the newspapers can be tossed, the plastic can be reused when wiped clean with distilled white vinegar, and the pillowcases can be washed in hot soapy water. The cost of these pads is minimal whereas purchased incontinent pads average more than a dollar each.

Tracheostomy Care Kits

When clean technique is used, gloves are not necessary; only good hand washing is required prior to suctioning or caring for a tracheostomy. Most of the supplies in a tracheostomy or "trach" care kit can be obtained from local tobacco or notion stores and can be made as follows:

- Regular ½-inch hemming tape is available at notion stores and can be used in place of the twill tape provided in disposable tracheostomy kits.
- Pipe cleaners or small brushes (available at local pipe or tobacco or variety stores) can be used to scrub the inner cannula.
- Gauze can be purchased in bulk from most pharmacies.
- Tracheal suctioning catheters can be cleaned and reused 8 to 10 times before they become too stiff and must be discarded. The catheters commonly become cloudy after the second or third cleaning but this does not affect their function. To keep the catheters "clean," store them in a plastic bag after each use. To clean tracheal catheters the following supplies are needed:
    - Hydrogen peroxide
    - Liquid dish detergent
    - Boiling water
    - Cotton balls
    - Isopropyl alcohol.
    - Self-sealing plastic bags

Urinary Catheter Care

Intermittent catheterization is a technique used frequently for patients with a neurogenic bladder or those who are continent between their catheterizations. Intermittent catheterization is used only if the patient or family accepts the procedure. In most cases, intermittent catheterization can be accomplished using clean technique. However, the final choice among clean versus sterile catheterization technique is made by the physician and depends on the patient's particular circumstances.

With clean technique, urinary catheters can be used up to seven days if they are cleansed properly after each use. To clean catheters used in intermittent catheterization, the following supplies are needed:

- Soap and hot water
- French rubber catheters (several)
- Receptacle in which to place urine (a toilet is OK)
- Self-sealing bags
- Clean towels and washcloths
- Tube of water-soluble lubricant
- If the patient is female and is catheterizing herself, a mirror

Catheters are collected after each use in a towel, basin, or self-sealing bag for bulk cleaning. Collected catheters are washed with hot soapy water, rinsed in clear water, and stored in self-sealing plastic bags or clean towels. As with tracheostomy care, if clean technique is used there is no need for gloves, only good hand washing.

General Tips

For patients confined to bed and without an open skin lesion, cornstarch spread on the lower sheet allows the patient to move about more easily and helps prevent "sheet burn."

To assist in keeping urine smells to a minimum, wipe mattresses, plastic sheeting, tubing, and urinary drainage bags with full-strength white distilled vinegar.

Self-Help Devices

When a person is disabled, whether with a short-term or long-term disability, it often takes more time and effort than usual to accomplish daily tasks. It may also require unnecessary dependence on others or pose safety problems. Therefore, evaluation by a therapist for the use of self-help aids is as necessary as an evaluation for the use of any DME. In some cases, the simpler devices can be homemade although the more technical ones cannot. Self-help aids or devices range from simple, large, or long-handled utensils to high-tech, breath-activated, or simple touch- or movement-generated electronic devices.

Despite the fact that commonly used self-help aids are readily available from most DME providers and specialized ones

can be ordered, the costs of all of them must somehow be reimbursed. Unfortunately, insurance coverage for self-help devices or aids is not common. Therefore, decisions about coverage are made case by case and are based on medical necessity, not convenience. Unfortunately, reimbursement from health care payers is frequently limited to the standard models, and the patient and family must be prepared to assume the cost difference if deluxe items are preferred.

Long-Term Care Equipment and Medical Supplies

The long-term care and post-acute arena has experienced a great deal of change due to the implementation of the prospective payment system. One area affected is coverage of DME and medical supplies while the patient is in a long-term care facility and has Medicare Part B coverage. In all cases, medical necessity *must be* documented and the physician *must complete* a certificate of medical necessity if the DME item or supplies are to be covered. Since many insurers follow Medicare guidelines, it is key to query the insurer for their stance on the following issues that are now allowable under Medicare Part B:

Enterals

Medicare does not cover enteral therapy, but it covers the following:

- Formula
- Plastics to administer the formula
- Pump rental, if applicable and deemed medically necessary
- Tubes for administering the formula
- Formula additives

Urologic Devices

Medicare covers urologic devices such as urinary catheters and external urinary collection devices used to collect or drain urine when the patient has permanent urinary retention or permanent urinary incontinence. These include the following:

- Catheter supplies
- Foley catheters
- Texas/condom catheters
- Insert trays
- Drain bags (bedside)
- Leg bags
- Irrigation supplies
- Leg straps
- Intermittent catheter

Ostomy Supplies

Medicare covers ostomy supplies for use on patients with a stoma to divert urine, feces, or ileal contents to outside the body. These include the following:

- Wafers
- Pouches (closed and drainable)
- One-piece and two-piece appliances
- Ostomy adhesive
- Skin preps
- Deodorant tablets
- Ostomy pastes and powders
- Ostomy belts
- Ostomy irrigation supplies
- Adhesive remover
- Appliance cleaners

Tracheostomy Supplies

Medicare covers tracheostomy kits following an open surgical tracheostomy if the site is expected to remain open at least three months. Included with the kits, coverage is allowed for tracheostomy cleaning trays or disposable cannulas.

Wound Care

Surgical dressings are covered when either of the following criteria is met:

- The dressing is medically necessary for the treatment of a wound caused by or treated by a surgical procedure.
- The dressing is medically necessary when wound debridement is medically necessary.

Medicare does not pay for wound irrigation supplies but does cover the following:

- Primary dressings

- Secondary dressings
- Tape

Effective February 1, 2001, Medicare began covering Apligraf (graftskin) for use in the treatment of venous leg ulcers and diabetic foot ulcers. However, coverage for this remains health-plan–specific.

Diabetic Supplies

Medicare limits coverage for diabetic supplies to Type I, insulin-dependent diabetics or Type II noninsulin diabetics. These items include the following[86]:

- Blood glucose monitors
- Test strips
- Lancets

Other Devices

Most CMs working with patients who will be home alone should educate them and their families of the benefits of a personal emergency response system (PERS). These devices have been around since the late 1970s. While used primarily by the elderly, any disabled person who is alone for any period of the day or at risk could possibly benefit from it.

An emergency response system works by the subscriber wearing a personal help device (either around the neck or like a bracelet) that contains an activation device called a personal help button (PHB). The PHB when pushed activates the emergency response system to indicate that an emergency situation has occurred. The system uses the person's phone, and when pushed submits a signal to the PERS's phone connection, which dials predesignated responders (neighbors, family, or professionals) to alert them of the situation. Emergency help is then dispatched to the individual's home.

Lifeline Systems pioneered the emergency response system, and they continue to be the largest supplier of such systems. However, there are now a number of national companies on the market that either rent or sell the equipment to users and then offer 24-hour monitoring. Although not always reimbursed through the patient's insurer (some Medicaid programs do cover), the monthly cost is often minimal.

Assistive Technology

Assistive technology devices are any mechanical aids that substitute for or enhance the function of a patient's physical or mental ability when it is impaired. Such devices include anything from homemade to purchased, whether off-the-shelf, customized, or modified. The main intent of assistive devices is to help an individual perform ADLs. The term *assistive technology* encompasses a broad range of devices from low-tech (e.g., pencil grips, splints, paper stabilizers) to high-tech (e.g., computers, voice synthesizers, Braille readers). These devices include the entire range of supportive tools and equipment from adapted spoons to wheelchairs and computer systems for environmental control.

Assistive technology is used to support access, learning, and the performing of ADL tasks. It is appropriate for CMs to recommend assistive technology when it can assist and compensate for disabilities and allow the individual to function as normally as possible. Assistive technology is appropriate when it does any of the following:

- Enables an individual to perform functions that can be achieved by no other means
- Enables an individual to approximate normal fluency, rate, or standards—a level of accomplishment that cannot be achieved by any other means
- Provides access for participation in programs or activities that otherwise would be closed to the individual
- Increases endurance or ability to persevere and complete tasks that otherwise are too laborious to be attempted on a routine basis

- Enables an individual to concentrate on learning or employment tasks, rather than merely on mechanical tasks
- Provides greater access to information
- Supports normal social interactions with peers and adults
- Supports participation in the least restrictive educational environment

IDEA provides the following legal definition of an assistive technology device: "any item, piece of equipment or product system that is used to increase, maintain or improve functional capabilities of individuals with disabilities." Under IDEA, assistive technology devices can be used in the educational setting to provide a variety of accommodations or adaptations for people with disabilities.

IDEA also lists the services a school district may need to provide in order to ensure that assistive technology is useful to a student in the school setting. The law defines assistive technology service as "any service that directly assists an individual with a disability in the selection, acquisition or use of an assistive technology device." This service includes all of the following possibilities[87]:

- Evaluation of the technology needs of the individual including a functional evaluation in the individual's customary environment
- Purchasing, leasing, or otherwise providing for the acquisition of assistive technology devices for individuals with disabilities
- Selecting, designing, fitting, customizing, adapting, applying, maintaining, repairing, or replacing of assistive technology devices
- Coordinating and using other therapies, interventions, or services with assistive technology devices such as those associated with existing education and rehabilitation plans and programs

- Assistive technology training or technical assistance with assistive technology for an individual with a disability or, where appropriate, the family of an individual with a disability.

Assistive Technology Accommodations and Adaptations

Accommodations are reasonable modifications that are made to compensate for skills or abilities when an individual lacks. It also refers to a way of modifying a task or assignment so that the person can participate in spite of whatever challenges the disability poses. In contrast, adaptation is the development of unique devices or methods designed specifically to assist persons with disabilities and allow them to perform daily tasks. Examples of adaptations include special grips to turn stove knobs or specially designed keyboards to operate computers.

Assistive technology includes any type of high-tech or low-tech device that allows a person with a disability to function:

- **High-tech items**—computers; touch screens; voice-activated devices; robotic arms; environmental and remote control systems that turn lights on and off, open doors, and operate appliances; and locational and orientation systems that give vision-impaired persons information about where they are, what the ground nearby is like, and whether there is a curb nearby
- **Augmentative communication devices**—symbol systems, communication boards and wallets, programmable switches, electronic communication devices, speech synthesizers, recorded speech devices, communication enhancement software, and voiced word processing
- **Assistive devices for hearing or auditory-processing impairments**—

hearing aids, personal FM units, sound field FM systems, Phonic Ear, TDDs, and closed-caption TV
- **Visual aids**—screen readers, screen enlargers, magnifiers, large-type books, taped books, Braillers, light boxes, high-contrast materials, thermoform graphics, synthesizers, and scanners
- **Mobility devices**—self-propelled walkers, manual or powered wheelchairs, and powered recreational vehicles such as bikes and scooters
- **Positioning devices**—side-lying frames, walkers, crawling assists, floor sitters, chair inserts, wheelchairs, straps, trays, standing aids, beanbag chairs, and sandbags
- Controllable, anatomic sites like eye blinks and head, neck, or mouth movements may be used to operate the equipment wen a person is unable to use his or her hands; once a controllable anatomic site has been determined, decisions can be made about the most appropriate input devices (switches, alternative keyboards, mouse, trackball, touch window, speech recognition, and head pointers)
- **Access devices or modifications**—ramps and door openers to enter buildings, rooms, and other facilities; and devices that allow persons to follow Braille directions
- **Recreational assistive technology**—drawing software, computer games, computer simulations, painting with a head or mouth wand, interactive laser disks, adapted puzzles, and modified sports equipment
- **High-tech self-care assistive devices**—robotics, electric feeders, adapted utensils, specially designed toilet seats, and aids for toothbrushing, washing, dressing, and grooming
- **Low-tech self-care assistive devices**—wrist splints, clipboards

for holding papers steady, or Velcro tabs to keep positioning pads in place

As wonderful as assistive technology can be, it is not always easy to acquire. It takes expertise and persistence to find the correct devices. Then one must face the challenge of who will pay for the devices if someone needs them other than a child with special needs. This is necessary as often these devices are classified as not medically necessary for the treatment of the medical condition. In contrast, if a child with disabilities needs the devices and is eligible for special education, the child has a legal right to such technology, as it will assist them with learning. Both the Individualized Family Service Plan (IFSP) and the Individualized Education Program (IEP) that are required by the Individuals with Disabilities Education Act (IDEA) are potentially powerful tools for incorporating assistive technology into the education of students with disabilities. However, if approved for use in school, the devices often are not allowed out of the classroom. The CM may be required to pursue other options for procurement of similar devices for use at home. The biggest battle for the approval of assistive technology centers around the fact that this technology does not become part of a student's special education plan unless parents are knowledgeable about technology and know what to do to ensure that it becomes an integral part of their child's program.[88]

Home Evaluations and Modifications

For most technologically dependent patients, a home evaluation is necessary before the equipment is actually ordered and delivered and the patient discharged. This is necessary to ensure the home can accommodate the equipment and supplies physically, structurally, and electrically. Unfortunately, in many instances an actual home visit by the health care team is not always possible. If a home visit is impossi-ble, it is wise to ask the family to measure and draw a replica of the space to be used and have it reviewed by the therapist at the hospital. If the drawing indicates the space is unacceptable, a visit by a local home health agency or even a local building inspector may be necessary. The physical dimensions are not the only factors that must be considered. It is important to ascertain the answers to the following questions:

- Is the house strong enough struc-turally to handle the weight of the equipment?
- Can the electrical panel accommo-date the peak amperage required by all of the equipment? Note that all equipment must be assessed and the total amperage noted because most homes require extra electrical panels or circuits if they are to accommo-date the equipment.
- Can the patient maneuver around the house? All doorways and hall-ways must be measured and any bar-riers found must be corrected.
- Can the patient enter and leave the home safely or are ramps or other accommodations necessary?
- Is the heating and cooling systems adequate to maintain temperature control since most technologically dependent patients have problems with body temperature regulation? Also, because of the heat generated by continuously operating equip-ment, adequate ventilation and air circulation is necessary.
- Where are supplies to be stored? Is there adequate space?
- Does the home provide hot water, and is there indoor plumbing?
- Is there enough space to designate one area as clean and another intended to hold dirty or used sup-plies?
- Physically where will the patient spend most of his or her day? If a

large portion of the day is to be spent in bed, then consideration must be given to relocating the patient area to the activity center of the home (e.g., the living room or family room).

- In all cases, the bathroom must be assessed for its ability to accommodate and contribute to personal care and toiletry activities.

If the home is to be universally usable, it must contain the following features:

- Wide and level entries
- 32-inch interior door openings
- Passage spaces of 32 inches or more
- Variable height counters in the kitchen and bath
- Supportive grab bars in showers, in bathtubs, and around toilets
- Bathrooms large enough to accommodate walkers and wheelchairs
- Accessible switches and controls at reachable heights
- In some cases other modifications may include ramps, handrails, or an elevator or chair lift
- A bedroom and full bath on the ground floor[88]

If barriers are identified, corrections must be made as soon as possible. Other than workers' compensation and the VA, few health care insurers reimburse the patient to correct barriers or modify the home for any of the foregoing reasons. This is an expense the family must incur. If the family cannot afford the necessary corrections, they must be encouraged to solicit assistance from a community volunteer, church group, or fraternal organization. Many such organizations are willing to make these repairs or corrections as a "service project."

SECTION XI—ALTERNATE FUNDING

Because of the many disabling conditions associated with the foregoing diagnoses and the possible lifelong consequences and continual need for health care services, it is imperative to evaluate such patients continuously and when possible link them with appropriate alternate funding resources. Why is this necessary? Because such resources can either assist with the payment for health care services or add needed income. CMs must develop a schedule and include it in the case management plan whereby the financial status of the patient or family is assessed regularly.

Such assessments are necessary because the patient's health care coverage may terminate at any given time during the illness or recovery period. Assessments are also needed when a request for services is denied or when services are excluded or limited by the patient's health care benefit coverage.

Because of the importance of linkage to financial resources, CMs must maintain current knowledge of the commonly used alternate funding programs in the immediate vicinity and also in regions where the majority of their patients receive care.

These programs undergo changes that result from budgetary constraints as well as from changes made in the laws or federal or state administrative codes that govern the programs. Each primary alternate funding program is discussed in greater detail in Chapters 5 through 9.

Alternate funding often used to augment insurance benefits or provide coverage when there is no insurance or limited income includes the following:

- Adults
  - Medicaid
  - Supplemental Security Income (SSI)
  - Social Security Disability Insurance (SSDI)
  - Single parents with children: Aid to Families with Dependent Children (AFDC)
  - Veterans or retired from the military: veterans' benefits or CHAMPUS coverage

- Dependent spouse of a person on active duty in any military service: Program for Persons with Disabilities (PFPWD), previously the Program for the Handicapped (PFTH)
- Healthy families

■ Children
  - Medicaid
  - State Children's Health Insurance Program (SCHIP)
  - Supplemental Security Income (SSI)
  - Title V/Children's Medical Services programs
  - State agency responsible for administering services for the developmentally disabled
  - Dependent child of a person on active duty in any military service: Program for Persons with Disabilities (PFPWD)
  - Dependent child of a person eligible for Social Security: any Social Security benefits to which he or she may be entitled

To remain knowledgeable about the resources available, CMs should keep current data on at least the referral processes, eligibility criteria, and appeal processes required by the public programs offered within the state or county.

Because of variations in the programs, their eligibility requirements, and the manner in which eligibility is linked to services, it is wise to refer patients to public programs as soon as they are identified as possible candidates. Delays in the eligibility referral and screening processes are common. These delays are frequently due to barriers such as resistance by the patient or family who must be counseled that alternate funding programs are not "welfare" but additional insurance; the need to secure all paperwork and receipts that may be required to establish financial need; the agency's investigational process required to screen clients for eligibility; and the agency's backlog in processing new requests.

Although many patients may be eligible for several programs at once, other patients will not qualify because of higher financial reserves, income, or assets despite a demonstrated need for the program. In the latter category are patients and families who have too much to qualify yet too little to pay for the services and care required. It is in these cases the CM must be as creative and innovative as possible for a plan that will meet the patient's needs to be established. Sadly, in some cases, there is no solution despite all efforts. The following are examples of funding for which patients might be eligible:

- Regardless of age, if the patient has end-stage renal disease, referral must be made to Social Security's End-Stage Renal Disease program.
- In rare cases in which the patient may be undergoing an experimental or investigational procedure or service, he or she may be eligible for coverage of a portion of care and services through a research grant or clinical trial. However, to be eligible, the patient must have the specific diagnosis for which the study is designed. Also, the research may be limited to patients in specific national university or tertiary care centers.
- Another source of possible assistance, particularly when the patient's health care coverage limits or excludes some benefits, are funds available from some fraternal organizations. These organizations are often willing to assist with services ranging from payment for the services to assistance by volunteers when specific needs have been identified.
- For active duty military dependents, retirees, or their dependents, an excellent resource for assistance

when funding is limited or excluded by TRICARE or the patient's other health care benefit package is the Armed Forces Family Service Agency programs. Information about the availability of such assistance can be obtained by calling a TRICARE health care finder or the nearest military treatment facility's health benefits advisor (HBA) or managed care or patient administration personnel. Also, any patient needing specialized services such as a transplant may be eligible to have the procedure performed in any of the military centers of excellence (e.g., Wilford Hall Medical Center, Brooke Army Medical Center, Walter Reed Medical Center). The military also has other programs available to assist with the care of patients. More information can be found in Chapter 8.

- If the patient is a veteran, contact with the nearest VA office or the local or regional Veterans Clinic or medical clinic can help the CM determine whether the patient is eligible for any services that will be paid.

Using Community Resources

Due to the complexity of care required by case-managed patients and the fact that not all care may be covered by health care insurance, CMs must be very knowledgeable about all community resources whether local, regional, or national that can be used to augment and enhance the proposed case management plan. Many patients may be eligible for services from several agencies. In all cases, the family should be encouraged to make contact with any agencies that can offer the assistance or information required.

Many disease-specific (e.g., American Cancer Society, United Cerebral Palsy Association), church (e.g., Catholic Social Services, Lutheran Social Services, Jewish Social Services), and ethnic agencies (e.g., Jewish Social Services, Asian centers, Hispanic centers) offer an entire array of services. Many disease-specific agencies are operational locally as well as nationally, and in many cases a toll-free telephone number can access their national offices. Services provided by such disease-specific agencies include at minimum information and referral, literature, educational classes, and support groups.

The power of the support received by patients and their families from these support groups cannot be overstated. Whenever possible, patients and families should be linked to the agencies designed to respond to the needs of patients with a particular disease. In addition to disease-specific, church, and ethnic agencies, patients commonly use the following community resources:

- County chore worker or homemaker service agencies
- County public health clinics and services
- Emergency response systems
- Easter Seals Society
- Fraternal organizations
- Handicapped sports and recreation associations
- Handicapped transportation services (generally offered by local transportation authorities)
- Independent living centers
- Meals programs (delivered to homes or congregate sites)
- Legal advice, either from the local legal center for the disabled and elderly or a private attorney
- Library services
- Medical alert identification bracelets
- Department of Rehabilitation or vocational rehabilitation services
- For the visually or hearing impaired, referrals may be necessary to a center for deafness or blindness as well

as to obtain assistance with such services as:

- Guide Dogs for the Blind
- Lions Eye and Tissue Bank
- For children with special needs, referrals may be necessary to obtain such services as the following:
  - Women, Infants, and Children (WIC) nutrition program
  - Services offered by the Department of Education and Special Education
  - Special Olympics or any agency designed to provide handicapped recreational activities
  - Special children's foundations (e.g., Make-A-Wish Foundation) for special projects or to fulfill a child's wish

Many communities offer art and play therapy as well as other programs designed to help children who have a terminal illness. Availability of these services can be ascertained by calling the local American Cancer Society or the nearest regional cancer center that specializes in pediatric cancer care.

For high-risk pregnant women, referrals to the following may be necessary:

- County public health clinics for high-risk mothers and infants, or with a diagnosis of AIDS to AIDS clinics
- Title V/Children's Medical Services programs for genetic screening
- Planned Parenthood
- Women, Infants, and Children (WIC) nutrition program

For organ transplant candidates, CMs should link the patient to the nearest local organ procurement agency for any assistance or guidance that may be required in addition to referring him or her to disease-specific groups and transplant centers.

Persons living alone may benefit from "visitor" or "telephone visitor" programs offered by the local department on aging.

These agencies are designed to serve seniors. Information about such programs can be obtained from the Department on Aging. This is an invaluable resource for information about any of its programs in the area that serve the senior population. As described earlier in this chapter, another excellent program is the emergency response system, which consists of a device worn by the patient that when activated during a time of medical need, links the patient electronically to the nearest emergency department, which then mobilizes according to a prearranged emergency plan.

Certainly the community resources listed in this section are not all-inclusive. Each community offers a unique combination of resources. What is the best source for locating information about resources when a community resource directory is not available? The answer is the Yellow Pages of the telephone book and eventually the CM's own Rolodex file.

SUMMARY

Managing complex cases requires multiple skills. However, nothing can be done in vacuum. Thus, the CM must work closely with the entire multidisciplinary team as the case is evaluated and assessed, and the eventual case management plan developed. In reality, there are often many CMs involved with the care of a complex case. Thus, it is critical to appoint one key CM as the primary CM. This ensures communication flows from the physician, family, and all CMs. Ultimately, frustrations, fragmentations, and duplications are minimized. Each case is individual, so that there is no single plan that fits any two patients. Case management plans must be individualized to meet the needs of the patient and his or her financial abilities and limitations. To prevent complications or unforeseen episodes, close monitoring is critical. At least 20% of the U.S. population (54 million) suffer from disabilities. Of this percentage, at least one-half have severe disabilities that affect speech, hearing, walking, or performing basic functions. Therefore, case management plans must be in place to ensure needs are met.[89] When the patient's needs appear to be long-term or chronic, equally as critical will be teaching the patient or family to become the CM as soon as possible.

Chapter Exercises

1. In a group setting, discuss the field of medicine you feel is best suited to case manage cases; state why you feel as you do, be prepared to give examples of cases, and state two reasons why you feel the field of medicine selected is appropriate for the role.
2. In a group setting, discuss the many types of patient management programs health plans are using in an attempt to contain costs. Identify at least four types of programs and list some of the key components for each.
3. List the various competencies required for case management and include at least two of the competencies not required by accreditors such as JCAHO and NCQA.
4. Take a new case, and perform at least two assessments listed in the text on the new patient. Explain to your colleagues your findings and what you feel their importance will be in managing a case.

Suggested Websites and Resources

Complex Medical Conditions

www.medscape.com—Provides the latest clinical updates on multiple issues
www.ama-assn.org—American Medical Association
www.aegis.com—AIDS global information system

www.centerwatch.com—Information on clinical trials
www.napbc—Information on breast cancer
www.cdc.gov—Centers for Disease Control and Prevention
www.cms.hhs.gov—Centers for Medicare & Medicaid Services (formerly the Health Care Financing Administration)
www.nlm.nih.gov—National Library of Medicine, based at the National Institutes of Health
www.cmsa.org—Case Management Society of America
www.nih.gov/nia—National Institute on Aging
www.merck.com—Online version of the Merck manual
www.needymeds.com—Helps patients who cannot afford medications to obtain them
www.StrokeFamily.org—Offers practice software for persons at home who need to practice their speech
www.katsden.com—Death, dying, and grief information as well as information on advanced directives
orders@nits.fedworld.gov—Offers videos for those who work with persons with developmental disabilities
www.info@conceptmedica.com—Offers videos for persons working with children aged 6 to 12 years

Wound Care

www.medicare.gov/Supplier/Home.asp—Medicare's website for wound care supplies and information
www.wound.net—American Academy of Wound Management, the national multidisciplinary certifying board for health care professionals involved in wound care

Caregiver Websites

www.caregiving.org/—National Alliance for Caregiving
www.caregiving.com/support—Information on local support groups and services

www.alz.org—The Alzheimer's Association, a national voluntary health organization, provides information and services to persons with Alzheimer's, caregivers, researchers, physicians, and health care professionals

www.interfaithcaregivers.org/—Interfaith Caregivers Alliance

www.aoa.dhhs.gov/aoa/dir/132.html or *www.nih.gov/nia/related/aoaresrc/*—National Association of Area on Aging

REFERENCES

1. Case Management Society of America (CMSA): *Case Management Society of America's definition and philosophy*, available on-line at www.cmsa.org/pdf/DefofCM.pdf.
2. Cohen EL, Cesta TG: *Nursing case management: from essentials to advanced practice applications*, ed 3, St Louis, 2001, Mosby.
3. Coleman JR: Integrated case management: the 21st challenge for HMO case managers, Part II, *CM* 10 (6):28–33, 1999.
4. Zalta E, Eichner H, Henry M: Implications of disease management in the future of managed care. *Medical Interface* 7(2):66–69, 78, 1994.
5. Moreo K: Newest case management strategies of managed care organizations, *J Care Management* 5(6):10–19, 1999.
6. Newell M: *Using nursing case management to improve health outcomes*, Gaithersburg, Md, 1996, Aspen.
7. Peterson C: Pharmacoeconomics: determining the value of drug therapy, *Healthplan* 39(3):46, 1998.
8. McCollom P: Life care planning 101: an introduction to the process, *J Care Management* 5(6):24–27, 1999.
9. Harrell TW, Bagwell DM, Coupland MW: Building a future teaming up for a life care plan, *Continuing Care* 16(7):26–32, 1997.
10. Vesmarovich S, Hauber R, Temkin A, Burns R: Phoning home, *Advance for Providers of Post-Acute Care* 2(8):18, 1999.
11. Southwick AF: The law of hospital and health administration, ed 2, Ann Arbor, Mich, 1988, Health Administration Press.
12. Faltermayer F: Why healthcare costs can keep slowing, *Fortune* 129:75–82, 1994.
13. Bartling A: Trends in managed care, *Healthcare Executive* 10(2):7–11, 1995.
14. Harris MD, Lynch SA: Working with managed care networks: strategies for success. In Flarey DL, Blancett SS: *Handbook of nursing case management health care delivery in a world of managed care*, Gaithersburg, Md, 1996, Aspen.
15. Flarey DL, Blancett SS: *Handbook of nursing case management health care delivery in a world of managed care*, Gaithersburg, Md, 1996, Aspen.
16. Johnson C, Birmingham J: How to use research information to improve case management practice, *J Case Management* 5(3):41–49, 1999.
17. Clowers M: Facilitating better patient care: a case manager's guide to improving physician-patient communication, *J Case Management* 5(5):24–27, 1999.
18. Motta G: Skin & wound care: collaborating to achieve positive patient outcomes, *Continuing Care* 16(8):12, 1997.
19. Feuer L: Collaborate for efficiency, *Continuing Care* 18(5):2, 1999.
20. Feuer L: Who's looking in our medical record now? *CM* 10(1):16–17, 1999.
21. Davidhizar R, Bechtel G, Giger JN: Model helps CMs deliver multicultural care, *Case Management Advisor* 9(6):97–100,105, 1998.
22. Edlin M: Literacy and good health, *Healthplan* 39(3):52–58, 1998.
23. Setting case management caseloads remains tricky business. AHC/CMSA caseload survey, *Care Manager* 12(4):53, 2001.
24. How many cases can a case manager manage? *Nursing Case Management* 2(3):96, 1997.
25. Kelly B: The continuum connection, *Advance for Providers of Post-Acute Care* 4(3):38–40, 2001.
26. Kauffman-Nearhoof C: This thing called HIPAA, *Advance for Providers of Post-Acute Care* 4(3):51–54, 2001.
27. Kauffman-Nearhoof C: HIPAA: a new protected species, *Case Management* 7(4):38–42, 2001.
28. Ward D: Instant accessibility enhances case management efficacy, *CM* 8(3):44, 1997.
29. Thomas RL: Computer potpourri—practical technology, *CM* 8(3):50–52, 1997.
30. Coleman JR: New challenges call for rewriting the rules for problem solving, *CM* 7(2):47, 1996.
31. Quality problem solving, decision making, type theory, and case managers, Part II, *Nursing Case Management* 2:109, 1997.
32. Llewellyn A: A common thread, *Continuing Care* 19(4):24–29, 2000.
33. Schielke C: Patient advocacy: the shield that empowers, *Continuing Care* 16(3):22–26, 1997.
34. Hirni B: 50 ways to improve networking skills, *Case Management Advisor* 8(8):141, 1997.
35. Shendell-Falik N: Tips, tools and techniques—the art of negotiation, *Nursing Case Management* 2(3):107, 1997.
36. Smeltzer CH: The art of negotiation: an everyday experience. In Hein D, Nicholson M, editors: *Contemporary leadership behavior*, Philadelphia, 1994, Lippincott.
37. Henry S, Zander K: Improving patient adherence, *Care Management* 7(4):14–17, 2001.
38. Aliotta S: Patient adherence outcome indicators and management in case management and health care, *J Care Management* 5(4):24–31,81–82, 1999.
39. Editorial. Scare healthcare resources require CMs to focus efforts on compliance, *Case Management Advisor* 9(6):93–96, 1998.

40. Highsmith C: Case management strategies for "difficult" clients, *J Case Management* 14(1):26–31, 1998.

41. Nichols R: Managing cancer pain in managed care, *CM* 8(2):50, 1997.

42. Curtis CP: Disease management digest—when the problem is pain, *Care Management* 7(3):6–7, 2001.

43. Vasudevan S: Physical rehabilitation in managing pain, *IASP Pain Clinical Updates* 4:1–4, 1997.

44. Herbert P, Rochman D, McAlary PW: Dealing with pain—treating the physical, psychological and emotional aspects of patients with chronic pain, *Case Review* 4(6):16–19, 1998.

45. Jamison R: Psychological factors in chronic pain, *J Back Musculoskeletal Rehabilitation* 1996, pp 79–95.

46. Bogduk N, Merskey H, editors: *Classifications of chronic pain syndromes and definitions of pain terms*, Seattle, 1994, IASP Press.

47. Meaney ME: Professional integrity: a commentary—case management in the bliss zone, *CM* 12(4):63–65, 2001.

48. Website for information on Eric Erickson stages of development: www.ship.edu/~cgboeree/erikson.html.

49. Van Genderen A: How to develop and manage a case management department, *J Case Management* 2(4):30–40, 1996.

50. Bright PA: Skills help to cope with change, *Case Management Advisor* 8(8):142–143, 1997.

51. Hall KM, Hamilton BB, Gordon WA, et al: Characteristics and comparisons of functional assessment indices: Disability Rating Scale, Functional Independence Measure and Functional Assessment Measure, *J Head Trauma Rehabilitation* 8(2):60–74, 1993.

52. Aliotta SL: Key functions and direct outcomes of case management. In Cohen EL, Cesta TG, editors: *Nursing case management: from essentials to advanced practice applications*, St Louis, 2001, Mosby.

53. Kirk R: *Managing outcomes, process, and cost in a managed care environment*, Gaithersburg, Md, 1997, Aspen.

54. Birmingham J: Medicare conditions of participation recognize discharge planning experts, *Continuing Care* 15(1):16,34, 1996.

55. Weissman JS, Gastonis C, Epstein AM: Rates of avoidable hospitalization by insurance status in Massachusetts and Maryland, *JAMA* 268(17):2388–2394, 1992.

56. Certified case manager news, *Care Management* 7(2):45, 2001.

57. McClinton DH: Oncology case management, *Continuing Care* 15(1):8–13, 1996.

58. Rantz MJ, Scott J: Promoting self-management of chronic illness. In Cohen EL, De Back V: *The outcomes mandate: case management in health care today*, St Louis, 1999, Mosby.

59. New poll reveals American concerns about living with chronic conditions, *Care Management* 7(2):52, 2001.

60. Larson DE: *Mayo Clinic family health book*, ed 2, New York, 1996, William Morrow.

61. Health care update—ambulatory care, treatment advances help stabilize hospitalizations, *Care Management* 7(3):58, 2001.

62. Davidhizar R, Shearer RA: Helping the elderly to adjust to change and loss, *J Case Management* 6(2):22, 2000.

63. Newell M: Patient contracting for improved outcomes, *J Care Management* 3(4):76–80,85–87, 1997.

64. Wolfe GS: Improving care at end-of-life, *J Care Management* 3(5):10, 1997.

65. Taylor C: Ethical issues in case management. In Cohen EL, Cesta TG, editors: *Nursing case management: from essentials to advanced practice applications*, ed 3, St Louis, 2001, Mosby.

66. Kaufman J, Blanchon D: Managed care for children with special needs: a care coordination model, *J Care Management* 2(2):46–59, 1996.

67. Managed care and children with special health care needs: a subject review (RE 9814), *American Academy of Pediatrics* 102(3):657–660, 1998.

68. Deming LM, Wolf JC: Case management for ventilator-dependent children, *J Care Management* 3(5):15–25, 1997.

69. Folks DG: Munchausen's syndrome and other factitious disorders, *Neurol Clin* 13(2):267–281, 19959.

70. McCahill ME: Somatoform and related disorder, delivery of diagnosis as first step, *Am Fam Physician* 52(1):193–204, 1995.

71. Wellman NS: A case manager's guide to nutrition screening and intervention, *J Care Management* 3(2):12–27, 1997.

72. Pomeriau B: Swallowing nutrition issues, *Advance for Providers of Post-Acute Care* 3(3):14–15, 2000.

73. Bradsher KB, Parker M: *Home nutrition support: management issues for case managers*, Mosby, MCMC XI Medical Case Management Convention, San Diego, September 1999.

74. Motta G: Skin and wound care: changes in wound care reimbursement, *Continuing Care* 18(3);18, 1999.

75. Resource center: help for caregivers offered, *Case Manager* 11(1):13, 2000.

76. Employee assistance, *Continuing Care* 18(8):12, 1999.

77. Powell SK: *Nursing case management: a practical guide to success in managed care*, Philadelphia, 1996, Lippincott.

78. Scott A: Walking a tightrope, *Advance for Providers of Post-Acute Care* 3(3):12–13, 2000.

79. Golodner LF: Consumer voice. In Cohen EL, De Back V, editors: *The outcomes mandate: case management in health care today*, St Louis, 1999, Mosby.

80. Aruffo S, Gardner C: The importance of patient education materials, *Care Manager* 11(2):58–62, 2000.

81. Feuer L: Company size may not matter, *CM* 8(3):41–42, 1997.

82. Parver C, Hildebrandt S: Pending legislation to affect home care and DME, *Continuing Care* 15(6):36, 1996.

83. Salerno S: Making accurate seating assessments, *Advance for Providers of Post-Acute Care* 2(8):21–22 1999.

84. Peischi D: Growing wheelchairs, *Advance for Providers of Post-Acute Care* 2(8):68 1999.

85. Visiting Nurse Association of Sacramento, 1995.

86. Winfree A: Billing for DME, *Advance for Providers of Post-Acute Care* 3(10):24–25, 2000.

87. Kelker KA, editor: *Family guide to assistive technology*, Federation for Children with Special Needs, www.pluk.org/AT1.html#2.

88. Home modification for better living, *Long-Term Care Interface*, 2(5):21, 2001.

89. Rubinger H, Gardner R: Tearing down the walls, *Continuing Care* 21(3):25–27,31, 2002.

BIBLIOGRAPHY

Adkins C: Family caregivers, *Advance for Providers of Post-Acute Care* 6(3):19, 2000.

Alexander TT, Hiduke RJ, Stevens KA: *Rehabilitation nursing procedures manual*, ed 2,. New York, 1999, McGraw-Hill.

Bateman WB, Kramer EJ, Glassman KS: *Patient and family education in managed care and beyond—seizing the teachable moment*, New York, 1999, Springer.

Bienkowski SL: Lighting the way, *Continuing Care* 20(1):18-21, 2001.

Brown P, Phelps-Maloy J, Oddo D: *Quick reference to wound care*, Gaithersburg, Md, 2001, Aspen.

Bryant RA: *Acute and chronic wounds nursing management*, St Louis, 1992, Mosby.

Buckman-Murray R, Proctor-Zentner J: *Health promotion strategies through the life span*, ed 7, Upper Saddle River, NJ, 2001, Prentice Hall.

Ellis JR, Hartley CL: *Managing and coordinating nursing care*, ed 2, Philadelphia, 1995, Lippincott.

Feuer L: Getting your act together: it's called efficiency, *Continuing Care* 18(1):12-14, 1999.

Flavo DR: *Effective patient education. A guide to increased compliance*, ed 2, Gaithersburg, Md, 1994, Aspen.

Geyman JP, Norris TE, Hart LG: *Textbook of rural medicine*, New York, 2001, McGraw-Hill.

Giger JN, Davidhizar RE: *Transcultural nursing: assessment and intervention*, ed 3, St Louis, 1999, Mosby.

Hoeman SP: *Rehabilitation nursing: process, application, and outcomes*, ed 3, St Louis, 2002, Mosby.

Holloway NM: Nursing the critically ill adult, ed 4, Redwood City, Calif, 1993, Addison Wesley.

Lo B: *Resolving ethical dilemmas: a guide for clinicians*, Baltimore, 1995, William & Wilkins.

Loewy EH, Loewy RS: *The ethics of terminal care orchestrating the end of life*, New York, 2001, Kluwer/Plenum.

Miaskowski C: *Oncology nursing: an essential guide for patient care*, Philadelphia, 1997, Saunders.

Miaskowski C, Buchsel P: *Oncology nursing assessment and clinical care*, St Louis, Mosby, 1999.

Nies MA, McEwen M: *Community health nursing: promoting the health of populations*, Philadelphia, 1997, Saunders.

Purnell LD, Paulanka BJ: *Transcultural healthcare: a culturally competent approach*, Philadelphia, 1998, FA Davis.

Schyman J: Old concept, new trends: a primer on life care planning. long term care interface, *Long-Term Care Interface* 2(2):26-28, 2001.

Sigardson-Poor KM, Haggerty LM: *Nursing care of the transplant patient*, Philadelphia, 1990, Saunders.

Simpson KR, Creehan PA: *Competence validation of perinatal care providers: orientation, continuing education and evaluation*, Philadelphia, 1998, Lippincott.

Smith CM, Maurer FA: *Community health nursing theory and practice*, Philadelphia, 2000, Saunders

Stanhope M, Lancaster J: *Community and public health nursing*, ed 5, St Louis, 2000, Mosby.

Stone JT, Wyman JF, Salisbury SA: *Clinical gerontological nursing: a guide to advanced practice*, ed 2, Philadelphia, 1999, Saunders.

Trofino RB: *Nursing care of the burn patient*, Philadelphia, 1991, FA Davis.

Wallace RB, Doebbling BN: *Public health and preventive medicine*, ed 14, Stamford, Conn, 2000, Appleton Lange.

Weissman JS, Gastonis C, Epstein AM: Rates of avoidable hospitalization by insurance status in Massachusetts and Maryland, *JAMA* 268(17):2388-2394, 1992.

Wise BV, McKenna C, Garvin G, Harmon BJ: *Nursing care of the general pediatric surgical patient*, Gaithersburg, Md, 2000, Aspen.

Wong DL, Perry SE, Hockenberry MJ: *Maternal child nursing care*, ed 2, St Louis, 2002, Mosby.

CHAPTER

15

Disease Management

Gay Raney, RN, MSN

OBJECTIVES

- To describe the differences between disease management and case management
- To define what disease management is and the populations it serves
- To be able to characterize at least three of the processes in disease management

Historically the initial focus of disease management as early as Pasteur's time was to eliminate or contain epidemics. Over time, however, and especially in the twentieth century, the U.S. public health care system has used disease management to address the escalating costs of care for specific diseases or segments of the patient population in an attempt to control health care expenditures. The term *disease management* was first officially developed in 1993 and was used by the Boston Consulting Group in reference to the approaches being taken by the pharmaceutical industry. Since then, disease management has grown and evolved as an impressive approach to managing specific disease and patient populations across the continuum.[1]

Population aging has immense implications for all countries. According to the National Center for Chronic Disease Prevention and Health Promotion, during the 21st century the aging of the population will present some of the biggest challenges for health care. These challenges will center on knowing how to prevent and postpone disease and disability while maintaining the health, independence, and mobility of an aging population.[2] Globally individuals are now surviving longer because epidemics of infectious diseases such as tuberculosis and respiratory disease were better controlled when they were children. Also, this longevity can be attributed to the successes achieved in the past 50 years against microbial and parasitic diseases, and to the creation of a healthier environment through improvements in hygiene and sanitation, treatment with effective, affordable antibiotic and antiparasitic drugs, and the availability of vaccines to prevent disease.

Life expectancy in the United States has increased dramatically from 47 years in 1900 to 76 years in 1990. Since 1900 the U.S. population has tripled. By 2030 the number of older Americans (those aged 65 years or older) will have more than doubled. This growth in both the number and proportion of older adults is placing increasing demands on health care systems. Thus, the United States is on the brink of a longevity revolution, and with it comes an increase in chronic diseases and health care needs. In general, noncommunicable diseases such as coronary heart disease, cancer, diabetes, and mental disorders are more common than infectious diseases in the industrialized world. As the population ages and longevity increases, chronic diseases will become more prevalent, and as they do, effective disease management programs must be in place to assist organizations in focusing on and establishing programs that will help stabilize and manage specific diseases and control the costs of care.

Over the last several years, there has been a strong incentive to develop different modalities of case management as a means of increasing quality and containing health care costs. These various methods are briefly described in the chapter in this text on complex care. Disease management, however, was one of the first methods introduced by many organizations as a potential solution to the increasingly expensive acute health care delivery system because it is a modality for providing early intervention before acute care is needed.

According to the 1994 annual report of the Robert Wood Johnson Foundation, in the United States escalating health care costs cannot be addressed without addressing the problem of chronic disease management. This report presented the following statistics:

- More than 90 million Americans live with chronic illnesses.
- Chronic diseases account for 70% of all deaths in the United States.
- The medical care costs of people with chronic diseases account for more than 60% of the nation's total medical care expenditures.
- Chronic diseases account for one third of the years of potential life lost before age 65 years.[3]

DEFINITION OF DISEASE MANAGEMENT

Although there is no standardized definition of disease management, most health professionals agree that disease management is a comprehensive and coordinated system of care that manages a disease state rather than an acute episode, with the goals focused on maximizing favorable outcomes and cost containment for the given disease entity. According to the Disease Management Association of America (DMAA),

disease management is a system of coordinated health care intercommunications for populations with conditions in which patient efforts are significant. Disease management:

- Supports the physician or practitioner/patient relationship and plan of care,
- Emphasizes prevention of exacerbations and complications utilizing evidence guidelines and patient empowerment strategies, and
- Evaluates clinical, humanistic, and economic outcomes on an ongoing basis while improving overall health.[4]

The DMAA supports the view that a disease management system can be recognized as a program only if it includes the six components listed below; without all six, a care system is providing nothing more than disease management services. The six components necessary for a program to be called a disease management program are as follows[1]:

1. Population identification processes
2. Evidence-based practice guidelines
3. Collaborative practice models that include physician and support service providers
4. Patient self-management education (may include primary prevention, behavior modification programs, and compliance and surveillance programs)

5. Process and outcomes measurement, evaluation, and management
6. Routine reporting and feedback loop (may include communication with the patient, physician, and ancillary providers, and practice profiling)

Disease State Management

Disease state management can be described as an integrated system of interventions, measurements, and refinements of health care delivery designed to optimize clinical and economic outcomes within a specific population. Although the term *disease state management* is used by many organizations, it is not entirely correct because the patient and not the disease is being managed. While other terms, such as *population-based care or continuous health care improvement*, are used to describe disease management programs, disease state management, or sometimes just disease management, is the term used by most in their program titles.

Whatever the term, properly designed disease management programs must rely on aggressive prevention of complications as well as treatment of chronic conditions. The program is created with a clear understanding of the natural course of a disease and the effect of interventions at critical points in delaying or preventing complications.

It also offers processes that accomplish the following:

- Focus on primary illness prevention, educating the patient in self-management of the disease while controlling symptoms with behavior modification and compliance with pharmaceutical regimens during times of disease exacerbation and remission.
- Improve the course of disease by preventing acute disease exacerbation, while controlling cost by decreasing the number of hospitalizations and outpatient and emergency department visits, which pose a significant burden in mortality, morbidity, and cost.
- Use an interventional form of case management that treats high-risk, high-cost patients who actively participate in maintaining an optimum state with regard to a specific disease component and forge a partnership with the patient and the physician to achieve desired clinical, financial, and quality-of-life outcomes.
- Use clinical practice guidelines, protocols, or pathways to standardize the care and treatment of a specific disease to influence health care outcomes and health care utilization costs; guidelines sequence and monitor a patient's progress, while treatments ensure that goals and outcomes are met for disease management.
- Use evidenced-based health care in conjunction with statistical analysis and adjustment to improve disease management based on the analytical findings; ensure that goals and outcomes are continually reviewed and evaluated from the perspective of the patient and the continuum of care of the disease.

In addition, properly executed programs allow their individual disease management services to do the following to ensure that outcomes are optimal[4]:

- Develop treatment care plans
- Implement treatment care plans
- Develop patient education programs
- Provide treatment monitoring and compliance assurance
- Foster full continuity of care
- Identify disease components and cost drivers
- Measure and assess outcomes
- Develop preventive care strategies
- Provide contract health care management services that result in optimal outcomes

- Serve as an intermediary between the pharmaceutical company and the managed care payer and between the payer and the health care providers
- Collect outcomes data to monitor the effectiveness of interventions
- Identify components of diseases and their cost drivers
- Develop and use patient education and compliance resources to encourage improved patient wellness and adherence to management regimens
- Encourage caregivers to focus on treatment plans based on the disease process rather than simply on reimbursement
- Emphasize disease prevention
- Encourage full continuity of care

According to an article in *Managed Care*, American Healthways, Inc., a leader in the establishment of disease management programs and one of the first organizations to receive accreditation by the National Committee for Quality Assurance, has found that disease management improves the health of patients with chronic diseases (diseases that are prolonged, do not resolve spontaneously, and are rarely cured completely) while lowering the associated health care costs. American Healthways has developed the first set of standards to ensure that chronic disease programs are improving the quality of care. The standards are divided into the following seven categories[5]:

1. Program organization, including medical leadership and coordination among physicians and other practitioners
2. Program staffing
3. Physician support
4. Outcomes measurements
5. Clinical practice guidelines
6. Patient self-management
7. Continuous quality improvements

Case Management and Disease Management

Literature supports the fact that case managers are often asked to assist in the development of disease management programs for their organizations because of their clinical expertise and their role in promoting delivery of cost-effective care to different patient populations.[6] According to U.S.-based researchers and an article in *Disease Management and Health Outcomes*, "case management may be the delivery approach of choice for implementing disease management programs and critical care pathways in the managed care environment."[6A] The role of the case manager is to apply preestablished criteria to a selected patient population, who are managed using a standardized treatment plan, regular follow-up to ensure that the plan is working, and ongoing statistical data collection to support outcomes. Another article declares that the case manager makes a difference in the health care system by implementing change and becoming a catalyst, that is, a stimulus bringing about or hastening a result.[7] Case managers are also viewed as the professionals who can make a difference in the health care system by bridging the gaps in understanding and knowledge with a commitment to measurable outcomes and comparing yesterday's findings with today's information.[8]

The definition of case management supports the concept of disease management, because case management is defined as a systems approach centered on the following:

Accountability, coordination, integration and achievement of outcomes within effective time frames, while promoting prudent use of resources and improving quality of patient care.[9]

Case managers play a pivotal role in the cost-effectiveness of disease management because they manage patients and their diseases throughout the continuum, improving the efficiency and quality of services, encouraging patient self-care, and coordinating the care team to create a seamless provision of services for patients and their families.[1] Effective disease management programs incorporate many of the same steps used in case management. These include the following[8]:

- Client identification
- Assessment
- Care planning
- Implementation
- Monitoring
- Reassessment

It is through case management that disease management will follow along the health care continuum, managing disease by medical protocols and assessing needs for community resources, with transition to appropriate services like palliative care and hospice care.

Case management is now being considered in many countries as a method of integrating and coordinating health and social systems that can benefit most complex health client groups. Case management assists and coordinates care for patients with long-term health problems, because many of these patients lack the knowledge or advocacy skills to obtain appropriate services.[8]

Ethics

Disease case managers must be imbued with strong ethical principles. They must find a balance and make decisions based on patients' outcomes, not just on cost containment. They must do the right thing for the community, for the patient, and for the organization. The ethical practice of disease case management is guided by the following principles:

- **Autonomy**—self-direction, the right to refuse or accept treatment; the basis of the concept of informed consent
- **Beneficence**—actions for the benefit of the patient, "doing good"

- **Nonmaleficence**—avoidance of harm
- **Justice**—fairness, equal treatment, appropriate distribution of benefits and burdens
- **Veracity**—truth telling

The information age has brought new challenging ethical situations. Different modes of communication have been developed via computer E-mail and voice mail, and with use of these new modalities, concerns for patients' confidentiality and privacy have come to the forefront. When one works with patients it is imperative to obtain a signed release of information at the case opening, and patients must also be informed of their rights. According to Medicare regulations and the Patient's Bill of Rights, patients must be given notice of their rights, including the right to receive or refuse care. These rights include the following[10]:

- The right to access emergency services and to be free from discrimination
- The right to file a complaint
- The right to informed consent
- The right to formulate advance directives
- The right to confidentiality
- The right to actively participate in care decisions, which includes the right to request or refuse treatment and the right to procure and donate organs
- The right to privacy and dignity
- The right to safety and the right to freedom from restraints and seclusion

Advance care planning is an important part of ethics and the ethical dilemmas that are often associated with chronic diseases. Case managers must communicate to patients the importance of making health care decisions and appointing an agent to speak for them when they cannot. Patients should discuss medical choices with their families and physicians. Case managers working with patients in any capacity must encourage patients to complete an advance health care directive, send a signed copy to their provider for inclusion in their medical records, and keep a copy of the document in their own medical care files.

MEETING THE CHALLENGE OF DISEASE MANAGEMENT

Promoting Healthy Lifestyles to Reduce and Manage Chronic Diseases

Research has shown that healthy lifestyles are more influential than genetic factors in helping older people avoid the decline and deterioration traditionally associated with aging. People who engage in healthy behaviors—especially getting regular physical exercise, avoiding tobacco use, and eating a healthy diet—reduce their risk of chronic diseases and have half the rate of disability of those who do not. To promote healthy lifestyles, case managers must emphasize the following:

- **Abstinence from smoking**— Avoiding tobacco use dramatically reduces the risk of premature death and disability. Almost a quarter of all deaths from coronary heart disease and nearly all deaths from lung cancer are due to cigarette smoking. In addition, smoking is responsible for most cases of chronic, debilitating lung diseases such as emphysema.

- **Exercise**—Being physically active reduces the risk of coronary heart disease, colon cancer, diabetes, and high blood pressure. Regular physical activity also helps older people decrease their risk of falls, reduce anxiety and depression, maintain a healthy body weight, and maintain joint strength and mobility. However, two thirds of older adults do not exercise on a regular basis. Loss of muscle tone and lack of upper body strength contribute to frailty.

- **Nutrition**—Eating a healthy diet lowers a person's risk for many chronic diseases, including coronary heart disease, stroke, some cancers, diabetes, and osteoporosis. Healthy nutrition provides the right ingredients for prevention and repair of disease.

- **Use of early detection methods**— Screening for diseases that can be effectively treated in their early stages can save lives and reduces health care costs. Such diseases and conditions include breast, cervical, and colorectal cancers; diabetes and its complications; depression and anxiety disorders; high blood pressure; and elevated cholesterol levels.

- **Injury reduction**—Falls are the most common cause of injuries in the older population. Physical inactivity and environmental factors can put older adults at increased risk of injuries. Simple home-based prevention measures such as removing tripping hazards, installing grab bars and handrails, and improving lighting can significantly reduce the risk of falls and associated fractures.

- **Adult immunization**—Pneumonia and influenza are responsible for more deaths among older adults each year. Immunizations can reduce the incidence of these diseases.

While much remains to be learned about other chronic diseases or conditions such as osteoporosis, Alzheimer's disease, urinary incontinence, Parkinson's disease, tooth loss and periodontal disease, and psychiatric disorders, as well as about the prevalence of these disorders, associated risk factors, and effective measures to prevent or delay their onset, the health care system must evaluate ways to respond to these conditions as well.[2]

PROCESSES OF DISEASE MANAGEMENT

Steps in Program Development

In establishing a disease management program, as indicated earlier in this chapter, not only are the six steps identified by the DMAA critical but the following steps will also be important as a program is developed.

Step 1: Analysis

The first step is to analyze the patient population served and identify the top diagnoses or patient populations affected and the physician leaders who will be instrumental in the program. As information is analyzed, additional elements to be studied include the following:

- All of the drugs, therapeutic devices, and therapies used in the treatment of the specified disease
- All hospital days and emergency department visits with *International Classification of Diseases, Ninth Revision* discharge codes for a specified disease, a particular diagnosis, or complication associated with the specified disease
- All laboratory and other diagnostic costs associated with the specified disease

Often the whole process starts with general education regarding disease management, determination of the diseases felt to have the greatest impact on the organization, and identification of the personnel who might be most interested in spearheading an effort.

Physicians should be encouraged to take a proactive leadership role in disease management program planning, discussions, development, and implementation. Physicians should act as facilitators and should participate in the distribution of treatment guidelines and the monitoring of patient outcomes. These elements are always essential components of a successful disease management initiative. The total success of a disease management effort will depend on the organization and the participation and cooperation of physicians.

One of the first actions taken is preliminary identification of the "champion partners" for the program. These often include the following:

- Interested health care professionals
- Pharmacists
- Family medicine physicians
- Specialist physicians
- Representatives of provider organizations

To assist in the implementation of this step, a key method might be to arrange for a speaker to present an educational session on the topic selected. This speaker can give a basic overview of the proposed disease management population and include a list of the special needs of those with the disease and the end points, tools, and processes that are expected be used to measure program outcomes.

Step 2: Disease Selection

After the review in the foregoing step, the next step is to select a disease that affects the organization and study the successes or failures of other organizations that have selected the same disease for target interventions. As the committee studies reports and findings from previous patient encounters, it is wise to select diseases that predominately influence drug costs and hospital and emergency department usage, as well as common diseases and issues examined by the organization's utilization review committees. This review must also determine the number of patients with a specific disease, the cost of their care, and the problem spots suggested by indicators of health outcome. It should be kept in mind when reviewing the literature on specific diseases that disease prevalence and spending and utilization trends may vary from state to state and often within a specific geographic region. This variation depends on patient and geographic demographics, treatment patterns, and other factors unique to that state or region. General criteria for selecting a disease to be intensely managed include the following:

- High prevalence of chronic disease state
- High dollar volume or high quantity of drug use
- Potential for wide variation in treatment and therapeutic approach
- Potential for lifestyle modification to improve outcomes
- High risk of negative outcomes

As a specific disease comes under consideration, questions the team needs to consider include the following:

- What portion of the disease population should be a priority for disease management?
- What demographic factors are important?
- Which disorders are the most prevalent in the population?
- Which disorders are the most expensive to treat?
- Which services, types of treatments, or sites of care are the most expensive for the most prevalent disorders (e.g., inpatient hospital stays, emergency visits, outpatient services, physician visits, and, prescription medications)?
- For which disorders is there the most variation in treatment patterns and the greatest opportunity for improvement?
- For which high-priority disorders is there likely to be a return on the investment from disease management and why?

Choice of Diseases to Manage

The disease entity to be targeted can often be chosen through the analysis of data. In most cases this will be the disease that has the highest costs of care, that drives patient encounters with the health care system,

and that has the highest prevalence among the patients served. Typical diseases for which there are unique treatments and interventions and unique cost patterns are the following:

- Respiratory diseases
  - Asthma
  - Chronic obstructive pulmonary disease
- Cardiovascular diseases
  - Angina
  - Cerebral vascular accident
  - Congestive heart failure
  - Coronary artery disease
  - Lipid irregularity (need for cholesterol management)
  - Hypertension
- Mental health diseases
  - Depressive disorders
  - Anxiety and tension
- Diabetes
- Ambulatory infectious diseases
  - Otitis media
  - Urinary tract infection
  - Community-acquired pneumonia
- Pain
- Upper gastrointestinal diseases
  - Peptic ulcer disease
  - Reflux esophagitis
- Women's and children's disorders
- Chronic illness
  - Complex chronic conditions
  - Fibromyalgia
  - Frailty in elderly patients
  - Hemophilia
  - Human immunodeficiency virus infection
  - End-stage renal disease
  - Ulcers and wounds

The key is to select the disease that is most prevalent and to implement the program for that disease and ensure its effectiveness before developing other programs.

Step 3: Development of Disease Management Guidelines

What do you think of when you hear the term *clinical guidelines?* These words elicit mixed emotions in many health care professionals, especially physicians, who often view guidelines as "cookbook" medicine or an insult to their skills. However, clinical guidelines are well developed and evidence based, and they are useful clinical tools that should teach everyone that not all care plans are as thorough or as scientifically grounded as they should be. Disease management programs focus heavily on clinical guidelines, which are used as an alternative approach—a treatment "blueprint" that is based on input from affected parties of what works and what does not work.

Thus, after partners are chosen and a baseline analysis is made of the diagnoses for possible study and the current care patients with these diagnoses receive, it is time to draft treatment guidelines (also known as clinical practice guidelines or practice parameters). Guidelines, when finalized, must show ways to improve outcome quality, reduce inappropriate care, and increase standards of care by reducing practice variability. Clinicians participate in the design of protocols they will be expected to follow.

Well-designed disease management guidelines encourage a continuum of care. These criteria can better ensure that appropriate diagnostic procedures are ordered, appropriate treatments are chosen, appropriate follow-up and monitoring take place, and appropriate patient education is conducted to achieve optimal outcomes.

Designers of disease management protocols work with clients and caregivers to develop treatment plans that optimize care, standardize diagnostic and treatment methods, integrate wellness and prevention measures, emphasize patient education, and monitor compliance without having the feel of cookbook medicine. Outcomes data should be collected and analyzed to measure the impact on the quality of care and costs. Also, as the program advances, it is critical to identify those physicians who fail to comply with treatment guidelines and to implement a process to ensure compliance. Without it, the program will not be able to change physicians' behavior.

Step 4: Establishment of Goals

As the program is developed, a key component is to identify goals—both short term and long term. These goals must be designed to measure success in areas such as the following[11]:

- Promotion of an understanding of the disease and coping strategies
- Teaching of techniques for the monitoring of disease progress, self-management, and avoidance of exacerbations
- Involvement of patients in support groups or organizations that provide continuing education, counseling, and fellowship
- Empowerment of patients to make appropriate decisions regarding therapy and identification of the symptoms that will trigger the need to call for help.
- Communication with care providers

Step 5: Pilot Phase

Once the disease has been selected, the team must develop and design the interventions that make the most sense for that disease. When these interventions are completed, conducting a pilot phase is wise so that the new systems that have been created or considered can be tested. Testing includes collection of new data (claims data, survey data, medical abstract data) and application of data analysis techniques to compare these new data with comparable older data. This data analysis can be used in the development of outcome measures and provides a mechanism whereby costs can be tracked. During this phase, time must be allowed to seek feedback from physicians and other health care team members.

Step 6: Implementation

Before entering the final phase or implementation step, one must ensure that the pilot phase allowed sufficient time for the development and testing of all systems for data collection, analysis, and feedback regarding health outcomes and costs. The final program should be implemented in phases. Otherwise costs and time are often underestimated. To ensure successful implementation, a dedicated and trained staff is a vital component. Within each step it is critical that all key decision makers be involved if changes are made in the initial design. An effective disease management program will incorporate all the elements of outcomes management, interdisciplinary teamwork, claims analysis and feedback, and medical treatment guidelines by the time it is implemented.

The Chronic Disease Educational Self-Management Program

Self-management is the ultimate goal of a disease management program. While there are a variety of successful programs in existence, one program that is highly successful is the one offered by the Stanford Patient Education Research Center. This center uses a community-based self-management program that assists people with chronic illnesses. Its program consists of the following:

- Techniques to deal with problems such as frustration, fatigue, pain, and isolation
- Appropriate exercise for maintaining and improving strength, flexibility, and endurance
- Appropriate use of medications
- Promotion of effective communication with family, friends, and health professionals
- Nutrition guidelines
- Education on how to evaluate new treatments

To complement the program, each participant receives a copy of the companion book *Living a Healthy Life with Chronic Conditions*, second edition, and an audio relaxation tape, *Time for Healing*.[12]

Measurement of Success

The primary measure of success for a disease management program is the outcomes produced. Well-designed studies are critical in documenting improvement in care and include such indicators as clinical and economic outcomes and surveys of quality of life and patient satisfaction. Performance can be compared with that recorded in national databases so that organizations can evaluate their own results as well as those achieved by others.

Successful disease state management uses continuous improvement programs to determine the ongoing changes necessary to provide the most cost-effective health care management through health education.

The key to any successful disease management program is to design programs that teach patients health promotion while creating an environment for behavioral changes. A program such as this allows patients to care for their bodies and empowers them to manage disease.

FUTURE TRENDS

As disease management programs are implemented and patients become more savvy, patients are demanding access to information they can understand. Therefore several trends are emerging, including the following:

Internet or E-Health

Patient access to electronic information via the Internet is becoming very popular with consumers. Patients use the Internet frequently to research disease information and treatment. While it is critical to warn patients of the importance of using valid Internet sites as they do their research, one should note that the health care industry is now producing web-based disease management systems for the layperson. To access this information, the patient needs only a standard web browser or a custom device that can interface to medical application servers and data repositories on the Internet.

Further studies will need to assess whether use of the Internet and the personal computer helps to improve the quality of life of chronically ill patients, reduce hospitalizations, and decrease health care costs. Web-based disease management systems monitor the condition of chronically ill patients and provide measurement of the entire disease management program.

Human Genome Project

The 21st century is a new era of disease management with the near-completion of the Human Genome Project—the sequencing of the 3.12 billion rungs on the double-helix ladder of the human genetic code—which will give scientists full access to the structure of the human genome. This will allow researchers to identify which genes are linked to a given disease state. These new tools will help researchers to define disease pathways. In the near future we will be able to turn on or turn off certain genes to prevent disease, which will make available a whole new world of disease management tools.

Telemedicine

Sophisticated systems use special telemedicine or other technologies to constantly monitor vital signs, compliance with the treatment regimen, or other health indicators. Home-based telemedicine technology can be used as a tool for the delivery of disease management care. The core definition of telemedicine is *tele* 'distance' and

mederi 'healing'; thus the term means '"distance healing." Telemedicine includes the use of interactive video for health care practice and the use of the Internet by both providers and patients. These means allow access to clinical information and expanded use of peripheral monitoring devices. Technologies are rapidly evolving that eliminate the need for a computer in the home. Interactive video devices that use a patients' own television set and the existing phone line in the home are today a technical reality. They are a user-friendly and low-cost means of providing home-based telemedicine care to patients.[13]

■ SUMMARY

Although a variety of modalities are used to offer case management and contain costs, one alternative that is possibly the most prevalent is the programs offered by organizations related to specific diseases. These programs are disease management programs. To be considered a valuable option and one recognized as a program, the services must have six essential components: population identification, evidence-based guidelines, collaborative practice models, patient self-management education, process and outcomes evaluation, and routine reporting and feedback. If these are not present, the services offered are strictly disease management services.

Most organizations that wish to develop disease management programs use existing data to identify the disease categories whose treatment they wish to influence. When a specific disease is selected, the choice is based primarily on the numbers of persons affected, the costs associated with their care, and the resources needed to operationalize a program. The ultimate goal of the program must be to teach patients self-management skills that will result in favorable outcomes for all involved.

Chapter Exercises

1. Discuss in a group setting the differences between disease management and case management.

2. In this same group discuss the meaning of disease management and the populations it serves, and again compare it to case management.

3. In this same group, define the six essential components of a disease management program and the processes that are key to any such program.

Suggested Websites and Resources

www.agingwithdignity.org/—Aging with Dignity

www.aarp.org/index.html—American Association of Retired Persons; nonprofit, nonpartisan membership organization for people older than 50 years of age

www.depts.washington.edu/druginfo/Disease/dm.html—Disease management and alternative products information

www.dmaa.org/—Disease Management Association of America

www.healthresourcesonline.com/managed_care/dis_man.htm—Disease Management Directory 2001 and Guidebook; source book for trends, tools, vendors, strategies, and outcomes

www.nucleus.net/dm/—Disease management forum and resources

www.mayoclinic.com/takecharge/self_manager/index.cfm—Disease Self-Managers

www.cms.hhs.gov—Centers for Medicare & Medicaid Services (formerly the Health Care Financing Administration)

www.healthcare-informatics.com/issues/2000/03_00/cover.htm—Healthcare Informatics

hstat.nlm.nih.gov/hq—Health Services/Technology Assessment Text (HSTAT): health information

www.lifemasters.net—LifeMasters Supported SelfCare, Inc.: interactive health management services

www.dmnow.org/—Medicaid Disease Management & Health Outcomes

www.cdc.gov/nccdphp/index.htm—National Center for Chronic Disease Prevention and Health Promotion

www.nationaljewish.org/diseases/d1.html—National Jewish Medical & Research Center

www.nlm.nih.gov/nichsr—National Library of Medicine, National Information Center on Health Services Research and Health Care Technology

www.partnershipforcaring.org/HomePage/—Partnership for Caring: end-of-life issues

www.eatright.org/adap0298b.html—Position of the American Dietetic Association on the role of nutrition in health promotion and disease prevention programs

www.stanford.edu/group/perc/cdsmp.html—Stanford Patient Education Research Center

www.thedailyapple.com/public/aboutUs.jhtml/—The Daily Apple: health information

www.who.int/home-page/—World Health Organization

dir.yahoo.com/Health/Diseases_and_Conditions/—Yahoo Health Index of Medical Information

REFERENCES

1. Lee SS: Case management resource guide: disease state management and case management—new horizons for healthcare, available on-line at www.cmrg.com/dmintroduction.htm.
2. Centers for Disease Control and Prevention, available on-line at www.cdc.gov/nccdphp.
3. The Robert Wood Johnson Foundation: *Promoting patient self-management of chronic illness*, available on-line at http://www.rwjf.org/reports/grr/027407s.htm.
4. Disease Management Association of America, *Definition of disease management*, 2000, available on-line at www.dmaa.org/definition.html.
5. Inside track, managed care. Company releases disease management guidelines, *Continuing Care* 19(5):10, 2000.
6. Goldstein R: Nursing case management: managing the process of patient care, *Nursing Case Manage-*

ment: *The Disease Management Approach to Cost Containment* 3(3):99-103, 1998.

6A. Case management: important delivery approach in managed care, *Disease Management and Health Outcomes* 1(3):165, 1997.

7. Mullahy C: The case manager is the catalytic collaborator, *J Care Management* 1(1):7-9, 1995.

8. Smith JE: Case management: a literature review. *Can J Nursing Administration* 11(2):93-108, 1998.

9. Zander K: *Managing outcomes through collaborative care: the application of care mapping and case management*, Chicago, 1995, American Hospital Publishing.

10. Murer C: Rehabilitation update; HCFA: focus on rights; Medicare hospitals face new regulations on patients rights, *Continuing Care* 19(5):12-14, 2000.

11. Gurnee MC, Da Silva RV: Constructing disease management programs, *Managed Care*, June 1997, available on-line at www.managedcaremag.com/archives/9706/ 9706.disease_man.shtml#conditions.

12. Stanford University, Chronic disease self-management program, available on-line at www.stanford.edu/group/perc/ cdsmp.html.

13. Brown AC, Garrison C: The emerging role of telemedicine in extended-care risk management, *Managed Care Interface* 3(1), available on-line at www.medicomint.com/ Search/SubjectDetails. asp? SUBJECT=The+Emerging+ Role+of+ Telemedicine+ in+ Extended%2DCare+ Risk+ Management.

BIBLIOGRAPHY

The American Medical Association (AMA) issues E-mail guidelines, *Managed Care Interface* 13(8):39-40, 2000.

Carneal G: The evolution of utilization management, *Managed Care Interface* 13(12):86-92, 2000.

Chan F, Leahy M, McMahon B et al: Foundation knowledge and major practice domains of case management, *J Care Management* 5(1):10,13-14,17-18,26-28, 30, 1999.

Chronic illness: subject of a successful program, *Hospital Case Management* 12(8):148-149, 2000.

Constructing disease management programs, *Managed care*, Yardley, Penn, 1997, Stezzi Communications.

Debusk RF, Miller NH, Taylor CB et al: Chronic disease management: treating the patient with the disease(s) vs treating the disease(s) in the patient, *Arch Intern Med* 15(9):2739-2742, 1999.

Gurnee M, Da Silva R: Constructing disease management programs, *Managed Care*, June 1997, available

on-line at www.managedcaremag.com/archives/9706/ 9706.disease_man.shtml#conditions.

Hodges LC, Hall-Barrow JC, Satkowski TC: Chronic disease management, *Medsurg* 7(4):226-234, 1998.

Jamison M: Chronic illness management in the year 2005, *Nursing Economics* 16(5):246-253, 1998.

Joch A: A much maligned movement finds new respect in the e-health age, *Healthcare Informatics*, March 2000, available on-line at www.healthcare-informatics.com/issues/ 2000/03_00/cover.htm pages.

Kirsh WD, Lee R: Decreasing cost and increasing patient satisfaction: the implementation of a cancer disease management program, *Managed Care Interface* 12(8):65-68, 2000.

Kozma CM: Case management: a tool for disease management programs, *Managed Care Interface* 12(8): 62,64, 1999.

Kozma CM: Why implement disease state management programs: cost, cost, cost, *Managed Care Interface* 13(8):60-61, 2000.

Lucas J: The ethics of managed care, *J Care Management* 5(1):56-57, 1999.

Martin R: Getting gung ho on guidelines, *Managed Care Interface* 13(5):68-69, 2000.

O'Reilly M: Is Internet-based disease management on the way, *Can Med Assoc J* 160:1039, 1999, available on-line at www.cmaj.ca/cgi/reprint/160/7/1039.pdf.

Poole P, Chase B, Frankel A et al: Case management may reduce length of hospital stay in patients with recurrent admissions for chronic obstructive pulmonary disease, *Respirology* 6(1):37-42, 2001.

Reeder L: Anatomy of a disease management program, *Nursing Management* 30(4):41-45, 1999, available on-line at www.nursingmanagement.com.

Rosenberger J, Wiemers N: Care maps in the medical rehabilitation, *J Care Management* 5(2):23-28,30-32,37, 1999.

Rossi P: *Case management in health care: a practical guide*, Philadelphia, 1999, Saunders.

Skinner N: The case report: who is the real case manager, *J Care Management* 5(2):56-60, 1999.

Staton MP, Walizer EM, Graham J, Keppel L: Nursing case management: managing the process of patient care, *Nursing Case Management* 5(1):37-45, 2000.

Todd W: New mindsets in asthma: interventions and disease management, *J Care Management* 1(1):37-52, 1995.

Whitfield A: Branching out: as disease management grows, it is taking root in new conditions & new technologies, *Continuing Care* 19(5):24-29, 2000.

CHAPTER
16

Case Management of the Transplant Patient

Patricia Ann Zrelak, RN, MS, PhD

OBJECTIVES

- To describe the role of the case manager in meeting the needs of the transplant candidate
- To explain the case manager's involvement in postoperative management of the transplant patient
- To discuss the importance of coordination between the payer's case manager and the transplant team case manager in directing care and meeting the needs of the patient and family

Over the last 40 years, remarkable progress has been made in transplantology. The quality of care is increasing, and the number of patients undergoing transplantation is growing; thus, it is one of the top ten diagnoses seen in case manager caseloads. Transplant care, both before and after surgery, is costly and complex. Because of the high risk, high utilization of resources, acuteness of the patient's medical condition, patient needs, and high costs involved, referral criteria for case management must include all transplant and potential transplant patients. Transplant-related referrals are high priority and must be dealt with promptly. Common organ and tissue transplants that the case manager may see include the following types:

- Heart
- Heart and lung
- Lung segment
- Single or double lung
- Liver
- Liver segment
- Pancreas
- Pancreas segment
- Pancreatic islet cells
- Intestines
- Stomach and intestines
- Kidney
- Kidney and pancreas
- Autologous and allogeneic bone marrow

This chapter focuses on the most complex transplant patients for the case manager, those undergoing solid organ and bone marrow transplantation.

EPIDEMIOLOGY

The number of patients in need of organ transplantation is dramatically increasing. On the other hand, the number of organs available is continuing to lag. According to the United Network for Organ Sharing (UNOS), as of September 21, 2001, there were approximately 78,241 patients awaiting solid organ transplantation in the

United States (Table 16-1). Yet in the previous calendar year (2000) only 22,953 organ transplants were performed (Table 16-2). Relaxation of organ donor criteria, better public education and understanding, utilization of minority requesters for minority donor recruitment, use of both non-heart-beating donors and nonrelated living donors, implementation of the principle of presumed consent, and increased procurement efforts by hospital and organ procurement organizations (OPOs) have

helped address this demand. The reality, however, is that many patients continue to die while waiting for a transplantable organ.

Because of improvements in mortality and morbidity rates for transplant patients, most transplantations are now accepted as standard medical care and no longer considered experimental therapy. The survivability and quality of life of organ recipients varies greatly depending on many factors. These include geographical

TABLE 16-1
United Network for Organ Sharing (UNOS) National Patient Waiting List for Organ Transplants, September 21, 2001

Type of Transplant	No. of Patients Waiting for Transplant
Kidney transplant	49,923
Liver transplant	18,411
Pancreas transplant	1,145
Pancreas islet cell transplant	248
Kidney-pancreas transplant	2,490
Intestine transplant	179
Heart transplant	4,181
Heart-lung transplant	212
Lung transplant	3,776
TOTAL*	78,241

*UNOS policies allow patients to be listed with more than one transplant center, and some patients may need more than one organ; therefore the total number of patients is slightly less than the sums listed.

TABLE 16-2
Number of Transplants Performed in 2000 based on Organ Procurement and Transplantation Network data, August 3, 2001

Type of Transplant	No. of Patients Waiting for Transplant
Kidney transplant (5,293 were from living donors)	13,372
Liver transplant	4,954
Pancreas transplant	1,145
Pancreas islet cell transplant	435
Kidney-pancreas transplant	911
Intestine transplant	79
Heart transplant	2,198
Heart-lung transplant	48
Lung transplant	956
TOTAL	22,953

Double kidney, double lung, and heart-lung transplants are counted as one transplant.

location, severity of the illness, age of the recipient, waiting time for an organ, and type of organ needed. New federal regulations require that performance data on transplantation programs be available to the public and that such data be updated at least every 6 months and be available no more than 6 months later than the period to which they apply.[1] Standardized definitions and criteria are to be used, and data are to include characteristics of individual transplant programs such as the number of transplants performed, survival rates, the number of organs not accepted for transplant, waiting times, and other data useful to patients, their families, and health care professionals. This information can be viewed on the UNOS website (see Suggested Websites and Resources at the end of the chapter). Other reliable websites of interest to both the case manager and patient include those maintained by governmental agencies with an involvement in organ transplantation (e.g., Department of Health and Human Services [DHHS]), search sites such as MEDLINE (National Institutes of Health), and the numerous organ and health care associations involved in specific disease processes and/or transplant care and health (see Suggested Websites and Resources for website addresses and/or contact numbers). The information on these websites along with insurance data and coverage, data for a specific transplant center, knowledge of the geographic location of the center, and general feelings about the individual center's care can be used in making transplant decisions. The performance data from UNOS are also a helpful resource for care managers interested in transplant research.

TRENDS IN TRANSPLANTATION

Greater experience and advances in surgical techniques along with the remarkable discoveries being made in medical science are leading to many promising new treatment modalities for organ failure. Trends with which the case manager should be familiar are grouped into the following categories:

- Organ procurement and preparation
- Molecular and cellular biology
- New medication and antirejection strategies
- Xenotransplantation
- Artificial organs

Organ Procurement and Preparation

Efforts to help increase the pool of available organs include the relaxation of donor criteria (as noted earlier), the use of nonrelated living kidney donors, the development of transplantation procedures relying on living related liver and lung donors, and the implementation of procurement reporting laws (e.g., the National Organ and Tissue Donation Initiative of December 1997, which requires all Medicare-participating hospitals to notify organ procurement organizations of all deaths and imminent deaths). Although payments to donors are currently illegal under the National Organ Transplantation Act of 1984, recommendations are being considered that would allow financial incentives to be paid to organ donors and/or their families. Suggested incentives include a death benefit paid directly to the organ donor's family, reduction in state or local income tax, payment of some or all costs associated with burial of the donor, or payment of some portion of the hospital costs incurred by the donor family.

In addition, there are ongoing advances in the preservation and management of donor organs prior to procurement and between procurement and transplantation. These advances are not only increasing the number of organs suitable for transplant but are prolonging the survival of both the organ and the organ recipient.[2]

Molecular and Cellular Biology

Advances in molecular and cellular biology are providing a new genetic basis for developing novel approaches in preventing and treating organ failure and in improving the success, safety, and availability of organ transplantation. Two of the more futuristic developments are the Human Genome Project and the advances in stem cell research. Although years away from clinical application, both promise to have far-reaching consequences not just in the prevention of organ failure but in the transplant process. Most diseases have a genetic component. The Human Genome Project is making it possible to start identifying the gene or genes that are responsible for or can modify a person's risk for certain disease conditions. Soon we may see mass genetic screening for inherited diseases and be able to treat inborn errors of metabolism by gene transfer or gene repair therapy. Genetic techniques are already being used in the development of new pharmaceutical agents and improved tissue typing methods.

Stem cell discoveries are quickly advancing the long-standing goal of human tissue regeneration. Great efforts are being made to isolate and identify the characteristics of stem cell populations of various tissues. Although research is still early in development, the use of stem cells may provide an almost limitless supply of cells for transplantation and organ development in the future.

One advance in regenerative medicine is the nontraditional transplant method of dividing single organs, such as the kidney. Successes in this area already include liver, pancreas, and lung transplantation.

New Medication and Antirejection Strategies

Acute and chronic rejection is still the leading problem in transplantation. The high failure rates due to rejection and/or the inability to control infection are being addressed partially by the advances in pharmaceutical immunology. Not only are newer immunosuppressive medications helping to increase longevity in all transplant cases, but they are improving the quality of life by lessening the side effects associated with past immunosuppressive regimens. Transplantations of organs such as small bowel that have not had the same success rates as have transplants of other organs are being greatly assisted by these efforts.[3] Approaches for targeted drug design include gene therapy and the use of monoclonal antibodies, peptides, and peptidomimetics.[4] New drugs include tacrolimus (FK506), mycophenolate mofetil (RS-61443) , rapamycin (RPM), brequinar sodium (BQR), and 15-deoxyspergualin (15-DS).

The case manager should expect to see greater achievements in pancreatic islet cell transplantation, so that transplantation will one day take place early in the diabetic disease process. To date, most pancreatic transplants in diabetic patients are of whole organs and are performed in conjunction with kidney transplant, since most patients with advanced diabetes have end-stage renal disease (ESRD). Newer strategies incorporate different methods of immunoalteration and immunoisolation. Several research groups are working on the transplantation of isolated hepatocytes. Efforts in these areas are targeted at disease caused by inborn errors of metabolism.[5]

The numerous breakthroughs in understanding the immune system are being used to induce immunologic tolerance in the host to prevent graft-versus-host disease and graft rejection (failure). Examples of these types of immune reduction strategies include the simultaneous performance of a bone marrow transplant or injection of bone marrow into the thymus gland when a solid organ is transplanted, the use of plasmapheresis and photopheresis to modulate the immune response in a less toxic and perhaps a more selective manner,[6] and experimental post-transplant infusion of donor splenocytes to induce peripheral tolerance.

Xenotransplantation

Advances in genetic engineering are allowing manipulation of the immune response in genetically modified or transgenic animals. These advances, along with the wider acceptance of liver and heart-lung allografts and tissues and the improved survival of patients receiving such transplants, is renewing interest in xenotransplantation (the transplantation of tissue from one species to another, such as from a nonhuman primate to a human). Besides the ethical issues, there are still many medical issues to resolve (such as organ size, compatibility, hormone and cytokine responses, autoimmunity, and the problems of opportunistic infections and the risk of unknown infectious infections), but gigantic leaps are being made in surmounting the many hurdles currently limiting this potential source of organs.

Mechanical and Artificial Organs

Promising advances are being made in the development of mechanical devices and organs. The first area of advance is in the development of assistive devices that perform highly specialized functions. Most case managers are well versed in the care of patients with simple assistive devices (e.g., pacemakers, internal defibrillators, and implanted insulin pumps). The more complex assistive devices that are used as a bridge until definitive surgical intervention, permanent implantation, or transplantation can be performed are commonly seen at tertiary medical centers. Examples of these include ventricular assist appliances, intraaortic balloon pumps, and intravenous oxygenators. Devices are becoming more sophisticated through the application of artificial intelligence, their biomembranes are becoming more effi-

cient and safe, and the devices are becoming smaller. Similar advances are being made in other types of support systems. For example, portable hemodialysis machines may soon be available.

Advances are also being made in developing complete artificial organs. The greatest success to date has been with the artificial heart.[7] Although several mechanical heart models have been approved by the Food and Drug Administration, so far they have been short-term solutions for those too sick for cardiac transplantation or for those for whom an organ has not been available. Other organs in development include the bioartificial pancreas and liver,[8] as well as an ex vivo liver perfusion system.[9]

CASE MANAGEMENT INVOLVEMENT AND PRETRANSPLANT CARE

The transplantation process begins when an organ or tissue transplant becomes a medical option for care. Although earlier referral is often indicated, patients are frequently not referred for transplantation until the more conventional medical and surgical therapies have failed. The earlier a patient is identified as a potential transplant recipient and can receive care from the transplant team, the greater the likelihood of a positive outcome. Once a patient is identified as a potential transplant recipient, it is extremely important that the referral to the case manager be expedient (if the individual is not already involved). The actual level of involvement by the case manager will depend on organizational policy and patient need, but at least two care managers are usually involved. The first case manager represents the health care payer and referring facility, and the second case manager represents the transplant program. The case manager for the transplant program may be a nurse with on-the-job experience in transplant nursing or an advanced practice nurse.

The organ evaluation process is complex and can be both physically and emotionally taxing. In addition to improving clinical outcomes and preventing delays in care, early case management referral allows the case manager time to explore the patient's eligibility for health care benefits (a prerequisite for most transplant referrals), as well as an opportunity to establish rapport with the patient and family. The payer case manager is usually the lead person in the initial pretransplant care. At the time of the actual transplant and during the immediately postoperative period, the case manager representing the transplant facility will take over this role. The importance of collaboration between both case managers cannot be over emphasized. Coordination is necessary to ensure that treatment is progressing as anticipated, that health care payer benefits are communicated, and that, as the discharge planning process approaches, referrals for postacute care or procurement of pharmaceuticals or other medical service needs are directed to the appropriate providers. If the patient is linked to a health care payer that specifies which providers must be used, it is critical for this information to be relayed to the transplant team. Otherwise, the patient may be directed to the wrong providers and then be held financially responsible for costs until the services can be transferred to the appropriate network provider.

TRANSPLANT CENTER EVALUATION

As of August 13, 2001, there were 260 transplant medical centers in the United States with a total of 874 different organ-specific programs (Table 16-3). Ten of these centers have in-house OPOs, and 97 have in-house histocompatability laboratories. Each transplant center requires an initial evaluation of the patient to determine if the patient is indeed a transplant candidate. Each individual center has its

TABLE 16-3
Number and Type of Organ Transplant Programs Within the 260 Transplant Medical Centers, August 13, 2001

Type of Transplant Program	Number
Kidney transplant program	245
Liver transplant program	122
Pancreas transplant program	137
Pancreas islet cell transplant program	32
Intestine transplant program	39
Heart transplant program	141
Heart-lung transplant program	82
Lung transplant program	76
TOTAL	874

own specific requirements and list of medical information they necessary for the initial evaluation. The health care payer's case manager must provide timely facilitation of this evaluation process. It is important that both case managers work collaboratively to prevent any delays in care and to ensure that the patient is linked to the appropriate transplant center within the health care payer's network.

It is important for the transplant evaluation to occur at a transplant center that is approved by the health care payer to avoid a denial of coverage. Most health care payers, to stabilize costs and ensure quality of care, have selectively contracted with specific provider networks for transplant services. These centers are sometimes referred to as centers of excellence. Likewise, patients with Medicare or Medicaid insurance must use facilities that meet the Medicare or Medicaid requirements and that have been certified by these programs to avoid possible denial of care.

In all cases, patient demographic and medical information must be shared. Copies of the patient's medical records must be submitted along with all pertinent laboratory tests. Despite the fact that many laboratory tests may have already been performed prior to the request for the evaluation, the transplant team may request that all or some of the tests be repeated to their specifications. If additional tests are required, it is again vital to coordinate and to obtain preapproval from the health care payer's case manager. If this is not done and it turns out that the laboratory test or other tests could have been performed within the health care payer's network, payment may be denied.

Once the patient is accepted for an evaluation, the initial transplant assessment requires at least the following[10]:

- Complete medical history and physical examination
- Routine laboratory testing and blood typing (including C-reactive protein levels)
- Electrocardiogram and cardiologic evaluation
- Pulmonary function tests with a baseline room air arterial blood gas measurement
- Prothrombin and partial thromboplastin time tests
- Twenty-four-hour urine protein and creatine clearance tests
- Radiologic studies
- Immunologic studies
- Cytotoxic antibody screen
- Infectious disease screen, including tests for hepatitis B surface antigen and core antibodies, third-generation hepatitis C virus antibody screen, test for human immunodeficiency viruses 1 and 2, screen for human T-cell lymphotropic viruses I and II, Epstein-Barr virus immunoglobulin G antibody test, screen for cytomegalovirus antibodies, toxoplasmosis antibody titer, Venereal Disease Research Laboratory test for syphilis, and negative results on tuberculin skin test for high-risk patients
- Dental evaluation and treatment of caries before surgery
- In women, Papanicolaou smear and mammogram if over 40 years of age

- In men, a prostate screen if over 45 years of age
- Colonoscopy if older than 50 years of age (or if guaiac stool test result was positive in a younger person)
- Other organ-specific tests
- Screening for preexisting active infection[11]
- Determination of immunization status and requirements[11]

In addition to an extensive patient medical workup, the patient and family must undergo psychiatric evaluation. The evaluation serves the following purposes[3]:

- To identify comorbid mental illness and plan interventions for this condition
- To determine whether the patient can be sufficiently educated for the transplant patient role and to ensure that the patient has an adequate understanding of the transplantation procedure in order to give informed consent
- To learn whether the patient will be able to form a collaborative relationship with physicians and comply with the medical regimen
- To assess substance abuse history and recovery, and predict the patient's ability to maintain long-term abstinence
- To help the transplant team know the patient better as a person in order to provide more effective clinical care
- To learn about the psychosocial needs of the patient and family, and plan for services during the waiting, recovery, and rehabilitation phases of the transplantation process
- To establish baseline measures of mental functioning so that postoperative changes can be monitored
- To ensure that the patient has adequate social supports available

At the time of this evaluation, the patient and family are given specific information about the transplant process, including the anticipated wait, the surgical procedure, the immediately postoperative management, and the long-term approach. In addition, the patient and family are given information pertaining to housing, transportation, and financial expectations. The most common reasons for denial of a transplant are the following[3]:

- Age (although most centers do not directly restrict age)
- Presence of multisystem disease not correctable by a transplant
- Presence of recent infections or infections refractory to treatment
- Presence of acute peptic ulcers or liver disease
- Presence of malignant neoplasms (centers require that patients be disease free for varying periods of time, but this is not an across-the-board exclusion)
- Current history of alcohol or drug abuse
- Repeated noncompliance and/or indications that the patient will not be compliant with required regimens in the future
- Psychiatric illness (i.e., organic mental syndromes, psychosis, and mental retardation)
- Presence of irreversible brain damage
- Lack of social support

Once a patient is accepted as a candidate, the patient's overall medical status must be assessed periodically to ensure that the patient remains suitable for transplantation. This assessment also keeps patients in active status on the organ waiting list. During this time, patients must become their own best advocates. This includes being diligent with regard to taking medications as prescribed and being sensitive to symptoms that may need to be reported to the primary or transplant team.[10] It is important that the referring providers and transplant team communicate regularly about any changes in the condition of the patient that may affect eligibility for transplantation. This will also improve management of the primary illness of referral and any comorbid conditions.

NATIONAL REGISTRIES

The federal government regulates transplant activities under the 1984 National Organ Transplant Act. This act created a national transplant system, the Organ Procurement and Transplantation Network (OPTN), to ensure an equitable system for allocating available organs. The DHHS, which contracts for services with UNOS, oversees the network. One of the many tasks of UNOS is to maintain the national list of all recipients waiting for an organ transplant and to supervise organ distribution. When a patient is accepted as a candidate for a solid organ transplant, he or she is placed on the organ transplant list and his or her name is entered into this national registry. Under UNOS, the United Stated is divided into 11 different regions. Within each region, there are OPOs that procure and allocate organs for transplantation according to policies that are agreed upon nationally, regionally, and locally. As of August 13, 2001, there were 59 operating OPOs in the United States. All hospitals that perform transplants are required to abide by the rules and requirements of the OPTN to be eligible to participate in the Medicare and Medicaid programs. The act has been amended twice to encourage the development of a fair national system of organ allocation.

When organs are donated, a complex sequential matching effort takes place based on a point system set forth in UNOS policies. The procuring organization accesses a centralized computer operated by UNOS, enters information about the donor organs into the computer, runs the match program, and coordinates the procuring and transplanting surgical teams. The computer program generates a list of potential recipients ranked according to medical and other criteria (e.g., blood type, tissue type, size of organ required, medical urgency of the patient, time already spent on the waiting list, and distance between donor and recipient). For each type of organ there is a specific matching algorithm based on successful markers for that type of organ. Under the current system, waiting patients are given first priority for most organs procured in their local areas. If a matching patient is not found locally, the search is broadened, first regionally, then nationally. An exception is the all-antigen or six-antigen kidney, which is always shared nationally. After the list of potential recipients is obtained, the transplant coordinator contacts the transplant surgeons caring for the top-ranked local patient to offer the organ. Additional laboratory tests designed to measure the compatibility between the donor organ and the recipient may be necessary. Often a backup patient is notified, because the first transplant surgeon may decline the organ. Once the organ is accepted, transportation arrangements are made and surgery is scheduled. A transplant center typically has 1 hour from the time an organ is offered to communicate acceptance. A primary determinant of organ viability for transplant success is a short "cold ischemic time," the period between the time blood flow to the organ is stopped in the donor and the time that blood flow to the organ is restored in the recipient. Therefore potential recipients must be ready to go at all times. It is important that they do the following:

- Keep their telephone numbers *current*
- Know how to use their pagers, keep them operational (it is good to keep a spare battery available at all times), and carry them at all times
- Keep track of their recent laboratory test results

Similarly, the National Bone Marrow Donor Registry coordinates unrelated allogeneic bone marrow transplants. The National Marrow Donor Program (NMDP) is a nonprofit organization that has a cooperative agreement with the Department of the Navy and a competitively renewed contract with the Health Resources and Services Administration. The mission of the NMDP is to identify hematopoietic stem cell donors and then procure and deliver stem cell transplants to patient who do not have a suitable matched family member donor. This organization has a clearly stated set of minimum performance criteria for both donor harvest and transplant centers. The NMDP has also developed criteria that govern allocation (e.g., donors must match at five or more of six specified histocompatibility loci).

It is difficult to predict how long the wait for an organ may be for a particular patient. Waiting times can vary from a few days to many years. Times vary based on the type of organ or tissue required, the patient's medical condition, disease stage at the time of referral, the center, and the medical urgency. The waits of patients who are taken off the list prior to receiving a transplant, such as those who die, those who decline a transplant, and those who lose eligibility, are not reflected wait time data.

TRANSPORTATION AND HOUSING

Since time limits the viability of solid organs, most transplant programs require patients to be no more than 3 hours away from the transplant center both prior to transplantation and in the immediately postoperative period. These 3 hours are inclusive (preparation, driving, parking, etc.). Therefore many patients need to relocate (at least temporarily) to be near the transplant center. Depending on the type of transplant, the speed with which an organ is recovered, and the patient's recovery, the required length of stay near the transplant center may be from a minimum of several weeks to many months.

Health insurance may cover some travel expenses. Some polices cover airfare but not lodging; others will pay a daily rate for food and lodging but will not pay for airfare. Depending on the patient's physical condition, the urgency of the transplant, and the distance to the transplant center, transportation needs for the time of the actual transplant may need be considered in advance. In most cases, patients are able to arrange for transportation via commercial or private means. If the patient's physical condition is critical, however, ground ambulance or air ambulance transportation may be necessary There are a number of volunteer pilot organizations that can help with air travel. Most require the patient to be ambulatory and have distance restrictions or limitations. Although many limit their services to organ and transplant activities, many do not. These services can be a valuable resource for case managers with patients with other types of complex disease processes. Wise case managers will develop or obtain a list of available air transportation services in their area to share with patients and their families. It is recommended that the first call be to the Mercy Medical Airlift's National Patient Air Transport. Other valuable air sources are as follows:

- Air Care Alliance
- AirLifeLine (for patients ambulatory at the time of transplant and for follow-up visit, up to 700 miles)
- Angel Flight
- American Red Cross (limited to military personnel with emergency travel needs)
- Corporate Angel Network
- Mercy Medical Airlift (MMA)
- Mission Air Transportation Network
- Mission Aviation Fellowship

Several commercial airlines have a donated air mile funds for transplant patients. It is best to work through MMA. On occasion, some commercial airlines have offered special fares or free tickets to people who must travel for medical care (this is a rarity, however).

Beneficiaries of the TRICARE program (previously the Civilian Health and Medical Program of the Uniformed Services or CHAMPUS), may be eligible for free transportation by the military's air medical evacuation system if an air ambulance is required. Information about this resource is available by calling any military treatment facility or Scott Air Force Base in Illinois.

For ground transportation the American Cancer Society and the Travelers Aid Society may be able to offer some assistance. The Greyhound Bus Company has been known to provide free bus transportation for transplant patients with financial need. Once the patient is at the transplant center, low-cost bus service or medical van assistance for after-care is often available.

In addition to arranging transportation, finding inexpensive lodging near the transplant center can be a problem, especially if the family and patient need to relocate for an extended period of time. Potential assistance may be obtained from the following sources:

- The American Cancer Society, which maintains the Hope Lodges, available in many large cities
- The National Association of Hospital Hospitality Houses
- The Ronald McDonald Houses
- The medical center, which may maintain low-cost apartments that are available to transplant patients (this is common but one usually needs to inquire)
- Local hotels, which may have reduced rates for transplant program patients; this information can usually be obtained from the transplant program coordinator or financial planner

For patients with Medicaid insurance, federal regulations require states to ensure necessary transportation for patients to and from the provider of care. Transportation is defined to include related travel expenses, such as meals and lodging en route to and from medical care and while receiving care, both for the patient and, if necessary, for an attendant. Payments for food and lodging are often marginal, however, and many states may restrict payment for transportation to the amount needed to reach the nearest available provider.

AFTER-CARE

Most transplant centers require that, immediately after transplantation, the patient receive care at the transplant center's outpatient clinic. Patients are seen daily or as often as required by the transplant team. Depending on the outcome of the procedure and the patient's medical course, some patients may require the services of a home health agency or infusion center on discharge. The transplant team monitors responses to the treatment and the progress of the transplant. For these reasons, most transplant centers have arranged to provide discounted housing and transportation, and use a specific home health agency or infusion agency.

Unfortunately, if after-care requires the services of a home health agency and these services are not included in the rate agreed upon between the transplant center and the health care payer, a separate rate negotiation may be necessary. Otherwise, reimbursement problems or a denial of coverage can ensue. This is especially true when the patient's benefits are linked to a specific provider network. To prevent such occurrences, close communication between the facility case manager and the health care payer's care manager is again critical. This ensures that claims will be paid and the family will not be responsible for the nonnetwork provider's charges.

PSYCHOSOCIAL ASPECTS OF TRANSPLANTATION

Many inherent psychosocial and emotional demands are made on both the patient and the family during the different stages of the transplant process that can have a significant influence on the patient's health and well-being. All patients and families experience some degree of emotional turmoil during this time. Many patients and families have been living with the stress of declining health for many years. This, coupled with the overwhelming stress of financial pressures, fears related to the organ transplant process, and changes in family structure, can be insurmountable. Often the patient, family, and health care team underestimate the amount of emotional stress present. Consequently, case managers must be diligent in their efforts to make sure that problems are identified and are adequately addressed.

Pretransplant Considerations

During the initial psychological evaluation, case managers need to be aware that many candidates want to prove their suitability for transplantation and may downplay their fears or uncertainties. This behavior is often motivated by the fear of being rejected as a transplant candidate. Even after the patient is accepted, a lot of stress is associated with the waiting process, especially if the organ failure is acute and there is no reliable backup medical support (such as with dialysis for ESRD). Patients who have been on waiting lists for a long time often feel forgotten or abandoned. Candidates may also feel guilt knowing that someone must die for them to live. Common defense mechanisms used by patients at this stage to help them cope of which the case manager should be particularly aware include denial, displacement, minimization, rationalization, isolation of affect, projection, and reaction formation. Cognitive deficits may manifest due to metabolic disturbances secondary to end-stage organ failure and polypharmacy. Adjustment disorders, depression, anxiety disorders, and encephalopathy are common psychiatric events in the preoperative period that need prompt referral to psychiatric services.[12] In addition, referrals for recreation therapy may be in order for acutely ill patients who need additional support and distraction.

Posttransplant Considerations

Although well-being is improved after surgery, the patient often has a new set of medical problems with which to deal. Stresses associated with organ transplantation includes the constant threat of rejection, dependency, and the side effects of immunosuppression; the need for painful posttransplant procedures (e.g., biopsy); and resumption of an independent role.[12] Psychosomatic integration of the new organ can also be a challenge for some. Discharge delays, body image distortions, depression, hirsutism, psychological rejection, sexual concerns, and pain management are all potential problems.[12] Common posttransplantation psychiatric symptoms include medication withdrawal, delirium, insomnia, anxiety, mood disorders, and hallucinations and delusions (especially in those with visual and auditory impairments).

Continuum Considerations

Stress related to the transplant process affects the entire family. The patient's medical needs frequently dominate what was once normal life. Family stressors includes changes in income, work, school, environment, internal processes such as family roles, and stability. Financial pressures are exacerbated when (1) the illness involves the primary breadwinner, (2) the transplant contemplated is considered experimental or investigational and the medical efficacy of the procedure and outcomes

have not been proven, (3) the patient is a child and one or both parents must quit a job or take a leave of absence, or (4) the transplant must be performed out of the area, and the patient and family must be relocated or separated. In cases in which the patient is the breadwinner and loses his or her job, the family's daily income vanishes and often their health care insurance as well. In such cases, the patient and family may not have sufficient financial resources or reserves to pay for continuation of the insurance benefits, even through the provisions of the Consolidated Omnibus Reconciliation Act (COBRA).

Depending on their personal assets, many patients may qualify for Medicaid. Unfortunately, if the patient has any financial resources at all, he or she may be disqualified from Medicaid until these resources have been consumed. Exhaustion of private assets brings additional stresses such as guilt about being on "welfare," divorce, or bankruptcy, which further exacerbate an already devastating situation. Another source of pretransplant and posttransplant stress is the presence of limited funds for procurement of medications. The patient's lack of financial resources to purchase his or her own medications after the transplant is a factor that must be considered when candidacy for transplantation is evaluated.

As stated earlier, not all kinds of transplants are done at every transplant center. Therefore, another stressor often seen in transplant patients is separation anxiety. Not only does the patient now face a life-and-death situation, he or she also faces separation from the family. The separation also places additional strains on the family, such as isolation and unexpected financial burdens. These stressors are magnified when the potential transplant candidate is a child, because frequently one parent stays with the child while the other remains at home working or caring for other children.

Considerations for Children

Children undergoing the transplant process have unique needs. Although the quality of life usually improves after transplantation, some children have been reported to experience delayed physical growth and development, and to have stunted psychosocial development. Although the effect is not well studied, lower nonverbal intelligence, lower academic achievement, and poorer scores on learning and memory tests have been reported.[12] Pediatric recipients may have difficulties with psychosocial adjustment, especially related to dissatisfaction with the cosmetic side effects of immunosuppressive therapy and a lack of socialization skills and social competence.[10] Common posttransplantation behavioral problems include depression, poor social adaptation, and/or noncompliance with the medical regimen. Each stage of growth and development has its own set of stressors for both the parents and child. It is important to work closely with the transplant team and child life specialist in meeting the short-term and long-term psychosocial needs of pediatric transplant patients and their families. An additional stressor for families with teenagers is potential loss of insurance coverage when the teenager comes of age. Young adults may also have greater difficulty achieving both financial and psychosocial independence from their parents due to stunted growth and development and possible limitations in educational achievements.

LIVING DONORS

Organ donations by living individuals are becoming more frequent. Living donors currently represent the source of about 25% of all kidneys transplanted in the United States. There are many ethical as well as other concerns with which the case manager may become involved in transplants with a living donor. These includes

subjection of a healthy person to the complications of an operation, loss of income if the donor is the primary wage earner in the family, unknown outcome for the recipient, guilt felt by the donor if the recipient dies and/or rejects the organ, and temporary abandonment of the donor's family while the donor is hospitalized and recuperating. Within families, there may be pressure or coercion that makes it impossible to obtain voluntary donor consent. The living recipient may also experience feelings of guilt or indebtedness to the donor. Use of a living donor is especially problematic if the donor is a sibling or a child. All potential living donors must go through a psychiatric evaluation to ensure that the prospective donors are acting in the absence of coercion and in the presence of accurate information regarding the consequences of their actions for the health of the recipients and for themselves. The psychiatrist or mental health professional conducting the psychosocial evaluation of the donor must have no previous clinical relationship with the potential recipient. The donor must make an independent decision under conditions of strict medical confidentiality. If a translator is used in making the evaluation, the translator must be a professional health translator and must be unknown to both donor and recipient.[3]

RESOURCES

Whenever the case manager identifies the presence of psychosocial stressors, it is vital that he or she make every attempt to provide the patient or family with some form of counseling, whether offered by a health care professional or a support group. Support may be obtained from sources such as the following:

- Support groups (church groups, organ-specific groups, and other community disease-specific agencies)

- Psychiatrists
- Psychologists
- Family counselors
- Clinical social workers
- Lay counseling services (such as those provided by a church or support organization)
- Internet support resources (E-mail lists, usenet newsgroups, real-time chat forums)
- Tapes and literature that deal with current issues related to organ failure and transplantation

PROVIDERS

Most patients are limited by their insurance coverage with regard to the transplant providers they are able to access. In an effort to assure quality, contain costs, and enhance the provision of organ and tissue transplantation services, many major private health insurers and health maintenance organizations (HMOs) restrict payment of transplantation procedures to designated programs, often referred to as centers of excellence. These programs are chosen based upon total annual transplant volume, 1- and 2-year patient and graft survival rates, and other criteria according to the type of procedure and recipient (e.g., pediatric versus adult).[13,14] If centers meet the minimum volume and outcome criteria, insurers negotiate discounted charges for the procedure. Discounts may be as high as 25%.[13] Patients are often offered incentives to use designated centers of excellence, with insurers frequently paying travel costs and reducing or waiving copayment amounts.

Medicare uses very stringent criteria to certify organ transplant centers, and consequently many health care payers adhere to the same guidelines in their coverage language. Thus, health care payers often specify that transplants are allowed only in those centers that are "Medicare certified." If the transplant is not done at such a facility, reimbursement may not be allowed. In these cases, the patient will be financially liable for the procedure if research funding is not available. Many health care payers make similar requirements with regard to bone marrow transplant centers. These centers are required at a minimum to be members of the National Bone Marrow Donor Registry.

To ensure that all providers used are appropriate, the facility-based case manager must coordinate all details with the health care payer's case manager. Similarly, the health care payer's case manager must know which types of transplants are performed at the most frequently used centers and which postacute care providers they may use. Just as important is a knowledge of the capabilities of other transplant centers, nationally and in other parts of the state. This information is necessary when, because of the patient's condition and the type of transplant, the procedure cannot be performed at a network provider and a nonnetwork center of excellence must be found.

If the transplant procedure cannot be done at the network transplant center, the case manager must be prepared to request approval through the extracontractual review process or negotiate a reduced rate for the actual services to be rendered. For instance, liver transplantation coverage is a benefit provided by most health care payers; however, not every liver transplant center may be certified to perform the procedure for every diagnosis. Likewise, not all facilities are certified to perform pediatric transplants. If the appropriate transplant center is not in the health care payer's network, the case managers on the case must collectively be prepared to guide the patient to the appropriate center, making the necessary arrangements for care and reimbursement. It is therefore wise for case managers to keep a current list of frequently used transplant centers in their reference files. At minimum, this list should include the following:

- The name of the transplant medical director
- The phone numbers of the center, financial coordinator, transplant coordinator, clinical nurse specialist, case manager, and social worker
- Specific details of what medical and patient demographic information are required at the time of referral
- The types of transplants performed and any information about the center's outcomes and transplant history

FINANCIAL ARRANGEMENTS AND ALTERNATIVE FUNDING CONSIDERATIONS

Transplantation is an expensive endeavor, and for most patients financing their transplant is a tremendous concern. Evidence of ability to pay is a criterion that must be met before the patient is accepting as a potential organ recipient and placed on the waiting list. In addition to the expense of the transplant, many patients have the stress of changes in employment due to their preexisting illness and/or anticipated recovery time. Case managers involved with transplant patients must work with patients and their families to explore and apply for all alternative funding programs to which patients may be entitled. This includes applying for alternative sources of income, health care benefit policies, and unemployment benefits. Most transplant programs have a social worker or designated finance person who is especially knowledgeable in transplant financing. It is important that the case manager work closely with the transplant center care manager and patient throughout this entire process.

COSTS

It is difficult to predict the actual out-of-pocket costs for an individual transplant.

Charges vary substantially based on the condition of the patient; the condition of the donor; the geographic location of the donor, patient, and transplant center; transplant center practices; changing health care costs; the type of organ; the type of posttransplant therapy; the required immunosuppressive therapy; and possible posttransplant complications. Most economic analyses of transplantation costs are based on the billed charges directly related to the surgery. When the cost of a transplant is analyzed, distinctions must be made between accounting costs, billed charges, estimated reimbursement, contracted prices, and actual reimbursements by third-party payers. In addition, a significant portion of the cost of a transplant is related to the pretransplant and follow-up care, which are not traditionally included in most financial analyses of transplant costs. The following are the direct and indirect costs associated with bone marrow and organ transplants that the case manager must keep in mind while assisting a patient with planning.

Direct Medical Costs

- Pretransplant disease management
- Pretransplant evaluation and testing
- Transplant surgery and associated hospital stay
- Organ procurement fees (procurement fees are paid by the recipient)
- Fees for surgeons, physicians, radiologists, anesthesiologists, and other specialists who may be involved in the transplant process
- Follow-up clinic and home health care
- Laboratory testing
- Antirejection agents and other medications
- Physical, occupational, and vocational rehabilitation
- Insurance deductibles and copayments
- Additional medical costs and hospitalizations related to management of complications

Nonmedical or Indirect Costs

- Transportation to and from the transplant center (including before and after transplantation); time is usually of the essence, and the cheapest route of transportation may not be available or feasible.
- Food, lodging, and long distance telephone calls; depending on the distance and weather conditions, the patient may need to live near the transplant center immediately before and after the transplantation.
- Child care.
- Lost wages for the patient and primary caregiver or significant other.

As a rule, if the transplant is a covered benefit, then the medical expenses associated with the transplant are covered. These expenses include human leukocyte antigen (HLA) and HLA DNA testing, which are necessary to determine whether the donor organ or tissue matches the recipient's. Health care payers vary in their policies on organ acquisition costs and testing. For example, many payers will not pay for any expenses related to the harvesting of the donor organ. In the case of an allogeneic bone marrow transplant, tests of living related donors may be covered whereas tests of unrelated donors and donor searches are not. In other cases, the costs of donor harvesting are covered if they are billed by the recipient's hospital but not by the donor's hospital. Other health care payers do not cover any donor charges.

TRADITIONAL INSURANCE

Almost all health insurance plans now cover at least a portion of if not all solid organ and bone marrow transplantation. Traditional insurance plans typically pay about 80% of the hospital charges, which leaves around 20% for the recipient to pay (up to a fixed or ceiling amount). Managed care and hospital organizations often pay 100% of the cost of a transplant with the exception of small copayments for office visits, medications, and such. Because of the multifaceted needs and great expense of transplant care, however, it is easy to exceed the "cap" or lifetime limit imposed by many companies. Insurance coverage must be verified not only to protect both the patient and the other parties involved, but also to provide for the best planning, especially when there are gaps in coverage. It is important that there be no exclusion clauses or disqualification clauses in the policy. If the patient has more than one insurance carrier, care must be coordinated to maximize overall coverage.

Many plans will not reimburse for transplants or medications considered to be investigational or experimental, although this is beginning to change. Medicare has recently expanded payment guidelines for experimental bone marrow transplants. While most solid organ transplants are no longer considered experimental, some insurance companies may refuse to accept them as part of the standard of care for specific disease conditions and may refuse to pay for some of the newer therapies associated with the transplant.

CONSOLIDATED OMNIBUS BUDGET RECONCILIATION ACT

Advanced heart, kidney, liver, or lung disease often prevents a person from working or from working full time. Often these changes can result in the loss of employer paid health benefits. It is important that the case manager work with the patient to obtain COBRA benefits as indicated in the funding section of this text. COBRA benefits also apply to those who have become disabled as defined by Social Security guidelines or who have had to change working hours due to the sickness of a child. Application for benefits must be made within 60 days of the employment change, however. Transplant coverage will be limited to the original terms of the policy. Some insurance companies will allow individuals to change to an individual policy after the COBRA time limits but usually at a less desirable rate. The case manager must keep in mind, while helping the patient and family maximize their benefits, that COBRA benefits may be terminated if the patient-payee joins another group health plan (unless it has limits because of a preexisting condition), the patient-payee cannot pay the monthly premiums, the original employer stops offering its employees a group health plan, or the patient-payee becomes eligible for Medicare. For patients who lose COBRA benefits, a "federal fallback" program may be an option.

MEDICARE, MEDICAID, AND MEDIGAP

Both Medicaid and Medicare offer solid organ and bone marrow transplant coverage for those who fulfill certain age and diagnostic criteria. Medicaid benefits are generally reserved for individuals with low incomes or those who are receiving other forms of governmental assistance, such as Aid to Families with Dependent Children or Supplemental Security Income (SSI). Medicare is available to people over the age of 65 years and others who are either disabled, have ESRD, or qualify for Social Security Disability Income (SSDI). Medicare offers two basic plans, Part A and Part B.

Medicare Part A is free to eligible members and covers a percentage of basic hospital care and follow-up treatment. Medicare's hospital insurance covers 100% of the costs of the hospital stay and transplant operation after the annual deductible is paid. Patients who need regular dialysis or have a kidney transplant are automatically eligible for Medicare Part A regardless of age if the patient, his or her spouse, or dependent children get Social Security cash benefits or have worked the required amount of time to qualify (usually 10 years).

Medicare Part B, an optional plan, covers additional outpatient services. People enrolled in Part B pay monthly premiums and a small annual deductible payment, and have a 20% coinsurance liability. This program covers physician services, outpatient hospital services (including dialysis), medical equipment, and other health services and supplies. Medicare pays for 80% of the cost of immunosuppressant agents needed within the first 3 years of solid organ transplantation; however, many patients cannot afford the remaining 20%. For renal transplants, the dosages, and therefore the costs, are significantly reduced after 3 years but can still be substantial. Medicare coverage can be extended if the patient is disabled or unable to work, or if the organ is rejected or lost during this time.

There are no deductibles or copayments for living donors. For patients with both employer group health insurance and Medicare coverage, Medicare will be their secondary payer (the group insurance pays first) for the first 30 months that they are eligible for Medicare coverage. After that period, Medicare becomes the primary payer and their group insurance pays second. Case managers who work with Medicare patients should obtain a free copy of *Medicare Coverage of Dialysis and Kidney Transplant Patients* from their local Medicare office.

Patients seeking predialysis or preemptive transplantation should clarify their health insurance status to ensure that the costs of their evaluation and the preparation of a living donor are covered. Medicare ESRD benefits do not commence before dialysis and transplantation. This waiting period, called a qualifying period, may be eliminated depending on the type of treatment chosen. Preemptive transplantation may offer improved patient and graft survival over conventional transplantation. Although it is not the standard of care, preemptive transplantation decreases or eliminates the complications and increased cardiovascular risk associated with long-term dialysis and is thought to decrease the incidence of acute rejection. Those who receive a transplant before the development of frank uremic symptoms or commencement of dialysis may not feel the improved sense of well-being typically enjoyed by dialysis patients after transplantation and should be warned of this.

Since Medicare does not always cover 100% of all medical needs, a supplemental private insurance policy, called a supplemental or "medigap" policy, may be purchased to help pay for some of the expenses not covered by Medicare. Usually, medigap policies must be purchased within 6 months of the effective date of Medicare Plan B. Information on the medigap insurance policies available in a state can be obtained from the state insurance department. This department can also advise regarding which insurance companies are selling different medigap plans. For the number of the state insurance department, call the National Insurance Consumer Hotline. Other resources include the local Social Security office; the Medicare hotline, and the transplant finance team member.

Since eligibility for both Medicare and Medicaid can depend on prior enrollment in Social Security's SSI or SSDI programs, a patient should enroll in these program, if eligible, as soon as possible. SSI is available low-income people who are over 65 years, are blind, or have a disability. People who are disabled and unable to do any substantial work may be eligible for SSDI. After receiving SSDI benefits for 24 month, one is eligible for Medicare.

TRICARE (CHAMPUS) AND THE VETERANS ADMINISTRATION

The TRICARE Standard program may share the cost of heart, lung, heart-lung, liver, kidney, and combined liver-kidney trans-

plants. Patients must receive preauthorization from the TRICARE medical director and must meet certain selection criteria. For further information, contact the nearest military health care facility or the TRICARE or CHAMPUS benefits service branch.

Honorably discharged veterans may be eligible for Veterans Administration (VA) benefits. It has become more and more difficult, however, to become eligible without a service-connected disability. Patients who first became ill while in the service or who are indigent may be eligible to receive a transplant at a VA medical center. Those without a service-connected disease may still be eligible for treatment at a VA hospital if the hospital has room in its program and chooses to provide treatment. Some veterans may also receive VA funding for medications. For more information, contact the local veterans hospital or VA office.

OTHER SOURCES OF HEALTH INSURANCE

Two other sources of health insurance for persons at high risk with preexisting conditions who have been denied insurance include high-risk pools and guaranteed issued insurance. High-risk pools are offered in only some states, and premiums can be higher (50% to 200%) than those of standard policies. Benefits are usually more restricted than in standard policies, and coverage for outpatient medication is generally limited. A directory of high-risk insurance policies available in each state has been compiled by the organization Communicating for Agriculture. Some states have a guaranteed issue law that requires insurers to offer individual coverage regardless of preexisting conditions. All individual policies are usually more costly in these states. Resources regarding coverage can be obtained from an employee's human resources department and their benefits officer or personnel, the

Pension and Welfare Benefits Administration, and the Department of Health and Human Services.

Other sources of funds include the following:

- Savings
- Retirement or pension accounts (many accounts allow early withdrawal or borrowing against the account for special hardship events)
- Second mortgage or reverse mortgage
- Life insurance (either a loan against insurance or a cash-in)
- Fundraisers
- Fraternal organizations
- Title V Children's Medical Services program (limited help with denied or uncovered medical costs for children)
- Grants (although limited in scope and very restrictive, research funds or grants may occasionally pay for transplants for patients who qualify)

The financial counselor at the transplant center is an excellent resource for information on specific alternative funding programs that may be directly associated with that center.

Several organizations specialize in helping people raise money for an organ transplant. This assistance may take the form of helping with fundraisers, providing direct financial assistance and emergency grants for medications and transplant-related expenses, and providing information on other financial resources. Examples of such organizations include the following:

- American Kidney Fund
- American Kidney Foundation
- American Liver Foundation
- Barbara Anne DeBoer Foundation
- William B. Dessner Memorial Fund (kidneys)
- Children's Organ Transplant Association

- National Foundation for Transplants
- National Transplant Assistance Fund

MEDICATION

Medications are a recurring expense. New and improved drugs are continually being developed, which keeps the costs high. There are several national mail-order pharmacies that specialize in the needs of transplant patients. Many insurance plans offer discounts for patients who use mail-order pharmacies. Examples of mail-order pharmacies are American Preferred Prescription, Inc., Chronimed, SangStat Medical Corporation, and Stadtlanders Pharmacy (see the list of websites and other resources at the end of the chapter). Several pharmaceutical companies provide drug-specific subsides to indigent patients. Examples of these are also provided in the list of websites and contact numbers. Another resource is pharmaceutical patient assistance programs (*www.needymeds.com*). These are clinical pharmacist-managed medication assistance programs that help patients procure immunosuppressant medications from pharmaceutical manufacturers. Closely related is the Pharmaceutical Research and Manufacturers of America (*www.phrma.org*), which provides a directory of prescription drug patient assistance programs for physicians that gives information on drug companies providing medications to physicians for patients who could not otherwise afford them. Their directory provides information on what medications are covered as well as eligibility criteria. Some transplant centers, such as the Medical College of Georgia, provide immunosuppressant medications to transplant patients who cannot afford to pay for them. In addition, there are a variety of state programs and private organizations (e.g., the American Kidney Foundation, National Organization for State Kidney Programs) that can assist in the procurement of needed medications.

DISABILITY INSURANCE FOR TRANSPLANT RECIPIENTS

Besides health insurance coverage, the case manager should work closely with the transplant patient to obtain disability coverage as needed. Most patients will be off work for at least 3 months following transplantation. Most disability plans do not compensate recipients for total lost wages, which adds to patients' financial hardship. Recipients who are receiving benefits under the Social Security Disability Income (SSDI) or Supplemental Security Income (SSI) program at the time of transplantation will continue to receive the same benefits posttransplantation, as long as they still are unable to work. State disability insurance (SDI) benefits vary from state to state. SDI is available to recipients who are employed and who pay state income taxes. SDI eligibility begins 1 week after the patient stops working and can possibly continue for up to 1 year. Not all states have SDI. Employed patients may be covered by a work-related disability program. The case manager should work closely with the patient and the patient's employment benefit office.

Many patients are eligible for SSDI. SSDI is long-term disability program for patients who are considered disabled for at least 1 year. Patients on short-term disability benefits should apply early for SSDI, since establishing eligibility can take several months. Social Security payments are monthly and are based on a patient's individual earnings in the highest earnings quarter. Patients with ESRD who are receiving dialysis or who have undergone transplantation are eligible for SSDI if they have paid Federal Insurance Contribution Act (FICA) taxes. Patients receiving SSDI may return to work on a limited basis without losing their Social Security benefits. They may still collect SSDI as long as they do not earn more than $500 per month for longer than 8 months.

SSI is a federally funded program administered by the Social Security Administration. This program provides monthly cash benefit to persons who have disabilities and limited income and resources. Patients must meet both financial and disability criteria. The disability must be a medically determined mental and/or physical condition that is expected to last 1 year or longer. Often patients receive this in addition to their SSDI benefits. The SSI amount varies from state to state, depending on the cost of living of the respective state.

FAMILY MEDICAL LEAVE ACT

Important to the family and patient is the Family Medical Leave Act (FMLA). FMLA requires employers to provide up to 12 weeks of unpaid of protected leave to eligible employees for certain family and medical reasons that make the employees unable to perform their work. Employees are eligible if they have worked for an employer for at least 1 year (minimum of 1250 hours over the previous 12 months) and if there are at least 50 employees within 75 miles. The employee may be required to provide advance leave notice and medical certification. For the duration of FMLA leave, the employer must maintain the employee's health coverage under any group health plan. Upon return from FMLA leave, most employees must be restored to their original or equivalent positions with equivalent pay, benefits, and other employment terms.

VOCATIONAL REHABILITATION

Many transplant recipients are not working at the time of the transplantation for various health reasons. These patients, together with patients who are unable to return to their prior employment because their job responsibilities are in conflict with transplant-related restrictions, may be eligible for vocational rehabilitation. The Social Security Administration can help people with disabilities get the vocational rehabilitation services they need. There are several work incentives to help people retain their current cash benefits (e.g., SSDI, SSI) and health insurance coverage during a trial work period. Some patients with ongoing needs may qualify as handicapped under the Americans with Disabilities Act.

TRICARE COVERAGE FOR ALLOGENEIC BONE MARROW TRANSPLANTATION

If a patient who needs an allogeneic bone marrow transplant has no other insurance and his or her primary health care coverage is through TRICARE (previously the Civilian Health and Medical Program of the Uniformed Services, or CHAMPUS), he or she must be referred to or evaluated by the transplant team of the Wilford Hall Medical Center in San Antonio, Texas. This referral or evaluation must be done prior to the performance of any evaluation or transplant procedure by a civilian transplant center. Referral to this center is necessary because, before reimbursement can occur, a nonavailability statement must be issued by the Wilford Hall Medical Center. This nonavailability statement stipulates that the services required by the patient were not available from Wilford Hall Medical Center. The nonavailability statement allows the patient to undergo the evaluation or have the transplant performed in a civilian transplant center. More importantly, it allows the transplant center to be paid.

A word to the wise: Wilford Hall Medical Center, like many military treatment facilities, is a state-of-the-art center of excellence. This facility matches or exceeds the standards set for any civilian center of excellence, and case managers should not underestimate its capabilities. If the patient has TRICARE coverage, the case manager should take a proactive role in advocating that the transplant occur at Wilford Hall Medical Center or the military transplant center designated. Not only will the transplant be performed in a state-of-the-art center, but also most services related to the transplant will be free, including most outpatient care and medications.

Commonly, many plans exclude any charges related to services rendered to the donor prior to brain death; these are paid by the donor's insurance. When a patient needs an allogeneic bone marrow transplant from an unrelated donor, much of the testing and search costs must be borne by the patient or family, and in many cases, the patient must rely on fraternal organizations and other groups that conduct fund raisers to assist in raising the money needed.

EXPERIMENTAL TRANSPLANT PROCEDURES

When a transplant procedure is one that is considered experimental, it is absolutely critical for all case managers to collaborate regarding the needs and details that arise. Thus, when a transplant referral comes to a health care payer's case manager from a transplant center and the requested transplant procedure is not the customary request for the given diagnosis or is known to be experimental, special precautions must be taken. Many health care payers exclude experimental or investigational services or items from reimbursement, and the patient and family must fully understand the potential financial implications of such a transplant. Consequently, for transplant procedures that are known to be experimental or about which doubts exist, all case managers involved must work closely together to make sure that all the information and medical facts justifying the transplant are made known. If they are not, coverage for the transplant procedure may be denied when it might have been allowed if all the facts had been presented at the time of the review and coverage determination. Many times treatments are very successful but, because of the small study sizes, they are not accepted as standard care.

If doubt is raised about the transplant procedure or if it is known to be experimental, there are several things a case manager can do. In addition to requesting the standard medical information about the evaluation or the transplant procedure, the health care payer's case manager must query the referral source regarding the standard-of-care status of the actual transplant procedure. In addition, a copy of the consent form the patient will sign should be requested. If the transplant procedure is known to be experimental, the patient must be informed of this fact and must acknowledge his or her awareness of it by signing the consent form. If the patient is not informed of participation in an "experiment," the facility performing the procedure may incur significant monetary fines and other penalties. Disease-specific treatment guidelines should be obtained from the payer's network as well as from an outside nonnetwork source.

If there is doubt about the transplant procedure and its status, the case manager or the health care payer's medical director must conduct research to find information from key national resource groups about the status of the transplant procedure. In many cases, the organization's legal counsel must be consulted for guidance. Appeals should be filed early, and patients should prepare immediately to go to the next steps. Good record keeping is essential. Patients should request specifics and ask to the have the denial in writing. It is recommended that patients stress in their

appeals that the procedure is medically necessary and that, without treatment, the condition will continue to get worse.

Sources that can assist with verification of the status of the transplant include the following:

- Center for Health Care Technology
- National Institutes of Health
- National Cancer Institute
- Office of Patient Advocacy
- Other major tertiary transplant centers throughout the country
- On-line computer services, such as MEDLINE

Although the research modalities used to evaluate whether a transplant procedure is experimental vary with the health care payer or organization, the primary reason for research is to validate that the procedure is indeed experimental. In many cases this research is conducted when the request for the initial evaluation for the transplant is submitted. In other cases it is conducted when the patient is deemed a candidate for transplantation and it is known that the outcome procedure, the transplantation, is experimental.

Second opinions can also be helpful. In most indemnity plans or preferred provider organizations, the insurance plan will pay for a second opinion (but it is always wise to check in advance). In an HMO, the doctor must refer the patient for the second opinion in order for the plan to pay. This becomes problematic when the plan has only one contract with a specific organ service. It is in the patient's interest, however, to pursue the matter. Second opinions can also be obtained independently. The patient will most likely have to pay out of pocket for this. The case manager can help in arranging a second opinion and in keeping the cost down by sending copies of the medical records, x-ray films, and laboratory results to the second opinion physician.

The actual approval or denial of the recommendation of the initial evaluation varies from payer to payer. For instance, some payers indicate that if the evaluation recommendation is approved, this approval sets up a "right of expectation" that the transplant procedure will be covered, even though it is experimental and excluded from coverage. In contrast, other payers view the approval of the evaluation recommendation as a second opinion. In either case, it is imperative for all case managers to be familiar with the requirements of the health care payers regarding the evaluation process. In all cases, both facility-based and health care payer case managers must work closely together to avoid delays in the approval process and to ensure that all information is submitted as expeditiously as possible. In addition, a formal grievance should be filed in cases of denial of coverage, and the patient should prepare to take the case to a state regulatory agency (such as the state insurance commissioner) and/or to take the plan to court (or to arbitration if the plan has agreed to that option). There are several patient advocacy groups in addition to individual organ societies that may be of help in negotiating for treatment.

If patients are part of an experimental therapy or clinical trial, they must first read, understand, and sign an informed consent form that clearly defines the nature of the experiment in which they are to be involved along with its potential risk and benefits. They must also receive a copy of the Patient's Bill of Rights, which should clearly define the nature of their commitment.

INDICATIONS AND CONTRAINDICATIONS FOR TRANSPLANTATION

The following subsections (although not all inclusive) offer guidelines regarding the indications, contraindications, and referral criteria recommended for the various types of transplants. It behooves each case manager to be familiar with this material and the processes required for approval or denial when requests are generated. Although the following transplants are commonly performed, the conditions for which they are considered a standard of care are limited. Each health care payer has its own list of acceptable conditions for which benefit coverage is allowed. The most common generic clinical reasons for denial of coverage for an organ transplant are given in the subsection on transplant center evaluation and are not restated here.

Heart Transplantation[10,12,15]

- Indications
  - Younger than 70 years (some programs will not consider candidates older than 65 years)
  - Systolic failure with diminished exercise capacity seen on a metabolic stress test with a maximal oxygen uptake of 14 m/kg/min or greater
  - Ejection fraction <20%, arrhythmia, serum sodium level <120 mEq/L, a left bundle branch block on electrocardiogram or a cardiothoracic ratio on chest radiograph >0.75
  - Healthy condition except for end-stage cardiac disease
- Absolute contraindications
  - Systemic illness that will limit survival despite heart transplant
  - Neoplasm other than skin (this includes low-grade prostate cancer that has not been "cured" or in remission for >5 years)
  - HIV infection or acquired immunodeficiency syndrome (AIDS) (in certain circumstances a waiver may be granted)
  - Systemic lupus erythematosus or sarcoid that has multisystem involvement and is still active
  - Any systemic process with a high probability of recurring in the transplanted heart

- Fixed pulmonary hypertension with pulmonary vascular resistance >5 Wood units, and/or a transpulmonary gradient >15 mm Hg (these are arbitrary values)
- Relative contraindications
  - Peripheral vascular disease not amenable to surgical or percutaneous therapy
  - Asymptomatic carotid stenosis >75% or symptomatic carotid stenosis of lesser severity
  - Ankle brachial index <0.7 or substantial risk of limb loss with diminished perfusion
  - Uncorrected abdominal aortic aneurysm >4 to 6 cm
  - Systemic infection that makes immune suppression risky (e.g., with HIV, hepatitis B virus, or cytomegalovirus)
  - Severe pulmonary disease
  - Diabetes mellitus with end organ damage (e.g., neuropathy, nephropathy, and retinopathy)
  - Psychosocial impairment that would jeopardize the transplanted heart
- Indications for referral
  - Systolic heart failure (as defined by ejection fraction of <35%)
  - Inclusive etiology: ischemic, dilated, valvular, and hypertensive
  - Exclusive etiology: amyloid, HIV, or cardiac sarcoma
  - Ischemic heart disease with intractable angina
  - Nonamenability to treatment by coronary artery bypass graft or percutaneous revascularization,
  - Ineffectiveness of maximal tolerated medical therapy
  - Rejection for direct myocardial revascularization or transmyocardial revascularization or lack of success if the procedure was attempted
  - Intractable arrhythmia uncontrolled with a pacing cardioverter defibrillator

- Nonamenability to electrophysiologically guided single or combination medical therapy
- Rejection for ablative therapy
- Hypertrophic cardiomyopathy
- Persistence of class IV symptoms despite maximal therapy as follows:
  - Alcohol injection
  - Myomectomy
  - Mitral valve replacement
  - Maximal medical therapy
  - Pacemaker therapy
- Congenital heart disease in which severe fixed pulmonary hypertension is not a complication

Heart-Lung Transplantation[10,12]

- Indications
  - Eisenmenger's syndrome with an irreparable shunt defect
  - Refractory right ventricular diastolic dysfunction (right ventricular end-diastolic pressure >15 mm Hg)
  - Severe intrinsic left ventricular dysfunction (left ventricular ejection fraction <45%)
  - Cystic fibrosis (CF)
  - Primary pulmonary hypertension
  - Severe end-stage pulmonary or cardiopulmonary disease
  - Life expectancy <6 months to 1 year
  - Age no older than 50 to 55 years (for heart and lung or bilateral lung) or 60 to 65 years (for a single lung)
- Contraindications
  - Active infection or systemic illness
  - Thoracic trauma
  - Life-limiting conditions such as renal or hepatic failure, or malignancy
  - Previous major thoracic surgery
  - Lack of compliance with supportive medical regimens or lack of rehabilitation potential
  - HIV infection or AIDS
  - Morbid obesity
  - Irreversible brain damage
  - Irreversible liver impairment

- Insulin-dependent diabetes with neuropathy, retinopathy, or peripheral vascular disease
- Indication for referral (not all inclusive)
  - Exhaustion of all other modes of conventional medical and surgical therapy

Lung Transplantation[10,12]

- Indications
  - Chronic obstructive pulmonary disease (bronchiectasis, emphysema, α_1-antitrypsin deficiency)
  - Primary pulmonary fibrosis
  - CF
  - Primary pulmonary hypertension
  - End-stage pulmonary disease in a mobile patient younger than the age of 65 years in the absence of other significant organ disease
  - Sarcoidosis
  - Eisenmenger's physiology (with progressive right ventricular failure, marked deterioration in functional capacity, hemoptysis, and worsening hypoxemia)
  - Lymphangioleiomyomatosis
  - Septic lung disease
- Contraindications
  - Insulin-dependent diabetes (not stipulated by all centers)
  - Active infection
  - History of malignancy within the past 5 years
  - Chronic pulmonary emboli
  - Systemic lupus erythematosus
  - Primary pulmonary hypertension
  - Myogenic respiratory disease
  - Renal insufficiency
  - Cor pulmonale with gross cardiomegaly
  - HIV infection or AIDS
  - Bone marrow failure
  - Hepatic cirrhosis
- Relative contraindications
  - Tobacco use within 6 months
  - Physiologic age >65 years for single lung transplant
  - Physiologic age >60 for bilateral lung transplant
  - Psychosocial instability
  - Weight outside of acceptable range (<70% or >130% of predicted weight)
  - Prednisone use >20 mg/day or 40 mg every other day
  - Mechanical ventilation
  - Major dysfunction of other organs, especially kidney, liver, and central nervous system
  - Coronary disease or left ventricular dysfunction
  - Significant peripheral vascular disease
  - Symptomatic osteoporosis
  - Severe chest wall deformity
  - Sputum containing panresistant bacteria or *Aspergillus*
  - Active hepatitis B or C infection
- Indications for referral (not all inclusive)[10]
  - For patients with CF
    - Initiation of supplemental enteral feeding by percutaneous endoscopic gastronomy or parenteral nutrition
    - Cycling IV antibiotic therapy
    - Noninvasive nocturnal mechanical ventilation
    - Increasing frequency of hospital admission
    - Increasingly severe exacerbation of CF, particularly an episode requiring hospital admission
    - Recurrent massive hemoptysis
    - Development of CO_2 retention
    - Worsening arterial-alveolar gradient requiring increasing concentrations of inspired oxygen
    - Decreasing forced expiratory volume in 1 second (FEV_1) or FEV_1 <30%
  - For patients with sarcoidosis
    - Presence of cor pulmonale or pulmonary hypertension
    - Stage 3 disease on chest radiograph (pulmonary infiltrates without hilar adenopathy)

- Nonpulmonary features of disease (lupus pernio, hepatomegaly, pulmonary osteoarthropathy, upper airway involvement)
- FEV_1 <50% or total lung capacity <80%
- Obstructive lung disease (chronic obstructive pulmonary disease, α_1-antitrypsin deficiency)[12]
- Postbronchodilator FEV_1 <25% of predicted, and/or
- Arterial partial pressure of carbon dioxide ($Paco_2$) ≥55 mm Hg, and/or
- Elevated pulmonary artery pressures with progressive deterioration
- Restrictive lung disease (idiopathic pulmonary fibrosis or other interstitial lung disease)
- Symptomatic progressive disease unresponsive to medical therapy
- Bronchodilator forced vital capacity <60% to 70% of predicted
- Resting hypoxia ($Paco_2$ <55 mm Hg)
- Hypercarbia ($Paco_2$ ≥45 mm Hg)
- Declining clinical course
- Bilateral bronchiectasis
- Increasing resistance of infecting bacterial organisms
- For patients with pulmonary vascular disease
  - Projected life expectancy <2 years
  - New York Heart Association class II or IV functional level

Liver Transplantation[12,16]

- Indications
  - End-stage liver disease for which other available medical and surgical treatments have been exhausted
  - Extrahepatic biliary atresia for which hepatoportoenterostomy has failed
  - Chronic active hepatitis with progressive liver failure and a life expectancy of <6 months (includes hepatitis C, the most common condition resulting in the need for liver transplantation)
  - Primary and secondary biliary cirrhosis
  - Hepatic vein thrombosis with progressive liver failure and ascites that has not responded to anticoagulants or portal decompression surgery
  - Sclerosing cholangitis with chronic nonsupportive inflammation of the bile ducts with no history of multiple surgeries, extrahepatic duct disease, or the presence of biliary infections
  - Imminent death
  - Inevitable irreversible damage to the central nervous system
  - Deterioration of quality of life to unacceptable levels
  - Primary hepatic malignancy confined to the liver but not amenable to resection
  - Alcoholic liver disease in patients who develop evidence of progressive liver failure despite appropriate medical treatment and cessation of alcohol abuse
  - Postnecrotic cirrhosis
  - Metabolic diseases such as the following:
    - Budd-Chiari syndrome
    - Wilson's disease
    - α_1-Antitrypsin deficiency
    - CF
    - Glycogen storage disease
    - Argininosuccinic acidemia
    - Oxaluria
    - Tyrosinemia
    - Ornithine transcarbamylase deficiency
    - Primary hepatoma
    - Fulminant liver failure
    - Hemochromatosis
    - Retransplantation
- Contraindications
  - Uncontrolled infection outside the hepatobiliary system

- Encephalopathy with edema or irreversible brain damage
- Congenital anomalies that prevent surgery
- Primary hepatic malignancies extending beyond the margin of the liver
- Secondary hepatic malignancy
- Metastatic hepatobiliary malignancy
- Severe hypoxemia due to right-to-left intrapulmonary shunt
- Severe renal or cardiopulmonary disease (may require dual organ transplantation)
- Lack of sufficient psychosocial stability to ensure compliance with required regimen
- Relative contraindications
- HIV infection or AIDS
- Age older than 65 years
- Portal vein thrombosis
- Renal failure not associated with liver disease
- Intrahepatic sepsis
- Prior extensive hepatobiliary surgery
- Indications for referral
  - In adults
    - Life-threatening and progressive irreversible liver disease
    - New-onset ascites in a cirrhotic patient
    - Ascites resistant to medical therapy
    - Spontaneous bacterial peritonitis
    - Increasing fatigue in a cirrhotic patient so that daily activities cannot be performed
    - Onset of hepatic encephalopathy
    - Progressive malnutrition and muscle wasting
    - Recurrent bacterial cholangitis
    - Symptomatic hepatopulmonary syndrome
    - Onset of hepatorenal syndrome
    - Fulminant hepatic failure
    - Worsening synthetic function in a cirrhotic patient

- Decreasing serum albumin level
- Rising prothrombin time
- Development of hepatocellular carcinoma within a cirrhotic liver
- In the pediatric population[10]
  - Intractable cholestasis
  - Portal hypertension
  - Multiple episodes of ascending cholangitis
  - Failure to thrive, malnutrition
  - Intractable ascites
  - Encephalopathy
  - Unacceptable quality of life
  - Metabolic defects for which liver transplantation will reverse life-threatening illness and prevent irreversible central nervous system damage

Simultaneous Kidney and Liver Transplantation

- Indications
  - Severe irreversible renal dysfunction due to:
    - Polycystic kidneys with massive hepatomegaly
    - Glomerulonephritis (typically immunoglobulin A nephropathy)
    - Failing kidney transplant with end-stage liver disease (typically due to hepatitis B or C virus)
    - Repeat orthotopic liver transplantation with cyclosporine nephrotoxicity
    - Oxalosis
    - Prolonged preorthotopic liver transplantation with dialysis dependence
    - Diabetic nephropathy
- Contraindications
  - Similar to those for a single liver or kidney transplant
- Indications for referral
  - Similar to those for individual organ transplantation

Simultaneous Kidney and Pancreas Transplantation[17]

- Indications
  - ESRD
  - Age younger than 50 years (generally 18 to 50 years)
  - Glucose control problems (e.g., frequent hypoglycemia or hypoglycemia awareness)
  - Absence of disabling advanced diabetic neurovascular complications
  - Insulin-dependent diabetes mellitus
  - Good understanding of the uncertain benefits of a successful pancreatic transplant beyond glycemic control
- Contraindications
  - Coronary artery disease manifested by poorly controlled angina, congestive heart failure, or ejection fraction <50%
  - Peripheral vascular disease manifested by leg ulcers or previous amputation
  - History of alcohol or drug abuse, or mental illness that would interfere with the recipient's ability to participate in a disciplined medical regimen
  - Stenosed or occluded renal veins or arteries
  - Congenital disorders such as hypoplasia, aplasia
  - Hereditary disorders such as Alport's syndrome, polycystic kidney disease, and pyelonephritis
  - Renal cell carcinoma
  - Multiple myeloma
  - Wilms' tumor
  - Hemolytic-uremic syndrome
  - Thrombotic thrombocytopenic purpura
  - HIV infection or AIDS
- Indications for referral
  - Similar to those for single organ transplantation

Pancreas Transplantation[12]

- Indications

- Insulin-dependent diabetes with the following:
  - Serious proteinuria
  - Diminished glomerular filtration rates
  - Evaluation of the patient for kidney transplant
  - Secondary complications more serious than the risks of major surgery and immunosuppression
- Contraindications
  - Metastatic cancer
  - Infection
  - Overwhelming immunosuppressive disease
- Indications for referral
  - Center specific—vary from early treatment of diabetes mellitus to diabetes with proteinuria and/or diminished glomerular filtration rate, diabetes in patients not yet on dialysis, to illness requiring both kidney and pancreas transplantation

Kidney Transplantation[10]

- Indications
  - Glomerulonephritis
    - Henoch-Schönlein purpura
    - Immunoglobulin A nephropathy
    - Focal glomerulosclerosis
    - Anti–glomerular basement membrane disease
    - Mesangiocapillary glomerulonephritis (type 2)
    - Membranous glomerulonephritis
    - Idiopathic and postinfectious crescentic glomerulonephritis
  - Chronic pyelonephritis (reflux nephropathy)
  - Congenital kidney disorders
    - Hypoplasia
    - Horseshoe kidney
  - Hereditary kidney disorders
    - Polycystic kidneys
    - Medullary cystic disease
    - Nephritis (including Alport's syndrome)
    - Tuberous sclerosis

- Metabolic disorders
  - Diabetes mellitus
  - Hyperoxaluria
  - Cystinosis
  - Fabry's disease
  - Amyloid disorders
  - Gout
  - Porphyria
- Toxic nephropathies
  - Analgesic nephropathy
  - Opiate abuse
- Obstructive uropathies
  - Tumors
  - Renal cell carcinoma
  - Incidental carcinoma
  - Wilms' tumor
  - Myeloma
- Trauma with resultant renal vascular disease
- Irreversible acute renal failure
  - Cortical necrosis
  - Acute tubular necrosis
- Irreversible chronic renal failure
- Multisystem disease
  - Progressive systemic sclerosis
  - Systemic lupus erythematosus (inactive)
  - Vasculitis
  - Macroglobulinemia
- Contraindications
  - Due to the increasing success of renal transplantation, there is no absolute contraindication to transplantation for ESRD.[12]
- Relative contraindications
  - Heart disease severe enough to create unacceptable risks during the surgical procedure or immediately postoperative period
  - Age older than 70 years; generally, persons older than 70 years or those who are intolerant of dialysis are considered on a case-by-case basis
  - Malignant disease within the last 5 years and no recurrence within a minimum of 1 year
  - History of noncompliance or psychiatric disease of such magnitude that postoperative compliance will be jeopardized
  - Active liver disease
  - HIV infection or AIDS
  - Obesity over 150% of ideal body weight
  - Unacceptability to the patient of potential complications from immunosuppressive medications
- Indication for referral
  - Ideally referral is prior to initiation of dialysis.

Bone Marrow Transplantation

- Indications
  - There are over 75 different diseases for which bone marrow transplantation is the treatment of choice. The most common are as follows:
    - Malignant disorders
    - Acute lymphocytic leukemia
    - Acute nonlymphocytic leukemia
    - Chronic myelogenous leukemia
    - Preleukemia
    - Hairy cell leukemia
    - Chronic lymphocytic leukemia
    - Hodgkin's and non-Hodgkin's lymphoma
    - Select solid tumors (i.e., breast cancer, lung cancer, testicular and germ cell tumors, neuroblastoma, primary brain tumors, melanoma, ovarian cancer and sarcoma)
    - Nonmalignant disorders (acquired and congenital)
    - Aplastic anemia
    - Severe combined immunodeficiency disorder
    - Myelofibrosis
    - Osteoporosis
    - Hematologic disorders
    - Wiskott-Aldrich syndrome
    - Fanconi's anemia
    - Diamond-Blackfan anemia
    - Cyclic neutropenia
    - Chédiak-Higashi syndrome
    - Chronic granulomatous disease
    - Thalassemia

- Mucopolysaccharide storage diseases
- Lipid storage diseases
- Lysosomal storage diseases
- Bone marrow transplantation is recognized as standard therapy for the diagnosis
- Contraindications
    - Age older than 55 years for allogeneic transplantation and older than 65 years for autologous transplantation
    - Active systemic infection
    - HIV infection or AIDS
    - Psychological disorder
    - Alcohol and drug dependence
    - Life-threatening conditions such as cardiac, renal, or liver failure
- Indications for referral
    - Life-threatening and potentially fatal outcome of the underlying disease
    - Potential cure of an otherwise incurable disease by the delivery of tumor-eradicating doses of chemoradiotherapy and/or reconstitution of diseased (or chemoradiotherapeutically ablated) bone marrow by normal lymphohematopoietic pluripotential stem cells

Small Intestine Transplantation

- Indications
    - Short bowel syndrome
    - Crohn's disease
    - Gardner's syndrome
    - Radiation enteritis
    - Superior mesenteric artery or vein thrombosis
    - Trauma to intestinal vasculature
    - Intestinal atresia
    - Gastroschisis
    - Volvulus
    - Necrotizing enterocolitis
    - Microvillous atrophy
    - Pseudoobstruction
- Contraindications

- Active drug or alcohol dependence
- Life-threatening condition such as cardiac, renal, or liver failure
- HIV infection or AIDS
- Malignancy
- Active infection (sepsis)
- Extensive atherosclerosis
- Advanced neurologic dysfunction
- Severe cardiopulmonary insufficiency
- Lack of need for permanent intravenous nutritional support
- Indications for referral
- Irreversible and chronic intestinal failure
- Inability to receive total parenteral nutrition (TPN)

ANTICIPATED TEACHING

Teaching varies with the organ transplanted and the transplant center. All case management plans, however, must provide for teaching the transplant patient. Education of transplant patients before discharge must cover the following areas, at a minimum:

- The importance of compliance with follow-up laboratory testing and biopsies, and any specific instructions pertinent to the transplant and clinic visits
- The medication regimen, including side effects and contraindications
- The importance of compliance with the regimen for immunosuppressants or antirejection medications
- Methods of coping with the psychological effects of having a transplant and the many lifestyle changes; when and where to seek help and available support groups
- All aspects of infusion, wound care, nasal gastric tube care, and/or other skilled care needs
- Exercise recommendations
- Activity restrictions including postoperative restrictions on activities such as lifting, strenuous exercise,

and sexual intercourse, driving restrictions; and long-term avoidance of activities that may place the organ at risk
- Dietary recommendations and restrictions, and special diets
- The need to maintain body weight within 10% of the ideal for age and height
- Prevention of accelerated graft atherosclerosis
- Methods of preventing infection (e.g., safe sex; good personal hygiene; precautions in gardening, travel, handling of pets; avoidance of persons with an illness)
- Importance of keeping both regular follow-up appointments and the annual posttransplant visit
- Importance of maintaining general health (especially by scheduling regular dental and ophthalmologic appointments and keeping immunizations up to date)
- Birth control and the need to avoid pregnancy (for at least 1 to 1.5 years after successful transplantation)
- Importance of not ignoring changes in condition or body cues and recommendations on when to call the physician. These cues generally include the following:
  - Signs and symptoms of rejection (and, for bone marrow transplant patients, signs and symptoms of graft-versus-host disease [GVHD])
  - Signs and symptoms of infection
  - Signs and symptoms of organ failure
- How and when to contact transplant personnel (routine and emergency)
- Importance of avoiding alcohol, tobacco, illicit drugs, and immunizations with attenuated virus
- Importance of avoiding over-the-counter drugs without physician approval
- Record keeping (indices such as blood pressure, weight, and others as needed)

DISCHARGE AND AFTER-CARE

As the transplant patient's condition stabilizes and the time for discharge approaches, arrangements are made for postacute care either by the center's outpatient transplant clinic or by the patient's own attending physician in his or her local community. The actual arrangements depend on the outcome of the transplant and any complications that may be present, the transplant center's criteria for immediate postoperative care, the patient's place of residence and accessibility to medical care in his or her local community, and the referring physician's willingness to assume responsibility for the care.

Depending on the type of transplant, some patients are required to remain near the transplant center for 2 to 3 months after discharge for close monitoring and care by the transplant staff. For this reason, a home health agency is rarely used to monitor the actual transplant. A home health agency may be required, however, for skilled care needs unrelated to the transplant.

All patients with transplants are at risk of rejection at any time. Consequently, they must take antirejection drugs indefinitely and require frequent blood studies, biopsies, and other tests to measure the toxicity of the drugs and detect symptoms of rejection. All patients require, at a minimum, annual follow-up examinations and tests by the transplant center. Thus, the after-care of a transplant patient is costly, since the cost of antirejection drugs (immunosuppressive agents) alone can exceed $1500/month.

READINESS FOR DISCHARGE

As the time for discharge approaches, the following criteria may assist in identifying which patients are ready for discharge:

All Transplants

- The patient's condition is stable with no signs of deterioration.
- There is no fever or signs of sepsis
- There are no signs of active rejection
- The patient is not receiving intravenous antibiotics or intravenous immunosuppressive medications (occasionally a bone marrow transplant patient may go home while receiving intravenous antibiotics, but this is rare).
- The patient understands the physical signs and symptoms of rejection (this includes GVHD for bone marrow transplant patients), the medication regimen including contraindications and side effects, and the importance of adhering to the schedule of posttransplant follow-up testing.
- Nutritional status is adequate; dietary restrictions are understood; and any nausea and vomiting or diarrhea has been controlled.
- A caregiver is available to assist with routine tasks, because many patients suffer from fatigue and have activity restrictions, at least initially.
- Hematologic, platelet, and other laboratory results are within the desired range.
- The patient is tolerating medication.
- Pain management is adequate.

Heart Transplant

Teaching of the family or caregiver regarding the following has been completed:

- The importance of a salt-restricted diet
- The need for daily monitoring of weight, blood pressure, and pulse rate
- The need to report chest pain to the physician or transplant coordinator immediately

- Specific characteristics of a denervated heart (e.g., need for prolonged warm-up and cool-down periods)

Lung Transplant

Teaching of the family or caregiver regarding the following has been started or completed:

- Home incentive spirometry, oximetry, and pulmonary function testing
- Use of home oxygen if needed
- Avoidance of fluid overload and fluid restriction
- Follow-up pulmonary rehabilitation and endurance exercising

Liver Transplant

Teaching of the family or caregiver regarding the following has been started or completed:

- Feeding tube or TPN line
- T-tube care
- Dressing changes
- Daily weight monitoring

Pancreas Transplant

Teaching of the family or caregiver regarding the following has been started or completed:

- Glucose monitoring
- The prevention of bicarbonate loss
- Urinary catheter care, if necessary (usually removed prior to discharge except when an anastomotic leak is present)
- The need to monitor urinary output and voiding patterns

Kidney Transplant

- No dialysis is necessary.
- There are no signs of acute tubular necrosis.
- The patient is aware of how to:
  - Promote normal urinary elimination patterns and prevent urinary tract infections
  - Monitor urine output and daily weight.

Bone Marrow Transplant

- Platelet transfusions have been discontinued or decreased or can be performed on an outpatient basis.
- Patient is out of protective setting.
- Teaching of the family or caregiver regarding the following has been initiated or completed:
  - The appropriate feeding method (TPN or enteral nutrition)
  - Infusion services, medications, and line care
  - Use of sunscreen lotion
  - Avoidance of crowds and the need to wear a mask in public (must be worn for several months after transplantation)
  - Avoidance of persons with known viral or fungal diseases
  - Recognition of GVHD (allogeneic transplant patients)
  - Recognition of signs and symptoms of other body dysfunctions or complications associated with long-term bone marrow transplantation

Intestine Transplant

- Intestinal graft is adequately functioning and the patient is able to tolerate an oral diet.
- No signs or symptoms of exit-site infection such as redness, warmth, and drainage are present.
- Teaching of the family or caregiver regarding the following has been started or completed:
  - Jejunostomy tube feedings (a jejunostomy tube is often left in place for short-term supportive nutritional therapy)
  - Reporting of intolerance to feedings and/or problems with gastrointestinal dysmotility (50% of cases), such as reflux esophagitis, pyloric spasm, and gastric hypomotility (usually during first 12 weeks).
  - Prevention of chronic diarrhea (medication, low-fat diet).

- Ileostomy care (reversal of the ostomy usually occurs 1 year after the transplantation)

Stomach-Intestine Transplant

Teaching of the family or caregiver regarding the following has been started or completed:

- Prevention of diarrhea
- Reporting of alterations in nutritional status such as the inability to retain fluids or food
- Colostomy care
- TPN and enteral feeds
- The signs and symptoms of pancreatitis

SERVICES REQUIRED FOR DISCHARGE (ALL TRANSPLANTS)

The services required at discharge for transplant patients depend on any transplant complications that may be present and the center's requirements for immediate and ongoing monitoring. Because most transplant patients must reside near the transplant center, however, the conditions that require continuous care or monitoring are generally managed through outpatient services offered by the transplant center. Nevertheless, this is not always true. The following services are commonly required:

- Many liver transplant patients require the services of an extended care facility, subacute care facility, skilled nursing facility, or home health agency for skilled nursing care such as dressing changes, T-tube care, or care of a feeding tube or TPN line until the family, caregiver, or patient has mastered the required techniques.
- Bone marrow transplant patients, if discharged with a TPN line, nasogastric tube, or enteral feeding regimen, require the services of a home health agency for care and continued teaching until the techniques have

been mastered by the patient, family, or caregiver.

- Social worker or psychological counseling or support groups frequently continue after discharge to help the patient and family learn methods of coping with the disease and necessary lifestyle changes.
- In many cases, the new transplantation patient is seen weekly at the transplant center for several weeks after the transplant for testing and evaluation to ensure that the organ is functioning well.
- If the transplant patient is discharged to his or her own community or lives a great distance from the transplant center and transportation costs are a problem, the patient's local attending physician will be required to perform any necessary biopsies and order laboratory studies. The biopsy specimen slides and results of these tests are then transferred to the transplant center for review and recommendations. If the transplant physician makes changes to the treatment regimen, the local attending physician will be the one to implement them. Arrangements must be made by the patient to be seen at least monthly by the transplant team or as often as specified by the team.
- If home health agency services are used, they are likely to be employed not for care and monitoring of the transplant but for care or retraining of other body systems that deteriorated prior to the transplant procedure, or for training in or performance of infusion procedures, TPN feedings, nasogastric tube care, enteral feeding care, or wound care. The home health agency must stay involved until the patient, family, or caregiver has mastered all care techniques. The services most commonly required from a home health agency are:
  - Physical and occupational therapy for strength, mobility, and endurance
  - Skilled nursing care for compliance with medication schedule, other identified specific skilled nursing needs, blood pressure monitoring, infusion services, wound care, or teaching or reinforcement of teaching of diabetic care to patients with new steroid-induced diabetes.

LABORATORY TESTING

For all transplant patients, laboratory tests must be performed once or twice weekly for 4 to 6 weeks after transplantation. Therefore, the case management plan must provide for this. The following list includes the most frequently ordered tests required by transplant patients after discharge:

- Blood urea nitrogen level
- Creatinine clearance
- Blood glucose level
- Complete blood count
- Cyclosporin level, in either serum or whole blood
- Screening chemistry panel
- Platelet count
- Ultrasonography and biopsies
- Blood pressure
- Lipid panel

In addition, weight and blood pressure must be closely followed, and the patient must undergo routine cancer screening, especially for breast, cervical, prostate, colorectal, and skin cancer. Following are additional requirements for specific transplant patients:

- Heart transplant patients require the following:
  - Heart biopsy, performed on a regular basis and at the frequency outlined by the transplant team. Frequency varies according to the

needs of the patient. However, this test is the prime means of monitoring rejection. If the patient is experiencing transplant rejection, the frequency of biopsy will increase.

- Any other tests specific for measuring heart function and signs of rejection, including chest radiography, cardiac catheterization, and electrocardiography.

- Lung transplant patients require the following:
  - Lung biopsy, arterial blood gas measurement, chest radiography, and pulmonary function tests

- Liver transplant patients require the following:
  - Frequent measurement of liver enzyme levels and other tests to measure liver function and signs of rejection

- Pancreas transplant patients require the following:
  - Laboratory monitoring of serum glucose, serum amylase, and lipase levels, plus urinary amylase level; select centers monitor serum anodal trypsinogen and pancreas-specific protein levels.
  - Follow-up biopsies and technetium scans.

- Kidney transplant patients require tests such as the following:
  - Urinalysis, urine cultures, and other tests specific for measuring kidney function and signs of rejection
  - Bone density testing[18]

- Bone marrow transplant patients require tests such as the following:
  - Serologic studies and bone marrow biopsy to measure bone marrow function and detect GVHD disease

- Intestine transplant patients require the following:
  - Ultrasonographic examinations and mucosal biopsy
  - Frequent endoscopic surveillance and intestinal function tests

- Pediatric patients have a higher incidence of graft thrombosis and will need must be followed more closely; they also need ongoing assessments of growth and development.[19]

EQUIPMENT COMMONLY ORDERED

Durable medical equipment is rarely needed for transplant patients. If it is required, however, the case management plan must identify what is necessary and where it will be obtained. If equipment is needed, it is often for disabilities that occurred prior to the transplantation or for postoperative complications. Commonly required equipment includes the following:

- All kidney-pancreas transplant patients require a glucose monitor and supplies if these were not purchased prior to the transplant.
- Any transplant patient discharged home while still receiving intravenous or enteral feedings requires the appropriate supplies and solutions as well as dressings for care of the site.
- Many liver transplant patients require dressings and related supplies for care of the abdominal wound.

MOST COMMON COMPLICATIONS

As preparations for discharge continue, the transplant team's teaching plan generally covers complications and how to deal with them. All patients must know what to do when the following occur:

- They have a fever of >100.5°F (38.5°C).
- Their nutritional status is altered or they are unable to keep down food, fluids, or medications.

- Their hematologic status is altered, as evidenced by the results of laboratory studies.
- Their liver function test results are elevated.
- They experience pain and tenderness over the transplant site (except in bone marrow transplant patients).
- An infection occurs (colds, pneumonia, wound infection).
- Cyclosporin toxicity or antirejection drug toxicity or reactions occur.
- An outbreak of shingles, herpes infection, or Epstein-Barr virus infection occurs.

In addition, although patient education varies depending on the organ transplanted, it must include what to do and whom to call when complications occur. The following lists for each type of transplant describe the specific topics that must be covered:

- Liver transplant
  - Nephrotoxicity and renal dysfunction
  - Neurotoxicity
  - Posttransplant lymphoproliferative disease
  - Hypertension
  - Hyperglycemia
  - Weight gain
  - Hypercholesterolemia
  - Gout
  - Signs and symptoms of aplastic anemia
- Heart transplant
  - Fluid overload
  - Arrhythmias other than those commonly associated with a heart transplant
  - Weight gain beyond desired limit
  - Hypertension
  - Obesity and hyperlipidemia
  - Gastrointestinal complications
  - Accelerated transplant coronary artery disease
  - Renal disease
  - Graft vasculopathy

- Lung transplant
  - Fluid overload
  - Weight gain beyond desired limit
  - Obliterate bronchiolitis
  - Drops in peak expiratory flow measures
- Pancreas transplant
  - Hematuria and cystitis
  - Bladder leak and metabolic complications of bladder drainage
  - Pancreatitis
  - Metabolic complications
  - Graft thrombosis
  - Lymphoproliferative disorders
- Kidney transplant
  - Weight gain beyond desired limit (3 kg)
  - Decreased urine output
- Bone marrow transplant
  - Diarrhea of >1 L/24 hr
  - Oral infections and candidiasis
  - Skin pigmentation changes
  - Dryness of mouth, eyes, vagina
  - Soreness, redness, or blisters of fingers and toes due to chemotherapy toxicity
  - Fungal infections
- Intestine transplant
  - Gastrointestinal dysmotility, including reflux esophagitis, pyloric spasm, and gastric hypomotility
  - Chronic diarrhea
  - Hemorrhage, thrombosis, and intestinal and biliary leaks
  - GVHD (rare)
- Stomach-intestine transplantation
  - Diarrhea
  - Alterations in nutritional status and inability to retain fluids or food
  - Pancreatitis

BARRIERS TO DISCHARGE OR ACCESS TO CARE

Barriers to discharge of a transplant patient vary with the particular patient. Also, postoperative complications and the complexity of care required to manage such complications present additional barriers to locating appropriate care resources. Typical barriers associated with the discharge of transplant patients include the following:

- Lack of a caregiver
- Limited or nonexistent access to required resources
- Unavailability of a local physician
- Inadequate home conditions (e.g., water, heat, and cleanliness)
- Lack of or inadequate transportation for follow-up care
- Uneducability of the patient, caregiver, or family

SUMMARY

Because transplant care both before and after surgery is costly and very complex, it is important for case managers to follow this category of patients. The services offered by a case manager are varied but often include linkage of the patient to the following:

- The appropriate transplant center within the payer's network
- Alternate funding sources (e.g., Medicaid, or if a child, the state's children's medical services program) to assist in payment of any out-of-pocket expenses for housing, transportation, and medications
- Psychologic or peer support groups for the patient and family
- The appropriate pharmacy for ongoing medications; this often means a mail-order pharmacy, from which a greater supply of medication can be obtained for a reduced out-of-pocket cost

Because financial hardships are a reality for transplant patients, the case manager must work closely with the patient and family to ensure that they are linked to any disability or other income programs offered by the state, by an employer, or through a privately paid disability policy. Depending on the patient's work history and the permanency of the disability, application for Social Security Disability Income might also be warranted.

All transplant patients have their own set of criteria for eligibility for candidacy as well as their own preoperative and postoperative requirements, services, and needs. As such, coordination and excellent communication between at least the transplant center and payer case manager are critical if gaps or duplications in care or services or payment are to be avoided.

Chapter Exercises

Case study: Ms. Wallace is a 48-year-old registered nurse with pulmonary hypertension in need of a heart-lung transplant. She is a single parent with two children, aged 17 and 18 years, who still live at home. Her physician has referred her case to the university transplant center, 200 miles away.

1. As the primary payer case manager, describe your role in preparing Ms. Wallace for her initial evaluation. Make sure to include all aspects of care.
2. Ms. Wallace has asked you for assistance in researching the outcomes of a heart-lung transplant and the outcomes obtained by the university transplant center. To what references could you refer her? Your list should include at least five specific websites or references.
3. Ms. Wallace has limited financial resources and is unable to work. As the primary payer case manager, describe how you will assist Ms. Wallace in dealing with her financial situation.

Suggested Websites and Resources

Education, Transplant-Related Organizations, Resources, and Government and Private Agencies

www.aircareall.org—Air Care Alliance

www.airlifeline.org or 800-446-1231—AirLife Line

www.aap.org—American Academy of Pediatrics

www.aapa.org—American Academy of Physician Assistants

www.aasld.org—American Association for the Study of Liver Diseases

www.aacvpr.org—American Association of Cardiovascular and Pulmonary Rehabilitation

www.aacn.org—American Association of Critical-Care Nurses

www.aadenet.org—American Association of Diabetes Educators

www.aakp.org—American Association of Kidney Patients

www.aans.org—American Association of Neurological Surgeons

www.aatb.org—American Association of Tissue Banks

800-726-2824—American Bone Marrow Donor Registry

www.cancer.org—American Cancer Society

919-932-7845—American Center for Transplant Resources

www.acc.org—American College of Cardiology

www.acg.gi.org—American College of Gastroenterology

www.facs.org—American College of Surgeons

www.diabetes.org—American Diabetes Association

www.eatright.org—American Dietetic Association

www.americanheart.org—American Heart Association

www.aha.org—American Hospital Association

www.ajn.org—American Journal of Nursing: top sites for nursing

www.akfinc.org—American Kidney Fund

www.liverfoundation.org—American Liver Foundation

www.lungusa.org—American Lung Association

www.ama-assn.org—American Medical Association

anna.inurse.com/—American Nephrology Nurses' Association

www.a-o-t-a.org—American Organ Transplant Association

www.aphanet.org—American Pharmaceutical Association

www.apprx.com—American Preferred Prescription, Inc.

www.redcross.org or 207-728-6401—American Red Cross

www.web742d8.ntx.net/—American Share Foundation

www.asaio.com—American Society for Artificial Internal Organs

www.asbmt.org—American Society for Blood and Marrow Transplantation

ashiamp@aol.com—American Society for Histocompatibility & Immunogenetics

www.amsect.org—American Society of Extra-Corporeal Technology

www.ash-us.org—American Society of Hypertension

314-991-1661—American Society of Minority Health and Transplant Professionals

www.asn-online.org—American Society of Nephrology

www.a-s-t.org—American Society of Transplantation (formerly American Society of Transplant Physicians)

www.thoracic.org—American Thoracic Society

www.amtrauma.org—American Trauma Society

www.auanet.org—American Urological Association

www.angel-flight.org or 703-365-7357—Angel Flight

www.aosw.org—Association of Oncology Social Work

www.aopo.org—Association of Organ Procurement Organizations

www.rehabnurse.org—Association of Rehabilitation Nurses

www.ast.org—Association of Surgical Technologists

BADFDN@aol.com—Barbara Anne DeBoer Foundation

www.beincharge.com—Be in Charge Program, Schering Corp.

www.bmtinfonet.org—Blood & Marrow Transplant Information Network

www.bonemarrow.org—Bone Marrow Foundation

www.liver.ca—Canadian Liver Foundation

www.cma.ca/cma/common/linkNavigate.do? skin=130—*Canadian Medical Association (CMA)*

www.cancercare.org—Cancer Care, Inc.

www.fda.gov/oashi/cancer/cancer.html— Cancer Liaison Program of the U.S. Food and Drug Administration

800-227-2732—Cancer Research Foundation of America

www.cdc.gov—Centers for Disease Control and Prevention (CDC)

www.phppo.cdc.gov/CDCRecommends/— Wonder Prevention Guidelines

305-547-5787—Center for Liver Diseases

www.centerwatch.com—Center Watch Clinical Trials Listings Service

www.cche.net/principles—Centre for Health Evidence: evidence-based practice

www.york.ac.uk/inst/crd/srinfo.htm—Centre for Reviews and Dissemination: systematic reviews

www.livertx.org—Children's Liver Alliance

www.classkids.org—Children's Liver Association for Support Services

www.cota.org—Children's Organ Transplant Association

www.tricare.osd.mil/beneficiary—TRICARE

www.shareyourlife.org—Coalition on Donation

www.cochrane.org/cochrane/newreviews.htm —Cochrane Library (Cochrane reviews)

800-445-1525—Communicating for Agriculture

914-328-1313—Corporate Angel Network

202-205-0396—Department of Health and Human Services

www.va.gov—Department of Veterans Affairs

www.hrsa.dhhs.gov/ops/dot/—Division of Transplantation (U.S. Health Resources and Services Administration)

www.herts.ac.uk/lis/subjects/health/ebm.htm —Evidence-based medicine

www.healthatoz.com—Health A to Z: health information

www.healthgate.com—HealthGate

www.hiaa.org—Health Insurance Association of America

www.text.nlm.nih.gov—Health Services/Technology Assessment Texts

www.hepc-connection.org—Hepatitis C Connection

www.hepfi.org—Hepatitis Foundation International

www.hepnet.com—HepNet: The hepatitis Information Network

www.insulin-free.org—Insulin-Free World Foundation

202-622-4695—Internal Revenue Service

www.umn.edu/~iptr—International Bone Marrow Transplant Registry

www.ishlt.org—International Society for Heart and Lung Transplantation

www.itns.org—International Transplant Nurses Society

www.jcaho.org—Joint Commission on Accreditation of Healthcare Organizations

www.jdfcure.com—Juvenile Diabetes Foundation International

800-893-1995—Kidney Transplant Patient Partnering Program

www.leukemia-research.org—Leukemia Research Foundation

800-955-4572—Leukemia Society of America

www.leukemia-lymphoma.org—Leukemia and Lymphoma Society

www.stadtlander.com or 800-238-7828—
  LifeTimes (Stadtlanders Pharmacy)
www.livingbank.org—Living Bank
www.Lymphoma.org—Lymphoma Research
  Foundation of America
www.mdchoice.com—MDChoice
www.themarrowfoundation.org—Marrow
  Foundation
800-638-6833—Medicare Hotline
www.medicinenet.com—MedicineNet
www.ncbi.nlm.nih.gov/entrez/query.fcgi—
  MEDLINE (for professionals)
www.nlm.nih.gov/medlineplus—
  MEDLINEplus (for consumers)
www.medweb.emory.edu/MedWeb—
  MedWeb at Emory University
*www.medwebplus.com/subject/Practice_Guide
  lines.html*—MedWebPlus
www.mercymedical.org or 800-296-1191—
  Mercy Medical Airlift
800-296-1217—Mercy Medical Airlift's
  National Patient Air Transport
  Helpline
*www.gla.ac.uk/departments/surgerywestern/
  transplant/ethnic.html* and
  *www.lifesharing.org/minority_communities.
  html*—Minority Organ/Tissue
  Transplant Education Program
www.miracleflights.org—Miracle Flights for
  Kids
416-222-6335—Mission Air
  Transportation Network
909-794-1151—Mission Aviation
  Fellowship
www.multiplemyeloma.org—Multiple
  Myeloma Research Foundation
www.nahhh.org and 800-542-9730—
  National Association of Hospital
  Hospitality Houses
www.napnap.org—National Association of
  Pediatric Nurse Associates and
  Practitioners
www.naswdc.org—National Association of
  Social Workers
800-627-7692—National Bone Marrow
  Transplant Link
www.ndri.com—National Disease Research
  Interchange

www.nci.nih.gov—National Cancer
  Institute
213-736-1455—National Cancer Institute
  Cancer Legal Resource Center
www.children-cancer.com—National
  Children's Cancer Society
www.kidney.org—National Donor Family
  Council
www.transplants.org—National Foundation
  for Transplants
www.guidelines.gov/index.asp—National
  Guideline Clearinghouse
www.nih.gov/health/—National Heart,
  Lung and Blood Institute, National
  Institutes of Health
www.nationalhlafund.org—National HLA
  Fund, Inc.
800-942-4242—National Insurance
  Consumer Hotline
www.nih.gov—National Institutes of
  Health
www.nih.gov/ninr—National Institute of
  Nursing Research, National Institutes of
  Health
www.kidney.org—National Kidney
  Foundation, Inc.
www.childrensleukemia.org—National
  Leukemia Research Association
800-654-1247—National Marrow Donor
  Program
202-865-4888—National Minority Organ
  and Tissue Transplant Education
  Program
www.rarediseases.org—National
  Organization for Rare Disorders
800-733-7345—National Organization
  for State Kidney Programs
www.nosscr.org—National Organization of
  Social Security Claimants'
  Representatives
www.npath.org or 800-296-1217—
  National Patient Air Transport
  Helpline
www.transplantfund.org—National
  Transplant Assistance Fund
www.ebmny.org—New York Academy of
  Medicine Evidence-Based Medicine
  Resource Center

904-798-8999—Nielsen Organ Transplant Foundation

713-790-3275—North American Society for Dialysis and Transplantation

www.applmeapro.com/natco—North American Transplant Coordinators Organization

www.nurseweek.com—Nurseweek

www.nursingworld.org—Nursing World

888-999-6743 (in the United States) or 612-627-8140 (outside the United States)—Office of Patient Advocacy

www.ons.org—Oncology Nursing Society

www.transweb.org/partnership—Partnership for Organ Donation

www.patientadvocate.org—Patient Advocate Foundation

202-219-8776 or 202-219-7222—Pension and Welfare Benefits Administration

www.needymeds.com—Pharmaceutical Patient Assistance Programs

www.pharmacyandyou.org—Pharmacy and You

www.pharminfo.com—PharmInfoNet

301-443-1886—Public Health Service

www.phassociation.org—Pulmonary Hypertension Association

312-836-7100—Ronald McDonald Houses

www.sangstat.com—SangStat Medical Corporation

www.sheffield.ac.uk/~scharr/ir/netting—ScHARR Netting the Evidence

www.2ndwind.org—Second Wind Lung Transplant Association

800-772-1213—Social Security Administration

www.sccm.org—Society for Critical Care Medicine

www.seopf.org—South-Eastern Organ Procurement Foundation

www.stadtlander.com—Stadtlanders Pharmacy

www.tppp.net—Transplant Patient Partnering Program (Roche)

www.primenet.com/~trio—Transplant Recipients International Organization

www.transweb.org—Transweb

800-638-2610—TRICARE

www.unos.org—United Network for Organ Sharing

800-892-2757, ext. 285—United Way/Delta SkyWish Program

202-219-8776—U.S. Department of Labor (nonpublic employment coverage)

www.house.gov—U.S. House of Representatives

www.senate.gov—U.S. Senate

www.4women.gov—Women's Health Resources

www.wctf.org—World Children's Transplant Fund

Drug Company Subsidies

www.rxassist.org/default.cfm—Volunteers in Health, a national program sponsored by the Robert Wood Johnson Foundation

www.rxhope.com/—Pharmacy program sponsored by PhRMA

www.needymeds.com/—Information website that links to pharmaceutical companies that have patient assistance programs for pharmaceuticals

State Pharmaceutical Assistance Programs

www.rxassist.org/pdfs/state_programs.pdf—Links to the states that offer free drug programs and lists the contact phone numbers and additional information

REFERENCES

1. Health Care Financing Administration: *Public use files on transplantation*, Washington, DC, 2001, The Administration.
2. Niklason LE, Langer R: Prospects for organ and tissue replacement, *JAMA* 285:573-576, 2001.
3. Trzepacz P, Dimartini A, editors: *The transplant patient: biological, psychiatric, and ethical issues in organ transplantation*, Cambridge, 2000, Cambridge University Press.
4. Hayry P: Chronic rejection: risk factors, regulation, and possible sites of therapeutic intervention, *Transplant Proc* 30:2407-2410, 1998.
5. Ambrosino G, Varotto S, Basso S et al: Hepatocyte transplantation: an experimental study to treat acute liver failure in pigs, *Transplant Proc* 33:62-65, 2001.
6. Barr ML: Photopheresis in transplantation: future research and directions, *Transplant Proc* 30:2248-2250, 1998.

7. Miyashita T, Enosawa S, Suzuki S et al: Development of a bioartificial liver with glutamine synthetase-transduced recombinant human hepatoblastoma cell line, HepG2, *Transplant Proc* 32:2355-2358, 2000.

8. Petersen P, Lembert N, Wesche J et al: Improved diffusion properties of a new polysulfone membrane for the development of a bioartificial pancreas, *Transplant Proc* 33:1952-1953, 2001.

9. Abouna GM, Ganguly P, Jabur S et al: Successful ex vivo liver perfusion system for hepatic failure pending liver regeneration or liver transplantation, *Transplant Proc* 33:1962-1964, 2001.

10. Steinman TI, Becker BN, Frost AE et al: Guidelines for the referral and management of patients eligible for solid organ transplantation, *Transplantation* 71(9):1189-1204, 2001.

11. Avery RK, Ljungman P: Prophylactic measures in the solid-organ recipient before transplantation, *Clin Infect Dis* 33(suppl):S15-21, 2001.

12. Ginns LC, Cosimi AB, Morris PJ: *Transplantation*, Malden, Mass, 1999, Blackwell Science.

13. Evans RW: Public and private insurer designation of transplantation programs, *Transplantation* 53(5):1041-1046, 1992.

14. Coulter CH, Fabius R, Hecksher V et al: Assessing HMO centers of excellence programs: one employer's experience, *Manag Care Q* 6(1):8-15, 1998.

15. Nolan MT, Augustine SM: *Transplantation nursing: acute and long-term management*, Norwalk, Conn, 1995, Appleton & Lange.

16. Arumugam R, Soriano HE, Scheimann AO et al: Liver transplantation in children for metabolic diseases, *Transplant Proc* 30:1993-1994, 1998.

17. Sutherland DER, Gruessner AC, Gruessner RWG: Pancreas transplantation: a review, *Transplant Proc* 30:1940-1943, 1998.

18. Loertscher R: Management issues in renal transplantation, *Transplant Proc* 30:1723-1725, 1998.

19. Harmon W: Pediatric organ transplantation, *Transplant Proc* 30:1952-1955, 1998.

CHAPTER

17

Case Management of the Mentally Ill Patient

Peggy A. Rossi, BSN, MPA, CCM, CPUR

OBJECTIVES

- To identify at least four reasons why mental health case management has been slow to evolve
- To describe the basic provisions of the Mental Health Parity Act (MHPA), to discuss its impact on mental health services, and to determine whether the reader's or the patient's state has a mental health parity law and, if not, what plans the state has to develop such a law
- To define the members of the treatment team as well as the most common treatment modalities and sites of care

Psychiatric case management has existed since the end of World War II, and in fact community psychiatric case management was the first documented model for case management. Psychiatric and mental health case management, however, has been slow to evolve and to match medical models. This slowness can be attributed to two primary causes: the models historically have not taken an outcomes-based approach, and many mental health care practitioners have viewed the case manager's role to be planning discharge and connecting the patient with community resources. Nevertheless, many newer models do focus on outcomes. This diversity of views of psychiatric case management has essentially made case management for mental health a meaningless term with no universally accepted definition. Here, we define mental health case management as any systematic program that coordinates individual patient care throughout the organizationally defined continuum of services and settings. Thus many mental health case management models include management of only acute-care services or only outpatient services, while others concentrate on management of community-based services. The primary focus of all models has been to minimize fragmentation, and even today, most psychiatric case management services are limited in scope to the services provided by a given health care organization.[1]

Smith, in his article "Shifting Gears: Moving to the Next Level of Psychiatric Disease Management," declares that a disease management approach is the best model for psychiatric case management. One must agree with his assessment, because, given the limited range of services covered by many organizations and their case management models, fragmentation continues, and no single individual is held accountable for the entire continuum of care. However, for case management to be successful in managing quality and costs, case managers must be given the authority and accountability for the entire continuum of care. In the end, mental health disease management has become the model that meets the foregoing requirements because it focuses on chronic mental illness and manages that illness based on predetermined quality and cost outcomes.[1]

As one looks at mental health and the need for a case management or disease management model, one must understand the implications of the following statistics with regard to the demand for mental health services. One must also understand that case management is needed for many of the more seriously ill and that case management, when offered, must not be confined merely to acute episodes of care or acute-care services.

- More than 54 million Americans have a mental disorder in any given year, although fewer than 8 million seek treatment.
- Depression and anxiety disorders—the two most common mental illnesses—each affect 19 million American adults annually.
- Approximately 12 million women in the United States experience depression every year—roughly twice the number of men.
- One percent of the population (more than 2.5 million Americans) has schizophrenia.
- Bipolar disorder, also known as manic-depressive illness, affects more than 2 million Americans.
- Each year, eating disorders such as anorexia nervosa and bulimia nervosa affect millions of Americans, 85% to 90% of whom are teens or young adult women.
- Depression greatly increases the risk of developing heart disease. People with depression are four times more likely to have a heart attack than those with no history of depression.
- Approximately 15% of all adults who have a mental illness in any given year also experience a co-occurring substance abuse disorder that complicates treatment.
- Up to one half of all visits to primary care physicians are due to conditions that are caused or exacerbated by mental or emotional problems.
- White adults who have either depression or an anxiety disorder are more likely to receive treatment than African American adults with the same disorders, even though the disorders occur in both groups at about the same rate when socioeconomic factors are taken into account.
- The rate of illicit drug use is 10.6% among Native Americans, 7.7% among African Americans, 6.8% among Hispanic Americans (all races), 6.6% among whites, and 3.2% among Asian Americans.
- About twice as many African Americans as whites were without health insurance in 1998 and 1999 .
- More than half of all African Americans and Native Americans are anticipated to use public insurance to pay for inpatient mental health treatment, compared to 34% of whites.
- Misdiagnosis and inadequate treatment often occur in minority communities. Factors that can contribute include a general mistrust of medical health professionals, cultural barriers, co-occurrence of other disorders, socioeconomic factors, and primary reliance on family and the religious community during times of distress.

- One in five children has a diagnosable mental, emotional, or behavioral disorder. Up to 1 in 10 may suffer from a serious emotional disturbance. Seventy percent of children with these disorders, however, do not receive mental health services.
- Attention deficit hyperactivity disorder is one of the most common mental disorders in children, affecting 3% to 5% of school-age children.
- As many as 1 in every 33 children and 1 in 8 adolescents may have depression.
- Once a child experiences an episode of depression, he or she is at risk of having another episode within the next 5 years.
- Teenage girls are more likely to develop depression than teenage boys.
- Children and teens who have a chronic illness, endure abuse or neglect, or experience other trauma have an increased risk of depression.
- Suicide is the third leading cause of death for 15- to 24-year-olds and the sixth leading cause of death for 5- to 14-year-olds. The number of attempted suicides is even higher.
- Studies have confirmed the short-term efficacy and safety of treatments for depression in youth.
- Alcohol, marijuana, inhalants, and club drugs are the most frequently used drugs among middle-school and high-school youth.
- Research has shown that the use of club drugs such as ecstasy and GHB (γ-hydroxybutyrate) can cause serious health problems and, in some cases, death. Used in combination with alcohol, these drugs pose even more danger.
- Children and adolescents increasingly believe that regular alcohol and drug use is not dangerous.
- Among middle-school and high-school students, fewer than 20% of young people between the ages of 12 and 17 report using alcohol in the previous month, and fewer than 4% report drinking heavily in the previous month.
- Young people are beginning to drink at younger ages. This is troubling, particularly because young people who begin drinking or using drugs before age 15 are four times more likely to become addicted than those who begin at age 21.
- Children of alcohol- and drug-addicted parents are up to four times more likely to develop substance abuse and mental health problems than other children.
- Twenty percent of youths in juvenile justice facilities have a serious emotional disturbance and most have a diagnosable mental disorder. Up to an additional 30% of youth in these facilities have substance abuse disorders or substance abuse disorders co-occurring with other disorders.
- Late-life depression affects about 6 million adults, but only 10% ever receive treatment.
- Older Americans are more likely to commit suicide than any other age group. Although they constitute only 13% of the U.S. population, individuals age 65 and older account for 20% of all suicides.
- At least 10% to 20% of widows and widowers develop clinically significant depression within 1 year of their spouse's death.
- Among adults age 55 and older, 11.4% meet the criteria for having an anxiety disorder.
- Alcohol abuse and dependence are four times as prevalent among men older than age 65 years than among women in the same age group.[2]

OVERVIEW

Because mental health is a specialty in itself, mental health case management (like pediatric and geriatric case management) should be performed by persons who specialize in the field. In reality, however, many case management organizations do not have separate mental health and medical case management programs. Therefore, this chapter is included as a means of assisting case managers who must assume a dual role. It also aims at educating case managers and senior management regarding the complexities associated with mental health case management and the reason this type of case management should be provided by qualified mental health professionals.

Although medical case management has existed for years, mental health case management as it is known today has been slower to evolve. As the venue for providing mental health care continues to shift, however, and as treatment modalities change from traditional inpatient care, physician office visits, and group therapy to other forms of outpatient care, so must the focus of mental health case management.

Due to the complexity of mental health, long gone are the days when "mental health case management" consisted merely of nurses' monitoring and limiting days of service through the utilization review or retrospective review of acute-care services, or social workers' linking mentally ill persons with basic resources. Why, then, has nursing case management taken so long to arrive in the mental health arena? The answers are many and varied. The reasons cited by Smith[1] and the other most obvious reasons are the following:

- For the most part, health care payers provided very few if any mental health benefits, and once the person exhausted his or her lifetime bene-

fits, care was shifted to the public payer—Medicaid. Medicaid was either unwilling or unable to invest the necessary resources to care adequately for the person.
- Psychiatry was exempt from the diagnosis-related group (DRG) payment system, or more commonly termed *DRG exempt*, so little scrutiny was applied to length of stay or treatment decisions.
- Insurance reimbursement methods provided little incentive for the provider to consider cost-effective alternatives or other forms of reimbursement.
- Like their counterparts in the medical-surgical arena, mental health providers have been reluctant to change from their traditional methods of providing care because the "new" ways are not consistent with their practice patterns, philosophies, or professional experience.
- Although deinstitutionalization occurred in the 1970s, alternatives to inpatient care have been slow to materialize.
- Many psychiatric mental health professionals have not believed that critical pathways are appropriate for use with the psychiatric population because of the psychiatric client's unique and varying needs and responses to treatment.

Also, during the past decade, new challenges to the mental health system have emphasized the fact that we have more persons in need of mental health care and that access to care has not always been ideal. When patients need care, someone must be able to serve as an advocate and assist these patients in gaining access to the services to which they are entitled. Other reasons for the changes seen in mental health care include the following:

- The erosion of family and social support systems

- Fragmentation and lack of resources due to budgetary cuts for many community programs or resources
- Destigmatization of mental illness, which allows more persons to recognize and accept mental health care
- Increased complexities and stresses of life and society in general, which have led to increased mental health symptoms and chemical dependency
- Advances in medication and psychologic therapeutic techniques and, thus, in the ability to treat more disorders effectively

Because mental illness is complex and many patients are chronically disabled (either by the dysfunction itself or because they have been unable to gain access to treatment), case managers assigned to mental health must be specialists in their field, and a primary goal must be to minimize fragmentation of services. Mental health case managers must have the following, at a minimum:

- Clinical knowledge of diagnoses and of applicable treatment modalities and options, as well as clinical interventions and medication management specific to the mental health disorder; this also includes the ability to assess the client's previous and current levels of physical and psychosocial functioning, symptoms, coping abilities, and support systems.
- A knowledge of community resources, services, and providers that can best serve the patient given the limited or nonexistent health care coverage, as well as the ability to play a coordinating role and ensure appropriate utilization of resources.
- The skills and expertise to serve as a discharge planner or teacher.
- The skills and expertise to assume responsibility for quality and cost outcomes and to establish clear,

measurable, and realistic outcome measures.
- A broad knowledge of patients' rights, confidentiality laws, and other mandates (e.g., Health Insurance Portability and Accountability Act, federal Privacy Act, the Comprehensive Alcohol Abuse Prevention, Treatment and Rehabilitation Act, and the Americans with Disabilities Act).

Case managers must be keenly aware of the requirements imposed by the acts mentioned earlier, since mental health information pertinent to the patient is closely regulated by these acts. Case managers must also possess a knowledge of the acts that are specific and pertinent to the release of information and the type of information protected by these acts, as well as knowledge of recent cases resulting in legal awards and outcomes that can affect the practice of mental health. One such case is that involving a man who was ridiculed at work because he had a neurologic disorder (*Lanni v New Jersey Department of Environmental Protection*). In this case, violations of the provisions of both the Americans with Disabilities Act and New Jersey's Law Against Discrimination were found. In his lawsuit, Philip Lanni alleged that he was constantly ridiculed for his neurologic impairments, which included dyslexia, during his 5-year tenure as a radio dispatcher for the New Jersey Department of Environmental Protection's Division of Fish and Wildlife. In this case, both the state and Lanni's two supervisors were found liable, and an award was made to Lanni.[3]

As mental health case managers develop their case management plans, they must focus on outcomes if the plan is to assure cost-effective, high-quality care. To accomplish this, they must identify clinical outcomes in the initial stages of development of the case management plan, because these outcomes drive the clinical processes, rather than the resources driving the outcomes. One primary way to ensure that this process occurs is to identify and set clear and measurable outcomes on the front end of care. The use of an outcomes-focused framework with valid and reliable measures will ensure the benchmarking of services and quality care across the continuum.[1] The continuum-of-care outcome measures include the following:

- Acute-care hospitalizations (includes assessments, stabilization, symptom management, and discharge planning)
  - *The outcomes measure must be symptom specific.*
- Home health care (includes connection to community resources, continued improvement in quality of life, and the practice and validation of coping skills)
  - *The outcomes measure must focus on quality of life and goal attainment.*
- Partial hospitalization or outpatient care (includes symptom management, coping skills development, psychoeducational processes, and crisis intervention and prevention)
  - *The outcomes measure must focus on a life skills profile.*
- Outpatient ambulatory care (includes issue-focused and specialty-oriented processes to develop and validate coping strategies, and relapse prevention)
  - *The outcomes measure must focus on the psychiatric outcome and functional assessment.*
- Continued community care (includes mental health promotion, mental illness prevention, and maintenance of stabilization)
  - *The outcomes measure must focus on functional skills and global clinical improvement.*[1]

DIAGNOSTIC FLAGS

What is mental illness? It is a disease that causes mild to severe disturbances in thinking, perception, and behavior. Unfortunately, if these disturbances significantly impair a person's ability to cope with life's ordinary demands and routines, then he or she must be directed to seek proper treatment by a mental health professional. Mental health professionals believe that many mental illnesses have biologic causes, just as do cancer, diabetes, and heart disease, whereas many other mental disorders are caused by a person's environment and experiences. Mental illness can be divided into five major categories:

1. **Anxiety disorders**—These are the most common mental illnesses. The three main types are phobias, panic disorders, and obsessive-compulsive disorders.
2. **Mood disorders**—These include depression and bipolar disorder (or manic-depressive disorder). Symptoms may include mood swings such as extreme sadness or elation, sleep and eating disturbances, and changes in activity and energy levels. Suicide may be a risk with these disorders.
3. **Schizophrenia**—This is a serious disorder that affects how a person thinks, feels, and acts. Schizophrenia is believed to be caused by chemical imbalances in the brain that produce a variety of symptoms, including hallucinations, delusions, withdrawal, incoherent speech, and impaired reasoning.
4. **Dementias**—These include diseases like Alzheimer's, which leads to loss of mental functions, memory loss, and a decline in intellectual and physical skills.
5. **Eating disorders**—These include disorders such as anorexia nervosa and bulimia nervosa, which are serious, potentially life-threatening illnesses.

As in medical case management, lengthy inpatient stays and diagnostic flags are not always the only criteria one uses to select a mentally ill patient for case management. Certainly flags are useful, but in cases appropriate for mental health case management the diagnoses and need for services are intertwined with other influences such as age, behavior patterns, family dynamics, past medical or mental health history, adequacy of the original treatment plan, compliance with the treatment plan, standards of care, availability of resources, and financial capabilities or availability of alternate funding programs. All of these variables may influence case selection. Nevertheless, the following diagnoses are frequently associated with mental health case management:

- Adolescent adjustment reaction
- Manic-depressive (bipolar) disorder
- Schizophrenia
- Sexual abuse
- Chemical dependency
- Major depression
- Dual diagnoses
- Dissociative identity disorder

The symptoms commonly associated with these diagnoses are also intertwined with case variables, and these symptoms may be the reason for a referral and not the actual diagnosis. Common symptoms associated with the many psychiatric diagnoses may include the following:

- Inability to perform from day to day in any capacity or role, or to conduct the normal activities of daily living
- Disruptive behavior and agitation
- Immobilizing symptoms
- Anxiety, panic reactions, or agitation
- Impulsive or overaggressive behavior
- Impaired sense of reality caused by hallucinations, delusions, or paranoia
- Vegetative symptoms of depression
- Parasuicidal, self-destructive behavior
- Homicidal tendencies
- Inability to interact with others
- Defiant behavior
- Explosive behavior

MENTAL HEALTH CARE PROFESSIONALS AND PROGRAMS

Specialized managed mental health care and substance abuse treatment are rooted in four key approaches to clinical treatment: use of alternatives to psychiatric hospitalization, use of alternatives to restrictive treatment for substance abuse, goal-directed psychotherapy, and crisis intervention.[4] Treatment of the symptoms or overall disorder is provided by any combination of providers and programs. If mental health case management is offered, it must include the following four components:

1. A mechanism to promote correct diagnosis and treatment
2. The ability to promote efficient use of resources
3. Mechanisms to prevent recidivism
4. Monitoring for and preventing substandard care

Traditional Types of Treatment

The following are treatment techniques that may be used with any one of the foregoing approaches:

- **Psychotherapy**—This is a method of treatment that involves talking face to face with a therapist to resolve issues.
- **Behavior therapy**—This is a treatment that focuses on stress management, biofeedback, and relaxation training to change thinking patterns and behavior.
- **Psychoanalysis**—In this technique long-term treatment is used to identify unconscious motivations and early patterns to resolve issues and make the patient aware of how those motivations influence present actions and feelings.
- **Cognitive therapy**—This type of treatment seeks to identify and

correct thinking patterns that can lead to troublesome feelings and behavior.

- **Family therapy**—This modality includes discussion and problem-solving sessions with every member of the family.
- **Movement, art, or music therapy**—This method of treatment includes the use of movement, art, or music to express emotions and is very effective for persons who cannot otherwise express feelings.
- **Group therapy**—This is a common treatment modality in which a small group of people, with the guidance of a trained therapist, meet to discuss individual issues and help each other with problems.
- **Pharmacotherapy**—This is a common treatment modality that is beneficial to some persons with mental or emotional disorders. Unfortunately, while medication should be taken in the prescribed dosage and at prescribed intervals, and adherence to this regimen should be monitored daily, this does not always occur. Thus, medication management programs often must be included in the overall treatment plan.
- **Electroshock therapy**—This modality is used to treat some cases of major depression, delusions, and hallucinations, or life-threatening sleeping and eating disorders that cannot be treated effectively with drugs and/or psychotherapy.

Traditional Mental Health Professionals and Facilities

Typically, the health care professionals who provide mental health care include the following:

- **Psychiatrist**—This is a medical doctor who has special training in the diagnosis and treatment of mental and emotional illnesses and who is qualified to prescribe medication.
- **Child or adolescent psychiatrist**—This is a medical doctor who has special training in the diagnosis and treatment of emotional and behavioral problems in children and who is qualified to prescribe medication.
- **Psychologist**—This professional has an advanced degree from an accredited graduate program in psychology, as well as 2 or more years of supervised work experience in the field of psychiatry. This professional is trained to make diagnoses and provide individual and group therapy.
- **Clinical social worker**—This professional has a master's degree in social work from an accredited graduate program and is trained to make diagnoses and provide individual and group counseling.
- **Licensed professional counselor**—This professional has a master's degree in psychology, counseling, or a related field and is trained to diagnose and provide individual and group counseling.
- **Mental health counselor**—This professional has a master's degree in psychology, counseling, or a related field and several years of supervised clinical work experience and is trained to diagnose and provide individual and group counseling.
- **Certified alcohol and drug abuse counselor**—This professional has had specific clinical training in treatment of alcohol and drug abuse and is qualified to diagnose and provide individual and group counseling.
- **Nurse psychotherapist**—This is a registered nurse who is trained in the practice of psychiatric and mental health nursing and is qualified to diagnose and provide individual and group counseling.

- **Marital and family therapist**—This professional has a master's degree in psychology, counseling, or a related field with special education and training in marital and family therapy and is qualified to diagnose and provide individual and group counseling.
- **Pastoral counselor**—This professional has a degree in clinical pastoral education and is trained to diagnose and provide individual and group counseling.

Some mental health and substance abuse programs are designed to treat both adults and children. In most cases, however, child and adult services and programs are provided by separate professional entities. If the program is designed to treat all age groups, case managers must be knowledgeable about the treatment modalities and levels of care provided, the fees charged, and the types of patients served by the various programs. Programs designed to serve the mentally ill include the following:

- **Acute-care inpatient psychiatric facilities**—As with medical and geriatric patients, not all mentally ill patients require inpatient care, and patients should be placed in the least restrictive environment possible consistent with their care and safety. Patients who show acute symptoms or who are suicidal, however, may require admission to an acute-care psychiatric hospital. Acute-care psychiatric facilities provide multidisciplinary care that allows daily visits by a psychiatrist as well as skilled nursing care and observation. Inpatient care also allows the entire multidisciplinary team to conduct assessments and implement therapy designed to stabilize condition of the acutely ill patient. Depending on the patient's diagnosis, an inpatient program offers one-on-one intervention or constant observation, seclusion, or restraints; pharmacotherapy and skilled observation of responses to drugs and other treatments; skilled interventions including any other tests or therapy necessary, such as electroshock therapy; and any combination of individual, group, and family psychotherapy sessions as deemed necessary.
- **Partial hospitalization programs**—During the past decade, partial hospitalization programs have arisen as a cost-effective alternative to inpatient care. In a partial hospital program the patient is treated by the same multidisciplinary team and provided with all the services normally associated with inpatient care. However, these patients are allowed to return home in the evenings and on weekends to maintain some normalcy in their lives. In addition to reducing costs, these programs have helped to decrease the stigma associated with mental illness. Thus, they have allowed patients to maintain more intact relationships with peers, family, and coworkers. Many health care payers use partial hospitalization programs in place of inpatient care and thus extend the mental health benefits they provide. In these situations, one inpatient day is frequently exchanged for two partial days of treatment. Partial programs vary from half-day to full-day programs. Partial programs are important for patients who require a step-down unit because they allow such people to make the transition from hospital to home in incremental moves. In addition, the programs are useful for persons who require continued care and consistent support to maintain the clinical stability they achieved while in the acute-care setting. People who are

unable to maintain stability even when receiving other types of outpatient services may also benefit from partial hospitalization programs.

- **Residential treatment centers (adolescents and children), public or private**—Residential treatment centers provide 24-hour care for adolescents or children who have a psychiatric illness that is too severe to be treated effectively at a less restrictive level of care. These centers are also intended for any child who cannot be treated at home within the family unit even with the help offered by other outpatient services. Patients entering a residential treatment center must be medically and psychiatrically stable and capable of participating in the program. To remain in the program, the patient must show clinical improvement, and the family must actively participate in the program as well. Such progress allows the patient to be discharged to a less restrictive level of care and eventually reintegrated into the family unit. The therapeutic program offered by residential treatment centers includes at least the following components:
  - A multidisciplinary treatment team
  - Active family involvement
  - Twenty-four-hour nursing assessments and skilled nursing care
  - Individual, group, and family psychotherapy
  - In some programs, other therapies, prevocational and vocational training, and regular or special education classes
- **Outpatient programs**—These are possibly the most common modality for the treatment of mental illness today. These programs are typically provided in the privacy of the therapist's office. However, some group and family sessions are conducted in outpatient facilities. Outpatient programs are designed to treat both acute and chronic illnesses. They consist of the following treatment methods in any combination:
  - Individual counseling, psychotherapy, and psychoanalysis
  - Diagnostic evaluation and testing
  - Group psychotherapy
  - Family psychotherapy
  - Pharmacotherapy and/or medication management programs
  - Diagnostic evaluations and psychologic testing
- **Home health agency care**—Traditionally, home health agency care has centered on services to medical-surgical patients; mentally ill patients have not had access to this level of care. As care has shifted from inpatient to outpatient settings, however, home health services for people with mental illness have evolved. Mental health clients receiving home health agency care must meet the same needs criteria for home-based or skilled nursing care as must any other patient in order for the agency to provide the care and receive reimbursement. Unfortunately, not all home health agencies provide mental health care. If they do, case managers must ensure that the care is delivered by licensed personnel who actively practice in the mental health field. Case managers assigned to serve mentally ill patients must familiarize themselves with the home health agencies in their area that provide this service.
- **State hospitals**—Placement in state hospitals is rare but is occasionally necessary for patients who are so severely impaired mentally that traditional mental health care is of no

avail. Although state hospital placement can be voluntary, entrance in most cases occurs through a court order and the conservatorship process. Because of the complex regulations regarding state placement, all case managers working with mental health patients must be very familiar with their state's laws and the requirements for admission to such hospitals. State hospital care is rarely reimbursed by health care payers because most patients require custodial care. Also, by the time state hospital placement occurs, any mental health benefits that were available generally have been exhausted. Therefore, the most common source of payment for state hospital care is Medicaid.

Substance Abuse Programs

When treatment for substance abuse or chemical dependency in either an inpatient or outpatient program is desired or recommended, benefits are often payable only under the patient's selected mental health benefit structure. This is unfortunate, because many health care payers use stringent guidelines for the type and length of program they will approve. As with other mental health benefits offered, many apply the same stringent day, dollar, or lifetime limits to the chemical dependency or substance abuse services they cover. Some health care payers offer "substance abuse programs" that cover nothing more than a 3-day detoxification regimen. The case manager must then help patients who want treatment to gain access to free services in the community, or patients must assume the costs of such treatment themselves. The programs offered when treatment is allowed can be divided into the following categories:

- Detoxification programs (both inpatient and outpatient)
- Inpatient rehabilitation programs

- Structured outpatient programs
- Day treatment programs
- Individual or group outpatient programs

In most cases, chemical dependency programs are offered in an outpatient setting. The actual treatment given depends on many factors relating to the patient's chemical dependency and the characteristics displayed by the patient. The following features are common among chemically dependent patients:

- They have used the substance over a prolonged period of time.
- They frequently are high or intoxicated and are unable to fulfill their obligations and duties.
- They have a marked tolerance for the drug or substance and show characteristic withdrawal symptoms when intake of the substance is stopped or reduced.
- They show manipulative or abusive behavior that seriously impairs their social, family, occupational, and educational functioning.

Inpatient admission of a substance abuse patient, if necessary, frequently results from the following:

- An unstable medical condition that was exacerbated by or resulted from the substance abuse behavior, withdrawal, or impending withdrawal
- An unstable psychiatric condition that places the patient at risk of self-injury or injury to others
- A life-threatening episode that results from drug or alcohol intoxication and overdose

When admitted as an inpatient, the substance abuse patient remains hospitalized until he or she is medically stable and the substance abuse problem can be managed at a lower level of care such as in a day treatment program. Most chemical dependency programs last for 4 weeks, and often the actual treatment program can be a combination of inpatient and outpatient care. Both inpatient and outpatient programs offer care by a multidisciplinary team composed of mental health professionals who specialize in chemical dependency.

Day and evening chemical treatment programs are designed to serve patients who cannot maintain abstinence during the transition back to the community. Evening programs allow the person to continue to work while he or she receives treatment after the normal workday. In a day program, the patient receives treatment during the daytime hours and returns home at night. These programs are like partial hospitalization programs only the focus is on substance abuse. The primary difference between the two programs is the time spent (per day or per week) in the program. Regardless of the setting, chemical dependency programs offer at a minimum the following components:

- Individualized treatment planning
- Assessments of patient's psychologic, physiologic, and psychosocial function
- Substance abuse counseling
- Skilled nursing care (but not according to the social model)
- Weekly individual, group, or family psychotherapy sessions
- Treatment planning for after-care and arrangements for services such as a half-way house, group home, or other community support services that help the patient remain sober
- Relapse prevention planning
- Active participation in an Alcoholics Anonymous or Narcotics Anonymous program

Programs designed for children have the same components but also include psychoeducation classes.

Management of Patients with Dual Diagnoses

The definition of dual diagnoses can be confusing because the term can apply to persons with some combination of a medical condition, mental health condition, and/or substance addiction. If dual diagnoses are present, the case manager often finds the case more complicated and treatment more prolonged. Also, historically mental health benefit plans have been very restrictive in terms of day and dollar limits, and if one is not careful benefits can be swiftly be depleted. To further complicate the issues related to accessing appropriate and timely mental health care, one often is confronted with two sets of players who authorize or case manage the services as well as two benefit structures with separate limitations and exclusions and different copayments.

Management of Patients with Severe and Persistent Psychiatric Disorders

Persons with severe and persistent psychiatric disorders (SPPDs)—such as schizophrenia, significant mood disorders, substance abuse, some personality disorders, and some phobias—experience a myriad of problems. These often include treatments with unpleasant side effects (such as medications that cause abnormal or involuntary movements) and a society that does not fully understand psychiatric disorders, in which discrimination is a likely outcome. Persons with SPPDs often become alienated from their communities because they are socially awkward and lack basic social and coping skills. These factors contribute to a vicious cycle that eliminates opportunities for social learning and the development of significant social supports. The end result is that many patients have a very poor quality of life.[5]

Thus, case managers working with SPPD patients must possess a broad repertoire of skills and have several characteristics that distinguish them as good case managers. These skills include the ability to do the following:

- Reinforce relationships.
- Be consumer oriented.

- Be assertive.
- Work within the patient's community and not in an office setting.
- Locate resources that address all need domains and are cross-sectional (i.e., locating housing, gaining access to health care, gaining access to financial resources, accessing vocational programs, locating transportation, building a social support network, finding ways for the patient to use free time).
- Serve on a long-term basis, since the person may need long-term services and care (this ensures that services will not be cut off for any reason).
- Work as a team member, since case management for this category of patients is often more effective when provided by a team of case managers who share responsibility for the ensuring that the patient's needs are met; use of a team approach also helps prevent case manager burnout.

Success in meeting various needs depends, in part, on the range of resources that individuals have available. Therefore, assessing resources, or the lack of resources, is imperative when determining the needs of the SPPD patient. As a rule, resources can be divided into three main areas: financial and material resources needed to purchase the necessary care and services, the repertoire of necessary social and coping skills, and a social network that can lend support in meeting the patient's needs. Many persons with SPPD are impoverished and therefore lack the financial or insurance resources required to obtain care. Although federal or state entitlement programs might be available, they are often not adequate to meet the needs of the SPPD patient. Fortunately, it is this category of patients that is affected by the new mental health parity laws. Therefore, it is critical that case managers working with persons in this category be very knowl-edgeable about the laws in their states that pertain to mental health parity.

Mental Health Carve-Outs

Changes in mental health care began to occur in the late 1970s and early 1980s, when insurers and self-insured employers began to apply general utilization management techniques to help control their indemnity plan health benefit costs. During this time these approaches were less effective in controlling the costs of mental health and substance abuse care than in controlling other medical costs. Thus, the scene was set for development of a niche industry of specialized managed care mental health and substance abuse organizations that contracted directly with health maintenance organizations (HMOs), indemnity insurers, and self-insured employers, and applied their special techniques in managing mental health and substance abuse costs.[4] Eventually, over the next few years, mental health benefits were transferred from HMO managed care through what was termed a "carve-out" process. Behavioral health services so carved out are now managed by specialized managed care organizations.

Case managers unfamiliar with the mental health system often find that coordinating the care of a patient with a mental illness is difficult because most behavioral health care in the United States is managed by specialized companies, known as managed behavioral health care organizations (MBHOs), under carve-out contracts with HMOs. As estimated 170 million Americans, or 68% of all persons covered by health insurance, are enrolled in some type of managed behavioral health program. Ten companies control approximately 76% of this market. Unfortunately, since only a small number of MBHOs dominate the market, dramatic changes have occurred in the practice of private psychiatry and psychology. This is partly because many of the MBHOs rely predominately on utilization review as a cost containment mechanism, rather than on disease management programs or case management services. Moreover, as a result of the carve-out relationship, many HMOs have become distanced from certain aspects of care and often lack the infrastructure necessary for the delivery of behavioral health care, which results in serious problems in service and claim payment.[6]

Thus, if the mental health patient requires a case management or disease management program, linkage may be exasperating as one attempts to work through the layers of who is actually responsible for the authorization of care and services or the payment of claims.

Mental Health Parity

Although the problem of mental health care coverage was not totally solved with the enactment of the Mental Health Parity Act (MHPA) of 1996 (Public Law 104-204, Title VII), in some states and for some health plans some restrictions on mental health benefits have now been lifted. The MHPA amended the Employee Retirement Income Security Act and the Public Health Service Act to require group health plans, if they choose to offer mental health benefits, to provide the same financial conditions for such benefits that they provide for medical and surgical benefits, including the same aggregate lifetime limits and the same annual limits, if any, for specific categories of mental health illnesses. The MHPA makes such parity requirements *inapplicable* to (1) substance abuse or chemical dependency treatment, (2) employers with fewer than 50 employees, and (3) any group health plan (or health insurance coverage offered in connection with such a plan) for which implementation of this provision results in a cost increase of at least 1%.

The act further amended Title XVIII (Medicare) of the Social Security Act to restructure the mental health benefit and provided for the following:

- Coverage under Medicare Part A (hospital insurance) of inpatient hospital services furnished primarily for the diagnosis or treatment of mental illness or substance abuse for up to 60 days during a year, as well as coverage of intensive residential services furnished to an individual for up to 120 days during a year
- Lower copayments for certain outpatient mental health and substance abuse services
- Waiver of copayment for case management services furnished to a seriously mentally ill adult, a seriously emotionally disturbed child, or an adult or child with a serious substance abuse disorder
- Case management services for an unlimited duration for such individuals
- Provision of items and services furnished under Medicare Part B (supplementary medical insurance) for the treatment of mental illness or emotional disturbances according to standards established by the Secretary of Health and Human Services
- Coverage of a new category of intensive community-based services including, among others, partial hospitalization services as well as psychiatric rehabilitation services, in-home services, and day treatment for substance abuse for individuals of any age and of other mental health services for individuals under age 19 years
- Requirement that intensive community-based programs (whether at another facility or freestanding) be authorized by state law or certified by an appropriate accreditation entity

- Supervision of individualized treatment programs by nonphysician mental health professionals to the extent permitted under state law[2]

Basically, the federal MHPA requires employers that offer mental health benefits to set annual and lifetime caps equal to those for medical and surgical benefits. The measure excludes businesses with 50 or fewer employees and allows all employers to be exempted from the law if their costs rise more than 1% as a result of complying with the act's requirements. The law allows health insurance plans to set different benefit levels for copayments, deductibles, inpatient hospital days, and outpatient visits.

If a state has a mental health parity law that requires more comprehensive coverage, the federal parity law does not weaken the state law, nor does the federal law preclude a state from enacting stronger parity legislation. More information on mental health parity can be found on websites such as *www.mentalhealth.org*, the National Mental Health Association website at *www.nmha.org*, and *www.insure.com*. For a listing of the states that have enacted mental illness parity laws, see the insure.com website.

Case Management Plan

Development of the mental health case management plan differs very little from development of plans for medical cases. Consequently, the same seven steps needed for development and monitoring of a case management plan are followed:

1. Assessment and collection of pertinent medical data
2. Organization of the data for planning
3. Coordination and linkage
4. Negotiation of discounts or reduced rates when nonnetwork providers are used
5. Implementation of the plan

6. Assessment of compliance with the plan at regular intervals and assessment of the clinical support system and initial and ongoing counseling and education
7. Reassessment and revision of the plan during periods of crisis or long-term illness, or throughout the time the case is open to case management

As with case management for any patient, the ultimate goals of mental health case management are as follows:

- To ensure that care is appropriate
- To provide care at the appropriate level
- To ensure that services and providers selected are effective in rendering treatment and that deterioration or rehospitalization is prevented
- To ensure that care is provided in the most cost-effective environment to obtain optimal cost savings

Mental health case management uses virtually the same implementation techniques that are used in medical case management. The aims are as follows:

- To help the patient gain access to appropriate resources for diagnosis and treatment
- To assist the patient and family in obtaining access to community resources that can augment insurance mental health benefits
- To monitor the patient's progress and make recommendations for alternate treatment modalities
- To assist the family in applying for guardianship or conservatorship, when applicable
- To advise the family on how to gain access to the support required to cope with the situation

Because many mental health conditions are chronic, many case management processes will be required sporadically throughout the patient's lifetime. Also, as in medical case management, there is no "cookbook" to follow. Although some of the techniques listed earlier may be applied only once, others may be used repeatedly throughout the case. As in medical case management, these processes occur in no specific order, and there is no set number of services or providers that may be used in the case at a given time.

Families dealing with the mental illness of a parent, spouse, or child react no differently from families dealing with a medical illness in the family. When psychologic problems or feelings of being overwhelmed arise or are identified, they must be dealt with, and the family must be linked to support groups or professional counseling. Because of the multiple problems associated with mental illness and the chronic nature of most such conditions, it is common for entire families to receive therapy. Reactions such as the following are frequent:

- Embarrassment or shame
- Feelings of frustration with the system
- Exhaustion due to sleeplessness caused by worry, fright, and fear of the unknown if the patient is abusive or violent
- Anger over depletion of financial resources due to lack of reimbursement, benefit limits, or exclusions by the health care payer
- Anger and frustration with the insufficient numbers of agencies or facilities that can adequately manage the patient
- Anger that the illness is occurring in their family

The key to the success of a mental health case management plan is establishment of a high level of trust by the patient in his or her case manager. Trust increases the commitment of the patient and family to the final plan. Depending on the severity of the dysfunction, the mental health case manager often assumes the role of advocate to ensure the provision of appropriate care, especially medication management.

MEDICATION MANAGEMENT

Often the primary culprit in the exacerbation of any illness is the poor management of medication usage, regardless of the patient's condition or the diagnosis. Although management of medications is important for all patients, it is imperative for mental health patients because medication is often the thread that keeps these patients out of more expensive facilities. Medication management not only allows patients better control and use of their mental health benefits, it also decreases the risk that their benefits will be prematurely exhausted by preventing frequent and costly inpatient admissions or treatments.

As most health care professionals know, historically most mental health benefits have been limited by health care payers and the benefit packages selected by employers. Although some changes have occurred with passage of the mental health parity laws, many policies, especially those offered by small employer groups, continue to impose day or dollar limits or a yearly or lifetime maximum on benefits; others exclude specific diagnostic categories such as learning disorders, eating disorders, attention deficit hyperactivity disorder, and autism from benefit coverage. Other benefit plans limit coverage to inpatient care and offer minimal coverage for outpatient treatments. Still others require that care be delivered by members of a select panel of providers or professionals.

ALTERNATE FUNDING AND COMMUNITY RESOURCES

Because of the long-term nature of mental illness, case managers must work closely with the patient and family or conservator to make sure that they apply for any alternate funding programs to which the patient may be entitled. These programs include the following:

- Supplemental Security Income
- Medicaid
- Social Security Disability Insurance and Medicare
- General assistance and food stamp programs if the patient is unemployed
- State unemployment or disability income, if applicable
- Special education if the patient is 21 years of age or younger and is still enrolled in school
- Title V Children's Medical Services program (some states offer assistance with treatment for mental illness)
- Programs of the state agency responsible for providing services for those with developmental disabilities
- Programs of the state agency responsible for mental health services

To assist persons without insurance coverage or to ensure that the mental health case management plan and physician's treatment plan are complete and that the patient receives the maximum benefits allowable under any insurance coverage, linkage with community resources may be necessary. These resources may include a local health department that offers some limited programs for persons with mental health disorders. Because these programs are state funded, however, the clinics are obligated to serve first individuals who meet "priority population criteria" as defined by a state's mental health department. Unfortunately, waiting lists may be lengthy, and not all individuals may be eligible for services. In some jurisdictions local funding is provided for additional services. Such services can be used to augment health care benefits that are limited or exhausted. The following are additional

resources one might wish to explore when insurance coverage is limited or absent:

- Community agencies whose mission is to serve persons with mental health disorders
- Clergy
- Family physician, if available
- Family service agencies; ethnic, church, or other support groups; or other community service agencies such as Catholic charities, family services, or Jewish social services
- School counselors
- Self-help support groups (i.e., groups for alcoholism, overeating, the loss of a child, codependency, grandparenting, various mental illnesses, cancer, parenting)
- Community hotlines, crisis centers, and crisis intervention programs
- Abuse and domestic violence programs
- Infant and foster care shelter programs
- State and county departments of mental health
- County department of social services
- Volunteers of America, Salvation Army, and similar programs
- Veterans Administration programs (for veterans only)

SUMMARY

This chapter offers a brief overview of some of the many programs available for mental health care if the patient's individual health care benefit package offers mental health care coverage. Unfortunately, mental health benefits are often severely limited. This limitation, combined with the fact that many mental health conditions are chronic, means that any health care benefits provided by the health care payer are often exhausted quickly if the patient is not covered by the provisions of the 1996 MHPA. This law requires that aggregate lifetime and annual dollar limits for mental health benefits be equal to those for medical and surgical benefits under a group health plan and stipulates that employers retain discretion regarding the extent and scope of mental health benefits offered to workers and their families (including cost sharing, limits on numbers of visits or days of coverage, and requirements relating to medical necessity).

Unfortunately, many patients with mental disorders fail to receive appropriate care because they have no money for treatments or medications. Thus, case management is as vital for mental health cases as it is for medical cases. Case management is necessary if the quality of care is to be maintained and the patient is to receive the care he or she requires.

Chapter Exercises

1. In a group setting discuss the various reasons mental health case management has been so slow to develop and obtain the group's opinions of what is happening locally in mental health care and how services and case management are handled by the large insurers or public programs in the local region.

2. Describe the basics of the MHPA and its impact locally on patients and their mental health benefits. If the reader's state is one that does not have MHPA laws, contact a local congressional representative and discuss the following: What are the state's plans for MHPA laws? Is the state taking action on such laws? If so, how long before they are enacted? If not, why not?

3. In a group setting describe the members of the mental health treatment team and the types of treatments anticipated,

the various sites for mental health care delivery in the local region, and the community agencies available to provide supplementary services.

Suggested Websites and Resources

www.nmha.org—National Mental Health Association Resource Center; offers information on mental illnesses and treatments, and referrals for local treatment services; the resource center provides the following services at no cost to the public:

- Toll-free line: 1-800-969-NMHA (800-969-6642)
- Network of more than 340 affiliates
- TTY line for the hearing impaired: 1-800-433-5959
- Referrals to more than 7000 organizations nationwide
- Sixty different brochures and fact sheets on a variety of mental health topics
- Staff of experienced, professionally trained employees

www.mentalhealth.org—National Mental Health Information Center of the Substance Abuse and Mental Health Services Administration

www.insure.com—insurance information

www.va.gov—Veterans Administration

www.tricare.osd.mil/—TRICARE

cms.hhs.gov—Centers for Medicare and Medicaid Services

www.samhsa.gov—Substance Abuse and Mental Health Services Administration

REFERENCES

1. Smith GB: Shifting gears: moving to the next level of psychiatric disease management, *Continuing Care* 5(10):20–21, 1996.
2. National Mental Health Association, Mental health information fact sheets, available on-line at *www.nmha.org/infoctr/factsheets/index.cfm*.

3. Employee wins groundbreaking claim for mental disability, *Case Management Advisor* 10(4):53–55, 1999.
4. Kongstvedt PR: *The managed health care handbook*, ed 2, Gaithersburg, Md, 1993, Aspen.
5. Corrigan PW, Garman AN: Case management for individuals with severe and persistent psychiatric disorders. In Blancett SS, Flarey DL, editors: *Case studies in nursing case management health care delivery in a world of managed care*, Gaithersburg, Md, 1996, Aspen.
6. Fox A: MBHO/EAP enrollment reaches 220 million in 2000, *Open Minds* 12(6):7–8, 2000.
7. National Alliance for the Mentally Ill, available on-line at *www.nami.org/policy/stateparitychart.html. www.nami.org/helpline/factsandfigures.html*

BIBLIOGRAPHY

Baker F, Intagliata J: Case management. In Liberman RP, editor: *Handbook of psychiatric rehabilitation*, New York, 1992, Macmillan.

Corrigan PW, Buican B, McCracken S: The needs and resources assessment for severely mentally ill adults, *Psychiatr Serv* 46:504–505, 1995.

Duffy J, Miller M, Parlocha P: Psychiatric home care, *Home Healthcare Nurse* 11(2):22–28, 1993.

National Alliance for the Mentally Ill:*www.nami.org/helpline/factsandfigures.html.*

CHAPTER
18

Geriatric Considerations

Molly Kostlan, RNC

OBJECTIVES

■ To list some of the many skills necessary to be a case manager serving the geriatric population
■ To define what *elderly* means
■ To list the components of a geriatric assessment

DEMOGRAPHICS

Although there are different ways to measure population dynamics and life expectancy, as the baby boom generation ages the bulge in the U.S. population will clearly move toward the end of the age spectrum. The implications for all enterprises associated with providing care and services in the public and private sectors are profound. Case managers are in an ideal position to benefit from the intersection of applied technology, creative financing, and consumer demand as geriatric care moves from the periphery to the center of health care services. Reducing mortality rates from heart disease, cancer, and stroke may still mean learning to live with their sequelae and adjusting to the chronic health conditions associated with aging. Given that the risk of having a chronic condition develop is predicted to double about every 5 to 7 years after age 50 years, clients at advanced ages are likely to have multiple comorbidities.[1] As the population ages, maintaining optimal health for those with disabling chronic conditions such as diabetes mellitus, progressive dementia, arthritis, heart failure, and Parkinson's disease will be the foundation of clinical practice.

This shift in life expectancy is accompanied by a change in other trends. As the number of older persons increases, the importance of this group as a political entity also emerges, a phenomenon that will undoubtedly drive resource allocation and public policy decisions and create long-term financing vehicles. For the first time in decades, there has been a reversal of migration patterns to urban centers.[2] Many rural areas are seeing a repopulation movement that is already altering the landscape of community needs and services. Alternative living and group housing options for retirees are increasingly more available in suburban settings near adult children who are juggling the responsibilities of caregiver duties, parenthood, and employment. The shift in reimbursement strategies rewards health maintenance, not costly, late-engagement health care services. The most recent trend requires providers to demonstrate positive patient outcomes and functional gain to collect Medicare reimbursement.[3]

Any case manager whose caseload includes elderly patients must have a working knowledge of Social Security, Medicare, and Railroad Retirement programs and be able to understand the structure of any retirement plans if a client has opted to not contribute to Social Security. Additionally, case managers must possess a knowledge of services provided to geriatric clients under any programs that operate in the local area, including Medicare risk programs, Medicaid, Area Agency on Aging, and Supplemental Security Income (SSI). This knowledge is essential to ensure that linkage with programs to which the client is entitled occurs as needed.

DEFINITION OF ELDERLY

The terms *geriatric* and *elderly* are usually applied to adults older than 60 years, when certain physiologic features become apparent. In the literature, however, 65 years is a marker for Medicare eligibility, and much of what we know about the aging process is drawn from this database. Although sometimes separated into young-old, middle-old, and oldest-old, age is a relative concept. The 58-year-old man with coronary artery disease, congestive heart failure, and chronic renal insufficiency who has been nonambulatory for 2 years after a dense stroke may be functionally dependent and already qualify for Medicare based on duration of disability. The 75-year-old man in vigorous health may work part time or even full time and exercise regularly, aging at a normal rather than accelerated pace.

CHARACTERISTICS OF THE ELDERLY: THE AGING PROCESS

Aging clients and their family members usually have some awareness of the loss of tissue elasticity that accompanies the normal aging process, having witnessed the gradual appearance of wrinkles and loss of muscle tone. What they may not realize is that this loss of tissue elasticity is a generalized phenomenon. The loss of flexibility also contributes to decreased cardiac muscle mass and cardiac output, decreased capillary flow control and reduced renal clearance, decreased lung tissue elasticity, and function and changes in visual acuity. Changes in collagen structure result in thickening of the eye's lens, decreased space between the vertebrae, decreased strength of ligaments, and stiffness in tendons.[4] The metabolic rate slows as well, and with it the assembly of proteins from food intake, bone formation and remodeling, and the rate of all new cell production. These phenomena are accompanied by a change in body composition with an increase in fat relative to muscle tissue. Taken singly and in combination, these changes may affect absorption, metabolism, and excretion of food and drugs. Reduced protein stores translate to reduced enzyme activity, including neurotransmitters, hormones, blood cells, and components of the immune response. When normal changes of aging are complicated by pathologic conditions, maintaining steady-state conditions is a daily challenge.

The high incidence of depression in older persons may have underlying biologic causes, but poor health, bereavement, and a deteriorating social network may influence the severity of the symptoms. Loss of flexibility within the body can be presented conceptually to clients and family members as an explanation of why the older person does not "bounce back" as quickly from illness or injury or adjust rapidly to changes in fluid balance.

REFERRALS

Referrals for case management services for geriatric clients originate from various points along the care continuum. At times, an aging client with foresight may contract for consultation services for himself or herself, allowing a case manager time to fully explore dimensions of care needs and develop some form of a care plan for life. Under less ideal circumstances, services are requested when deterioration of a chronic condition or an abrupt change in health precipitates a decline in functional status that calls for a higher level of clinical sophistication, a greater amount of physical assistance, or both. In some cases, an individual with multiple conditions may be monitored by a patchwork of agencies in addition to a health maintenance organization or primary provider. High-risk diagnoses or flags mentioned in preceding sections serve as the most common reasons for referral for case management. Variables such as age, medical history, level of care required, resource availability, family involvement and interest, and reimbursement for the case management services influence the final decision to open a case.

Most elderly patients require maintenance or custodial care, a level of care not covered by Medicare. Most older insurance policies sold over the past 30 years cover skilled, not custodial, care and sometimes only after the policyholder has exhausted a Medicare benefit. Consumer demand has since created a market for a variety of long-term care policies. Complete understanding of coverage guidelines is imperative to determine exclusions and limitations. For example, skilled or custodial care might be covered only within a licensed skilled nursing facility and not in a private home or assisted-living facility. Medicaid does cover custodial care in facilities licensed for intermediate or skilled care. Exploring financial assets and liabilities with the patient and family is considered part of the overall assessment process and no less significant than any other portion. Determining if or when the client may be eligible for Medicaid or SSI when funds are limited is important. Because many patients require custodial care and the patient and family must pay privately for these services, families must be informed about the potential cost outlays and the alternate funding programs available the patient may be eligible for once financial reserves are depleted.

The search for resources to meet any patient's needs, through either private or public programs, creates its own set of challenges. Even with adequate financial resources, acquiring assistance, modifying the home, procuring supplies, and securing transportation may be hindered by inadequate community and caregiver resources, safety hazards, and geographic barriers that disrupt continuity of the plan. As long as elders and citizens in need are marginalized by the economic structure, services to assist them in maintaining autonomy will continue to be imperiled by greater demands, budgetary constraints, ignorance, and oversight.

ASSESSMENTS

The process for conducting the assessment will vary depending on the vantage point of the person acting as case manager. The private case manager will need to access records before the initial interview. Before conducting the initial interview and assessment, the case manager, with the patient's or conservator's permission, must collect as much pertinent medical, social, and cultural information as possible to establish and predict progressive physical, functional, and cognitive impairment. This information may include the following:

- Current medical records and medical history
- Family structure, history, and dynamics
- Occupational and social history
- Emotional and psychosocial history and evidence of memory
- Pattern of any alcohol, tobacco, or drug use

- Family or caregiver availability, capability, and limitations
- Resources previously used
- Patient and family financial status and insurance policies

Demographic information about the patient can come from a variety of sources, but the four most common are:

1. Questionnaires
2. Medical records
3. Consultation with physician or other health care professionals
4. Visual and interactive assessments of the patient

INTERVIEWS

Interviewing a geriatric client in his or her own environment, to the extent that organizational policy allows on-site assessment, is helpful. As much information as possible must be gathered and pertinent records thoroughly reviewed before the initial interview. Armed with a current record of the health and social history and an understanding of disease process, the case manager should approach the interview prepared to use assessment skills and imagination to identify where on the life continuum a client currently is and what sentinel event may have prompted a request for case management services.

The home visit offers several advantages. Not only does it eliminate the logistical problems of transporting a client, but the risk of distracting or disorienting the client may be reduced in a familiar environment. The client, any caregiver, and as many family members as practical should be available during the interview period to allow for individual and collective questioning and observation of family and group dynamics. A skilled case manager demonstrates the ability to listen, adjusts the rhythm of the questions to allow pauses, and poses questions that are often not asked.[5] The initial assessment interview must be of reasonable length, usually no longer than 2 hours, with additional phone contact and visits scheduled later for clarification if necessary.

As mentioned in other sections, formal assessment tools to determine functional or cognitive impairment (e.g., the Katz Adjustment Scale or the Folstein Mini-Mental Status Exam) or to detect symptoms of depression (e.g., Yesavage Geriatric Depression Scale) are readily available and easy to use. But a case manager whose style is interpreted as too "clinical" risks altering the tone of the interview and alienating a client. If the client cannot be candid in the presence of others, the value of the instruments is negligible. The case manager should be familiar with any assessment tools used by providers in the community to be able to interpret scores and changes from baseline as well as understand what to look for. The home visit allows an opportunity to view or evaluate:

- How the patient moves about in his or her own surroundings and conducts activities of daily living
- The need for any mobility aids or other adaptive equipment
- Any structural barriers (both interior and exterior) that, if not corrected, might affect the final plan
- The client's and family's cultural or religious beliefs, customs, or practices
- The actual home conditions and environment, compatibility with the client's needs, and geographic distance to resources and sites of medical care
- Interactions between the client and family
- All medications and their storage
- Food, food storage, and preparation area
- Accessibility to and from the home
- Geriatric case management plans

Designing a comprehensive care plan tailored to the current needs of a client while providing for future needs is always challenging. Case management plans for a geriatric client must factor in multiple layers of comorbid processes, how they interact, and the progressive nature of aging and pathologic conditions. The case manager must have an accurate clinical picture to create a model that can forecast disability and decompensation for a given client. The more complete the assessment, the better the client and the family will know how to predict disability and decompensation, what interventions delay or minimize them, and what options can be taken when needs change. Because a case manager may only be involved long enough to establish the plan and close the case, the final plan must be specific, reflect individual circumstance, and cover the entire spectrum of care anticipated for the client.

In most cases, an array of resources is necessary if the patient's needs are to be met in the least restrictive environment. Executing this type of planning requires time and individual consideration. Locating resources is time consuming. Much of the care required is custodial in nature and therefore less likely to be covered by insurance plans, limiting access to care and resources for the financially strapped. Contrary to popular belief, most patients can and should remain at home, with placement as the last resort. Thus the case management plan must limit alternative placement recommendations to those that require the fewest restrictions as the patient moves through the continuum of care.

The plan itself must contain provisions that allow revision by the family or significant other as the patient's condition changes and a method to reestablish case management services if the need arises. More importantly, the patient and family should be familiar with conditions that may trigger reevaluation of which resources or alternative care sites are appropriate for the next step. Including approximate costs for each level of care

along with recommendations for financial avenues and options for the family to explore is wise. As with all plans, the geriatric case management plan involves mutual agreements about problems and goals, identification of resources, and alternatives. The final plan must address:

- The patient's and caregiver's physical, functional, social, educational, spiritual, and cultural needs
- Financial abilities and alternate sources of assistance
- Level of care and resources that allow the patient to function at the highest level of independence
- Provision for the health and safety of both the patient and the caregiver
- Informal community resources that can be used to support or augment any formal health care provider benefits
- Problems and recommendations for nonmedical needs, including nutrition, transportation, architectural renovations of the home, assistive devices, and durable medical equipment
- Alternative care arrangements in case the home plan becomes unfeasible or ceases to adequately meet care needs
- Alternative arrangements for providing skilled care and for obtaining respite for the caregiver
- Nutrition and use of medications

Two areas to highlight in the final case management plan are nutritional needs and medication use. These are two of the most common causes of problems seen in the elderly. Although problems in both areas may be related to the specific factors listed in the following sections, one major underlying cause of these problems is lack of money. Most elderly people live on fixed incomes, which may or may not meet their everyday expenses. When illness strikes, the additional costs of medications or unexpected outlays for special diets can create a financial deficit, forcing the patient to make a choice between basic necessities or treatment of the medical condition. In any event, details of these two important aspects must be included in the final case management plan.

NUTRITIONAL CONCERNS

Nutritional needs are affected by the normal physiologic changes associated with aging as well as psychosocial and environmental factors. Factors that affect nutrition and may explain why the elderly person may not eat properly include:

- Cultural preferences
- Religious observances
- Behavioral patterns, depression, and grief
- Special dietary needs
- Vision problems
- Decreased taste sensation and therefore decreased food appeal
- Little motivation to cook for self and eat alone
- Inability to shop because of mobility problems or lack of transportation
- Limited financial ability to purchase food, especially food needed for a special diet
- Limited or nonexistent food preparation or food storage area or lack of cooking or eating utensils
- Limited geographic area served by the local home-delivered meal program
- Limited or nonexistent group meal sites
- Dental problems
- Reduced or limited activity

Some of the problems caused by nutritional needs in the elderly can be illustrated by the following example. One elderly gentleman lived alone in a downtown hotel. Although he really was a candidate for placement, he flatly refused to be discharged anywhere other than to his room. Arrangements were made for the necessary equipment, home health agency services, and delivery of meals. During the assessment interview, however, questioning never elicited whether he had eating utensils. The meals were delivered, but he was unable eat them until an observant home health agency nurse discovered that he lacked utensils. After this incident, a simple question was added to the discharge questionnaire used for patients being discharged home, especially to a hotel.

MEDICATIONS

The use of medications by the elderly is another major problem area that must be carefully assessed and addressed in the final case management plan. Physiologic changes associated with aging, including low serum protein, fewer metabolic enzymes, slowed digestion, and reduced renal clearance, predispose the elderly client to adverse reactions and overdosing. The chance of this occurring increases with the number of medications being taken. Proper treatment of one or multiple chronic conditions is a balancing act; intolerance of the plan or failure to adhere to it is likely to lead to problems. A treatment plan that includes a medication component must consider the logistics of the client affording, procuring, storing, and taking medications as prescribed. Expecting a client to understand the purpose of each medication and how each drug benefits optimal health is a lofty goal.

Reasons why the elderly client may not adhere to the recommended medication regimen are numerous and vary according to circumstance, including:

- Limited finances
- Complexity of the drug regimen
- Poor access to a pharmacy
- Inability to open containers
- Fear of drug dependency or desire to avoid unpleasant side effects
- Failure to discard outdated or discontinued medications

- "Pill sharing" (e.g., patient 1 has a medication that he or she is no longer taking, and patient 2 has similar symptoms as patient 1, so patient 1 gives patient 2 his or her medication)
- Conflicts with religious or cultural beliefs
- Depression and feelings of hopelessness or despair
- Poor vision
- Inadequate supervision
- Forgetfulness or confusion
- Failure to report use of over-the-counter drugs

Case managers must assess all prescription and nonprescription medications currently in use. This is best accomplished by using preliminary questionnaires, interview techniques that ask the patient to describe the process of checking blood sugars or preparing insulin, for example, and a home visit for visual confirmation when possible. The keys to managing medication use in the elderly include taking a detailed drug history and establishing a way to ensure that the patient is monitored for drug use and drug reactions as well as for adherence to any regimen established by the physician.

Monitoring and compliance with drug regimens is a critical element of care for the elderly, and provisions for this must be included in all geriatric case management plans. Monitoring can usually be accomplished by soliciting the assistance of family members or friends. In addition to the patient, the families and caregivers must be educated about the importance of medications and schedules. Creating a structure for dispensing medications on a time schedule is ultimately the most reliable way to monitor drug use. A proper structure provides its own reinforcement in addition to opportunity for monitoring use and timing drug reorders.

Successful management of chronic health conditions may depend on one or more medications taken at regular intervals, in the proper sequence, and at specific times to avoid interaction and achieve positive results. When a condition worsens, knowing that the current regimen is being followed is important to the medical provider, who might otherwise suggest additional drugs or increased dosages, both of which may create added expense and new problems. In older persons cognitive impairment may fluctuate over time, and confusion may be the first sign of an infection. For this reason calendars, check-off lists, and pill dispensers help even the high-functioning client. If a family member cannot reliably do so, many visiting nursing agencies will establish a medication regimen by prefilling syringes or containers with drugs and posting reminders of when the drugs must be taken. More elaborate means of medication reminders include phone reminder services and technology aids such as "smart" medication dispensers that can transmit digital information to a pharmacy over phone lines.

FAMILY INVOLVEMENT

A family caring for an older parent can feel as overwhelmed and confused as one caring for a child with special needs. One major difference exists, however, in the area of finances. Although younger patients often have health care coverage for their medical needs, the elderly often do not. Most elderly people need custodial care rather than skilled care, which is not covered by most health care payers. Financial worries only add to the strain.

Families of the elderly can benefit from being linked with support groups and services. Support groups strengthen families and allow them to cope better with their situation. These groups vary in quality, but a properly structured one can offer a legitimate forum to vent frustration and to gain expertise, confidence, and with luck, perspective. Sometimes adult children promise their parents that they will never place them in a nursing home, but promises fall to the wayside when reality strikes.

The involvement of the family is essential. Their level of participation plays a key role in determining the relevancy and success of the case management plan. Their complete cooperation in developing and implementing the plan hinges on several factors and seems to revolve around their reactions to the illness or injury, their general regard for the patient, and their geographic distance from the situation. Educating the family about the specific details of the disease and the resources available is one of the best ways to alleviate their fears. This may be the time to remind patients and their families that regular, modest levels of physical activity may slow the progression of disability and enhance quality of life. Care must be taken to avoid making an environment too soft (*too soft* refers to the inclusion of unnecessary services or supplies in a care plan to the point where the patient relies on these and loses self-motivation to care for himself or herself); timing of assistance is critical. Amenities such as in-room meals or recliner chairs with mechanical lifts may seem like gestures of kindness, but developing dependence on them deprives the patient of the opportunity to maintain muscle tone, stretch hip flexors, and practice balance and sequencing skills needed for transferring and walking. Relying on these amenities may increase the risk for falls in the future.

In discussions with the family, the case manager must take a proactive approach to alleviate the stigma of Medicaid and nursing home placement. Every effort should be made to describe Medicaid as insurance and to portray nursing homes as institutions where the quality of care can be maintained and the relationship between client and family can be preserved—not as a step in the final process of dying. The

case manager's ability to overcome the family's fears and bias depends on the family. However, if their behavior remains adamant or they are reluctant to accept information, the case manager may be required to close the case if alternatives cannot be found that satisfy their needs and demands.

COMMUNITY RESOURCES

Levels of Care

If facility-based care is included in the case management plan as an alternative, the patient, family, and caregiver must be made aware of all the various levels of care within the patient's given community. Case managers must also keep in mind that just because a patient is elderly does not mean that he or she automatically requires a skilled nursing facility or equivalent. Care for the elderly, or any patient for that matter, must be found in the least restrictive environment that can meet their needs. If out-of-home placement is required, facilities that may be explored include the following:

- Senior housing (assisted or independent)
- Residential care home
- Community board and care home
- Intermediate care facility
- Skilled nursing facility (frequently referred to as nursing homes), locked psychiatric facility, or Alzheimer's facility
- State institution (this is rare and should be the last resort)

The most expensive choices are skilled nursing facilities and state hospitals, where care provided ranges from skilled nursing to custodial care. Although some patients in skilled nursing facilities could conceivably be cared for at home, the costs associated with the care or supervision required are often far higher than the daily or monthly rates charged by a facility. Skilled nursing facilities are the largest provider of long-term institutional custodial care. Staffing in these facilities consists of professional nursing and rehabilitation staff as well as nursing aides. Costs for care in skilled nursing facilities range from $3000-$6000 per month or more and vary according to region. State hospital costs run even higher.

For patients who require an intermediate care facility, board and care facility, or residential care home, admission is specific to the licensure. Admission criteria are usually based on the patient's functional mobility, bowel and bladder control, physical care needs, and medication requirements. Although requirements may vary from state to state, supervision by licensed nurses is generally required in the intermediate care facility and optional in the other settings. In both settings the bulk of care is delivered by unskilled aides or nonlicensed staff.

Transportation is usually provided for medical appointments and other outings. These settings may not be able to accommodate a temporary infirmity that jeopardizes functional status or requires extra supervision. Average costs vary significantly for all levels of care and from region to region.

Costs for home care vary greatly depending on the patient's actual care needs. When all the costs of home care are tallied, home care may be far more costly than facility-based care. As the medical complexity of the client increases, therapeutic interventions necessary to correct imbalance or infection may themselves become complex, swamping even the most devoted caregivers. Facility-based care is designed to provide services to meet all the client's care needs while maintaining quality of care and safety. Personalization, however, may be compromised. Families must be informed of all alternatives and allowed to make their own choices about home care versus facility-based care.

Adult day care centers can be a wonderful resource for an adult who needs care or socialization during part of a day or week or while the caregiver is at work and out of the home. Adult day care centers generally operate from Monday through Friday and are separated into two categories: the medical model, which provides some skilled nursing and rehabilitation services along with socialization, and the social model, which provides services primarily designed to meet the social needs of the elderly. Many centers offer transportation to and from the facility. Charges for adult day care vary and are usually based on a sliding scale pegged to the patient's or family's income.

OTHER COMMUNITY AGENCIES ASSOCIATED WITH THE ELDERLY

Besides home health agency services, attendant care services, durable medical equipment services, adult day care, and skilled nursing facility care, resources that can augment any case management plan for geriatric patients may include some combination of the following:

- Meal programs, whether delivered to the home or at group sites
- Friendly visitor programs
- Telephone reassurance programs
- In-home supportive services (usually housekeeping or chore worker services provided either through community programs or through private pay resources)
- Emergency response systems
- Handicapped transportation services
- Church, ethnic, or social service agencies
- Senior housing units
- Legal services for the elderly and disabled
- Library services (e.g., home delivery of books for the visually impaired)
- Respite services
- Disease-specific agencies for support groups or literature

- Services provided to individuals of certain retirement groups

Certainly this list is not limited to these resources because each community varies in the types of services provided. Also, access to some services is directly linked to the patient's financial assets and ability to pay.

ALTERNATE FUNDING

Because most elderly people receive Social Security and Medicare, the most common alternate funding sources areas follows:

- Medicaid
- SSI
- Private health policies (e.g., for cancer treatment, custodial care, nursing home care)
- Agencies with a sliding scale
- Medicare Part B, for those who have not previously applied

OTHER ISSUES AFFECTING THE ELDERLY

The case manager is in a prime position to detect such unfortunate occurrences as neglect and abuse. The elderly person living at home is at risk for targeted abuse and, more frequently, benign neglect. Case managers have an ethical obligation and, in many states, a legal obligation to report suspected abuse or neglect to the nearest adult protective services agency, which is then charged with investigation. The case manager is well advised to learn the county or state reporting requirements for the area in which the client resides; reporting responsibility is voluntary in some states and mandatory in others.

Advocacy groups and professionals working with elders generally agree on what might constitute abuse and consider the following to warrant further investigation:

- **Active neglect**—intentional failure to provide care by denying food, medicine, or personal hygiene

- **Passive neglect**—unintentional failure to fulfill caregiver duties
- **Psychologic abuse**—infliction of mental anguish by insulting, demeaning, ignoring, making threatening remarks, or isolating the patient
- **Financial abuse**—illegal or unethical exploitation of a person's funds, property, or assets
- **Physical abuse**—intentional infliction of pain or injury

More obvious signs of neglect or abuse include the following:

- Bruising, lacerations, or skin sores
- Frequent broken bones
- Unmet medical needs
- Excessive clutter or filth
- Few or no social contacts
- Feces or urine not properly disposed of
- Rotting or molding food in refrigerator or on counters
- Reported use of frequent emergency room services for anxiety attacks or difficulty in breathing
- Claims history of multiple emergency services at various emergency departments or urgent care centers

Other signs that may be recognizable by an alert case manager include:

- Depression or depressive behavior
- Withdrawn behavior or extreme passivity
- Anxiety
- Hostility
- Excessive weight loss
- Physical injuries
- Recent impoverishment

End-of-life care is an important part of any patient's plan and should reflect the patient's wishes for intensity of treatment and resuscitation in the event he or she can no longer speak for himself or herself. To support these wishes, the patient may create a living will or request that a do not resuscitate (DNR) order be drawn up. If the patient has been declared incompetent, the appointed conservator may be responsible for these documents on the patient's behalf. The case manager must be familiar with the laws and regulations pertaining to these two documents. If a valid living will or DNR order is known to exist, this information must be included in the final case management plan.

Mental competence and decision-making capacity figure into many aspects of planning for elders. Many times patients cannot speak for themselves or are not competent to make informed decisions. Although the patient may be consulted, a third party—the conservator or family member—may make decisions for them. This situation intensifies the need for the case manager to consider all consequences and available alternatives and document all actions. This documentation is necessary to substantiate the ethical soundness of the case manager's actions if situations arise at a later date that challenge the final plan.

When the patient is incompetent but has not been declared thus and no conservator or guardian has been established, the case manager must be familiar with the laws and regulations pertaining to establishing the conservatorship process in the area where the patient lives, the time frame required for this process, and which agencies or professionals are responsible for implementation. In many states the conservatorship process, which usually involves a thorough search for personal and financial assets, can take several months from the time of application to assignment of a temporary conservator. If this situation occurs, often no action can be taken until the final conservator is appointed. This situation requires patience, diligent follow-up, and careful monitoring of the case to ensure continuity during a forced waiting period because a patient often may not be moved and money cannot be accessed to establish care at an alternate site until the conservatorship process is complete.

SUMMARY

Improper or inadequate case management planning for the elderly can lead to adverse conditions, readmissions, or admission to an inappropriate level of care. If the case management plan is not specific and the client, family, or caregiver are not educated about availability of community resources, patients may inappropriately use the emergency department for minor problems. Because resources are often limited for this category of clients, case managers must familiarize themselves with the community resources that serve the elderly. The goal of any case management plan must be to maintain or enhance the client's level of function and allow him or her to function in the least restrictive environment.

Despite the fact that the elderly client often needs help and assistance, this level of care is rarely considered skilled. In reality, it is nothing more than maintenance or custodial care or assistance with activities of daily living. Unfortunately, custodial or maintenance care is not reimbursable by the elderly person's primary health care payer—Medicare. Therefore geriatric case management planning involves finding appropriate resources that are cost-effective and financially affordable. Because the elderly are often vulnerable to exploitation or abuse, case managers who work with geriatric clients must be constantly alert for the signs and symptoms of abuse and neglect.

Chapter Exercises

1. List some of the many skills it takes to serve as a geriatric case manager.
2. Define what elderly means.
3. List the many components to a geriatric assessment and why this depth of information is important.

www.governmentguide.com—Government guide to services for seniors

www.aoa.dhhs.gov/aoa/stats/profile—Department of Health and Human Services Administration on Aging

www.agingstats.gov/chartbook2000—Federal Interagency Forum on Aging

www.fda.gov/oc/olderpersons—FDA website on information for the elderly

www.health.org/govpubs/mpw002/index. htm—National Clearinghouse for Alcohol and Drug Information

www.loaa.org—the League of Older Americans Area Agency on Aging

www.aarp.org—American Association of Retired Persons

www.nal.usda.gov/fnic/pubs/old.htm—Food and Nutrition Information Center

www.usgovinfo.about.com and then *http://usgovinfo.about.com/blssaprimer. htm*—Provides the reader with social security information

www.ssa.gov—Social Security Administration

www.census.gov/Press-Release/www/2000/cb00-187.html—U.S. Census Bureau

www.seniors-site.com/home/sitemap.html—Provides a variety of links to services for seniors or caregivers

www.cdc.gov/ncidod/eid/vol7no2/ strausbaugh.htm—CDC website with information about infections in the elderly

www.gericongress.com/—Links professionals to websites that are related to information pertinent to older persons as well as on-line courses for education related to older persons

www.nlm.nih.gov/medlineplus/seniorshealth general.html—National Library of Medicine website for senior health care information; this website also links to the National Institute of Health for Seniors (*www.nihseniorhealth.gov/*)

www.macmcm.com/ags/ags4.htm—Medical Association Communications on pain management in the elderly population

REFERENCES

1. Cassel CK: Why physicians need to know more about aging, *Hosp Pract (Off Ed)* 35(10):11, 2000.
2. Cuellar N, Butts J: Caregiver distress: what nurses in rural settings can do to help, *Nursing Forum* 34(3):24, 1999.
3. Kinsella A: Telehealthcare under PPS: tools to make it work, *Home Healthcare Nurse* 19:579, 2001.
4. Hill C: Caring for the aging athlete, *Geriatric Nursing* 22(1):43, 2001.
5. Davidhizar R, Shearer R: Helping elders adjust to losing autonomy, *J Case Management* 6(1):53, 2000.

Pharmaceuticals and Enteral Therapy

Marilyn Stebbins, PharmD, and Gregory Speicher, PharmD

OBJECTIVES

- To understand the differences between hospital and outpatient prescription drug benefits and formularies
- To recognize the different sources for drug information and determine which source is appropriate for specific drug information queries
- To identify strategies that the case manager can use to decrease out-of-pocket prescription expenses
- To identify the criteria that determine whether enteral therapy is medically necessary and therefore a covered benefit

PHARMACEUTICALS

Over the past two decades a significant portion of the technological advances in health care has involved pharmaceuticals. Not only have an increased number of new medications come on the market but also many new indications have been identified for older medications. In fact, over the past decade the Food and Drug Administration (FDA) has increased substantially the number of new drug approvals and has created a fast-track system for pharmaceutical manufacturers so that the approval process can be expedited. This has not come without a price, however, in terms of both cost and utilization. From a financial perspective, we have seen double-digit increases in pharmaceutical expenditures, while at the same time prescription drug coverage for individuals appears to be shrinking and out-of-pocket expenditures are increasing. From a utilization perspective, we have seen more drugs available and more indications for drugs, and therefore an increase in polypharmacy, which can place the patient at risk for adverse drug reactions and drug interactions. This chapter includes information that will be useful to the case manager in both the acute and nonacute settings. Discussed are the different types of drug coverage and formularies for oral, injectable, and experimental drugs; evaluation of medication histories; drug information resources; and strategies to assist in the war against rising drug costs.

Prescription Drug Coverage
Formularies

Prescription drugs are a covered benefit for most health insurers (including Medicaid) but not for Medicare, which has never covered outpatient prescription medications. The drug benefit varies among and within health insurers, however, and usually the drug choices are limited to those on a list of covered medications called a formulary. The patient's financial responsibility for the purchase of medications on the formulary takes the form of a copayment that is either a percentage of the actual cost of the drug or a fixed amount. Interestingly, two patients may be the same age and have the same health insurer and the same doctor, yet have very different drug benefits. This can make the case manager's job very difficult, as he or she may be dealing not only with patients with different health insurance plans but also with a vast number of different formularies.

As drug expenditures have increased, they have come to represent a much larger proportion of the total health care dollars spent by health insurers. To remain financially solvent, insurers have chosen different tactics to contain drug costs. Two of the most common strategies are to limit the formularies and to increase copayments. If the insurer chooses to limit the formulary to contain costs, a case manager may find that many medications a patient is taking are no longer covered. Several things can be done to help patients when this occurs. Most health insurers have an appeals process for drugs that are not covered. To get coverage for a given medication (when it is medically necessary and other alternatives have been exhausted), the physician is required to obtain prior authorization. This prior authorization process typically is frustrating for physicians, but the case manager can serve as facilitator. All health plans have medication prior authorization departments, and the case manager, on the behalf of the physician, can obtain the criteria for prior authorization. When the criteria are known and are considered in framing the appeal, the chances of receiving prior authorization are increased.

Another strategy that appears to be gaining acceptance is the elimination of formularies and the institution of tiered copayment structures. When a tiered structure is in place, the patient's access to drugs is no longer limited by whether or not the drug is on the formulary. Most drugs are available but with variable copayments. An example of a three-tier copayment structure is shown in Table 19-1.

Under this tiered structure the patient bears a greater financial burden but is not denied access to medications. The need for prior authorization is eliminated. Of note, some medications still are not covered in the tiered structure, such as medications to enhance life-style and cosmetic agents.

Medicare

As stated previously, Medicare does not provide an outpatient prescription drug benefit. The exceptions to this include coverage of pain medications for patients in hospice programs, coverage of immunosuppressive agents after organ transplantation, and coverage of some oral chemotherapy agents. Because Medicare lacks an outpatient drug benefit, many older persons supplement their Medicare benefits with Medicaid or supplementary insurance such as "medigap" policies, or turn to Medicare HMOs to obtain drug coverage. Unfortunately, the qualifications for Medicaid participation are quite stringent, medigap policies that offer drug benefits have become prohibitively expensive, and Medicare HMOs have either capped

TABLE 19-1
Three-Tier Copayment Structure

Tier	Drugs	Copayment
1st	Generic drugs	$5
2nd	Preferred brand-name drugs	$15
3rd	Nonpreferred brand-name drugs	$35

their drug benefits at a low rate, instituted generic-only drug benefits, or completely pulled out of specific counties. This lack of drug coverage for Medicare patients poses particular challenges for case managers, because the case-managed elderly population tends to be taking more medications than are younger cohorts. Alternative funding sources to assist patients are discussed later in this chapter.

Inpatient and Outpatient Formularies

The distinction between outpatient drug formularies and inpatient formularies is important. These two most often are very different. Hospitals purchase drugs independently of the health care insurer and have their own formularies. This becomes significant because, as a patient transitions to and from the outpatient setting and the acute-care setting, medication use can be interrupted, often at a time when it is most critical. This interruption occurs when the patient belongs to a health plan that has a specific formulary which determines the outpatient drug regimen, but upon hospital admission the patient is prescribed agents different from those in the outpatient regimen that comply with the hospital formulary. Therefore, the patient's regimen may potentially change twice in association with one hospitalization, once on admission and once again on discharge, when the patient returns to the original outpatient regimen. Another potential problem that can occur is that the patient may be sent home with prescriptions for medications that were on the hospital formulary but are not on the formulary of the outpatient health plan. If these agents are not covered by the patient's health plan, the patient must pay the full price of the medication, return to the hospital to get prescriptions for medications that are covered, or simply go without the medications. Case managers in the acute-care setting can facilitate a seamless transition of care by ensuring that

discharge medications are covered by the patient's health insurance.

Investigational and Experimental Drugs

Investigational or experimental drugs (those drugs not yet approved for widespread use by the FDA) are generally not covered by insurers. As a rule the FDA requires drugs to go through four phases of trials to prove the drug's safety and efficacy in treating a particular clinical condition. Three of these phases must be completed before the FDA approves a drug. The fourth phase occurs after the drug has been approved and marketed, and these latter trials are generally performed to obtain more safety and monitoring data. A case-managed patient may very well be taking an investigational drug in a phase III clinical trial. Typically the medication and laboratory costs are covered by the study. The case manager must assist the patient once the study is complete, however, to ensure that the patient's medication needs are being met once administration of the investigational drug is stopped. Often the drug may have received FDA approval by the time the study is complete. In this situation, the case manager may need to work with the health care payer to ensure that the drug can be continued and will be covered. This can be a challenge because, as stated previously, the fact that a drug is approved for a given indication does not guarantee that the health care payer will cover its use. In the event that a case-managed patient needs an investigational drug and is not eligible to receive it through a clinical trial, the health care payer may allow reimbursement for the drug. This reimbursement may be possible either through outright approval, through special approval granted by the medical director, or through use of an extracontractual process. The key to obtaining coverage is to provide sufficient data on clinical efficacy and cost-effectiveness to support the use of the drug.

Off-Label Use

Another situation that the case manager may encounter is the off-label use of medications. Off-label use of a medication differs from investigational use of a medication because a drug being used off label has been approved by the FDA; however, it has not been approved for the specific indication for which it is being administered. This is not an uncommon practice, yet it can present obstacles when the case manager is trying to get the medication covered by the health insurer. An example of a drug that was commonly used off label is captopril. The FDA originally approved the administration of this drug for hypertension; however, it was being used off label to treat congestive heart failure long before it was approved for this indication because there was good clinical evidence in support of this use. To get a medication covered for off-label use, it is necessary to present clinical evidence (studies) to the payers that supports the drug's safety and efficacy for the given indication or to prove that it is the community standard to use the medication for that indication. The approval process for off-label uses may involve obtaining prior authorization and is similar to the process for obtaining approval for use of an investigational drug.

Injectable Medications

With recent advances in biotechnology and the advent of the Human Genome Project, there are notably more injectable medications approved for use. Injectable medications can be divided into two classes: self-injectable drugs and office-injectable drugs. Self-injectable medications are those injectable drugs for which a prescription is written and filled at a pharmacy for administration at home by the patient or a caregiver. The classic example of a self-injectable medication is insulin. This class of medications is rapidly expanding to include drugs such as Imitrex (sumatriptan), Peg-Intron (interferon-α_{2b}), Lovenox (enoxaparin), Betaseron (interferon-β_{1b}), Avonex (interferon-β_{1a}), Copaxone (glatiramer), Enbrel (etanercept), Epogen (epoetin-α), and Neupogen (filgrastim). These drugs have revolutionized the management of migraine headaches, hepatitis, deep venous thrombosis, multiple sclerosis, rheumatoid arthritis, anemia, and neutropenia. The costs of self-injectable medications far outweigh the costs of oral medications, however, so the use of these drugs is heavily restricted by health care payers. Interestingly, most of the self-injectable drugs (insulin is the exception) are not covered by the pharmacy benefit. Of note, although self-injectable drugs are considered outpatient medications, Medicare covers a select few of these drugs. These include Miacalcin and Calcimar (calcitonin salmon), osteocalcin, erythropoietin (for end-stage renal disease), and low-molecular-weight heparin (Lovenox, Fragmin [dalteparin], and Innohep [tinzaparin]). Case managers will find that many health care payers have contracted out self-injectable drug services to specialty companies that determine the guidelines for approval, manage the prior authorization process, and handle distribution of the drugs. Although these medications represent a small volume of prescription drugs, they account for a large portion of the cost. Case managers may find that a large number of their patients are taking self-injectable drugs because these medications are used to treat conditions often encountered in case-managed patients. Because this is an evolving category of medications, the rules regarding them are also changing, and the coverage may be quite different among different health care payers. Each health care payer also has different mechanisms for the distribution of these medications. Most of the companies with whom the payers have contracted provide the self-injectable drugs to the patient's home via overnight mail delivery; however, through contracts with local pharmacies, all have provisions for patients who may need the medications immediately. The case manager may need to facilitate the procurement process when the patient has an urgent need for self-injectable medications. See the case study in Box 19-1.

Familiarity with Drugs

Drug Names

In dealing with pharmaceuticals, a source of confusion for health care providers as well as the lay public is the naming of drugs. The reason for the confusion is that many drugs carry multiple names. A patented brand-name drug has not only a trade name given it by its manufacturer but also a chemical name or generic name. Brand name medications have generic names even if the drug is not available in a generic version. One example is the drug Prilosec. Prilosec is the brand name of the medication; however, the drug was developed under the generic name omeprazole. The fact that it has a generic name does not mean that it is manufactured by a generic drug company and is available for a lower price. Generic drug manufacturers can produce the generic compound of the drug only after the patent of the brand-name manufacturer has expired. Only then will many different companies make and market the drug (which will be available under the generic name, such as omeprazole, but will be manufactured by many different generic drug companies). When there is competition in marketing the generic compound, the price of the drug falls.

Drug Information

Since the advent of direct-to-consumer advertising, the public has become increasingly inquisitive and educated about drugs. This makes it important for health care providers to become familiar not only with the names of medications but also with the indications for them, the standards of care for their administration, and their costs. Unfortunately, it is very difficult to find all of this information in one resource. Many drug information pocket guides are available. A guide should be found that is arranged in a way that makes it easy to find the particular type of information desired. Information that is available

---

BOX 19-1
Case Study of Self-Injectable Medication Procurement

A case-managed patient with a severe disease goes through the process to qualify for participation in a clinical trial involving a self-injectable drug that is FDA approved. However, the drug is not FDA approved for this particular indication. The patient is not accepted into the trial because the patient's condition is not severe enough to meet eligibility requirements. The case manager tries to assist the physician and the patient in obtaining prior authorization for the investigational use of this medication. Because this self-injectable drug does not appear on the health plan's list of covered self-injectable medications, the health plan advises the physician and the case manager to try to obtain authorization through the medical group's utilization management department (the medical group is a capitated group and may bear responsibility for the cost of self-injectable drugs not covered by the HMO). An authorization request comes to the medical group's utilization management department. The physician is asked for clinical evidence (results of clinical trials) proving the drug's efficacy. The cost of the drug is $50,000 per year. The available clinical evidence involves eight patients (case studies). The case study results were promising and prompted the clinical trial. The medical director of utilization management for the medical group denies the request, citing lack of clinical evidence. The case manager then works with the study coordinator to see once again if the patient might be eligible to enroll in the study. The patient goes to the study site for testing, and it is determined that the patient's condition has deteriorated and that the patient is now eligible for inclusion in the study. The cost of the drug is now the responsibility of those managing the clinical trial.

in most drug references includes the following:

- Drug name(s)
- Indications for use
- Mechanism of action
- Drug interactions (as well as other interactions, such as those involving food, laboratory tests, and diseases)
- Adverse effects
- Contraindications and precautions
- Dosing and administration

The *Physicians' Desk Reference (PDR)* is one of the most commonly used drug information resources. The information contained in this book is similar to that in drug package inserts. Not all drugs are listed in the *PDR*. Drug manufacturers pay to have their package insert information included in this reference guide. The *PDR* contains color pictures of drugs as well as the names, addresses, and telephone numbers of drug manufacturers. Another frequently used resource is *Drug Facts and Comparisons*. This reference not only has specific drug information but also provides comparative information about drugs within specific classes. It also includes important patient education information that may be valuable to the case manager. The publisher Lexi-Comp is another useful drug information source for health care providers. Lexi-Comp has a suite of drug information resources called the Clinical Reference Library. This library includes, but is not limited to, a drug information handbook for the health care practitioner, a handbook for nurses, and other specialty-specific drug information handbooks. In deciding which resource book is preferable, the most important considerations are that it contain the information important to the individual case manager and that it be arranged in a manner that makes sense to the user.

Unfortunately, most drug resource guides do not contain drug pricing information. If drug pricing information is important, the case manager can obtain monthly updates on commonly prescribed drugs from the *Drug Topics Red Book Update*. The most direct way to obtain drug pricing information for patients is to call the patient's pharmacy and request the information. Most pharmacies are happy to look up the prices of medications and contact the case manager or the patient with the information.

Another way to obtain drug information is via the Internet. Individual drugs can be looked up by brand name or generic name using a search engine. Search results will usually link to the pharmaceutical manufacturer's website. On this website can be found the drug's package insert information. Also available on the Internet is electronic drug information that can be downloaded to handheld devices such as the Palm Pilot. Most of these databases can be purchased for an annual fee; some are available at no charge. The software program ePocrates Rx is a drug information resource that is free to health care providers and can be downloaded to handheld devices. It is also one of the few resources that provides comparative pricing information.

In some instances the case manager may have a drug information query that is not easily answered from a drug information handbook. If a school of pharmacy is located in the area, it may have a drug information center that is open to health care providers either through a local number or a toll-free number. These centers are designed to answer more complicated drug information questions and generally provide referenced answers.

The FDA can also serve as an important drug information source for the case manager. If questions arise about whether a drug has been approved, the case manager can call the FDA's toll-free number. The FDA not only approves drugs for general use, it also approves other items, services, and devices. Thus, it is an excellent resource for information and clarification on therapeutic interventions.

Useful drug information resources are listed in Table 19-2.

Polypharmacy

The term *polypharmacy* implies misuse of multiple medications. The dilemma of polypharmacy is one that case managers face daily. With the advent of direct-to-consumer marketing and the increased availability of new prescription, herbal, and over-the-counter medications, the chance for polypharmacy increases. The aging of the population has contributed to the problem, because older people experience more health problems and consume more medications. The addition of even more medications to combat the effects of existing medications also exacerbates the situation. The consequences of polypharmacy are serious and numerous and include emergency department visits and hospitalizations due to inappropriate dosing, drug interactions, and duplicate therapy, all of which lead to escalating yet avoidable health cares costs. A solution to this complex problem cannot be achieved by any one health care discipline, and a multidisciplinary approach is required that tackles medication misadventures where they occur, in the hospital and in the home. The case manager is in a position to serve as the facilitator in combating polypharmacy. Several steps can be suggested by the case manager:

TABLE 19-2
Drug Information Resources

Resource	Information Available
Physicians' Desk Reference (PDR) Website: www.PDR.net	Manufacturer and product category Phonetic spelling for each listing Warnings Usage information Dosage Adverse reactions Clinical pharmacology Key to controlled substances FDA use-in-pregnancy ratings Drug interactions Contraindications Full-color photographs cross-referenced to the drug Manufacturers' telephone numbers and addresses All other FDA-required information
Drug Facts and Comparisons 2002 Pocket Edition Drugs listed by therapeutic class Websites: www.factsandcomparisons.com and www.drugfacts.com	Therapeutic class Drug name Product table Black box warnings Indications Administration and dosage Actions Contraindications Warnings Precautions Drug interactions Adverse reactions Various comparative tables

Continued

TABLE 19-2
Drug Information Resources—cont'd

Resource	Information Available
Lexi-Comp's Clinical Reference Library *Drug Information Handbook for Advanced Practice Nursing*, ed 3, 2000-2001 Drugs listed in alphabetical order Website: www.lexi.com	Drug name Drug interactions Therapeutic category Food/alcohol interactions Generic availability Effects on laboratory values Pregnancy risk factor Adverse reactions Use during lactation Overdose/toxicology Administration Related information Oral drugs Intravenous drugs Various comparative tables and guidelines
ePocrates Rx 6.0 Available for download to handheld device Website: www.epocrates.com	Use Pharmacodynamics/kinetics Warnings/precautions Mechanism of action/effect Formulations Contraindications Dosage for adults, children, elderly patients, patients with renal impairment Monitoring laboratory tests Monitoring and teaching issues Restrictions
FDA Website: www.FDA.gov	Information on products the FDA regulates Drug information Drug approvals Generic drug availability

FDA, Food and Drug Administration.

- Have the patient or a family member count the number of medications (prescription and over the counter) that the patient is taking regularly or as needed. If the patient is taking multiple medications or sees more than one physician, recommend that the patient or family member ask a pharmacist to perform a medication regimen review. This review should cover drug interactions, duplicate therapy, and recommendations for simplification of the medication regimen to drugs that can be taken once or twice daily, if possible.
- Ask the patient's primary physician to function as a gatekeeper for all medications, even those prescribed by other providers. Ask the primary care provider to consider the pharmacist's recommendations.
- Suggest that the patient use a single pharmacy that employs a computerized program to scan for drug interactions, duplicate therapy, and allergies. The pharmacy should also offer medication counseling and support in adherence to drug regimens as mentioned earlier.
- Be sure that the patient carries a comprehensive medication list at all times and presents it when any new medication is prescribed. The list should be presented if the patient is

hospitalized and should be updated with any changes that might be made upon discharge from the hospital.

Drug Utilization Review

In addition to utilization review for medical and mental health conditions, many health care organizations have a drug utilization review (DUR) process. The DUR process was originally designed to look at drugs with high utilization and/or cost. Of late, however, DUR has come to incorporate drug safety data such as adverse reaction reporting. DUR data are collected and analyzed, and findings are reported. Typically DUR reports include the following:

- Overall drug utilization and cost
- Reports of adverse drug reactions
- Patterns of drug utilization, drug costs, and physician prescribing practices
- Opportunities for physician and health care provider education
- Information on the timing of and targets for re-review

The ultimate goal of DUR is to develop cost-effective drug education programs that are focused on quality.

War Against Rising Drug Costs

Many different approaches can be taken in waging the war against rising drug costs. Throughout this process it is important for the case manager to act as an advocate for the patient. Being a patient advocate takes patience, attention to details, and a genuine interest in the patient's well-being. Without an advocate, most patients are lost and often will stop taking an expensive medication if it puts undue strain on their finances.

The first step in this endeavor is to determine the patient's budget, medication expenses, and insurance status. The case manager should obtain information on the patient's household income (including wages, Supplemental Security Income benefits, and pension), liquid assets, and the manageable medication budget. A complete list of the patient's medications should be compiled, including the actual out-of-pocket costs for each medication. When the case manager investigates the patient's insurance status, the patient's drug benefits should be documented, including covered medications, formulary, associated copayments, and potential dollar limits on drug benefits. Typically, patients will fall into one of three categories: those who have recently had a change in their drug coverage, those who have reached their benefit maximum, and those who have little or no drug coverage. Patients should also be screened for supplemental drug coverage by other sources such as TRICARE or Medicaid. Occasionally, patients have drug coverage that they are not using or that they do not know they are entitled to receive.

The case manager should determine the amount of savings needed for the patient to meet his or her budget. It should be evident which medications are accounting for the majority of the patient's medication expenses, what types of interventions will be ideal in the given case, and for which patient assistance programs a patient might qualify. Each strategy offers a different return on investment, so the case manager must decide how much time to allot for each case. Some strategies take very little effort to implement, while others are extremely time consuming. Knowing what savings are necessary, what areas to target, and what the patient's income is, the case manager can develop an appropriate strategy. Fortunately, most patients, regardless of income, will benefit from maximizing the use of generic medications, splitting pills, and using a mail-order pharmacy.

As prescription benefits shrink and patients' out-of-pocket expenses increase, the use of generic medications becomes an important strategy. Maximizing the number of generic drugs in any regimen can save patients with and without drug coverage 50% to 70% of drug costs. Unfortunately, many brand-name drugs do not have generic equivalents. When considering a switch to a generic drug, a case manager may consult a pharmacist to determine equivalency. The final switch must be made by a physician.

For patients without drug coverage, splitting pills of brand-name medications can save up to 50% of the price of the drug. Many drugs are priced at a flat rate for all available strengths and can be easily split using a pill splitter. These devices are inexpensive and safe, and can be purchased at any pharmacy. Pill splitting will provide cost savings even for medications that are not flat-priced as long as the higher-strength formulation of the medication is less than twice the cost of the lower-strength formulation (Table 19-3).

The important point is that the case manager must know where to obtain pricing information for medications. One source of this information is the *Drug Topics Red Book*. Also, all pharmacies have pricing information that is available upon request and which they must provide by law. The case manager must determine whether the patient is capable of splitting pills. Pill splitting requires that the patient be fairly highly functioning or have reliable caregiver support. Some pharmacies presplit medications when they are dispensed. The case manager must confirm with the patient that he or she has a reliable means for splitting the medication if this route is chosen (i.e., the patient has a pill splitter and can operate it). This type of intervention may require the help of a pharmacist, and a physician must rewrite the prescription to accommodate the change.

For patients with a drug benefit offering mail-order services, automatic savings of 30% can be obtained on covered medications. This 30% savings is due to the fact that mail-order pharmacies offer patients a 90-day supply of medication for two copayments instead of three (one copayment per 30-day supply is usually required by conventional pharmacies). This can provide significant savings if patients have high copayments. Health insurers require the use of specific mail-order companies, however. All health insurers require completion of special forms to initiate this process, but the forms are easily obtained from their respective customer service departments. Patients may have problems adjusting to this new system, but most embrace it in time and find it to be a convenient way to obtain their medications. This approach does require planning and forethought by the patient or caregiver, however, and may not be suitable for everyone. Also, to be a prime candidate for these programs, patients must be taking medications long term. Another way for patients to save even more is through Canadian mail-order services. The favorable exchange rate and price fixing by the Canadian government can provide significant savings on brand-name medications.

Patients with limited incomes are likely to be eligible for assistance pro-

TABLE 19-3			
Example of Pill-Splitting Cost Savings			
Drug	Strength	Signature	Cost/mo
Monopril	40 mg	Take 1 tablet daily #30	$26.43
Monopril	80 mg	Take 1/2 tablet daily #15	$13.21

grams. To determine qualification, the patient's income is compared with the federal poverty guidelines (Figure 19-1).

Patients with incomes less than 1 to 1.5 times the federal poverty level may qualify for Medicaid. It is important to ask if the patient has ever enrolled in or been eligible for Medicaid coverage. Some patients may be eligible but may be unaware of the program. The qualification process is slow at best and is complicated by confusing forms and legal technicalities that often deter patients from applying. Patients often need support and help from an advocate throughout this process to ensure completion. Patients may also need a source of affordable medication during the time the application is being processed. Patients eligible for Medicaid either will be covered in full or will have a share-of-cost benefit. Share of cost means that the patient has a deductible that must be met each month before Medicaid coverage begins. This share of cost varies and can be substantial.

Often the working poor are uninsured for prescription drugs and are unable to afford necessary medications. The pharmaceutical industry has provided assistance for these cases in the form of industry-sponsored patient assistance programs (PAPs) that furnish free medications to qualified patients otherwise unable to afford the medication. These programs may provide an emergency drug source for patients who are uninsured and unable to afford retail medication prices.

Each industry-sponsored PAP is different and has its own intricacies that must be learned. The more the programs are used, the easier they are to understand and the less work they require. The best programs provide an immediate supply of medication to patients and either enable them to continue to use their local pharmacies or send the medications directly to the patients' homes. The forms are simple and easy to complete, and can be photocopied and faxed to the company. The best programs permit the patient to obtain a 90-day supply of medication and allow a year's worth of refills. These programs usually require minimal documentation and have generous, clearly defined eligibility requirements.

The more labor-intensive programs have complicated forms that are obtainable in limited supply only by special

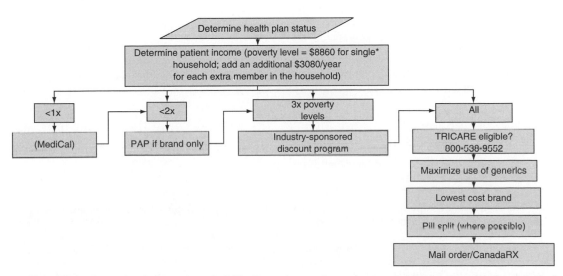

Figure 19-1 Chart for determining eligibility for patient assistance programs (PAPs). *Poverty levels based on 2002 figures.

request to the company. The medication is sent directly to the physician's office after several weeks of processing and shipping. The office must then contact the patient for pickup after the drug is received. Challenging programs require continued, unprompted follow-up by the patient and advocate, and require detailed documentation of income, medical expenses, and insurance eligibility. These programs often have very stringent or undefined eligibility criteria as well.

Participation in PAPs can be time consuming and frustrating for patients and physicians. Patient advocates are the key to the successful use of these programs. Acting on the patients' and physicians' behalf, advocates serve as mediators with the drug companies to ensure that all the necessary forms and documents are completed properly.

Some useful approaches to reducing the patient's drug costs are illustrated in the case study in Box 19-2. Figure 19-2

BOX 19-2
Case Study of Drug Cost Management

A 66-year-old woman complains that she is unable to afford her medications each month. Upon review of her medications you note that she takes the following drugs and purchases them for the listed prices:

Pravachol 40 mg qd	$124
Ramipril 10 mg bid	$79
Premarin 0.625 mg qd	$21
Levoxyl 0.075 mg qd	$8
Flovent 110 fg 2 puff qd	$85
Albuterol prn	$8
TOTAL	$325/mo

This patient states that she has no brand-name drug coverage but that generic drugs are covered with an $8 copayment. She has a monthly income of $957 and feels that she could afford to spend only $100 a month on medications, because rent and car payments consume a significant portion of her income. What suggestions do you have as a case manager?

Levoxyl and albuterol are generic medications covered under her benefit. Upon review you find that Ramipril and Premarin could be replaced with the generic substitutes enalapril and estropipate, respectively. Pravachol has no generic substitute but is one of the most expensive medications in its class. A less expensive alternative might be Lipitor, which could be split for even further savings. Finally, Flovent, manufactured by GlaxoSmithKline, is available through a PAP you have worked with before, and you know that she may qualify for the program.

After talking with a pharmacist you arrive at conversions to keep the patient's medications as close as possible to the original regimen. You then discuss these changes with her primary care provider. The physician writes new prescriptions and signs the required paperwork for the PAP. Her new medication regimen is as follows:

Lipitor 20 mg ss qd	$54
Enalapril 10 mg bid	$8
Estropipate 0.625 mg qd	$8
Levoxyl 0.075 mg qd	$8
Flovent 110 fg 2 puffs qd	$5 (PAP copayment)
Albuterol prn	$8
TOTAL	$91/mo

You and the patient complete the forms for the PAP and discuss the planned changes. The patient is concerned, but you assure her that you will work closely with her in the coming months and that you can resolve any new issues as they arise. You then discuss the possibility of the patient's using a mail-order pharmacy for her medications, because under her health plan she can obtain 90 days' worth of generic medication for two copayments instead of three. This could save her an additional $11 a month. For now she declines because she has used the same pharmacy for 50 years. But she is happy with her new medication costs.

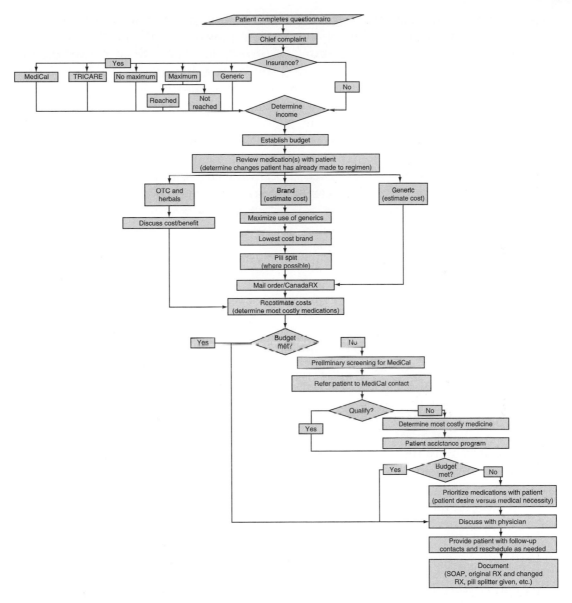

Figure 19-2   Processes and strategies to decrease drug costs. *OTC*, Over the counter; *Rx*, prescription; *SOAP*, subjective data, objective data, assessment, and plan.

details processes and strategies to decrease drug costs.

ENTERAL THERAPY FORMULAS

Because of the nature or severity of their illness or injury, many patients in case management require enteral therapy. In enteral therapy, a liquid nutritional product is administered into the gastrointestinal tract via a nasogastric, jejunostomy, or gastrostomy tube. Many health care payers cover enteral therapy as a benefit, but many others do not. Health care payers that do allow the therapy as a benefit cover it if documentation supports its medical necessity. This therapy is medically necessary if one of the following situations applies:

- The patient has an anatomic reason for an inability to swallow.

- The patient has a disease or pathologic lesion that prevents him or her from maintaining weight despite oral feedings.
- The patient requires the formula as the sole source of nutrition.

As a rule, enteral feedings that are excluded from coverage are those used for nutritional supplementation to boost protein or caloric intake. This exclusion also covers formulas that are the mainstay of a dietary plan, but for which no pathology exists to support their use. Unfortunately, formulas are also frequently excluded from coverage because they are over-the-counter items, and regardless of the mode of administration or the purpose of the formula, the general argument is made that "the patient needs to eat and groceries are not a covered benefit."

When enteral therapy is needed, the case manager must seek approval for coverage through the extracontractual process or procure funding for the formulas from alternate sources (e.g., Medicaid, the Title V Children's Medical Services program, or the local Commodity Supplemental Food Program of the Women, Infants, and Children [WIC] program). Coverage is necessary because far too often the cost of the formula exceeds the amount that the family, regardless of income, spends monthly for food.

Costs and Procurement

Because enteral therapy formulas can be costly, it may be necessary to negotiate discounts or per diem rates if the health care payer has agreed to pay for the formula and a nonnetwork provider is used. As with pharmaceuticals, if the health care payer's network pharmacies or infusion companies can supply the formula, the patient may be required to use these providers. If reimbursement for the formula is denied because its use does not meet the criterion of medical necessity, the patient and family can purchase it from any provider they desire.

When the formula is not available from providers in the health care payer's network and the patient receives the formula via a pump or by gravity flow, case managers must strive to ensure that reimbursement for the formula and all related supplies is made at an all-inclusive rate. Such a rate covers not only the formula but also all equipment and supplies, as well as any nursing visits needed for direct patient care or education of the family or caregiver in how to administer the formula and use the equipment.

Services Required

Patients receiving enteral therapy frequently require the skilled services of nurses from a home health agency or infusion therapy company. Such services are necessary until the patient and the family can demonstrate competence in administering the formula and changing the tube. The frequency and number of visits vary depending on the circumstances of the individual case. In most instances, however, this type of skilled nursing care is required only during the first 7 to 14 days; rarely are visits necessary beyond this time. If more visits are required, the actual notes relating to the need for skilled care must be reviewed carefully, and continuation of coverage is determined on a case-by-case basis.

Other services that must be incorporated into the case management plan include radiologic services, which are necessary to monitor tube placement. Depending on whether or not the patient is homebound, use of a local company offering portable radiologic services may be required, which raises costs.

For infants for whom the feeding tube is inserted and removed with each feeding, families or caregivers must be taught not only how to insert the tube but also how to recognize the signs and symptoms that the tube has been placed improperly. In such cases, skilled nursing visits from a home health agency or infusion company may be required (and are considered medically necessary) for a longer period than the initial 7 to 14 days typical in other cases.

Most gastrostomy feeding tubes or gastrostomy feeding buttons require little maintenance once the wound heals. Naturally, patient variables can affect the frequency of services. After the techniques of wound care and formula administration have been mastered, however, the care required may no longer be considered skilled. Care of such patients may then be classified as custodial. Also, because gastrostomy tubes are inserted directly into the stomach, little skilled care is actually required for enteral therapy via this route, even when the formula is administered through a pump. Because of these factors, the care required for gastrostomy tube feedings is rarely classified as skilled care, and rarely is this level of care reimbursable by health care payers.

The most common methods of enteral therapy administration are mechanical feeding pumps or feeding bags with gravity flow. Although most formulas are over-the-counter items, their bases vary—some have a powder base and must be mixed with fluid, whereas others are already prepared as liquid products. Likewise, the formula constituents vary for different reasons and depending on the diagnosis. For instance, Pulmocare liquid is a lactose-free product that is frequently used for patients with respiratory problems, whereas TraumaCal liquid is frequently used for patients sustaining multiple injuries or burns. Infants and children with chronic diarrhea, malabsorption, cystic fibrosis, short gut syndrome, and other symptoms related to allergies or sensitivities to corn or cow's milk may require Soyalac, Isomil, or Alimentum. Although case managers are not involved in writing the orders for the formulas, they must be aware of and have contact with procurement sources and nutritional counseling experts if families

are to be linked with the most cost-effective supplier of the formulas.

In rare instances, formulas can be homemade. This is the least desirable method of procuring formulas, however, and its feasibility depends on the specific requirements of the case. If costs are an issue and access to alternate funding is nonexistent, the case manager may wish to explore this option with the attending physician. If home preparation of the formula is possible, then it is critical to link the patient and family with a qualified dietitian who can calculate the nutritional needs accurately and assist the family in assembling the correct formula ingredients.

With few exceptions, administration of enteral formulas can be accomplished using clean technique rather than sterile technique. Switching to a clean technique as soon as the patient is deemed medically stable by the attending physician is a method of achieving cost savings, because it eliminates the costs of gloves and sterile water. Naturally, if a patient is confined to a facility, sterile technique is required, but the associated services are included in the overall daily rate.

■ SUMMARY

Prescription drug costs represent one of the fastest growing shares of the health care dollar. Although many payers provide prescription drug coverage, medication use and costs must be carefully monitored and tracked in the case management plan. It will benefit the case manager to be familiar with commonly prescribed drugs and to have good drug information resources available.

Medication costs for case-managed patients can become exorbitant, because the need for pharmaceuticals is often long term or lifelong. As payer and patient resources become less available, it is important for the case manager to be familiar with cost-effective medication strategies and with any PAPs that may be available.

Because of the nature of their disease or injuries, many patients require enteral feedings. Although many health care payers allow reimbursement of the costs of enteral products, equipment, and supplies if the formula is administered by tube and there is documentation supporting its medical need, other payers do not. In contrast, the cost of formulas administered by mouth and those used primarily as a nutritional supplement may not be reimbursed by any health care payer.

Although many formulas are considered over-the-counter products, they may also be available from infusion companies; if they are, the family has a "one-stop shop" for all their feeding supplies. While many formulas are over-the-counter products, they are costly and vary in price, so if their use is to be covered by the health care payer, the case manager must be prepared to negotiate a discounted rate or a per diem rate. When the patient requires enteral feedings after discharge home, the services of an infusion company or home health agency are commonly needed until the caregiver can demonstrate competence in administering the formula and changing the tube.

Chapter Exercises

1. Explain why pharmaceutical industry–sponsored patient assistance programs do not provide free brand name medications to all Medicare-eligible patients.

Suggested Websites and Resources

www.rxassist.org—Contains information about the federal poverty level and detailed information on individual

PAPs (including eligibility requirements, contact and processing information, and forms that can be downloaded)

www.phrma.org—Provides an annually updated PAP directory and some useful links

www.canadarx.net—Easy-to-use Canadian mail-order company; site contains pricing information as well as all the required ordering information

www.needymeds.com—Catalog of available programs listed by drug name and manufacturer; also has some useful references to several information resources that could be convenient to use; overall it has a format similar to that of rxassist.com but might be easier to navigate

Drug Topics Red Book Update—Published monthly by Medical Economics, $99 for a 1-year subscription (800-783-4903); a comprehensive reference for current packaging and new information on high-volume prescription and over-the-counter drugs

www.rxassist.org—RxAssist Plus; a useful patient and medication tracking software program that interfaces with the Internet so that the appropriate patient assistance forms can be completed quickly; also has a tickler feature that reminds the case manager to provide the patient with timely refills and reenrollment into programs when due; the software is provided free to nonprofit organizations, governmental agencies, and individual clinicians who care for the uninsured

BIBLIOGRAPHY

Beers MH: Explicit criteria for determining potentially inappropriate medication use by the elderly, *Arch Intern Med* 157:1531-1536, 1997.

Bertram GK, Katzung BG: *Basic and clinical pharmacology*, ed 6, Stamford, Conn, 1995, Appleton-Lange.

Block SS: *Disinfection, sterilization and preservation*, ed 4, Philadelphia, 1991, Lea & Febiger.

Depiro JT, Talbert RL, Yee GC et al: *Pharmacotherapy: a pathophysiologic approach*, ed 4, New York, 1999, McGraw-Hill.

Fisher JE: *Total parenteral nutrition*, ed 2, Boston, 1991, Little, Brown.

Food and Drug Administration: *FDA consumer from test tube to patient: new drug development in the United States*, Pub No FDA 95 3168, Washington, DC, 1995, U.S. Department of Health and Human Services.

Kaiser Family Foundation: *Prescription drug coverage for Medicare beneficiaries by Health Alternatives Inc.*, Menlo Park, Calif, 2001, The Foundation.

Koda-Kimble MA, Young LY: *Applied therapeutics: the clinical use of drugs*, ed 7, Baltimore, 2001, Lippincott Williams & Wilkins.

Lehne RA: *Pharmacology for nursing care*, ed 2, Boston, 1994, Little, Brown.

MacLeod SM: *Pediatric pharmacology and therapeutics*, St Louis, 1993, Mosby.

Pinnell N: *Nursing pharmacology*, Philadelphia, 1996, Saunders.

Rice R: *Manual of home health nursing procedures*, St Louis, 1995, Mosby, pp 3–12.

Rombeau T, Coldwell MD: *Clinical nutrition, parenteral nutrition*, ed 3, Philadelphia, 1993, Saunders.

Stanhope M, Knollmueller RN: *Handbook of community and home health nursing*, St Louis, 1992, Mosby.

Williams SR: *Nutrition and diet therapy*, ed 8, St Louis, 1997, Mosby, pp 447–478.

Postacute Care

CHAPTER
20

Introduction to Postacute Care

Peggy A. Rossi, BSN, MPA, CCM, CPUR

OBJECTIVES

- To identify at least four areas of the postacute arena used when discharge from an acute-care setting approaches
- To identify the key criteria for entrance into acute rehabilitation
- To distinguish between skilled and custodial care and cite examples of each
- To distinguish the two key payers for long-term care
- To identify the primary reimbursement methods for the postacute care arena as well as what coding mechanisms are used

As stated earlier many patients followed by case management will be in the acute stages of their illness. By its definition of case management, the American Nurses Association supports the fact that the case manager identifies and facilitates options for care across the continuum:

Dynamic and systematic collaborative approach to providing and coordinating health care services to a defined population. It is a participative process to identify and facilitate options and services for meeting an individual's health needs, while decreasing fragmentation and duplication of care and enhancing quality, cost-effective clinical outcomes. The framework for nursing case management includes five components: assessment, planning, implementation, evaluation, and interaction.[1]

Facilitating and managing the vast array of alternative levels of care within today's health care system can be daunting.

The variety of continuum of care services available across the United States is immense. Although some areas of the country offer a full continuum of care—acute-care hospitals, acute rehabilitation facilities, subacute units, skilled nursing facilities (SNFs), long-term acute-care units, home health agencies, hospices, and outpatient services—other parts of the country are less fortunate. In these less fortunate areas even the nearest acute-care hospital is miles away, and so are the other levels of care. Thus the challenge of case managers, utilization managers, and discharge planners to facilitate appropriate care in the most cost-effective setting begins with the resources available in the patient's geographic location (Figure 20-1).

Not surprisingly, some postacute care plans will go very smoothly and others not so smoothly. In the latter cases, patients or families often:

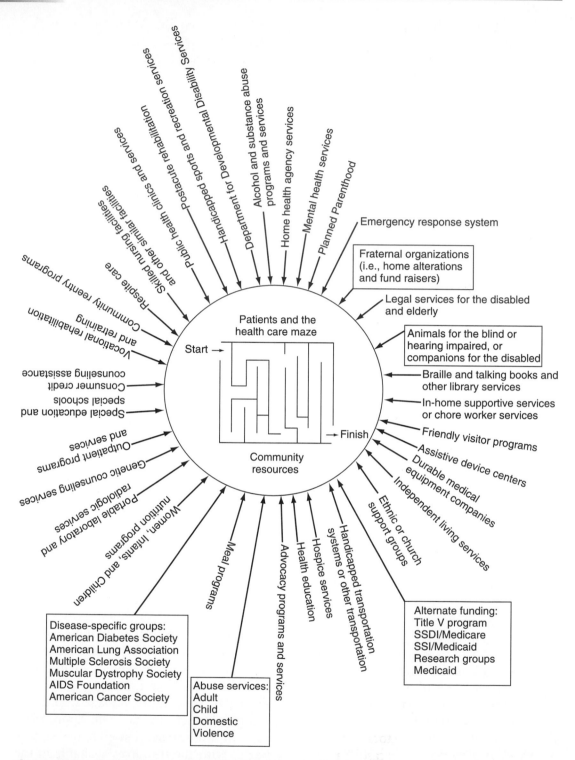

Figure 20-1 The health care maze. *SSDI,* Social Security disability income; *SSI,* Social Security income.

- Want more than can be provided (either by the provider or what their insurance will pay for)
- Refuse alternative options when first choices are not available
- Are unwilling to accept the fact the patient may be as doing as well as can be expected

Unfortunately, planning cannot always go smoothly because the patient's care needs are too great for the available resources or, worse yet, the funding is not there to pay for what is needed. Funding is one limiting factor that is encountered by most patients or families. They often fall into the "gray area"—not enough money to pay for services but too much to qualify for Medicaid or other public funding programs.

In general, when planning for ongoing care families want assurance that their loved one will be well cared for. To ensure the plans go smoothly, one must make every effort to ensure the patient and family are part of the planning process and that they are provided as much information as possible. Although many discharge planners and case managers may have given descriptions of the following to their patients or families, these reasons are those most often given for dissatisfaction with SNF care:

- They expect the level of care and level of staffing to be comparable to that of the acute-care facility.
- They want a private room when one is not available.
- They are unhappy when the facility cannot accommodate a separate telephone line into the patient's room.
- They are unhappy when visiting hours are limited to specific times of the day or evening.

Any or all of these factors may have been communicated as the case manager worked with the patient and family, but because patients and families are often in crisis, they do not always hear all that is said. Therefore it is wise to have brochures or other written literature available as a handout to validate what has to be communicated.

Many reasons exist for why discharges or transfers to the next level of care falter. There are also times when even the most experienced case managers will be thwarted in their efforts to implement an effective plan. If case managers are not careful and do not evaluate every detail, care may be improperly implemented and the whole plan can be destabilized. Experience does allow for the ability to overcome many obstacles, regardless of what they are or when they occur.

As cases are readied for discharge or transfer to another level of care, always assess the case for the following points:

- Were all needs identified and addressed?
- Were the patient and family involved with the care planning, were they pressured or coerced, or did they go along with the plan simply because of a lack of understanding?
- Were the patient and family realistic about the care plans? If not, were they in denial or unrealistic of expectations and options?
- Were interventions effective, or were there areas that might require revision at the next level of care? If so, was this communicated to the accepting provider?
- Were goals met?
- Did the patient and family get as much information and guidance as could be given for the situation?
- Were all services implemented and delivered as planned?
- Were problems with the implementation of the patient's care plan identified that could be barriers or issues that could affect other patients? If so, what steps are necessary to correct the situation?
- Was a suboptimal discharge plan arranged because of a lack of funding or available resources?

- Did the patient or family refuse the options given? (Remember that if the patient or family makes "bad choices," that is their decision if they are legally competent to make such choices.)
- Did case management efforts provide an opportunity to improve or optimize the outcome or quality of life for the person or family?

HOME PLACEMENT VERSUS OUT-OF-HOME PLACEMENT

In the United States, more than 12 million people need assistance with everyday activities because of a chronic condition such as heart disease, mental retardation, or AIDS. Although the majority of this population is approximately three fifths elderly, about 5.1 million working-age adults and 400,000 children with long-term care needs live in institutions or communities. Most live at home or in small community residences. The majority of caregivers are female relatives. With the graying of America these statistics may support the doubling of the need for long-term care. Estimates are that the number of elderly needing assistance could reach 14 million by 2020 and 24 million by 2060. In 1994, one in eight Americans was 65 years or older. By 2030, one in five will be a senior citizen. But the graying of America is not the only reason for this growth. Technology has meant that premature babies survive in greater numbers, children born with severe defects live, and people survive catastrophic accidents in greater numbers.[2]

Ensuring safe linkages and transfers to the various levels of care as the patient progresses or regresses is one primary function of case management. When working with patients and their families for the next level of care, all levels of care, alternative options, and financial resources for payment must be explored. Although the goal is usually to keep the patient at home, this is not always possible or realistic.

Goals

The first stage in coordinating and developing care planning is to establish realistic goals. The goals established should include what is to be accomplished and within what time frame. As goals are established it is important to create both short-term and long-term goals. Keep in mind that most goals are composed of many small goals and tasks that must be met for successful completion of the main goal. Missed details can delay or hinder success. Also, what might be a priority to the case manager or health care team may not be a priority to the patient or family. Always seek patient and family input as goals are established.

Planning

Before long-term placement is considered many caregivers continue to provide care far beyond their limits—physical, emotional, or realm of knowledge (e.g., a spouse who has never cooked or cleaned may be faced with new tasks for which he or she is totally unprepared). Even when moving to a residential care or other long-term care facility is the most realistic avenue to take, many people have a difficult time with such decisions. The biggest reason lies in "giving up their independence." Regardless of reasons, one of the most heart-wrenching experiences for all parties involved is considering or actually making a move from home to a facility. Unfortunately, many people do not plan ahead for such moves. Moves often occur in the worst possible environment—one made during a crisis event.

If planning and the move can occur in a noncrisis atmosphere, the confusion, emotional trauma, volatility, and upheaval of a sudden move can be avoided. When planning for a move to long-term care, a meeting with all persons or family members involved is by far the best technique to use. This meeting allows an opportunity for all to discuss their feelings about the move. Depending on the volatility of the decision, involvement of a third party or counselor may be required. Although this may be necessary for the impaired person, in most cases it is needed to alleviate the feelings of guilt associated with putting a loved one in "one of those homes." Education about placement allows quality to become foremost for all parties—the caregiver as well as the person being placed.

When exploring options for patients ready for discharge from an acute hospitalization, the first option should always be home. However, in some cases this is not possible or even medically appropriate or safe. The final selection made will hinge on many factors. If home cannot be an immediate alternative, a subacute care facility or an SNF may be appropriate. The decision will naturally depend on the availability of the facility and the patient's actual level of care and skilled need requirements.

If a case manager plans accordingly he or she could begin the process for patient care in a subacute facility, subsequently moving the patient to home care. It was this leveling of care that allowed the U.S. health care system to adjust to the otherwise major challenges created by diagnosis-related groups for hospitalized patients. Some health care professionals believed the federal government created—or at least provided—a loophole to permit providers to care for patients in some level of care. This concept resulted in the growth of subacute care programs. In addition, home health care boomed in the 1990s as a service for hospitals and permitted hospitals to move patients into their homes earlier than before. Different levels of reimbursement also defined different levels of care. Unfortunately, the service lines that case managers became comfortable with have now deteriorated under the Balanced Budget Act of 1997 (BBA) and the changes the act created for reimbursement.[3]

Although the case manager still has to evaluate what must be explored and implemented for postacute care, many more factors should be considered, especially with the changes in admission practices for postacute care agencies and facilities. This situation is further compounded by the critical shortage of nurses at all levels of care. Instead of having various levels of care and benefit reimbursement levels available, case managers today no longer have a smooth path to move patients along the continuum of care. Case managers must figure out when an SNF can be used, when a much more limited home care benefit can be used, or when hospitalization remains the appropriate answer. All this must be done while trying to ensure professional licensure is not affected and avoiding lawsuits.[3]

Today a case manager working for an insurer must be more alert to the needs of the patient because patients can now sue their health care insurers. Case managers have a duty to discover what level of service an organization can provide before using the service. Thus from a legal perspective, the case manager must know that providers have differing abilities to serve the patient. This knowledge requires the case manager to delve into the matter and identify the different levels of care patients require and match them to what each organization can provide.

The case manager can no longer safely assume such a comparison of service levels exists before directing patients to use a particular service. He or she must be prepared to develop a comparison of service levels, both from an inquiry and persona experience, to qualify a provider in relation to the patient's needs. This is necessary because the landscape of reimbursement has also changed and has placed increased responsibility on the case manager to identify whether any given agency selected can provide the level of care required. As a case manager gains experience in his or her community's postacute care resources, this knowledge will validate the varying levels of quality of care provided by various health care providers. Case mangers should document these levels to justify their decisions regarding what level of care was required and what provider was used.[3] From a legal perspective, a case manager has the duty to know the capabilities of the providers used and to document quality issues so appropriate changes can be made. Case managers who use poor judgment and fail to recognize quality issues while still using the agency for referrals will most likely find themselves with legal problems.

Case management companies must construct guidelines for use by their case managers that can help evaluate the overall situation as it relates to patient care. The judgment the case manager uses in rendering care to patients is foremost. The patient's care and safety are the focus and cannot be lost.[3]

After Medicare's prospective payment system took effect, the long-term care industry soon identified areas where reimbursement failed to cover expenses. In some parts of the country local facilities found that they could no longer provide complex medical care at the rate paid by Medicare under what is called the resource utilization group (RUG) system. Many SNFs now turn away the sickest Medicare patients who require postacute care. Consequently these patients are unable to access care when needed in their own communities. If care is found, it is often in a facility outside their own communities.[4]

Before any move for out-of-home placement, it is wise to encourage families to visit all appropriate facilities and make notes. A practice such as this allows the family to compare available options and gain insight into finding the most appropriate setting for their loved one. However, because managed care requires contracted providers and shorter length of stays, family members are often not given an opportunity to visit or select an SNF of their choice. These situations often arise when the impaired person requires the following:

- A ventilator
- Extensive wound care
- Special rehabilitation needs
- Intravenous feedings
- Isolation because of an infection
- Special equipment such as a pressure sore bed
- Care for dementia or behavior problems

Selecting any postacute care facility depends primarily on four elements:

1. Costs and the ability to pay
2. The level of care required and the facility's ability to provide it
3. Functional capabilities of the impaired person
4. Behavioral issues

The worksheet in Figure 20-2 is designed to assist a case manager in capturing patient-specific care needs as well as serve as a guide for determining the appropriate level of care.

Skilled Versus Custodial Care

Many payers use Medicare's criteria for determining skilled or custodial care. Medicare's criteria are possibly the most recognized and used of all criteria for such purposes. As in the determination of skilled versus custodial care, many insurers will only reimburse providers when care is provided in a Medicare-certified facility. To qualify for reimbursement, the patient must have daily skilled care at least 5 days per week. Because most skilled facilities offer services only 5 days per week, this frequency constitutes "daily skilled care" under Medicare criteria.[5]

Skilled Care

Under Medicare's criteria, decisions for coverage of skilled care must not be based on diagnosis, number of diagnoses, type of condition, degree of functional limitations, rehabilitation potential or prognosis, or the fact that someone is living with the patient. Decisions must be based on medical necessity, the complexity of prescribed service, and whether it can be performed

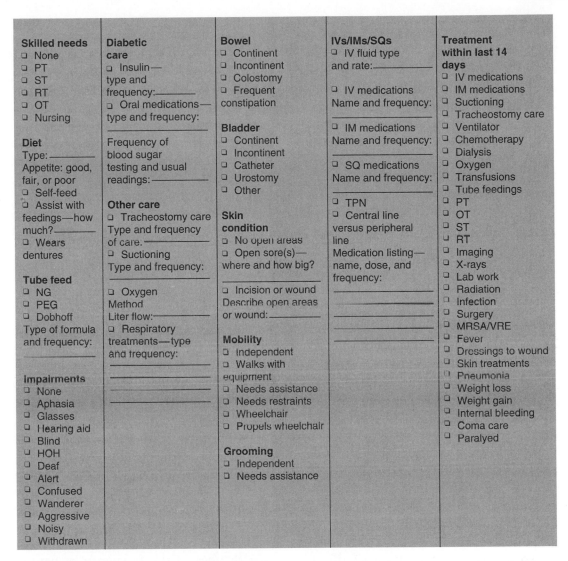

Skilled needs
- None
- PT
- ST
- RT
- OT
- Nursing

Diet
Type:_____
Appetite: good, fair, or poor
- Self-feed
- Assist with feedings—how much?_____
- Wears dentures

Tube feed
- NG
- PEG
- Dobhoff
Type of formula and frequency:
_____

Impairments
- None
- Aphasia
- Glasses
- Hearing aid
- Blind
- HOH
- Deaf
- Alert
- Confused
- Wanderer
- Aggressive
- Noisy
- Withdrawn

Diabetic care
- Insulin—type and frequency:_____
- Oral medications—type and frequency:
_____

Frequency of blood sugar testing and usual readings:_____

Other care
- Tracheostomy care Type and frequency of care._____
- Suctioning Type and frequency:
_____
- Oxygen Method
Liter flow:_____
- Respiratory treatments—type and frequency:
_____
_____
_____

Bowel
- Continent
- Incontinent
- Colostomy
- Frequent constipation

Bladder
- Continent
- Incontinent
- Catheter
- Urostomy
- Other

Skin condition
- No open areas
- Open sore(s)—where and how big?
- Incision or wound Describe open areas or wound:_____

Mobility
- Independent
- Walks with equipment
- Needs assistance
- Needs restraints
- Wheelchair
- Propels wheelchair

Grooming
- Independent
- Needs assistance

IVs/IMs/SQs
- IV fluid type and rate:_____
- IV medications Name and frequency:
_____
- IM medications Name and frequency:
_____
- SQ medications Name and frequency:
_____
- TPN
- Central line versus peripheral line
Medication listing—name, dose, and frequency:
_____
_____
_____
_____
_____

Treatment within last 14 days
- IV medications
- IM medications
- Suctioning
- Tracheostomy care
- Ventilator
- Chemotherapy
- Dialysis
- Oxygen
- Transfusions
- Tube feedings
- PT
- OT
- ST
- RT
- Imaging
- X-rays
- Lab work
- Radiation
- Infection
- Surgery
- MRSA/VRE
- Fever
- Dressings to wound
- Skin treatments
- Pneumonia
- Weight loss
- Weight gain
- Internal bleeding
- Coma care
- Paralyed

Figure 20-2 Worksheet to determine appropriate level of care. *PT,* Physical therapy; *ST,* speech therapy, *OT,* occupational therapy; *RT,* radiation therapy; *NG,* nasogastric; *PEG,* percutaneous endoscopic gastrostomy; *HOH,* hard of hearing; *TPN,* total parenteral nutrition; *IV,* intravenous; *IM,* intramuscular; *SQ,* subcutaneous; *MRSA/VRE,* methicillin-resistant staphylococcus/vancomycin-resistant enterococcus.

safely or effectively under general supervision or direct involvement of licensed nursing or rehabilitation professionals.

Skilled care involves services that are so inherently complex they can only be performed safely and effectively by, or under the supervision of, professional or technical personnel. Licensed professionals include registered nurses, licensed vocational or practical nurses, and physical, occupational, or speech therapists. Skilled nursing care or skilled rehabilitation therapy involves observation, assessment, judgment, supervision, documentation, teaching, or direction of specific tasks and procedures necessary to establish and execute the treatment plan. For coverage to continue, the patient must make steady and significant functional improvement. In addition, Medicare and health care payers impose the following constraints on services or treatments:

- They must be performed in accordance with a physician's written order.
- They must be reasonable and necessary for the illness or injury.
- They must be consistent with the nature and severity of the client's illness or injury.
- They must be provided according to acceptable standards of medical practice.
- They must be reasonable in terms of duration and quantity.

The purpose of this section is to highlight the basic issues that help a case manager determine whether a service is skilled or custodial (Figure 20-3). In many cases the answer will not be clear-cut. As a result all factors of the case must be considered before a final determination of skilled or custodial care is made. When in doubt, always review the case with the medical director or a physician advisor from a related specialty (e.g., a neurologist for neurology cases).

In making the determination that a patient requires skilled or custodial care, case managers must examine the current level and complexity of care and whether the patient needs medical supervision or direct care. Next, if these services were discontinued, would there be a significant probability (as opposed to possibility) that the patient would be at risk for complications or further need for acute care? Just because a patient has a caregiver who is trained to provide the care does not necessarily mean that the care is not skilled. Similarly, just because a patient has a spouse or other relative or significant other does not mean that person can provide the required care. In both cases, skilled professionals may be required indefinitely for either supervision or actual provision of direct care.

Custodial Care

Custodial care is a classification health care payers use to denote the point at which coverage is terminated. At this point, coverage from the payer ceases. Custodial or personal care is defined as "the services or personal care necessary to assist the patient in meeting activities of daily living (ADL)." Assistance with ADLs does not require trained medical or paramedical personnel. Most health care payers cover only short-term skilled care and no custodial care. If termination occurs for other reasons (e.g., exhaustion of benefits, patient reaches maximum day limit), other funds must be sought to continue payments for required services. ADLs include such activities as:

- Getting into and out of bed or a chair
- Turning over in bed
- Exercising to enhance overall fitness
- Toileting
- Bathing, dressing, and other personal hygiene activities
- Feeding (including gastrostomy feedings) or preparation of special diets
- Supervising or administrating medications that normally could be self-administered

The custodial care level can also be appropriate when a patient has ceased to make functional improvements for whatever reason or when there are no longer any changes in the frequency or type of care for a technology-dependent patient. The greatest confusion in reimbursement arises when a patient's care moves to the maintenance level or the caregiver has mastered the care techniques.

Unfortunately and often erroneously, health care payers often view any skilled care that has been mastered by caregivers to be custodial; benefits for this care are then usually terminated. The designation of custodial care in no way implies that the care being rendered is less than skilled; it means only that such care is not reimbursable because it is maintenance care. When termination of benefits occurs, the case management plan must include some form of monitoring to ensure that family

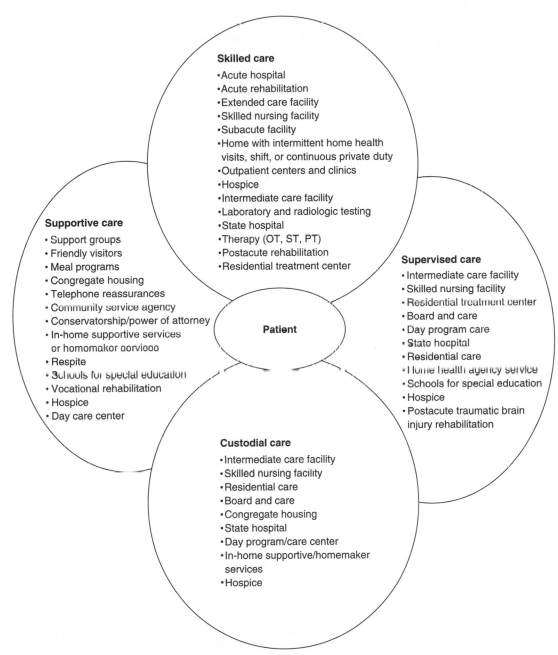

Figure 20-3   Levels of care. *OT,* Occupational therapy; *ST,* speech therapy, *PT,* Physical therapy.

members or other caregivers stay abreast of the skilled care techniques that may have to be implemented as the patient's condition changes. As a rule, a custodial care determination is not precluded by the fact that the patient is under the care of a physician or that services are ordered to support the patient's condition.

Custodial care can be further defined as the care rendered to a person who is mentally or physically incapable of providing the care to himself or herself. It is also appropriate for any person who requires a protected, monitored, or controlled environment, whether at home or in an institution.[6] In most cases, custodial care is the care required to support or sustain a person and allow the person to have ADLs provided (Box 20-1).

Authorizations

Regardless of the provider's name and reputation, if the case manager's organization does not allow on-site case management to ascertain firsthand the actual care rendered and responses to care, alternative measures to monitor care levels must be in place. This alternate mechanism for monitoring care is to have policies and procedures in place that set limits on the number of visits per authorization and, more importantly, the required documentation that medically justifies skilled need. Payment should be made only for the level and intensity of skilled care required.

A case manager's caseload will contain a variety of patients with varying skilled care needs and the resultant hours required for each. Although some patients will require daily or twice daily skilled visits from the home health agency, others will require 24-hour care. Even others will require a mixture of skilled and custodial care. The decision of the amount, frequency, and level of skilled care must be based on the intensity and severity of the illness or injury and the intensity and complexity of needed services. A key element that supports ongoing authorizations will be documentation that outlines intensity and severity.

Most insurers use a variety of nationally recognized criteria from which to base coverage determinations. Additionally, some insurers also apply their own internally developed criteria (generally developed with the insurer's network specialty providers). The three most widely recognized and nationally accepted criteria are as follows:

1. Interqual
2. Milliman Care guidelines
3. Medicare

As a coverage determination is made, the reviewers apply the criteria to the information (usually documentation obtained from the professional providers) they have been able to gather on the patient and his or her care needs.

DOCUMENTATION: THE KEY TO SUPPORT DECISIONS

Although the Centers for Medicare & Medicaid Services dictates the use of reporting tools such as Minimum Data Set (MDS), RUGs, and Outcome and Assessment Information Sets to support payments, private insurers and managed care

---

BOX 20-1

Examples of Custodial or Unskilled Care and Supportive Services

Services related to ADL are considered custodial, unskilled, or supportive and include:
- Administration of routine oral medications, eye drops, and ointments
- General maintenance of ostomies
- Routine care of indwelling bladder catheters and self-catheterization
- General maintenance and methods for treating incontinence, including use of diapers
- Wound care for uninfected postoperative or chronic conditions
- Prophylactic and palliative skin care, including bathing, application of creams or lotions, and repositioning
- Use of heat for palliative purposes
- General administration of oxygen and other inhalation treatments after the initial phase of teaching and treatment adjustments are completed
- General supervision of exercises including ROM
- Assistance with eating, dressing, and toileting

organizations use other documentation to support decisions. Documentation needed includes:

- Diagnosis and all existing conditions relevant to the care plan
- Level of need, frequency of visits, and by which discipline (e.g., special care, need for special dressings or supplies, laboratory testing, observations, teaching, long- and short-term goals)
- Any changes in condition and related physician's orders and changes in the care plan
- Responses to treatments and recommendations for changes in the care plan
- Referrals and coordination with other community agencies and reasoning
- Medication type, frequency, and any side effects
- Type of diet, hydration, and response
- Rehabilitation plan and ADLs

Documentation is the key to coverage when services might be considered skilled. In such cases the medical complication and special services required must be performed, supervised, or observed by a professional and documented by the physician's orders and in the nursing and therapy notes. Without it, there is nothing to support and justify skilled care. *(If it's not documented, it didn't happen!)*

When documentation is poor and continued benefit coverage or coverage for the next level of care is in question, it may be helpful to interview staff. Additionally, on-site evaluation of the patient may be needed to observe firsthand what the patient can and cannot do.

Barriers to Discharge or a Move Through the Continuum

For optimal results of any move, the patient and family must be involved in the process. With any patient, but especially one who will be admitted to a facility outside the immediate area, communication must be open and as frequent as necessary to educate the patient and family of the positive aspects of the placement. If the discharge or move is to be to a facility (other than acute rehabilitation), the family must be encouraged to visit, evaluate, and report back to the case manager or discharge planner. Because most facilities require admission paperwork to be completed before admission, the family must take the time to do this.

In reality the biggest barrier to discharge or transfer to other levels of care in the continuum is the fact that funds and benefits are frequently limited, exhausted, or just not available. Following are other barriers that a case manager must continually face.

Developing a case management plan for the discharge or move of a patient through the continuum of care, especially for patients who require complex care or depend on technological equipment, requires considerable lead time (several days to weeks). This time frame is necessary for a variety of factors:

- The patient and family must gain full acceptance of the plan.
- Training must be adequate and at least started.
- Resources must be located and ready to assume responsibility for the patient's level of care.
- Barriers must be identified.

Locating an appropriate facility or agency is often a labor-intensive process. Many facilities or agencies must be called before an appropriate one is located. When care is complex, placement will likely be outside the patient's immediate home area. Regardless of the event that lead to the barrier, case managers must be familiar with the levels of care available in a given community, throughout the state, and sometimes nationally.

Finding Other Funding

One of the biggest barriers to discharge planning or move of a patient through the continuum will be the lack of funding. Few patients need skilled services over the long term. Depending on any number of factors, a patient may move quickly from skilled to custodial care. When this happens the health care payer terminates coverage. Consequently, the family must be prepared to pay privately or enroll in Medicaid to ensure continued payment of long-term care costs.

The wisest plan approach to use in preparing patients and families for long-term care is openness and honesty. An open discussion of actual costs of care and what the family's financial responsibilities are likely to be is vital. Although some case managers will find this a difficult process, the easiest way is to open the discussion with comments such as, "because the costs of care are not always covered by the insurance benefit package, we need to discuss seriously your financial abilities to pay for the excluded or limited services. Although you do not need to tell me what you have in the bank, I want to give you some costs of services. From this discussion you can tell me if you can afford to pay for the care, how long you can pay, or if we need to work on a referral and application to Medicaid." Then proceed in telling them approximate costs of the services and supplies that are excluded or limited. Another way to start the conversation is to say, "The costs of _____ (e.g., SNF care) will be _____ (give them a global local range of costs). With these costs in mind, do you think you can pay for the services, or will a referral for Medicaid be necessary?" This is a "nitty-gritty" speech. It has to be done and is a part of good planning.

Unfortunately, those hardest hit when care is long term or out-of-pocket costs are high are those in the income bracket of "too little and too much." When this occurs, the patient or family must exhaust the majority of assets before possibly qualifying for Medicaid. Even then, some families continue to have "too much." Families who have too many assets to qualify but not enough to pay privately are the ones who really struggle.

If the patient remains eligible for health plan benefits, entitlements obtained as a result of eligibility for public funding or other entitlement programs will be used as the "payer of last resort." Under this premise, any benefits available from the health care payer must be used or exhausted or the other program is used for paying applicable copayments or deductibles.

ACUTE REHABILITATION

When evaluating a patient for discharge, one of the first considerations for patients with ongoing skilled therapy needs will be the potential for rehabilitation. Rehabilitation aims to restore functional capacity—mental or physical—to the highest level consistent with a patient's illness or injury. Rehabilitation can be provided at various levels of postacute care depending on the person's level and type of injury, level of cognitive ability to follow directions, functional abilities and disabilities, and support systems. Rehabilitation consists of treating and training a patient to maximize the potential for normal living physically, psychologically, socially, and vocationally.

Not all health care payers offer acute rehabilitation as a benefit, and others have strict day and dollar limits. Thus case managers from both the facility and the health care payer must collaborate to ensure that rehabilitation is available. The earlier rehabilitation is started, the greater the likelihood the patient can regain some function and avoid institutionalization or dependency. The overall course of rehabilitation varies with the patient, the premorbid personality, intelligence, education level, and community resources for follow-up care.

The patient's insurance benefit package is key as to whether an ongoing inpatient rehabilitation program will be paid for by the insurer (not all employers or policies cover rehabilitation). Most insurers follow Medicare's coverage guidelines for reimbursement of rehabilitation services. These basic guidelines require a patient to tolerate and participate in therapy for 3 hours per day. If the person has insurance coverage for rehabilitation, admitting diagnoses generally recognized when *recent functional loss* has occurred include:

- Stroke or cerebrovascular accident
- Multiple trauma
- Spinal cord injury
- Traumatic or acquired brain injury
- Amputation
- Other neurologic disorders
- Congenital disorders
- Musculoskeletal disorders
- Chronic pain (generally a specialized program)
- Cardiac disabilities (generally a specialized outpatient program)
- Respiratory disabilities (generally a specialized outpatient program)

Examples of skilled rehabilitation therapy can be found in Box 20-2.

BOX 20-2
Examples of Skilled Rehabilitation Therapy

- Services directly and specifically related to the patient's condition
- Services so technical or complex and sophisticated that they require the judgment and expertise of a licensed professional therapist
- Services that cannot be carried out by therapy aides or other unlicensed personnel

---

Documentation must support the fact that the person was independent in the functions before the insult or injury. Additionally, the physician must likewise document that significant improvement in functional ability is expected within a reasonable time frame.

The key to coverage is when the patient is medically stable, has the mental ability to follow one- to two-step commands, and is able to withstand at least 3 hours of therapy (occupational, physical, or speech) per day at least five times per week. If the patient's only need is occupational therapy, most insurers will not cover an inpatient rehabilitation program. Coverage ceases when the following occur:

- The goals have been met.
- The patient (or family) is noncompliant with the program.
- There is no progress after an adequate trial (if the person's status is questionable at the time of consideration for admission, a trial period of 1 to 2 weeks may be allowed).
- Complications develop and the patient must be transferred back to the acute-care facility.
- A complication develops that prevents participation in the rehabilitation for at least a week but the condition is not serious enough for acute admission. These patients are generally discharged to a lower level of care (e.g., subacute facility, SNF, or home).

The importance of rehabilitation was not recognized until recently. Consequently, many seriously compromised patients were moved to an SNF or a state hospital without benefit of a proper evaluation for the formal structured environment and intensive training an acute rehabilitation program offers. These patients were never afforded the benefit of any attempts at rehabilitation.

Disabled persons constitute a significant proportion of the U.S. population and case managers' caseloads. Because not all disabling conditions are handicapping or permanent, every patient's potential for recovery of some degree of independence must be considered. Naturally not every patient is appropriate for acute rehabilitation. If the patient is not an appropriate candidate for rehabilitation, then consideration must be given to SNF care or care at home. Many patients in this category have had trauma or a severe neurologic insult (e.g., stroke, subarachnoid bleed, hemorrhage) in which their cognitive level of functioning or medical care needs preclude immediate entrance into a rehabilitation center.

Case managers must be familiar with all phases of rehabilitation and with the availability and capability of local and regional rehabilitation facilities. Not all hospitals have a separate licensed rehabilitation unit appropriate for acute rehabilitation. Also, many freestanding rehabilitation units offer specialized care and accept only persons with certain levels of neurologic involvement or spinal cord injury.

Assessments for Rehabilitation

The cornerstone of rehabilitation medicine is a thorough assessment that goes beyond the traditional medical workup. As such, the patient is assessed for the following variables:

- Motivation
- Premorbid functional level and pertinent medical history
- Perception of illness, injury, and expectation for recovery
- Current physical and cognitive functional limits and capabilities, medical condition and stability, dependence on support for feeding, breathing and swallowing, seizure activity, pain, and mobility
- Psychosocial and socioeconomic factors, personality, values, coping skills, and attitudes that figure importantly in affecting the desired outcomes
- Ability to tolerate at least 3 hours of therapy per day
- Prognosis for recovery
- Plans for corrective surgery or reconstruction

During this time the family is also assessed for:

- Premorbid and postmorbid dynamics
- Expectations
- Legal and financial concerns
- Willingness to be trained as caregivers (if one is needed)
- Coping skills
- Attitudes toward the rehabilitation process

Although the primary focus of rehabilitation is the patient, the family must not be forgotten. For many reasons the family will be a key participant in processes and decision-making. When working with the family the team will observe a variety of reactions (e.g., anger, guilt, depression, helplessness and hopelessness, anxiety, denial, and withdrawal or the making of unreasonable demands).

Families need support to help them deal with their initial and ongoing reactions. To help alleviate fears and concerns, the team must maintain open, honest, and frequent communication. It is imperative they know or have the following:

- Resource information
- Advice on placement
- Discharge options
- Alternative funding for long-term care
- Other local community or health plan resources

As the reality of the situation sets in, or as the patient approaches discharge and the prospect of long-term care looms, many other fears and anxieties surface that must be addressed.

Assessment Tools

Measurements of functional health status have long been used in medical rehabilitation to justify the care rendered. Although standard measurements have not yet reached wide acceptance, they are slowly making their way into the assessment processes used by medical case managers. As in the past, many measures used focus on evaluating the degree of assistance patients require to perform ADLs. Common measurement or assessment tools include:

- The Expanded Disability Status Scale as it focuses on mobility
- Two tools used to focus on the effectiveness of the rehabilitation program are as follows:
1. The Level of Rehabilitation Scale used for communication
2. The Patient Evaluation Conference System used for interpersonal skills
- The Functional Independent Measures is used to measure:
  - Self-care
  - Sphincter control
  - Transfers
  - Locomotion
  - Mental cognition
  - Communication
  - Comprehension
  - Expression
  - Social cognition
  - Social interaction
  - Problem solving
  - Memory
- The Pediatric Functional Independent Measures (used for children aged 6 months to 7 years)

Other assessment tools include:

- Karnofsky Performance Status Scale (rates a patient's ability to carry on normal activities)
- Functional Assessment Staging
- Rancho Los Amigos levels of cognitive function
- Glasgow coma scale

Regardless of the tool used, it must also be age specific.

Evaluating Rehabilitation Outcomes

One challenge in evaluating outcomes is determining what consumers consider to be valid measures. The following, although included in Rehabilitation Accreditation Commission standards, appear consistent with consumer requests for postacute rehabilitation and produce a lasting difference in people's lives[7]:

- Length of stay
- Cost
- Functional status, including ADLs (e.g., household, community) and cognitive skills
- Patient/family satisfaction
- Living arrangement
- Level of assistance required
- Employment status
- Psychosocial adjustment, including social and emotional behavior, neurobehavioral functioning, measures of social value, and quality of life

SUBACUTE FACILITY CARE VERSUS SNF CARE

Subacute care facilities, extended care facilities, and step-down units are generally affiliated with an acute-care hospital. All facilities in these categories offer more intensive skilled care than does a general community-based SNF. Subacute care is an alternative for patients who are medically stable but do not require continuous availability of the diagnostic and therapeutic services of an acute facility. However, such patients do continue to require more technical skilled services that can be provided by an SNF. Table 20-1 can assist in determining the appropriate facility for postacute care.

Two years ago subacute care facilities were all the rage. Hospitals enjoyed reim-

Text continued on p. 637

TABLE 20-1
Comparisons of Levels of Care and the Services Provided

Care Requirements	Acute Rehabilitation	Subacute	SNF	Intermediate Care Facility	Assisted Living or Custodial Care
Ongoing medical care but stable for care outside acute facility	Therapy can be complex. Can tolerate 3 hours therapy per day	Treatments or therapy is complex; although therapy might be a part of treatment plan, other medical issues are the primary cause for subacute level of care; treatments are more complex or frequent than can be managed in an SNF; patients often have multiple medical problems that requires ongoing monitoring by registered nurse	Treatment complexities vary but as a rule are no more than once per shift or day. Patients generally are accepted if care skills require less than 3 hours per day to administer.	Patient is medically stable and only requires no more than 1 hour of nursing or medical services daily to maintain medical stability.	Persons in this category are stable. Although this category of patients can require some care, it is maintenance care, supervised care, or care that consists of ensuring ADLs are performed.
Rehabilitation	Patient can tolerate physically and mentally at least two therapy disciplines and at least 3 hours of therapy per day.	Patients can obtain therapy while undergoing treatments for other medical problems.	Therapy is generally limited to daily depending on SNF.	Generally not performed at this level but if so, therapy is administered by trained therapy aides under the supervision of a licensed therapist.	If patient requires therapy, generally this is not a level of care to consider because of safety reasons.
Mobility	Depending on level of injury or reason for rehabilitation, may require complex assistance with any transfers or mobility.	Depending on level of injury or reason for rehabilitation or complexity of other medical treatments, may require complex assistance with any transfers or mobility.	Depending on reason for SNF, may require assistance with any transfers or mobility.	Person able to transfer and ambulate about unit; can use walker or wheelchair.	Depending on the facility, patient can use a walker or wheelchair and can require some assistance with transfers. In most places, patients must be fairly independent.

Respiratory treatments	Some rehabilitation units will accept ventilator-dependent patients for either weaning purposes or for rehabilitation; long-term ventilator dependence is anticipated.	Some rehabilitation units will accept ventilator-dependent patients for either weaning purposes or for rehabilitation; long-term ventilator dependence is anticipated. If without a ventilator but with a tracheostomy, may accept for continued care of tracheostomy and suctioning needs. Suctioning and respiratory care treatments can often be more than four times per day. Can accept persons on oxygen or with inhalation therapy.	Generally limited to persons without treatments more than once per shift. Can take oxygen and some respiratory inhaler therapies.	Generally do not accept persons requiring oxygen or respiratory treatments.	Some facilities may allow portable oxygen units if patient can independently operate unit.
Suctioning with suctioning	Generally can handle persons with needs of more than once per shift.	Generally can handle suctioning if suctioning needs of more than once per shift.	Nonsterile or sterile limited to once per shift.	No suctioning	No suctioning persons
Wound care or dressings	Some facilities may accept patients with wounds that require dressing changes more than once per shift. If patient has complex wounds, unit may require subacute care before admission for acute rehabilitation.	Can perform complex dressing changes and do them more than once per shift.	Some facilities may perform complex dressing changes if not more than once per shift.	Generally limited to simple dressing changes if wound is noninfectious.	May allow, if home health agency nurse does dressing changes and dressings are simple and person is not infectious.

Continued

TABLE 20-1
Comparisons of Levels of Care and the Services Provided—cont'd

Care Requirements	Acute Rehabilitation	Subacute	SNF	Intermediate Care Facility	Assisted Living or Custodial Care
Medications	Can handle complex medications as well as frequent changes to regimen.	Can handle complex and multiple medications as well as frequent changes to regimen.	May be able to accommodate complex medicines as well as changes in regimen. In most facilities, because of the infrequency of physician visits, if medicine regimen contains frequent adjustments to program, admission will depend on facility and staffing capabilities. Can do oral, intramuscular, and subcutaneous delivery; may take persons with IVs.	Generally limited to oral medications and some subcutaneous (e.g., insulin).	Generally limited to only oral medications, which the person can self-administer with supervision.
Invasive tubes	Can accommodate Foley catheters and feeding tubes if multiple tubes may require patient to be at subacute level of care.	Can accommodate Foley catheters, G tubes, J tubes, ileostomies, colostomies, and feeding tubes as well as some wound vacs and other invasive treatment modalities.	Can accommodate Foley catheters and feeding tubes; may be able to handle other tubes, including wound vacs.	Generally persons with tubes and care are not accepted.	Persons with tubes are not allowed. Some may allow if person is self-sufficient with tube care and use.

Nutrition	Can accommodate total parenteral nutrition, IV fluids, feeding tubes, and total feeding-dependent patients.	Can accommodate total parenteral nutrition, IV fluids, feeding tubes, and total feeding-dependent patients.	May or may not accommodate any IVs or total parenteral nutrition.	Persons must be able to go to central dining room and feed self. No feeding tubes.	Persons must be able to go to central dining room and feed self. No feeding tubes. Some may provide meals in person's room short term after an illness.
Mental-cognitive-behavioral	Level of confusion or disorientation admission generally dependent on Rancho Los Amigos or Glasgow coma score.	May be confused or disoriented and require chemical or physical restraints. If psychotic or with a history of alcohol or drug abuse, then not accepted.	May be confused or disoriented and require chemical or physical restraints. If psychotic or with a history of alcohol or drug abuse, then not accepted.	Can accept persons who are confused or forgetful.	May be slightly forgetful but generally not accepted if confused and not a unit designed for Alzheimer's patients.
Education	Teaching needs are identified at admission and are ongoing throughout program because goal of programs is to ensure patient and family self-sufficient in care or at a point the home health agency can continue teaching program at discharge.	Teaching needs are identified at admission and are ongoing throughout program because goal of programs is to ensure patient and family self-sufficient in care or at a point the home health agency can continue teaching program at discharge.	Teaching needs are identified at admission. Goal at discharge is to ensure patient and family are taught the skills needed for ongoing care or at a point the home health agency can continue teaching program at discharge.	Generally little if any training occurs at this level because most care is performed by nonlicensed personnel who are under the supervision of a licensed professional nurse.	Generally no teaching occurs at this level.
Personal hygiene	Can take total care patients. Depending on person's capabilities, as much personal care as needed is provided. Goal is to teach patient self-care skills.	Can take total care patients. Depending on person's capabilities, as much personal care as needed is provided. Goal is to teach patient self-care skills.	Can take total care patients. Depending on person's capabilities, as much personal care as needed is provided. Goal is to teach patient self-care skills.	Personal care can be provided but patients often require minimal help with ADLs. May or may not accept in continent persons.	Many will take persons who require some help with ADLs and personal care. May or may not take incontinent persons.

Continued

TABLE 20-1
Comparisons of Levels of Care and the Services Provided—cont'd

Care Requirements	Acute Rehabilitation	Subacute	SNF	Intermediate Care Facility	Assisted Living or Custodial Care
Equipment needs	Equipment is provided by facility, including arrangements if specialized equipment is needed. If patient needs customized equipment, it will be ordered at that time or before admission.	Equipment is provided by facility, including arrangements if specialized equipment is needed.	Equipment is provided by facility, including arrangements if specialized equipment is needed.	Wheelchairs and walkers might be provided.	Person must bring or have their own.
Ongoing or intermittent testing or imaging	Depending on testing or imaging ordered and frequency, may require patient to be at subacute care before admission for acute rehabilitation.	Depending on testing or imaging ordered and frequency and whether unit is facility based or community based, may require patient remain at acute care until testing or imaging schedule at less frequency.	If testing or imaging at a frequent basis, may require subacute care before admission. If infrequent, generally performed by mobile laboratory or radiation unit.	Generally performed by mobile laboratory or radiology unit or the person might be taken to such units by any mode of transportation.	Person is responsible to obtain from clinic or local laboratory or radiologic unit; may be responsible for arrangements for own transportation.
MD visits	Daily	At least every 7 days	At least every 30 days.	At least every 60 days.	Patient needs to go to physician office or clinic for any medical care.

bursement rules that allowed them to maintain subacute facilities with the cost of care ranging between 40% and 60% less than acute-care settings. Thus, by using subacute facilities, patients could be discharged sooner. Then came the prospective payment system (PPS). PPS, which pays providers on a per diem rate and according to the patient's acuity, changed the game for many providers; subacute care was no exception.

With PPS, subacute facilities have been forced to examine their operations both internally and externally. Some are modifying services and admissions, and others are improving internal operation to improve efficiency and save money. But despite all the negative effects of PPS and the fact that acute hospitals continue to discharge patients sooner and with more complex conditions, the underlying need for subacute care will remain. Subacute facilities will remain economically and clinically attractive as well as a needed link in the continuum of care.

In a report by the Office of the Inspector General in 1998, 58.9% of patients were discharged home, 15.3% to SNFs, 9.8% to home care, 2.6% to intermediate care, and 13.4% to other places. From 1996 to 1998, discharges to SNFs increased by 1.6%, whereas discharges to home health fell 1.2% and to home 1%. Discharges to intermediate care and to other places increased by less than 0.5% each according to the study. Also, according to discharge planners surveyed by the Office of the Inspector General, facilities are requiring more detailed clinical information about patients and are more often coming to the hospitals to assess patients before deciding on admission. Because of additional regulations and paperwork, case managers working with patients who require a subacute facility have to be more diligent in determining if patients are in the correct facilities.[8]

Cuts in subacute reimbursement are driving the growth of long-term care hospitals. Long-term care hospitals are independent facilities in which the patient's average length of stay exceeds 25 days. This is in contrast to hospital-based subacute facility stays, which average 16 to 20 days, and freestanding subacute facilities, with even greater lengths of stay. Although there is some overlap between subacute facilities and long-term care hospitals, the types of patients cared for in each are not identical. As a rule, long-term care hospitals specialize in ventilator-dependent care, complex wounds, and certain cardiac problems.[9]

Because there is very little room for error with PPS, facilities will increasingly rely on case managers to keep cases under funding caps. Slight errors will mean the difference between making a profit and going out of business. As such, case managers, in addition to providing an appropriate discharge plan, will play a key role in final reimbursement. Case managers will be key on the front end by helping determine the process for admission and whether the facility will want to take the patient; they will also be vital during the patient's stay by ensuring monitoring occurs and the length of stay does not exceed the allotted days.

Despite the fact Medicare reimbursement will continue to be their primary payer, many facilities may shy away from the shrinking Medicare reimbursements. In so doing, they will place greater emphasis on accepting only privately insured patients. This is necessary because facilities will have no choice but to adjust their practices to make up lost revenue. They will be required to evaluate the larger picture when determining their target mix. To do this and survive, they must reevaluate their admission criteria, and clinical and administrative practices. The real key will be in their ability to attract high-acuity, private-pay patients if they are to increase

Medicaid reimbursement while offsetting any Medicare losses.

Under the rate structure laid out, subacute facilities will find themselves unable to admit certain kinds of patients. PPS classifies each subacute patient into 44 RUG levels, which determine patient acuity based on the Minimum Data Set (MDS). Facilities receive reimbursement for each patient according to his or her RUG level. The daily reimbursement figure includes both routine and ancillary care. When a patient enters a subacute facility, the clinical staff completes the MDS, which scores acuity and determines the RUG level. The first MDS score and the resulting RUG level determine the reimbursement for the first 14 days. After the 14th day, another MDS is completed, which then determines the score for the 15th through the 30th day. The cycle is repeated until discharge. All staff must be educated about MDS and RUG level importance and its score relative to reimbursement.[9]

Placement

If the patient's care is too complex or is affected by any case variables that preclude home care, facility placement is the appropriate option to consider. Health care professionals involved with discharging patients must be keenly aware of the multitude of postacute care facilities and the care levels provided by each. More importantly, these same professionals must be aware that the patient should be placed in the least restrictive environment that meets his or her needs. With this in mind, the following is a list of postacute care providers (which can be used in whatever sequence responds to the patient's needs) when out-of-home placement is required:

- Acute rehabilitation facility
- Subacute, extended care, or acute facility step-down unit
- SNF
- Intermediate care facility

- Postacute care rehabilitation facility
- Day treatment facility or care center
- Board and care home

As one works with patients and families, the following suggestions will help facilitate the move of a patient when out-of-home placement is required:

- Proximity of the facility to the family to prevent social isolation; as a rule, 30 to 40 miles is the accepted distance, but this must not interfere with placement if the only facility that can provide the needed level of care is farther away.
- Capability of the staff to provide the needed level of care to ensure they can manage care on all shifts.
- Adequacy of staffing to manage the level of care (and willingness of the administration to add additional or specific licensed staff when warranted); this factor must be evaluated before admission.
- Willingness of the administration to train staff when special training is necessary.

Licensure of a facility is also a key element that must be evaluated. To ensure compliance with Title XVIII of the Social Security Act and Medicare's federal conditions of participation, each state has developed administrative codes. These codes set minimum criteria and standards for the various levels of care provided. The state's regulating bodies use these for licensure and standardization of service.

Admission Criteria

What is the difference between an SNF and a subacute care facility? An SNF can be used for long-term placement and care. In contrast, a subacute care facility is designed for short-term care until the patient stabilizes further and can safely be discharged to a lower level of care. An SNF provides care for patients who do not need the full range of services available in an acute-care hospital but who may need

24-hour services or daily treatments provided or supervised by professional nursing or rehabilitation staff.

Centers for Disease Control and Prevention statistics reveal that nursing home residents in 1997 were more disabled and received more services than they did in 1985. This may reflect the availability of alternative services such as home health care, which allows people to postpone or avoid a nursing home.[10]

Once the patient is ready for discharge, one of the first questions will be, "Can the patient be discharged to home, or must placement in a facility occur first?" Unfortunately, placement in an SNF frequently carries a stigma. Many patients and families regard these "nursing homes" as the last resort, a place to die, and a warehouse for the elderly. This reactions often delays placement, and the case manager must take the time to educate everyone regarding the pros and cons of placement.

Case managers have several options to help families get past their fears. First and foremost is to be familiar with local facilities and their special features. Families must be encouraged to visit several facilities, make notes, visit favored ones at various times of the day, and stay attuned to their senses of smell, sight, and hearing as they make their placement decisions. Another technique is to collaborate with a social worker trained in counseling to educate the family in the benefits of placement.

In working with patients needing a subacute facility or SNF, case managers are charged with the enormous responsibility of knowing:

- All the different requirements
- The purposes of every venue
- What facility can best meet the patient's care needs
- The availability of reimbursement
- The legal requirements
- The availability of the facility

- The capacity of the facility
- The patient and family's desires

Staying Abreast

Returning to home is the goal for most case management planning. However, not all patients can go home. Case managers must stay abreast of local facilities, agencies, and other providers of care as well as the levels and types of care each provides. Knowledge of licensure laws and state administrative codes for health care providers is equally important. This knowledge is critical if quality of care is to be maintained. Most placements (except state hospital care and certain SNFs) should always be regarded as temporary, moving the patient from one level of care to another depending on how his or her condition progresses or regresses.

Many levels of care are excluded from the patient's benefit package and from payer coverage. Because care levels can plateau or change to custodial, families must be prepared to assume responsibility for payment. If they are unable to pay, public funding such as Medicaid or other resources must be sought.

HOME CARE

Home health care remains the primary choice of patients and families at discharge. This is often true even when high-technology home care arrangements must be made. Theoretically, if funds are available, a "mini intensive care unit" can be set up in the home.

Health care professionals hear it said repeatedly that home is the best place for patients because they do better in their own surroundings and environment. However, when patients are discharged sicker and sooner and require more complex care, home care can be more expensive than placement. More importantly, it is not always appropriate for every patient. Therefore, when home care is contemplated, five basic factors must be considered. These factors can serve as a decision-making guide. They can serve to assist in determining whether the patient can benefit from home care, whether the cost for such care is reasonable and acceptable to the health care payer, and whether the out-of-pocket expenses for the patient and family are manageable. The five factors are as follows:

1. The patient is ambulatory and can seek care provided by specific outpatient services, programs, or providers.
2. Whether the patient meets the criteria for homebound care and home health care providers can adequately provide the level of care required.
3. The patient's medical, psychological, or psychosocial needs for continued care or supervision can be provided in a home setting.
4. The home environment is conducive to the treatment plan, maintaining quality of care and achieving the desired goals.
5. The costs of the home care plan are comparable to or less than inpatient alternatives (e.g., continued hospitalization in an acute-care facility, SNF, subacute care facility, or rehabilitation unit).

Finding the Right Home Care Provider

Home health, infusion, and durable medical equipment agencies focus on the insured population that requires short-term episodic care and services (e.g., dressing changes, teaching, observation, chemotherapy, respiratory therapy, short-term equipment support). Consequently, finding a qualified agency to accept the technology–dependent patient can be a barrier to establishing a home care plan. This is true when cases are anticipated to require intensive care and services; the care will be costly and possibly long term. If the case manager is not careful in the selection process the provider may see the case as an opportunity to make money.

If an agency is found and the final decision is made that care can safely be rendered within the home setting, the following questions must be addressed:

- What level of care is required? Does the patient's care needs meet skilled or custodial criteria, or will it be a combination of both?
- If custodial, what care and services will be needed and by whom? More importantly, do the patient and family understand they will be financially responsible for this level of care?
- Whether skilled or custodial, what teaching must be given to the patient or caregiver before discharge?
- If the patient and family have selected home care because of guilt (they want to attempt care so they can say they tried), what contingency plan is in place in case of home care failure?
- What other agencies will be needed?
- What equipment and supplies will be needed?
- What other community support services will be needed?

Criteria for Skilled Home Care

Skilled home care is covered when the skill and proficiency of a professionally licensed health service provider is required to achieve the medically desired results. The patient must also be homebound, and care must be required on a daily and intermittent basis (generally this is several times per week). For reimbursement to occur most insurers require the agencies to be Medicare certified.

PPS and Home Care

As required by law, Medicare began paying all home care agencies under PPS as mandated by the BBA and as amended by the Omnibus Consolidated and Emergency Supplemental Appropriations Act of 1998. The new payment system completes the transition from the pre-BBA cost-based system, which encouraged inefficiency, waste, and abuse, according to the Centers for Medicare & Medicaid Services. It will replace the BBA-mandated interim payment system that has been in effect since October 1997 and has dramatically affected the home care industry. Under the proposed system the following will occur:

- Medicare will pay home health care agencies for each covered 60-day episode of care.
- Beneficiaries can receive an unlimited number of episodes of care.
- Medicare will pay home health agencies at a higher rate for those beneficiaries with greater needs.
- Agencies will receive additional payments for an individual beneficiary if the cost of care is significantly higher than the specified payment rate.
- The payment system will use national payment rates and adjustments to reflect area wage differences and the intensity of care required for each beneficiary.
- The payments will encompass Medicare-covered home health services for a 60-day episode of care, including skilled nursing and home health aide visits, covered therapy, medical social services, and supplies.
- Medicare will pay home health agencies separately for medically necessary durable equipment provided under the home health plan of care.
- Payment rates will be adjusted to reflect significant changes in the patient's condition during each Medicare-covered episode of care.
- Medicare will require agencies to provide at least five visits to benefi-

ciaries to receive the full payment for each Medicare-covered episode of care.[11]

With the changes in health care brought on by PPS, the home health care industry has found itself faced with a predicament—consolidated billing. Because the government wants to receive only one bill for all services rendered, home medical equipment companies and home health agencies must work closely together. This requires excellent communication between the case managers if processes are to be streamlined to ensure coordination occurs between all vendors and the physician. Why is one rate important? With high-tech home care it is common for patients to require a minimum of three different providers—a home health agency, an infusion agency, and a durable medical equipment company—meaning three different companies and three different rates.

Setting Up the Home Care Program

When setting up a home care program, case managers must understand that for many patients the costs of basic nursing care and the equipment necessary can exceed thousands of dollars per month. Not included in these costs are other charges (e.g., physician home visits, outpatient laboratory or radiologic services, pharmacy charges) for services that will be necessary if the patient's needs are to be met. When evaluating all costs, home care can be far more expensive than placement. Numerous daily visits by professionals (e.g., nursing, physical therapy, speech therapy, occupational therapy, laboratory, radiologic services) requiring multiple out-of-pocket copayments by the patient can make home care financially impossible for many patients. Consequently, out-of-home placement until the patient's condition is medically stable and can be managed more easily at home is usually the best plan.

Types of Services

When setting up home care, there are no set rules as to what type or variety of services a patient may require. For example:

- Arrangements for intermittent skilled services at home may vary (e.g., they may require skilled nursing as well as rehabilitation therapy, or they may require twice-daily dressing changes).
- Some patients will require infusion services that may consist of initial teaching and then ongoing delivery of the necessary supplies. In other cases, if the family cannot be taught or if the drug is complex or requires licensed professional administration, the agency remains responsible for the duration of the infusion therapy.
- Patients receiving skilled care may also need to hire unlicensed staff to assume personal care or homemaker duties (e.g., cleaning, laundry, cooking, shopping).
- Patients, whether skilled or custodial, may need to hire hourly, shift, or live-in professionals.
- Terminally ill patients may need hospice services in any combination of skilled or palliative care modalities.

The key to payment for home health care rests in the patient's homebound status and the level and amount of skilled care required.

Referrals to a Home Health Agency

When the case manager is unfamiliar with a home health agency, the following questions will be helpful to discern the appropriate provider:

- Is the agency certified by Medicare and Medicaid?
- What services does the agency offer?
- What are the costs of services per discipline?
- Is the agency willing to consider a rate negotiation?

- Is the agency willing to bill the insurer, or will the patient be required to pay for services and then submit the claims or bill?
- What are the professional training requirements of the nursing and rehabilitation staff? How many additional hours of training does the agency provide?
- What are the requirements for the home health aid staff? How many additional hours of training does the agency provide?
- What are the geographic distances covered?
- What are the agency's operating hours, and how are emergencies, weekends, and holidays covered?
- Who oversees the staff?
- Are the agency and staff bonded?
- Will the agency maintain communication with the physician? If so, how frequently and by what means?

USE OF VOLUNTEERS

One key element of caregiver failure is burnout. Burnout is generally related to the lack of funds for respite or the fact the caregiver is not given adequate periods of rest. If the case management plan requires extended periods of care, case managers must identify and include respite care or the use of volunteers. Unfortunately, although making use of volunteers can be a good idea, in reality it does not always work out. They are first and foremost "volunteers"—so in most cases their needs and wants will take priority.

If volunteers are included in the case management plan, they must receive training. Although their volunteer time might be spent on custodial care or companion functions, they must have the necessary training to perform even the most basic of tasks. (In addition, if the patient is confined to bed, care is far more difficult to provide than if the patient were up and about). This training must include tasks, proper body mechanics, and how to manage the patient to ensure safety. In some cases training for cardiopulmonary resuscitation or the handling of simple equipment might be needed.

Scheduling will be a key component of the planning. Volunteers need to know their schedule just as those who are employed do. By using a calendar to schedule the volunteer's time, the case manager can quickly identify gaps in coverage. In addition, volunteers are community specific. As a rule volunteers can be found from friends, churches, ethnic groups, and community organizations.

OUTPATIENT SERVICES

Community outpatient services are one of the biggest health care arenas handling postacute skilled care and other health care services. Outpatient services, whether hospital or community based, are varied and include the following:

- Diagnostic screening and testing
- Radiologic services
- Surgery
- Dialysis
- Therapy services (physical, speech, and occupational)
- Infusions or other medications that are not considered self-injectable or self-administered (including blood or chemotherapy)
- Emergency and urgent care
- Other outpatient services, including public health clinics, neighborhood and primary care centers, drug detoxification centers, mobile laboratories and clinics, and counseling centers

Upon discharge, if a patient is not homebound and ongoing skilled care and services are required, linkage with the local or nearest outpatient programs is critical.

A key component to getting outpatient services and compliance is transportation for the patient. Arrangements for transportation, the schedule, and the responsible entity are an important part of the case management plan. If the patient must rely on public transportation, the case manager may need to take an additional step and work closely with the outpatient provider to ensure that the provider will be able to accommodate the patient, regardless of the time.

Appointment availability and the type of services required are other barriers to the establishment of outpatient services. For some patients, inability to pay outpatient copayments is a primary culprit affecting plan implementation and compliance.

Patients discharged from a tertiary care center or center of excellence must often remain nearby to continue treatments as an outpatient. They must find affordable housing in the immediate area, which is not a covered expense allowed by health care insurers. If housing is required, the patient and family must work with the center's social services staff. Fortunately, in most cases this issue will have been discussed long before, during the preadmission workup. By preplanning, the patient and family have an idea of what additional expenses they can anticipate.

A challenge faced by case managers working with the elderly covered by a Medicare + Choice managed care organization will be the new ruling that allows these patients to be "temporarily out of the service area." The patient can be out of the service area for up to 12 months before disenrollment from the managed care plan. In these cases the case manager should have an established relationship with the client before he or she leaves the service area. This allows, at a minimum, proactive arrangements for any required routine care (e.g., dialysis) as well as prearrangements and negotiations for payment for the services.

TELEMEDICINE AND HOME CARE

Although telemedicine has traditionally been a product used by large tertiary and rehabilitation centers, this is no longer true in today's world of technologic advances. Telemedicine uses information and telecommunications technology to transfer medical information for diagnosis, therapy, and education. The information may include medical images, live two-way audio and video, patient medical records, output data from medical devices, and sound files. The telemedical interaction may involve two-way live audio and video visits between patients and medical professionals, patient monitoring data sent from the home to a clinic or transmission of a patient medical file from a primary care provider to a specialist. The American Telemedicine Association (ATA) uses the following broad definition of telemedicine:

Telemedicine is the use of medical information exchanged from one site to another via electronic communications for the health and education of the patient or health care provider and for the purpose of improving patient care.[12]

Additional information on telemedicine can be obtained by contacting the American Telemedicine Association or by visiting their website at www.american-telemed.org/.

ASSISTED LIVING FACILITIES

The service of assisted living is based on a Scandinavian model of serving the elderly that made its way to the United States in the mid-1980s. Today, 26 names in the United States alone refer to the concept, including the terms residential care, foster home, congregate care, and board and care. In assisted living, using the term *patient* is frowned upon.

Statistics related to assisted living facilities from an American Health Care Association (AHCA) survey showed that 58.1% of residents come from their own home and stay an average of 34 months. Approximately 14.1% come from nursing facilities, 9.4% from other assisted living facilities, and 11.7% from the hospital. The majority of persons leave the assisted living facility as they require a higher level of care; 44.4% go into a nursing facility. This progression has lead to a new term—"aging in place." In some assisted living facilities, wings of the building offer different levels of assistance ranging from assistance with ADLs to skilled nursing care. Thus, instead of going from facility to facility, people can remain in one place for care without the trauma associated with being taken from familiar surroundings.[13]

Many older adults who can no longer take care of their homes or themselves will not be candidates for SNFs, adult day service centers, or other similar facilities. However, they may be appropriate for an assisted living facility. These facilities differ widely in accommodations, services, staffing, admission policies, resident retention efforts, and price. Most people who go to assisted living facilities do not need nursing home care or services. They need access to health care professionals 24 hours a day, but not necessarily nursing care.[14]

The ACHA defines assisted living as a part of comprehensive long-term care that provides the necessary services to dependent elderly or disabled populations in the appropriate environment. These facilities, according to the ACHA, are "rendered in state-licensed facilities and include 24 hour protective oversight, food, shelter and the provision of a range of services to promote the quality of life of the individual." Additional common services include emergency response systems, three meals a day in a group dining room, personal care, social and religious activities, exercise and recreational activities, transportation, laundry, housekeeping, and general maintenance.[13]

Many assisted living facilities also provide care for patients with dementia. These patients are placed in a locked unit where they can roam freely within a homelike atmosphere. Residents in these units have similar living quarters and personal care and assistance, but more safety measures are in effect because they are allowed to roam freely.

Most assisted living facilities offer consumers a range of options in terms of private or shared accommodations as well as the size of the space (e.g., shared, studio, or one- or two-bedrooms units), but only 27% of facilities have all-private accommodations. Nearly all facilities provide or arrange 24-hour staff; housekeeping services; three meals a day; and help with all medications, bathing, and dressing. Approximately 52% of the facilities surveyed have either a full- or part-time registered nurse or licensed practical nurse on staff, and 25% arrange for nursing care with an agency. One in five (21%), however, do not provide or arrange for care or monitoring by a licensed nurse. Many facilities admit residents with moderate physical limitations such as wheelchair use (71%), but fewer than half (44%) admit residents who need assistance with transfers (e.g., in and out of bed, chair, or wheelchair). Fewer than half (47%) have residents with moderate to severe cognitive impairment. In most assisted living facilities, residents whose functional limitations necessitate help with transfers, whose cognitive impairment progresses from mild to moderate or severe, or who exhibit problematic behavior will be discharged from the facility. The same is true for a resident who needs nursing care for more than 2 weeks. Only about 5% of the residents leave because of financial reasons.[14]

If a move is to be made to an assisted living facility, it is important, when feasible, to include the patient in any on-site visits. If the patient cannot be included in a visit, taking pictures and bringing back enough information about the new environment will help to alleviate fears of the unknown.

Facility Checklist

When families have a choice of facilities case managers should advise them to make an initial visit to as many facilities as possible. They must make initial comparisons and register their first impressions of all facilities. As they tour each facility, they should ask for brochures, rate sheets, the activity schedule, menus, resident newsletters, and any other documents that will be helpful as they narrow their search. They must always ask to see the facility's license and any survey results from the state licensing agency. State licensing surveys should be posted in a central place for the public to view. Although an actual copy may not be available to take home, patients and caregivers can make notes of any deficiencies, especially those that center around patient care, food, and cleanliness. Once visits are completed, they can then seriously narrow the list down to a few facilities for the final selection process.

OTHER POSTACUTE CARE OPTIONS

As the patient is readied either for discharge or for a change in level of care within the continuum, many other options will need to be considered and are discussed on the following pages. The key element for any program, service, or facility will be the funding source; traditional health insurance does not cover many services if care is other than skilled care.

To assist with postacute care options or local services, many communities have what are called "information and referral" services. These are special programs designed to provide information about and referral to available services in a community. These services are available by telephone and are primarily sponsored by:

- The Older Americans Act
- The United Way
- Disease-specific agencies
- Community or ethnic agencies
- Other health-related service agencies

Respite Care

Respite care is the "break" or short-term care arrangements made to allow the caregiver time away from providing care to the severely disabled or frail elderly. Because respite care is rarely funded by health care payers, the caregiver or family pays for it from their own funds. Respite care can occur by having people come into the home or by placement in a facility (SNF or other facility). If the patient is terminally ill and receiving hospice care paid by the health plan or Medicare benefit, however, respite care is included in the patient's hospice benefit package.

Intermediate Care Facilities

Many states allow licensure of what are known as intermediate care facilities. These are similar to SNFs, but they offer fewer care hours. In many cases skilled care is minimal—often an hour or less per day (or week). However, in some states intermediate care can be offered at a higher number of hours per day for skilled care, especially when it is used for developmentally disabled persons as an alternative to state hospitalization.

Most patients cared for in an intermediate care facility are ambulatory and fairly independent. The principal criteria for persons entering this level of care will be bowel and bladder control and sufficient mobility. This level of care is rarely covered by health care payers.

Board and Care Facilities

Before the advent of assisted living facilities, the only options patients had for custodial care outside the home were SNFs, intermediate care facilities, and board and care homes. In most communities board and care facilities are licensed under community or group home licensure. Most will only accept ambulatory, fairly self-sufficient persons. However, some board and care facilities can take patients with a higher level of care (ones who might be confined to bed or even hospice patients); this will depend on their licensure.

Community board and care facilities are often used for patients with:

- Dementia
- Alzheimer's disease (depending on the facility, its licensure, and disease severity)
- Alcohol or drug abuse
- Varying degrees of mental illness
- Varying degrees of developmental disabilities
- TBI or ABI
- Varying degrees of ADL assistance needed

The principal services provided by a board and care facility are a room and meals. A few offer recreational activities. Others are designed for clients with specific disorders (e.g., alcohol or drug addiction, head injury). Some offer medical assistance such as medications and personal care; others do not. Depending on the facility, patients who need intermittent nursing care may be monitored by nurses from a home health agency. Patients see their physicians as often as necessary in the physician's office.

Domiciliary Care Homes

Domiciliary homes are traditionally run by the Veterans Administration and are similar to board and care or assisted living facilities in that they primarily provide custodial care. A Veterans Administration domiciliary is a residential center that offers a therapeutic, homelike environment for veterans. These veterans do not require hospital or nursing home care but are unable to live independently because of medical or psychiatric disabilities. Persons receive necessary medical and psychiatric care, rehabilitative assistance, and other therapeutic interventions on an outpatient basis from the nearby veterans hospital. Entrance into a domiciliary home is limited to eligible veterans who meet admission criteria. For more information see the Veterans Administration website at www.va.gov/facilities.

Alzheimer's Disease Facilities

Historically, if a patient with Alzheimer's disease could not be cared for at home the primary option for care was an SNF, ideally one specializing in Alzheimer's care. Unfortunately, these facilities were few and far between. Placement was typically at a facility ill equipped to meet the needs of the patient or at a facility far from loved ones and often outside the patient's community.

Fortunately, over the past few years care for patients with Alzheimer's needing placement has improved. Now many communities have board and care homes as well as large assisted living facilities that specialize in Alzheimer's care.

Depending on the patient's medical and physical needs and behavioral issues, most assisted living or board and care facilities will offer a secure and homelike environment where the person is allowed to wander around. Although these two levels are now available, the unfortunate fact remains that many facilities specializing in Alzheimer's care cater to private-pay clients. When money is exhausted or the patient's physical or medical needs or behavioral issues change, placement in an SNF is required because this is often the only level of care available.

More information on referral and other issues related to Alzheimer's care can be found at the Alzheimer's Association website (www.alz.org), the National Institutes of Health (www.nih.gov), National Institute on Aging (www.nia.nih.gov), and the National Institute of Mental Health (www.nimh.nih.gov).

Transitional Care Unit or Program

Community-based housing units are used primarily for patients with brain injuries and the developmentally disabled. The emphasis in these units is on retraining of the individual to allow him or her to care for personal needs and on providing vocational or educational skills that will allow the person to reenter society. These units offer varying levels of supervision and often do not provide the conventional medical model for care. These units are usually excluded from health care benefit coverage.

Domestic Violence Units

Facilities of this type offer temporary shelter and support to battered women and their children who need a safe place to stay in crisis situations. These shelters offer counseling, social service advocacy and referrals, emergency transportation, food and clothing, identification and intervention in child abuse situations, legal information and referral, and, when requested, assistance with relocation. Information on domestic violence services can be found in larger cities. Information is also available on the National Domestic Violence Hotline website (www.ndvh.org) or by calling 800-799-SAFE (7233) or 800-787-3224 for the hearing impaired.

Homeless Shelters

Dealing with the homeless is a reality in today's health care world because of their lack of health insurance. Additionally, many of the homeless will be youths younger than 18 years. The public health clinics and other free community "safety net" providers generally serve as the providers of care for this category of patients.

Although the reasons for homelessness are many and varied, they can be linked to:

- Unemployment and underemployment (many businesses only hire part-time workers at minimum wage)
- Poverty
- Domestic violence
- Runaways and throwaways
- Evictions
- Deinstitutionalization
- Major mental health illnesses
- Drug and alcohol abuse

Although many of the resources mentioned earlier in this section will be available to those with insurance, many of the homeless will be referred to public health clinics, safety net providers, or to providers that offer free services. Because many will be without insurance or ineligible for alternate funding programs, case managers must be savvy as to how to deal with this category of patients.

Homeless shelters are typically found in larger cities, with many run by volunteer organizations or churches. The most well-known volunteer organizations that run homeless shelters are probably the Salvation Army and Volunteers of America. As a rule homeless shelters offer temporary housing (1 day to 1 week) and meals. Because of the large numbers of homeless persons, many have strict admission criteria and require the person to be available at a specific time for screening. Most homeless shelters offer social worker services who can assist with counseling, social service advocacy and referrals, emergency transportation, food and clothing, and other county or state programs for which the homeless person might be entitled.

Day Hospital or Partial Programs

Day hospital or partial programs offer medical or psychiatric nursing or reha-

bilitation services to persons who generally spend only the day at the facility, returning home at night. Patients who need this type of care do not require 24-hour care but could require an inpatient stay if a day program were unavailable. For the most part, insurance policies pay for this level of care because it is often used in lieu of inpatient care. Many insurers recognize two outpatient hospital days for one inpatient day.

Residential Treatment Centers

Residential treatment centers provide a 24-hour therapeutic planned group living and learning environment to children or adolescents. Most children using such centers have a mental health disorder but have sufficient intellectual potential to respond to active treatment. Centers such as these provide individualized psychotherapy and other psychiatric services. Depending on the facility and its capabilities along with the patient's diagnosis, some coverage might be available under a mental health benefit package. Locating a resident treatment facility is often a difficult task because not every community offers such a level of care. Some funding may be available from the child's local school district if the center offers any academic activities. This funding is available through use of special education and the Individuals with Disabilities Education Act (IDEA) of 1991 (and as amended in 1997) that mandates a free education for all children.

Developmental Centers

Developmental centers are institutions that provide care to persons with more severe developmental disabilities (e.g., disabilities attributable to mental retardation, cerebral palsy, epilepsy, autism, or other neurologic disorders that originated before the individual reached the age of 22 and are expected to last indefinitely). These institutions are often referred to as state hospitals or state schools; the actual name for this type of provider varies from state to state. Entrance to such centers is gained through the state agency responsible for providing services to the developmentally disabled; often this agency is the state department of mental health or mental retardation. In California, the local regional center assumes this responsibility. Because care in such centers is long term, coverage from traditional health care insurance is rare. Most payments for care are from private funds or Medicaid.

Long-Term Psychiatric Facilities

Placement in long-term psychiatric facilities (which may include state hospitals or state schools) should be reserved for the mentally ill or very severely handicapped persons. Although this level of care may be covered on an interim basis by a health care payer if care is skilled, coverage is rare. Most patients in state hospitals need long-term care. Thus most patients must resort to Medicaid because the required care is custodial and needs a protective setting. State hospital care costs for a patient run $40,000 to $50,000 per year. These units are primarily nursing facilities designed to treat persons with severe mental illness or severe developmental delay (e.g., those with severe cerebral palsy or profound mental retardation) over an indefinite, possibly lifelong, period. These facilities are licensed by the state Department of Health. To be placed a long-term psychiatric facility, a person must either enter voluntarily or involuntarily under conservatorship.

Homemaker or Choreworker Options

Choreworker, attendant care, and homemaker services are intended for chronically ill or incapacitated individuals. Services are available from private homemaker agencies on a fee-for-service basis, local social service programs (e.g., in-home supportive service programs) for low-income persons

eligible for welfare benefits, or the state agency handling services for the developmentally disabled. To be covered by a state agency, the patient must be a client of the agency and the required services must be included in the individual program plan. The goal of homemaker service programs is to maintain the patient in the least restrictive environment. Homemaker service is not covered benefit allowed by health care insurers.

An in-home supportive service program is a state-funded county-administered program offered to low-income persons and those eligible for Supplemental Security Income. The intent is to enable elderly, blind, or disabled individuals to remain and function in a home environment of their choice. Services vary from state to state. To calculate the number of hours to be paid by the program, the client must undergo an assessment of need. Typical services include meal preparation, shopping, cleaning, transportation, and personal care. Hours granted for care are usually limited to a few per day, week, or month.

Meal Programs

Congregate meal programs are offered by church groups, social service agencies, and low-income housing complexes. Such meal programs allow joint dining by participants and are designed to facilitate socialization while ensuring participants receive a healthy meal. Most programs serve one meal per day from Monday to Friday, primarily to ambulatory or independent wheelchair bound persons. Costs for this program are nominal and many are based on a person's ability to pay or a sliding scale.

Meal delivery programs such as Meals on Wheels are operated by social service or ethnic-specific agencies, church groups, or other community-sponsored agencies. Meal programs are designed to meet the nutritional needs of the homebound. Most offer, at minimum, one hot meal and possibly one cold meal per day, Monday to Friday. Income, age, and the actual location of the residence are frequently the most common barriers to access. Many of these meal programs are funded through the Older Americans Act and are restricted to the low-income elderly.

OTHER PUBLIC SERVICES

Public Health Clinics

Although public health clinics and services are generally reserved as a "safety net" provider for the poor, these clinics may also be a source of care when patients have limited benefits or when benefit coverage has been exhausted. Public health clinics offer a variety of services, including maternal and child health, treatment for communicable diseases, and adult primary health.

Although contact with the public health department will probably be infrequent, case managers must be familiar with the services provided by this department and the location of clinics if patients or families wish to obtain access to care. Similarly, if the case manager needs information, especially about communicable diseases, these clinics and their staff can be invaluable aids.

Safety Net Providers

Some case managers will have clients using what are called "safety net" providers. Safety net providers are community providers who organize and deliver significant levels of health care and other related services to the uninsured, Medicaid, recipients, and other vulnerable populations. The vulnerable populations most often using safety net providers are those persons without insurance, the underinsured, migrant workers, or patients with special health care needs. Safety net providers are characterized by two distinguishing features: they serve all patients regardless of their ability to pay, either by legal mandate or through explicitly adopted mission statements, and a substantial number of their patient mix consists of the uninsured and other vulnerable patients.

According to the senate testimony given by Claude Earl Fox, MD, on March 23, 2000, to the Senate Committee on Health, Education, Labor, and Pensions and the Subcommittee on Public Health and Safety, as well as his speech on "The Role of Our Safety Net Providers and the Uninsured," safety net providers consist of:

- Community health centers, including specific public hospitals and local public health clinics
- Migrant health centers
- Health care centers for the homeless
- Health care programs for residents of public housing

These providers collectively offer primary and preventive health care services and case management with a family-oriented, culturally competent approach to more than 9 million people nationwide, including 3.5 million children. These patient populations consist of approximately the following:

- 86% Below 200% of the poverty level
- 40% Uninsured (health center uninsured patients have increased at twice the national rate since 1990)
- 34% Medicaid recipients
- 65% Minorities
- 40% Children
- 30% Women of childbearing age

Safety net providers are essential, effective, and efficient. They are located in low-income and minority neighborhoods, underserved rural communities, and in communities with a disproportionate number of at-risk people (e.g., children with special needs, people with serious mental illness, people with HIV/AIDS, the homeless, and those whose legal immigration status is unknown). Safety net providers have demonstrated their effectiveness with[15]:

- Improved health outcomes
- Increased preventative services
- Improved management of chronic disease
- Reduced number of avoidable hospitalizations
- High patient satisfaction

The Women, Infants and Children (WIC) Program

The Special Supplemental Nutrition Program for WIC is a government safety net provider. WIC offers short-term services designed to assist young families or mothers and children at nutritional risk because of low income and nutrition-related health conditions. WIC programs are available in urban areas and offer a variety of programs to promote education, a monthly food prescription package, and assistance with access to maternal, prenatal, and pediatric health care services.

Indian Health Service

Indian Health Service is a health program provided directly and through tribally contracted and operated facilities on reservations and in urban areas of the United States. This program is designed to serve any American Indian or Alaskan Native. Indian Health Service networks are composed of:

- **Contract Health Services**—These are health services purchased under contract from community hospitals and practitioners.
- **Health Center**—This is a facility that is physically separated from a hospital and offers a full range of ambulatory and outpatient services that include primary care physicians, nurses, a pharmacy, laboratory services, and radiography.
- **Health Station**—This is a facility that is physically separated from a hospital and health center but offers primary care physician services on a regularly scheduled basis.

OTHER COMMUNITY PROVIDERS

Community Agencies

A key component to case management plans is the ability to link patients to community resources or ethnic-specific or disease-specific agencies. In general, the names, eligibility criteria, and type and level of services provided by community agencies vary from state to state and even from county to county within a state. Community agencies are a wonderful addition to the case management plan and an invaluable resource for the patient and family. Community agencies are excellent sources of:

- Information
- Assistance with referrals
- Education through literature, classes, or public speaking forums
- Support groups where patients and families can share tips on how to use and navigate the system, how to perform tasks better, and how and where to obtain supplies
- Opportunities for social outings
- Opportunities for peer support from others who have experienced similar events or emotions
- Specialized services (e.g., transportation, advocacy, crisis intervention)

Although many resources are community specific, others are affiliates of national groups. Although many agencies are listed in local phone directories, national organizations may not be.

In most cases, national agencies concentrate their efforts on developing educational programs and literature and participating in research studies for the development of better techniques. As a rule, both local and national organizations provide information and referral services. Many agencies also offer the emotional support and socialization opportunities patients, families, and caregivers require. Most national organizations can be reached by a toll-free telephone number or by visiting their websites.

Telephone Reassurance Services

If local telephone reassurance services are available, they are offered through local senior organizations or volunteer agencies designed to serve seniors. Telephone reassurance programs are designed to have a volunteer call the subscriber (usually an older person living alone) each day at a predetermined time to chat and make sure the person is all right.

Victims or Witness Programs

Victims and witness programs are programs that offer crisis and short-term counseling and referral to private or public agencies to victims of violent crimes. Depending on the county, some money might be available for temporary assistance to victims who have necessary or unexpected expenses. Because the application process is lengthy and funds are not always available when the need is most critical, these programs are often not used in case management plans. However, case managers must be familiar with the programs to educate patients of their availability and purpose.

Utility Services

Most utility companies are willing to work with the disabled or persons with low income and offer discounted utilities or universal lifeline rates. Many have other programs and devices for the physically challenged or hearing or sight impaired. Electric companies, for example, are willing to work with patients and families when the patient is ventilator dependent and a high consumer of electricity. Also, local phone companies offer

adaptive equipment and services for the hearing impaired and physically challenged. Patients and families must be encouraged to make contact with their local utilities to ascertain the level and type of services for which they might be entitled.

Abuse Agencies

In all likelihood, many cases will involve suspected or known abuse. Health care professionals are mandated by law to report known or suspected abuse. Case managers must also be familiar with the processes necessary to ensure safety as well as the time frames for reporting.

Any patient, regardless of age, who is found during case management intervention to be in an abusive situation must be referred to the appropriate agency mandated by the state to investigate such cases. If this situation is discovered while the patient hospitalized, discharge often cannot occur until clearance is obtained from the appropriate agency handling the abuse issue.

In most states a verbal report must be made within 24 hours of notification of the abuse, followed within 24 more hours by a written report. Abuse or neglect can occur in a variety of forms, but it typically appears in one of the following five categories:

1. Emotional or verbal abuse accompanied by threats of violence or harassment
2. Sexual abuse involving inappropriate touching, fondling, or sexual acts that occur when the patient is forced, unable to understand, or threatened
3. Physical abuse that is witnessed or is apparent by unexplained bruises, welts, fractures, abrasions or cuts, or burns from cigarettes, ropes, or other hot surfaces
4. Physical and mental abuse involving the patient being confined or

locked in a room or tied to a bed or chair

5. Financial exploitation when family members or others misuse, steal, or withhold funds; do not purchase food, clothing, personal items, or medical care and supplies; or grossly overcharge the patient for services

Neglect is also reportable and includes such situations as:

- Filthy, unsafe, or hazardous housing environment or patient hygiene
- Lack of medical care or failure to administer prescribed medications or treatments
- Unexplained weight loss, malnourishment, or failure to thrive
- Absent parents or caretaker and inappropriate supervision
- Irregular school attendance

Canine Companions

Many patients might be eligible for a specially trained dog to assist in keeping the patient as independent as possible. Specially trained dogs are used for patients with vision or hearing impairments or developmental or physical disabilities. The most recognized vendor for such animals is Canine Companions for Independence. This organization provides assistance dogs to those whose independence or quality of life will be enhanced by a dog. If the person qualifies, animals are provided at virtually no cost. All expenses of breeding, raising, and training a Canine Companion are funded through private donations. More information on Canine Companions can be found on their website at www.caninecompanions.org.

Financial Counseling

Because many patients and their families caught in a catastrophic or long-term care situation are faced with tremendous unforeseen or unplanned out-of-pocket expenses, case managers should encourage referrals to local financial counseling agencies when needs are identified. In most states, this agency will be the Consumer Credit Counseling agency, and the National Consumer Credit Counseling website is www.nccs.org. Also, case managers should educate eligible clients regarding general assistance, food stamps, and other public programs.

PROGRAMS FOR CHILDREN WITH SPECIAL NEEDS

Infant Stimulation Program

Infant stimulation programs are designed to provide consistent and repeated stimulation to infants or small children younger than age 3 years with exceptional needs. The program trains parents or caregivers to provide appropriate stimulation. The goal of the program is to assist these children in reaching the developmental milestones established for their age group and disability. Stimulation may be offered in the areas of touch, sight, hearing, smell, taste, and motor control (movement, coordination, and sucking).

Special Education Programs

Specially designed instruction is for children with exceptional educational needs (physical or mental) that cannot be met by the regular school program, even if modified. This instruction is provided at no cost to the parents and is mandated by federal law (public law 94-142 and, more recently, the Individuals with Disabilities Education Act of 1991 and as amended in 1997). Special education programs provide a full range of options to meet the educational and service needs of children in the least restrictive environment. Children with exceptional needs are grouped for instructional purposes according to their instructional needs. Special education will be discussed in further detail in the funding unit of this text.

TRANSPORTATION

Transportation to and from the postacute care setting is often the primary culprit for noncompliance with outpatient services for all age categories. Although some public funding programs such as Medicaid or Children's Medical Services might pay the cost of postacute care transportation, traditional health insurance rarely covers the costs. This is true even when the person is receiving skilled services from an outpatient setting (e.g., dialysis, chemotherapy, physical therapy, or psychotherapy). Thus, while the patient is receiving outpatient care and services, transportation to and from will be his or her responsibility for payment.

DIALYSIS

Patients undergoing dialysis are often the most labor intensive of all cases followed by case managers. The discharge process often involves calling multiple facilities and dialysis centers and then arranging necessary transportation. If the patient is already linked to a dialysis center and has transportation, or the family can be trained in other dialysis techniques, the discharge can be simple. However, if the patient does not already use a dialysis center or has no transportation, or in some cases both, problems and delays in discharges are encountered. Unfortunately patients who need dialysis and other skilled care needs present the greatest challenges. Even greater challenges can be encountered when the patient's payment source is Medicaid. Dialysis within the home is possible. However, lead time will be needed to ensure adequate training occurs and the necessary supplies are procured.

Home peritoneal dialysis is the most rapidly growing form of dialysis. It addresses patient concerns about the costs associated with the dialysis itself and transportation. Peritoneal dialysis is often the choice for persons residing in rural communities because:

- It eliminates the need for transportation and the costs associated with transportation
- Patients can self-administer this drug at home
- Patients can maintain physical independence and go to work or travel as long as they have the solutions needed for the treatment
- It offers ease of access for the dialysis because new technology allows simple surgery for placement of the dialysis catheter in the abdominal wall

Because dialysis does require a large amount of supplies, case managers working with insurers should make every effort to obtain at least a 6 to 12-month authorization time frame. This decreases the need for continual authorizations (which are time consuming for all parties). Key to issuing such authorizations will be coordination of benefits with Medicare if the patient has private health care insurance. An authorization in increments also allows smaller quantities to be kept on hand and helps eliminate storage issues.

OTHER PROGRAMS

Adult and Pediatric Day Service Centers

One often overlooked and underused level of care is adult day service centers (ADSCs). ADSCs are a growing component of the continuum of care. This is true because ADSCs are a cost-effective alternative to nursing home care (e.g., many have an average cost of $50 per day). Unfortunately, ADSCs are not designed, staffed, or licensed to accept high-technology–dependent patients, but they are ideal for those who require minimal care. ADSCs promote independent functioning for adults in a safe, structured, and homelike environment. The primary clientele served are elderly and those with cognitive or physical impairments who need supervision. They also meet the health, personal care, and social needs of chronically ill adults.

If a daycare center is used, care plans are tailored to the needs of each person, incorporating the patient's and family's goals in an attempt to achieve optimal independence and function. The care plan offers detailed information about nursing care, physical exercise, therapeutic (e.g., physical or speech therapy) and recreational activities, and personal care.[16] As a rule the daycare center staff meets on a regular basis to monitor the progress of the participants and compliance with regulations and care plan goals. Additional monitoring is provided through established utilization committees and by customer satisfaction surveys. In most facilities the staff meets monthly to describe and rate each participant's status by using several different assessment tools that measure functional ability and mental and physical health.

Daycare centers are useful for families who elect to care for their loved one at home but who must continue working. They are also used as an option when a person with a head injury who does not need a nursing facility is unable to participate in vocational rehabilitation programs but needs socialization. Unfortunately, very few communities have ADSCs, and even fewer have them for children with special needs. Some daycare centers do provide care for high-technology–dependent children.

Nonprofit organizations, churches, and some nursing homes run most ADSCs. Costs vary from state to state and often from city to city. As a rule, health care payers exclude this level of care from reimbursement. Most costs are paid privately or by the state Medicaid program; if the person is developmentally disabled, the

state's developmentally disabled agency may pay.

All licensed adult and pediatric daycare centers must meet state, local, and federal guidelines. Case managers working with families who wish to use daycare centers must educate the families of the importance of using appropriately state licensed centers as well as the centers' role in providing respite, if nothing else. Case managers should encourage them to visit the center and view current state inspection reports and records as well as any complaints lodged against the center.

Inpatient Versus Outpatient Pain Programs

Possibly the most difficult patients case managers deal with are those patients with severe pain. Pain can be acute or chronic. Acute pain can be alleviated, in most cases, by modern technology or drugs, but it cannot be dismissed as not a challenge. Chronic pain, however, presents significant challenges.

Unfortunately not all physicians and health care professionals are well versed in pain and appropriate treatments. If treatment of pain is inadequate case managers must advocate on behalf of their patients for pain relief.

If the case manager sees that pain is not being managed adequately, consultation with the health care organization's medical director, pharmacy director, and the patient's primary treating physician may be in order. Professionals such as these afford an opportunity to discuss treatment options and educate the patient's treating physician.

Although many conditions can cause acute pain, two common conditions frequently seen in the postacute care setting are multiple trauma and terminal cancer. These patients must be kept as comfortable as possible. For patients with terminal cancer, every attempt must be made to spare them from a painful death.

Similarly, pain associated with multiple trauma or another medical condition or injury must not be allowed to progress to chronic pain.

The first program for pain management was established at Emory University in 1983 as an inpatient program.[17] Significant advances have been made over the past several years. Inpatient and outpatient, or a combination of the two, treatment programs are now available. Several hundred programs exist today throughout the United States.

Pain Management Goals

Treatment, whether inpatient or outpatient, must be flexible, individualized, and goal oriented. Both types of programs are useful for treating the psychological problems and behavior manifestations commonly associated with pain and dysfunction.

Generally, admission to either type of pain program is based on the patient's ability to understand and follow instructions as well as the motivation level of commitment for compliance with the program and the treatment regimen. Patients who are disruptive or aggressive or who have a severe psychiatric disorder frequently are not considered candidates because they are too disruptive to the treatment setting. The principal objectives of both inpatient and outpatient pain programs are as follows:

- To provide detoxification
- To relieve or decrease pain
- To restore the person to an appropriate functional level
- To eliminate use of assistive devices by restoring physical abilities and conditioning and to correct gait and posture
- To return the patient to work and leisure activities
- To educate the patient in prevention of reinjury, weight control, ergonomics, body mechanics, energy-saving techniques, wellness, and alternatives for pain relief
- To provide modification through biofeedback, family and group therapy, relaxation techniques, assertiveness training, and stress management
- To provide vocational retraining when applicable

Pain Program Costs

Pain management is an evolving specialty. Many providers offer a variety of pain management programs. These can be anything from an individual provider that offers one or more treatments to clinics and facilities that offer inpatient , outpatient, and multidisciplinary approaches to treatments. As a result, the following services in a pain management program are common:

- Patient education and lifestyle adaptations
- Acupuncture
- Physical therapy
- Passive therapies
- Manipulation and mobilization
- Pool therapy or aquatics
- Individual counseling or psychotherapy
- Group counseling
- Family counseling
- Instruction in biofeedback and relaxation
- Medication management
- Case management services
- Social worker services
- Steroid injections
- Nerve blocks
- Vocational counseling
- Nutritional counseling
- Transcutaneous electrical nerve stimulation

The efficacy of a program depends largely on the thoroughness of the initial evaluation, the patient's symptoms, and the final treatment plan. Average costs vary from program to program and from region to region but can range from several hundred dollars a day to $1000 or more per day.

Using Medical or Mental Health Benefits for Pain Programs

Because pain management is primarily a medical measure, the most effective approach is to make every attempt to allow coverage under the traditional medical benefit structure rather than a mental health benefit. However, this practice varies by health care payer. What are the advantages of coverage under the medical portion of the health care benefit package? At a minimum, they include avoidance of who should authorize and pay for the care (medical payer and mental health payer). It also eliminates a case manager and two case management plans.

Case Manager Involvement

The involvement of case managers in the actual pain management program depends on case variables and from which organization (e.g., facility-based case manager, health care payer) the case manager represents. Involvement by case managers outside their facilities does not cease while the patient is in the program. Nor should case managers be excluded as part of the team. The involvement of an outside case manager is critical if the team is to be kept apprised of health care benefits and limitations or exclusions. It is also needed to ensure if ongoing care is required at discharge, approvals are received, and coverage is extended and goals reached.

HOSPICE AND PALLIATIVE CARE

In a 1995 study, the National Hospice Organization reported that hospice has been a significantly underused health care service. Although hospice can be used for 6 months or more, the national average time for hospice care is between 35 to 50 days. Unfortunately, fewer than 20% of eli-

gible patients ever access their hospice benefits.[18]

The use of palliative care has increased in this country and is used to take care of the whole person—body, mind, and spirit. Both palliative and hospice programs involve pain control and the management of pain and its symptoms. Palliative care also focuses on other symptoms, such as nausea and breathlessness, spiritual care, emotional support for both the patient and family, social support, and help in obtaining equipment. Hospice care, on the other hand, has provisions for nursing and skilled care.

Similar to hospice, the palliative care team is provided by an interdisciplinary team of doctors, nurses, social workers, and clergy. The five principles of palliative care are as follows[19]:

1. Respect the goals, likes, and choices of the dying person.
2. Look after the medical, emotional, social, and spiritual needs of the dying person.
3. Support the needs of the family members.
4. Help gain access to needed health care providers and appropriate care settings.
5. Build ways to provide excellent care at the end of life.

PEDIATRIC PATIENTS

For many case managers chronically ill or technology-dependent children are a special challenge. Case managers must often deal with the needs of the patient's family as well as their own emotions about children with long-term, high-technology needs. In addition, technology-dependent children consume large amounts of case management time and resources and are usually known as high-dollar cases.[20]

When working with a chronically ill or technology-dependent child, one of the first tasks should be to encourage the child's family to apply for the state Children's Medical Services program. Also, depending on the child's disabilities and developmental needs, referral to the state agency responsible for developmental disabilities and the Department of Education may also be in order. These referrals are necessary because in many cases the child's health care benefit coverage only covers acute episodic periods of the illness or injury and rarely covers duplicate equipment and long-term care. Because of differences in these programs relating to eligibility factors and treatment options (e.g., for acute care versus chronic care), case managers must at minimum be familiar with referral criteria for local and state agencies.

Because community resources in the pediatric postacute care arena are sparse, many children with special needs are discharged home. When this occurs, family and caregivers should be fully trained in all areas of the child's care. In addition, if the family lives in a remote location and has limited access to community resources, the parents must fully understand the child's illness and know what to do in an emergency. In addition, they must be able to:

- Operate and clean all necessary equipment
- Be able to troubleshoot their own problems
- Know when to seek help
- Demonstrate proficiency in all areas of care, including knowledge of what to do when the equipment fails, all relevant medical issues, and how to administer cardiopulmonary resuscitation when necessary

A child with a chronic illness or injury often has special needs for the remainder of his or her life. Consequently, the family must be taught how to be the case manager for the child. In this capacity they must know:

- What community resources are available and whether and when the child will be entitled to these resources and programs
- How to navigate the system and barter for services
- How to file a formal appeal when services are denied
- What services can be provided by special education programs and other public funding programs and how each of the processes work
- When and how to obtain access to a professional case manager when difficulties are encountered

Teaching

The teaching required for the family of a child with special needs is often an ongoing task and is primarily influenced by the child's growth and development. For teaching to occur the family (and in some cases the child as well) must be assessed for their level and style of learning. Although the case manager is often not responsible for the actual teaching, he or she should monitor the teaching process to ensure goals are met and the case management plan proceeds as planned.

Just as critical is the need to monitor the teaching/learning cycle. This simple task is necessary to ensure that all aspects of care are taught and to evaluate the patient's needs. It is also necessary to ensure changes are made in the case management plan when the physician makes changes in the treatment plan. Keep in mind that monitoring of the teaching/learning cycle must be included in all case management plans—not just those relating to children with special needs.

Stresses and Emotional Responses

When children with special needs require services, lifelong, multiple stressors are commonly present for all involved. This includes the parents, the child, and siblings. When stressors are identified families should be encouraged to seek support from professionals or peer support groups. The case management plan must include a mechanism for assessment of stressors as well as an action plan linking the patient and family with appropriate resources.

Although some families have no resilience, others have an abundant supply. Families without resilience frequently require professional counseling if they are to meet the demands of their duties. When this need is identified appropriate resources must be immediately coordinated and implemented. If support and counseling are unavailable or inadequate from free community resources and the caregiver has mental health benefit coverage, coordination with the health care payer's mental health review staff is vitally important.

Many of the foregoing problems could be dealt with if health care benefit coverage and community resources were available. Lack of community resources is the biggest hurdle to obtaining care for families of children with special needs. Some families need help, whereas others just need to get away for a period of time and experience some normalcy in their lives.

Although barriers to discharge were discussed earlier in this section, it is important to understand the barriers that affect care of a pediatric patient:

- Providers or facilities that specialize in pediatric care are limited to larger cities.
- Fragmentation of care exists among providers.
- There is a lack of understanding by the general public (including health care workers) of pediatric diagnoses and needs and the family's frustrations in dealing with a system that cannot meet the child's needs.
- The programs, services, and funding programs (e.g., special education, Children's Medical Services, or state developmental disability services) are inconsistent in quality and vary

from state to state and from county to county. Families face endless bureaucratic obstacles in gaining access to them.
- Poor coordination and lack of joint development of the case management plan among providers, agencies, and the health care payer's case manager lead to fragmentation, duplication, and sometimes denial of services.
- Caseloads are heavy because the sheer number of children with special needs places limits on the ability of the case manager to work individually with patients and their families.
- Programs may be staffed by poorly or inadequately trained personnel who are insensitive to the needs of families.
- Because these children have special needs and many have skilled care needs, respite care is often lacking.

Some general barriers to lack of care and services for children include:

- High use of emergency department services for primary care
- Poor follow-up care for preventive services (e.g., tracking of immunizations when a child moves from health plan to health plan or to and from public programs)

Because there are so many variables case managers must be as creative as possible as they establish case management plans. This creativity is needed to make use of any combination of services from the various agencies to create a package that meets the needs of the child. Thus the importance of networking with other case managers who specialize in pediatric case management cannot be overstated. This simple task is extremely helpful as case managers research community resources and create an individualized case management plan for the child.

Neonatal Patients

Neonatal births often result in high dollar expenditures for the health care payer and the family. This category of patients must be automatically included among the referral flags used by health care organizations that offer health care benefit coverage to a younger population. The high costs associated with neonatal births are attributable to the anomalies of the baby, the complexity of the required care, the fact these babies are cared for in regional centers specializing in neonatal care, and the length of time it takes to stabilize the child for discharge. Not only do neonates consume enormous amounts of health care resources while they are hospitalized, similar consumption may continue after they are discharged. As a result, case management of neonates may be more labor intensive than other cases.

Discharges

Because few postacute care facilities are available for neonates, many are discharged home. Training of the caregiver or health care professionals who will be providing the care must be started as soon as the baby starts to stabilize if discharge delays are to be avoided. The actual training required is related to the intensity of services needed, the complexity of the care, and the severity of the illness. It also depends on the maturity and capabilities of the parents as well as the community resources available.

Adding to the difficulties of establishing services for a neonate is the fact that most communities lack the resources necessary to manage the child. This factor can be the primary culprit that precludes an earlier discharge.

The criteria used to gauge the neonate's readiness for discharge depend on the individual case as well as the particular neonatal center. However, for most neonates, readiness for discharge is related to such factors as those shown in Box 20-3.

BOX 20-3
Readiness for Discharge

- Ability to control the head
- Ability to maintain body temperature in an open environment
- Increased weight gain, or weight stabilization on the feeding regimen used
- Follow-up care by physician available
- Maintenance schedule for medications and feedings established; adjustments not required daily or weekly
- Home evaluation or assessment completed by public health nurse or home health agency nurse
- Teaching of parent, caregiver, or professional and any backup caregivers adequate; or family has successfully completed a 12-hour trial period of full care if they are to be the primary caregiver for any period of time
- Follow-up care by medical resources or other health care agencies available

---

Anticipated Teaching

It is impossible to list each test and service a child or neonate with special needs may require on discharge. This section merely outlines some of the considerations that must go into planning for the care of a technologically dependent child or a child with special needs. It also outlines some of the basic resources case managers may wish to explore when establishing the care and resources required by either the child or the family.

One of the most common barriers other than of a lack of providers that specialize in pediatrics is the prevalence of untimely referrals to funding programs, such as the state Children's Medical Services program or the state agency responsible for the developmentally disabled. When this occurs, the child may be denied access to programs for which he or she is eligible in the time of greatest need.

The chronically ill or injured child often becomes the chronically ill or injured adult. As a result services and care may be needed for the person's entire life. Therefore it is important to train families to be their own case managers and teach them how to negotiate the system, calling on the professional case manager only when they encounter obstacles.

When working with pediatric patient and their families, planning requires nothing less that total family-centered care, teamwork, and skilled professionals who understand that children are different than adults. In addition to providing expert medical care, an important element in caring for the critically ill child is keeping the family unit together and helping to maintain as normal a family environment as possible. When a child is stricken with a catastrophic illness, this becomes even more important.[71]

SUMMARY

Planning for postacute care or a move through the continuum takes expertise regarding the various levels of care and what each can or cannot do. Planning can be a labor-intensive process if the patient is stable at the present level of care but care needs are too great for the next level. Planning for discharge or the move through the continuum must start the day of admission for hospitalized patients and at case opening when the patient is identified as requiring long-term care.

With the BBA, PPS has come into play for postacute care services. As such, agencies and facilities have had to learn a whole new way of documenting needs to ensure reimbursement. This has affected the ability to move a patient rapidly from one level to another; now the agency or facility must rethink the types of patients they can care for if they are to be reimbursed appropriately.

Home care remains the primary choice for discharge. However, with today's sicker and more complex patients this is not always realistic. The case manager must therefore take a proactive role as he or she attempts to educate or sway the patient or family into more realistic planning.

With the fact patients are living longer, several modalities for care have arisen over the past several years. Such

care now includes assisted living facilities, homelike facilities for patients with Alzheimer's disease, and telemedicine. However, the greatest area of postacute care need in most communities, especially when home care is questionable, continues to be services for children or young adults.

Chapter Exercises

1. Identify at least four areas in the postacute field that can provide either short-term episodic or long-term care for patients.
2. True of false: When a patient is ready for rehabilitation, any patient can be admitted. If false, what is the primary guiding factor for readiness for PM&R rehabilitation?
3. List at least five differences between skilled and custodial care.
4. What are the key payers for skilled and custodial care?
5. Since the enactment of the BBA, what has been the primary method for reimbursement? Explain this payment method and list some of the requirements of SNFs and home health agencies for billing for the patients they admit.

Suggested Websites and Resources

www.ashp.org/longtermcare—American Society of Health-System Pharmacists long-term care and chronic care information

www-hsl.mcmaster.ca/tomflem/chronic. html —Links to chronic care websites

www.longtermcareprovider.com/content/home page/default.asp—Long-term care provider website

www.rwjf.org—Robert Wood Johnson website

www.medicare.gov/nhcompare/home.asp— Medicare's site to compare nursing homes in any given area *www.cms.hhs.gov/providers/*—CMS website for Medicare Conditions of Participation for all Providers

www.medicare.gov/publications/pubs/pdf/hh. pdf—Medicare publications

www.cms.hhs.gov/main—CMS website

www.access.gpo.gov/su_docs/—U.S. Government Printing Office and official federal government information at your fingertips

www.medicare.gov/Coverage/Home.asp—Medicare website for coverage questions

www.cms.hhs.gov/manuals/—CMS website for manuals, transmittals, and memoranda

www.cms-kids.com/—Florida's Children's Medical Services

www.acf.dhhs.gov/programs/add/—Administration on Developmental Disabilities

www.ed.gov/offices/OSERS/—Office of Special Education and Rehabilitation Services

www.ed.gov/offices/OSERS/Policy/IDEA/—U.S. Department of Education and the Individuals with Disabilities Education Act

www.naric.com/—National Rehabilitation Information Center

www.ed.gov/offices/OSERS/NIDRR/—National Institute on Disability and Rehabilitation Research

www.carf.org/—Rehabilitation Accreditation Commission

www.caninecompanions.org/ and *www.tagsys.com/Ads/CCI/*—Canine companions

www.dmoz.org/Society/Disabled/Service_Ani mals/Dogs/—Society Disabled Service Animals for dogs

Coma Recovery Association
807 Carman Avenue
Westbury, NY 11590
office@comarecovery.org
www.comarecovery.org
Phone: 516-997-1826
Fax: 516-997-1613

Brain Injury Association of America
105 North Alfred Street
Alexandria, VA 22314
publicrelations@biausa.org
www.biausa.org
Phone: 703-236-6000 or 800-444-6443
Fax: 703-236-6001

Family Caregiver Alliance
690 Market Street
Suite 600
San Francisco, CA 94104
info@caregiver.org
www.caregiver.org
Phone: 415-434-3388 or 800-445-8106
Fax: 415-434-3508

National Rehabilitation Information Center
1010 Wayne Avenue
Suite 800
Silver Spring, MD 20910-5633
naricinfo@kra.com
www.naric.com
Phone: 301-562-2400 or 800-346-2742
Fax: 301-562-2401

National Stroke Association
9707 East Easter Lane
Englewood, CO 80112-3747
info@stroke.org
www.stroke.org
Phone: 303-649-9299 or 800-STROKES (787-6537)
Fax: 303-649-1328

www.blvd.com—Disability Resource Center; devoted to accessible devices and options for the physically challenged and elderly

www.cmrg.com—Case Management Resource Guide

www.nichcy.org—National Informational Center for Children and Youth with Disabilities *www.dssc.org/frc/oseptad.htm*—National website sponsored by the U.S. Department of Education and other organizations that offers information for children with special needs and who need special education

www.tr.wou.edu/dblink—National Information Clearinghouse on Children Who Are Deaf-Blind (funded by the U.S. Department of Education)

www.ahcpr.gov—Agency for Healthcare Research and Quality, a department of the U.S. Department of Health and Human Services; offers information for both professionals and consumers

REFERENCES

1. American Nurses Association: *Modular certification examination catalog*, Washington, DC, 1999, American Nurses Credentialing Center.
2. Retzlaff K: Assisted living, *Continuing Care* 15(8):31, 1996.
3. Schaffer CL: Case management law. Reaching the right level, *Continuing Care* 19(1):16-18, 2000.
4. Motta GJ: Reimbursement relief, *Continuing Care* 19(4):4, 2000.
5. *St. Anthony's complete guide to Medicare coverage issues*, Reston, Va, 1999, St. Anthony's Publishing, section 214, pp 6-9.
6. *CHAMPUS code of federal regulations*, U.S. Government Printing Office. Title 32, Volume 2. July 1, 2001. pp 63-84
7. *CARF standards manual and interpretive guidelines for medical rehabilitation*, Tucson, Ariz, 1995, Rehabilitation Accreditation Commission.
8. Steinhauser EK: From wealth to welfare: PPS tightens rope on subacute care, *Continuing Care* 17(10):26-31-42, 1998.
9. Steinhauser EK: After the dust settles, *Continuing Care* 18(10):20-25, 1999.
10. National Center for Health Statistics, CDC website: www.cdc.gov/nchs.
11. Inside track. Medicare announces PPS rules for home health, *Continuing Care* 19(1):8, 2000.
12. American Telemedicine Association website: www.atmeda.org/news/guidelines.html.
13. Retzlaff K: Assisted living, *Continuing Care* 15(8): 30, 1996.
14. Rescigno SM: The nursing home-assisted living interface, *Long-Term Care Interface* 2(1):30-35, 2001.
15. Fox CE: *Senate testimony. The role of our safety net providers and the uninsured*, Washington, DC, March 2000, Administrator Health Resources and Services Administration, available on-line at www.hrsa. dhhs.gov/Newsroom/speeches/safetynettest.htm.
16. Reever KE: Adult day services, *Advance for Providers of Post-Acute Care* 3(10):30-31, 2000.
17. Chapman S: Outpatient pain management. In Tollison CD, editor: *Handbook of pain management*, ed 2, Baltimore, 1988, Williams & Wilkins.
18. Hamilton M, Thomsen T: Removing the label, *Continuing Care* 17(9):26-29,40, 1998.
19. LTC Newsfront: The utilization of palliative care gains ground, *Long-Term Care Interface* 2(1):20, 2001.
20. Deming LM, Wolf JC: Case management for ventilator-dependent children, *J Care Management* 3(5):15, 1997.
21. Kilinski R: Redefining the meaning of home care, *Continuing Care* 16(1):24-27, 1997.

BIBLIOGRAPHY

Bontke CF, Boake C: Principles of brain injury rehabilitation. In Braddom RL, editor: *Physical medicine and rehabilitation*, Philadelphia, 1996, Saunders, p 1027-1052.
Cope ND: The rehabilitation of traumatic brain injury. In Kottke FJ, Lehman JF, editors: *Krusen's handbook of physical medicine and rehabilitation*, ed 4, Philadelphia, 1990, Saunders, pp 1217-1251.
Cyte J, Gleason MB: *The care and rehabilitation of the patient in a persistent vegetative state*, Gaithersburg, Md, 1986, Aspen.
Glacino JT, Zasler ND: Outcome after severe traumatic brain injury: coma, the vegetative state, and the minimally responsive state, *J Head Trauma Rehabil* 10(1):40-56, 1995.
Hinnat DW: Psychological evaluation and testing. In Tollison CD, editor: *Handbook of pain management*, ed 2, Baltimore, 1988, Williams & Wilkins, pp 18-35.
Horn LJ, Zasler ND: *Medical rehabilitation of traumatic brain injury*, St Louis, 1996, Mosby, p 71.
Hosack KR, Roccbio CA: Serving families of persons with severe brain injury in an era of managed care, *J Head Trauma Rehabil* 10(2):57-65,1995.
Long CJ, Ross LK, editors: *Handbook of head trauma: acute care to recovery*, New York, 1992, Plenum Press.
Matthews J: Eldercare: choosing and financing long-term care, Berkley, Calif, 1990, Nolo Press.
McCaffery M: The scientific method, *Continuing Care* 15(3):18-20, 1996.
McPeak LA: Physiatric history and examination. In Braddom L, editor: *Physical medicine and rehabilitation*, Philadelphia, 1996, Saunders, pp 3-65.
Poretz DM: High tech comes home, *Am J Med* 91(5): 453-454, 1991.
Roth EJ, Harvery RL: Rehabilitation of stroke syndromes. In Braddom RL, editor: *Physical medicine and rehabilitation*, Philadelphia, 1996, Saunders, pp 1053-1081.
Sinaki M, editor: *Basic clinical rehabilitation medicine*, St Louis, 1993, Mosby.
Waldman SD, Winnie AP: *Interventional pain management*, Philadelphia, 1996, Saunders, pp 119-127.

Skilled Nursing Facility

Peggy A. Rossi, BSN, MPA, CCM, CPUR

OBJECTIVES

- To understand the impact of the Balanced Budget Act and the prospective payment system on nursing facilities
- To list the most common reasons for delays in discharge related to placement of patients into nursing homes
- To understand the new classifications and new forms required for skilled nursing facility residents

When a patient no longer needs acute care, the first question to be asked is whether the patient needs skilled or custodial care. The case manager must also examine the following:

- Does the patient require services intermittently rather than daily?
- Can the patient manage safely at home between nursing visits?
- If the patient is a rehabilitation candidate, is the patient at a point at which he or she can benefit from an intensive course of rehabilitation or is an alternate plan required until the patient can tolerate and benefit from intensive rehabilitation?

If the answer to each of these questions is No, then plans must be initiated for possible placement in a care facility, and often the first one considered is a skilled nursing facility (SNF).

Much has changed over the past few years regarding nursing facility admission and care due to passage of the Balanced Budget Act (BBA) of 1997 and implementation of a new payment methodology known as the prospective payment system (PPS). The BBA was passed during the Clinton administration for the primary purpose of reducing federal Medicare spending on SNF care.

Under PPS, a new reimbursement system for SNFs was slowly phased in and was fully implemented by the year 2001. Changes in reimbursement to SNFs were necessary because, according to a report issued by the Office of Inspector General (OIG) of the Department of Health and Human Services, nursing home costs were rapidly depleting Medicare funds. The report compared SNF costs in 1989 with those in 1997. The report indicated that, in 1989, Medicare paid $2.8 billion to nursing homes, or about 4.7% of the Medicare budget; in 1997 this amount increased to $12.2 billion, or about 5.9% of the Medicare budget.[1]

To better understand some of the difficulties case managers face in placing patients into SNFs, whether they are covered by Medicare, Medicare + Choice, or private health care insurance, it is important to understand the effect of Medicare's PPS requirements on the SNF process as a whole.

In contrast to the old payment system, in which payments were retrospective, based on reasonable cost and on the Medicare patient's actual medical needs, PPS is based on a consolidated payment or per diem payment that is prospective and case-mix adjusted. Under PPS the nursing home is paid a higher rate to treat patients requiring more resource-intensive care than to treat healthier patients. Overall, the payment rate is designed to reimburse facilities fairly while encouraging efficient, quality care. The PPS reimbursement is designed to cover the costs of the SNF stay of a patient requiring "skilled" care, including routine care, ancillary care, medications, therapies, capital equipment, and most other items, treatments, and services, such as transportation to appointments with a physician or other provider, previously paid for by Medicare Part B.

As in the past, for the patient to qualify for coverage (including coverage under a Medicare + Choice managed care organization plan) and for the SNF to be allowed to bill the government for services, the patient must meet Medicare's criteria of need for "skilled" care and must be certified by a licensed medical doctor as requiring an SNF inpatient level of care. Under PPS, however, when a Medicare patient is deemed by a physician to require care in an SNF and is admitted to the facility, the SNF must generate and complete a form called a minimum data set or MDS form. Briefly, information about the care needs of the patient are extrapolated and entered onto the MDS form, and the form is transmitted to Medicare within a specified time.

To meet the demands of the government for billing for Medicare patients, many SNFs have created the position of MDS coordinator. This person's primary job duties are to gather the required information, determine into which resource utilization group (RUG) the patient's care needs fall, and complete and submit the MDS form. A set schedule for form completion and SNF electronic transmittal of data to Medicare must be strictly followed. If not, the SNF receives a lower rate of reimbursement than would otherwise be granted.

There are seven major RUG categories, with patients requiring more complicated care classified into the higher RUGs. Therapy is not reimbursed per module or per service as in the past but is categorized into levels that must accurately reflect the patient's therapy needs. The accuracy of the data is critical when the patient is placed into a RUG category, as this is the primary means of determining the level of reimbursement for that patient.

Currently, Medicare continues to pay 100% of SNF costs for patients requiring "skilled" care for the first 20 days of a stay. If the patient remains beyond the initial 20 days, Medicare pays 80% of the SNF costs and the patient or a secondary health insurer assumes financial responsibility for the remaining 20% (copayment) of the SNF daily costs.

RESOURCE UTILIZATION GROUPS AND MINIMUM DATA SET

Under PPS two new terms were added to the vocabulary of the long-term care industry—*resource utilization group* and *minimum data set* (RUG and MDS). Both terms are employed by the SNFs and the government to determine the case-mix index used for reimbursement. MDS was in use prior to PPS but was employed primarily for care planning.

After initially assigning residents to 1 of the 7 major RUG categories, SNFs are required to further classify residents into 1 of 44 minor RUG categories. When the SNF classifies residents, it is allowed to take into account the different levels of care residents require. The seven major RUG categories are as follows:

- Special rehabilitation
- Extensive care
- Special care
- Clinically complex
- Cognitively impaired
- Behavior problems
- Reduced physical functions

Each of the RUG categories is associated with a payment rate that is based on a number of factors, such as the need for therapy and the patient's level of functioning as determined by the ability to perform the activities of daily living. Medicare typically reimburses SNFs only for the care of patients coded into the first four categories.

To classify a patient, the SNF must fill out the MDS assessment form. This is a standardized set of clinical and functional status measures that an interdisciplinary team from the SNF completes for every resident by the 5th, 14th, 30th, 60th, and 90th days of stay.

Full information on Medicare RUGs and MDS can be found on the website of the Centers for Medicare & Medicaid Services (CMS, formerly the Health Care Financing Administration) at www.cms.hhs.gov/pubforms.

MEDICARE CRITERIA

To certify providers, many payers employ the most widely recognized and widely used criteria for defining skilled and custodial care—those developed by Medicare. Although not every patient admitted to a facility is elderly or disabled, or covered by Medicare, health care coverage and payments generally are allowed when services are performed in Medicare-certified facilities. Most insurers also allow coverage only for the same services that Medicare would have covered.

For Medicare patients who are not a member of a Medicare + Choice plan, SNF care is covered under Medicare Part A, under three specific conditions:

1. The patient must have been hospitalized for 3 consecutive calendar days or longer in an acute-care facility within the previous 30 days for the condition for which he or she will be treated in an SNF.
2. The physician must certify that the SNF admission is medically necessary.
3. The patient must require daily skilled nursing or rehabilitation services.

If the patient is covered by a Medicare + Choice plan, the 3-day qualifying acute-care hospital stay does not apply.

Medicare Definition of an SNF

Medicare defines an SNF as an institution or a distinct part of an institution such as a skilled nursing home or rehabilitation center that meets all of the following criteria[2]:

- It has a transfer agreement in effect with one or more participating hospitals.
- It is primarily engaged in providing skilled nursing care and related services for residents who require medical or nursing care, or rehabilitation services for injured, disabled, or sick persons who need rehabilitation.
- It meets the requirements for participation listed in Section 1819 of the Social Security Act and in Title 42 of the *Code of Federal Regulations*, Part 483, Subpart B.

PPS

Since the advent of PPS, concern has grown that SNFs have altered their admissions criteria. This concern has arisen primarily because of the inadequacy of the payments allowed by PPS and the effect of PPS on patients and nursing facilities in general. In the year 2000, the CMS asked the OIG to conduct a study to determine whether the new PPS for SNFs was causing decreased access for Medicare beneficiaries. To address these concerns, the OIG's staff surveyed a random sample of 180 hospital discharge planners in eight states. These discharge planners were responsible for coordinating nursing facility care for patients being discharged from hospitals. Contrary to this author's experience, the report concluded that there were no serious problems in placing Medicare patients in nursing homes; however, it did find that nursing homes had changed their admission practices in response to the PPS.[1]

According to the OIG report, most discharge planners (66%) reported no difficulty in placing patients, 32% reported that placement was somewhat difficult, and only 1% reported it to be very difficult. Two thirds of the discharge planners interviewed reported that the total number of Medicare patients they discharged to nursing homes increased over the previous 2 years. Most of the respondents suggested that the cause was an increase in the number of patients who are elderly and who require skilled care. They also noted that patients are staying in the hospital for shorter periods of time and that some are leaving sicker and sooner and are more likely to need skilled care. As indicated earlier, some of the findings of the study are contrary to the author's experience while managing the discharge planning unit at a Sacramento acute-care hospital and while currently serving as director of a large medical group that uses four major hospitals, also in the Sacramento area. Here, although the number of admissions per 1000 generally has not changed much, daily placement delays are noted, and the SNF length of stay, bed days per

1000 SNF residents, and admissions per 1000 are constantly increasing. Many of the delays encountered now involve patients who are younger and are sicker or have more complex illnesses (often patients covered by Social Security Disability Income Medicare or Medicare for end-stage renal disease). Also affected are patients whose care is anticipated to be long term and to extend beyond the coverage limits allowed by Medicare Part A, and patients who will require Medicaid for payment of the SNF. Although some patients can be placed in SNFs further away from home and for some a home care plan can eventually be developed, most remain hospitalized at the acute-care hospital until they can be placed in a nursing home or a home care plan can be arranged. This experience in Sacramento in placing patients who are sicker and require more complex care is mirrored in the results of the OIG study, which found that, among the discharge planners who did report placement problems, the majority (58%) identified difficulties involving patients requiring extensive services.[1] The patients who are most difficult to place and who require extensive services include the following:

- Patients taking expensive medications
- Patients who need special supplies or equipment that will require expenditures by the SNF
- Patients on dialysis (especially those who require transportation to and from dialysis facilities, since transportation costs might exceed the amount of reimbursement the facility receives under PPS)
- Patients with complex or open wounds
- Patients with infections, including antibiotic-resistant infections
- Patients who require intravenous feedings or intravenous medications
- Patients who need complex direct nursing care

- Patients who have a tracheostomy, are receiving ventilatory assistance, or require other respiratory care
- Patients with multiple diagnoses
- Patients with behavior problems

CUSTODIAL CARE

Custodial or personal care is not a covered benefit of either Medicare or private health insurance (except when the patient has a private long-term-care insurance policy). However, as a result of many factors (e.g., the cost of home care, the absence of caregivers or family to provide care), many patients are in SNFs because they need long-term custodial care that cannot be rendered in another setting (due either to costs or to the level of care required).

The custodial level of care can be appropriate when a patient has ceased to make functional improvements for whatever reason or when there are no longer any changes in the frequency or type of care necessary for a technology-dependent patient—in other words, when the care required is maintenance care. In many cases patients who need custodial care require a protected, monitored, and controlled environment, and although nursing home care is costly, it is cheaper than 24-hour care in the home.

BARRIERS TO PLACEMENT

Barriers to placement are case specific. However, in addition to the conditions causing delays in placement cited in the OIG report mentioned earlier, other conditions raising barriers to placement include the following:

- The patient's illness is related to human immunodeficiency virus or acquired immunodeficiency syndrome.
- The patient has a stage 3 or higher decubitus ulcer.

- The patient weighs over 200 pounds.
- The patient has a contagious disease.
- The patient is a child.
- The patient is an adult younger than 50 years.
- The patient lacks family or another party responsible for financial follow-through once insurance coverage terminates.
- The patient needs total care (often depends on the type, intensity, and frequency of care).
- The patient has psychiatric problems in addition to physical ones.
- The patient abuses alcohol or drugs.
- The patient shows combative or physically or verbally abusive behavior.
- The patient needs more hours of nursing care per day than the facility is licensed or staffed to provide

When any of these conditions is present, it is common for the discharge planner or case manager to call many facilities before an appropriate one is located. It is also not uncommon to have to place the patient outside the immediate area. Case managers must be familiar with the levels of care available not only in the local community but also throughout the state and must have access to information on facilities throughout the nation.

SOURCES OF PAYMENT FOR NURSING HOME CARE

Depending on the insurer and the facility, if the patient requires subacute care, the costs are most likely covered through insurance. For nursing home care, however, the payment sources are many and varied. If the patient requires skilled care, the private insurer or Medicare will pay the costs for the most part. Unfortunately, for care at an SNF to be reimbursable, the patient must have a health care policy that specifically covers this level of care. If the policy has an SNF benefit, then like Medicare it may set day or dollar limits; once these limits are reached, if continued care is required, the patient must pay privately, must be eligible for Medicaid, or must make arrangements for an alternate level of care.

According to the American Association of Retired Persons, the average cost for SNF care is close to $50,000 a year.[3] Although a few people have private long-term-care insurance, almost one third pay all the costs of care out of their own pockets. Another 70% receive help from Medicaid or other government health care safety net programs for lower-income people or those impoverished by high medical expenses.[3]

According to the NursingHome Reports.com website, sources of payment for the $72 billion spent on nursing home care in America can be broken down as follows[4]:

- Out of pocket = 33%
- Medicare = 9%
- Medicaid = 52%
- Other government programs = 4%
- Private health insurance = 2%

SUMMARY

Case managers must be keenly aware of available SNFs, their capabilities, and any problems or licensing issues. For questions about licensing and care, the best source of information is the state agency responsible for licensing and certification of health care facilities.

Not every patient requires the services of an SNF, but for those who do, care must be carefully coordinated to ensure that the patient is placed appropriately and that rehospitalization is avoided. For optimal results the family must be involved in all aspects of the placement, especially facility selection. Planning must begin as soon as the patient is identified as a candidate for placement.

Finding an appropriate facility is often a labor-intensive process, and the patient may be placed on several waiting lists until a vacancy is found. Also, because some patients have a multiplicity of conditions or illnesses, or need intensive or complex care, not all patients are candidates for placement in an SNF. In some situations, the patient may require short-term placement in a subacute-care facility. In other cases, care may be possible at home. All families must be counseled and prepared for the financial impact (and often guilt feelings) associated with long-term placement in an SNF. They also must be assured that such placement is frequently the only alternative to home care and that there is nothing wrong in admitting that they are not capable of caring for the patient at home.

Chapter Exercises

1. Visit a local SNF and discuss with the administrator the impact of the BBA and PPS on the nursing home industry in general. Discuss many of the pros and cons as well as the changes made in the way the nursing home now does business compared with how it did business in the past.

2. In your discussion with the SNF administrator, ask him or her to list the most common reasons they can or cannot accept patients.

3. While at the nursing home spend time with the MDS coordinator and ask him or her to review the data elements and requirements for the completion of the MDS form, the use of the RUGs, and the time guidelines and mandates the nursing facility must follow to be in compliance with the government's requirements for payment.

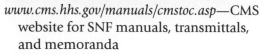

Suggested Websites and Resources

www.cms.hhs.gov/manuals/cmstoc.asp—CMS website for SNF manuals, transmittals, and memoranda

www.cms.hhs.gov/providers/—CMS website for SNF providers

www.cms.hhs.gov/cop/—CMS site for Medicare Conditions of Participation for SNFs

www.medicare.gov/—Medicare website for consumers

www.medicare.gov/Library/PDFNavigation/ PDFInterim.asp? Language=English&Type=Pub&PubID=021 74— Medicare guide to choosing a nursing home

www.medicare.gov/Library/PDFNavigation/ PDFInterim.asp? Language=English&Type=NonPub&Title= Nursing+Home+Checklist&Size=19+KB& Filepath=%2Fnursing%2Fchecklist%2Epdf —Medicare nursing home checklist

www.americanaging.org/—American Aging Association

www.n4a.org/—National Association on Area on Aging

www.aahsa.org/public/consumer.htm— American Association of Homes and Services for the Aging

www.aahsa.org/public/sh.htm—American Association of Homes and Services for the Aging

www.aarp.org/confacts/health/medicaidnurse. html—information on paying for nursing home care through Medicaid, maintained by American Association of Retired Persons

www.aahsa.org—American Association of Homes and Services for the Aging

www.medicareed.org—Center for Medicare Education

www.aahsa.org/public/consumer.htm#gen— American Association of Homes and Services for the Aging consumer website

REFERENCES

1. Brown JG: Executive summary. In *Early effects of the prospective payment system on access to skilled nursing facilities,* OEI-02-99-00400, August 1999.
2. Health Care Financing Administration, *Skilled nursing facility manual,* Pub No 12, available on-line at www.cms.gov/manuals/12_snf/SN00.asp.
3. American Association of Retired Persons, Medicaid: paying for nursing home care, available on-line at www.aarp.org/confacts/health/medicaidnurse.html.
4. National eldercare referral systems, Inc., NursingHome Reports.com, available on-line at www.nursinghomereports.com/paying_for_care/who _pays.htm.

BIBLIOGRAPHY

St. Anthony's Medicare coverage manual, Reston, Va, 1999, St. Anthony's Publishing, Section 201, p 6-4.

Civilian Health and Medical Program of the Uniformed Services: *Code of federal regulations,* Washington, DC, July 1, 2001, U.S. Government Printing Office, Title 32, Vol 2, pp 63-84.

Home Health Agency Care

Patrice Hilgendorf, BSN, MHS, and Elizabeth M. Akers, RN, BSN, PHN

OBJECTIVES

- To be familiar with the various types of home health agencies and the services they provide
- To differentiate skilled home care from custodial or nonskilled home care
- To describe some of the jobs the home care case manager is expected to perform

Once a patient no longer requires acute care, the case manager must decide, based on the chart findings and physician's orders, whether or not the patient can return home. During the review the following questions may be asked: Can the patient be managed safely at home with part-time, intermittent visits by skilled personnel? Are the needs of the patient custodial? If placement in a facility is necessary, which facility affords the least restrictions but can provide the required level of care? Can safe care in the home be arranged?

The home health agency will also assign a case manager to the patient. The home care case manager performs the same functions as do case managers in the hospital or outpatient setting. The main difference is that he or she is also responsible for the overall assessment of the patient's needs at home and the establishment and evaluation of a care plan to meet those needs. The home health case manager may be a nurse or a therapist and, like case managers in other settings, is accountable for the achievement of desired outcomes. He or she coordinates the care given by the personnel in various disciplines to prevent duplication and promote the attainment of goals established by the home care team in a given episode of care or a certification period (i.e., physician must initially certify that home care is required and must continue to recertify the need until the patient is stable and can be discharged from home health care). The home care case manager also provides education, advocacy, discharge planning, resource management, and outcomes management.

Public health visiting nurses have been familiar with case management concepts for over 60 years and were the pioneers of today's home care industry. Insurance case managers as well as hospital discharge planners rely on information shared by the home health case manager when patients require readmission to acute-care facilities or transfer to other programs, agencies, or levels of care.

TYPES OF AGENCIES AND SERVICES PROVIDED

Home health agencies may be public, private, proprietary, or nonprofit; may or may not be licensed; and may provide skilled or nonskilled care, or both, in patients' homes. Most health care payers require, at a minimum, that the home health agency be licensed by the state department of health services, and many require that an agency be Medicare certified; others require the agency to be accredited by the Joint Commission on Accreditation of Healthcare Organizations (JCAHO). Some agencies may also be Medicaid certified or may be certified only by JCAHO and Medicaid. Other accreditation organizations exist as well. To be certified by both Medicare and Medicaid, however, agencies must comply with both the Medicare home health conditions of participation and state licensing regulations. A complete copy of home health conditions of participation can be found on the website www.cms.hhs.gov/providers/hha/.

No set rules exist regarding the types of services a patient may need, but great variation may be found in what services will be reimbursed by the patient's health insurer. For example, some patients may require intermittent visits from skilled professional staff (registered nurses, physical therapists, etc.) for hands-on treatments or health education. The same patients may also need to hire unlicensed staff to assume personal care or homemaking duties (i.e., cleaning, laundering, cooking, shopping). Yet other patients may need the services of hourly, shift, or live-in professionals to create a safe residential environment.

Skilled Intermittent Home Care

Skilled intermittent home care is provided by agencies that are, at a minimum, licensed by the state. Most are also Medicare certified and accredited by the JCAHO or Certified Hospital Admission Program. Skilled intermittent care is what most payers and most people have in mind when they think of home care or visiting nurses. Visits are made by professional staff to provide treatments or instruction to the patient. Such services may include wound care, disease management education (e.g., after cardiac surgery), establishment of a home exercise program by a physical therapist, and so on. Visits may be made as often as daily to perform wound care or as infrequently as monthly to change a Foley catheter. The frequency varies depending on the patient's needs. Agencies are increasingly using standardized, diagnosis-based care plans or clinical pathways that give recommended frequencies for services in addition to the clinical guidelines for the services to be rendered. Several versions of home health clinical pathways with recommended care plans and visitation frequencies have also been published. Use of such pathways can help assure that all patients with a particular diagnosis receive standardized care, which is modified to their unique needs.[1]

Skilled intermittent care agencies generally base their care-delivery models on the Medicare certification requirements. As stated earlier, the agency assigns its own case manager, who is responsible for coordinating the patient's care and interacting with other involved parties, such as the insurance case manager and community agencies. Caregiver visits generally last between 30 minutes and 2 hours, depending on the care being provided. Services include skilled nursing (by registered nurses and licensed vocational nurses), rehabilitative services (physical, occupational, and speech therapy), and social work services. Home health aides may also be provided for assistance with personal care, such as bathing.

The cost of skilled intermittent home care varies depending on the type of services needed and the location of the agency (rural agencies often have higher charges because of longer driving distances between patients). Currently, charges vary from $85 to $120 per visit for skilled professionals and from $50 to $90 per visit for home health aides. Agencies may request a higher rate for complex care requiring longer visits, such as administration of intravenous infusions. In rural areas, they may levy mileage charges or request an hourly fee for the care of patients who live more than a 30- or 40-minute drive from the agency.

An example of low-cost care is the care of a patient who has had a total knee replacement and needs physical therapy for four to six visits but has no other medical problems and does not need any other services. On the other hand, a patient with multiple medical conditions who experiences a cerebrovascular accident may need the services of a registered nurse, physical therapist, occupational therapist, speech therapist, and social worker as well as those of a home health aide. Another example of a case requiring costly care is that of a patient who lives alone, needs twice-daily wound care, must receive infusions, has many social and emotional problems indicating a need for social work services, and requires the help of aides for bathing.

Private Duty Care

There are two broad categories of private duty nursing—skilled and unskilled. Skilled private duty nursing is provided by a state-licensed agency to patients with complex medical needs who require several hours of care daily. A registered nurse or licensed vocational nurse provides such care. Examples of patients requiring such care are those who are ventilator dependent, have tracheostomies, and require frequent suctioning, and those who receive intravenous infusions that require monitoring. Unskilled care is

provided by nursing assistants or attendants. Unskilled care may include assistance with activities of daily living, housekeeping, and meal preparation. Typically such care is provided for 4 or more hours per day for patients who are not yet ready to enter an assisted-living situation or who cannot safely be left alone in their homes.

Skilled Private Duty Care

It is common for mechanically dependent patients to require private duty nursing. This is especially true on the patient's initial discharge and during periods of crisis, or when the caregiver needs respite. The following are examples of patients who need private duty nursing:

- Ventilator-dependent persons
- Patients with new tracheostomies who require frequent suctioning and instruction
- Terminally ill patients with multiple skilled nursing needs
- Patients with multiple skilled care needs who require professional nursing interventions for several hours per day or a medical condition that requires continuous skilled care

The need for private duty care must be assessed individually. The necessary number of hours of skilled nursing is based on the frequency and duration of care required (e.g., care may be needed several times in each 8-hour shift, sporadically, or instantly at any time during a 24-hour period). If private duty nursing is allowed, the number of hours requested or approved should be contingent on the family's or caregiver's competence in providing the care and on other case variables such as the intensity and complexity of the care required. In some cases private duty nursing is arranged to provide the skilled care the patient needs and to allow the caregiver time to sleep or attend to personal matters or business. Many insurance companies require that the family perform the necessary care for at least one 8-hour shift per day.

It is common on discharge of a technology-dependent patient or patient requiring complex care to provide continuous private duty nursing for a few days. Family caregivers begin learning the necessary skilled care techniques in the hospital but may require some observation and coaching as care in the home begins. As the caregiver develops proficiency, or the patient's needs become less intense, the nurse's hours can be reduced; however, this schedule is case specific.

NEGOTIATION OF COSTS WITH PAYERS

Costs for private duty and skilled nursing vary from region to region, but case managers should expect a quote of approximately $30 to $50 per hour. Many agencies are willing to negotiate a daily or shift rate discount, but some are not. Despite the cost, private duty nursing is appropriate for the following patients:

- Technology-dependent patients whose physician agrees to home care and whose family, once trained, can assume a portion of the responsibilities for care
- Patients unacceptable for placement in a subacute-care facility owing to the complexity of skilled care needs
- Patients at risk of frequent readmission to an acute-care facility or frequent emergency department use and whose intermittent or daily home health agency care is insufficient

Private duty nursing is also useful for technology-dependent patients who refuse any option except home care. If such a patient is competent, out-of-home placement cannot be forced, as it violates the patient's rights.

NEGOTIATION AND APPROVAL OF EXTRACONTRACTUAL CARE

Because of the limitations many health care payers place on home care benefits, care in a skilled nursing facility is often the most cost-effective alternative. If this level of care is not possible, approval may have to be obtained for private duty nursing or some combination of home health services.

It is common for many technology-dependent patients to require 16 to 24 hours per day of private duty nursing for several weeks, or until the family or caregiver is proficient in all the skilled techniques required for care or the patient's medical condition has stabilized. Once ventilator-dependent patients are stabilized and comfortable in their homes, private duty nursing can eventually be decreased to 8 hours per day or discontinued altogether. Maintaining private duty nursing for one shift affords the primary caregiver respite to sleep before resuming a normal 16-hour shift of care.

When an extracontractual process is used, the case manager may have to seek weekly approval for ongoing private duty nursing. This allows better case control and monitoring of the situation. It also avoids the expectation that care will continue indefinitely. Obtaining approvals in this way takes more of the case manager's time, but in the long run it is the best way because the case manager stays apprised of problems and progress. More importantly, it allows gradual decrements in the level of care.

One technique to use in seeking continued home health care or hourly skilled care is to obtain 5 to 7 consecutive days of nursing or therapy notes and include them with the request. This gives the reviewer a better idea of the skilled level of care required and of the patient's response to treatment, and expedites approval.

MEDICAID-FUNDED PRIVATE DUTY NURSING (IN-HOME WAIVERS)

When benefits are exhausted or the extra-contractual process fails, the case manager may wish to consider applying for patient acceptance into a Medicaid in-home waiver program, Medicaid's version of private duty nursing. Unfortunately, application for a waiver program is an arduous process, and unless application is made months earlier, such a program may not be a viable option. Case managers must be familiar with the Medicaid programs and waiver programs, including eligibility requirements and the appropriate procedures in their state. This is especially true if it appears that the patient will require 24-hour care and this level of care is excluded by the health care payer. Application must be made as early as possible.

If the patient is eligible and appropriate for a Medicaid in-home waiver, the health care payer retains responsibility for all other services or benefits not related to the services provided by the waiver (i.e., for benefits to which the patient is entitled by virtue of the health plan coverage). For instance, if the Medicaid waiver covers skilled care for a ventilator-dependent patient who requires gallbladder surgery, the surgery is covered by the patient's health care payer, not by Medicaid. Medicaid is the payer of last resort, and if the patient is eligible for the Medicaid waiver, the waiver covers only services the payer disallows.

ALTERNATIVE FUNDING PROGRAMS

For technology-dependent children with special needs, the case manager must work closely with the state's Title V Children's Medical Services program and with the agency responsible for administering services to persons with developmental disabilities to gain broader benefits. This is especially true when hourly private duty nursing is required but is excluded from the child's health coverage. Hourly private duty nursing coverage varies from state to state, and as such, case managers must be familiar with coverage allowances and the application process for their state.

The key to providing a cohesive, nonredundant, and thorough care plan is to develop the child's case management plan jointly with the health care payer and each agency providing an alternative source of funding for which the child might be eligible. Alternative funding or entitlement programs are payers of last resort, so any benefits available from the health care payer must be exhausted before other funding is activated.

Another key element in working with alternative funding programs to deliver coherent care is to use their vendored private duty registries or home health agencies. Often the vendored or paneled providers are not in the health care payer's network, and the case manager may need to request approval for their use, either through the normal review processes or extracontractually.

MEDICARE HOME HEALTH CARE ELIGIBILITY REQUIREMENTS

Home health care provided by a Medicare-certified agency is required when the skill and proficiency of a technical or professional health service provider is necessary to achieve the medically desired results for a homebound patient. To qualify for coverage for services, the agency must be Medicare certified; the patient must require primarily the skills of a registered nurse, physical therapist, or speech therapist; and the services must be ordered by a physician. Home health agencies may provide the services of some or all of the following skilled technical and professional personnel:

- Registered nurse
- Licensed practical nurse or licensed vocational nurse

- Physical therapist
- Speech or language pathologist or audiologist
- Occupational therapist
- Medical social worker
- Home health aide
- Registered dietitian
- Specialty care professional (e.g., enterostomal therapy nurse or wound ostomy–certified nurse, psychiatric nurse, chemotherapy nurse, infusion nurse, pediatric nurse, diabetic or cardiac clinical specialist, respiratory therapist)

Definitions

Case managers must be familiar with common Medicare home health terminology such as the following:

- **Confined to home** or **homebound**—Medicare defines a homebound person as one who is essentially confined to the place of residence due to illness or injury and who can be ambulatory or otherwise mobile but is unable to safely be absent from the residence except for periods of relatively short duration. Leaving the home may require the assistance of one or more persons and entail a considerable and taxing effort on the part of the patient. The patient is allowed some short absences from home, which may now include absences for the purpose of health care treatment, including adult day health care, or for religious services, without jeopardizing homebound status. Many of the following definitions can be found in the Medicare manuals, which are available on-line at www.medicare.gov/publications/pubs/pdf/hh.pdf.
- **Intermittent** or **part-time skilled care**—This care is defined as the services of licensed professionals that is required daily (i.e., a daily visit or several times per week). Skilled home care can also be provided by more than one licensed professional, and in some cases may require two or more visits from different licensed professionals in one day. Still, these constitute intermittent, or part-time, care.
- **Reasonable and necessary**—This concept relates to the idea of medical necessity and is hard to define. Generally, reasonable and necessary services are consistent with the given diagnosis, are standard practice for the treatment of the diagnosis or functional problem, and are likely to result in the desired outcome most of the time.
- **Place of residence**—The Medicare Home Care Guidelines define place of residence as wherever the patient makes his/her home. This may be the patient's house, apartment, or trailer; a relative's home; a board-and-care facility or other residential facility; and so on. There are exclusions for facilities at which skilled care is provided.[2]
- **Unduplicated**—This term applies to services not duplicated between disciplines or provided by another agency.
- **Skilled care**—Skilled care is defined as those services for which the knowledge of a professional is required to exercise a skill, render judgments, and evaluate process outcomes.[3] A task defined as skilled (e.g., complex wound care, insulin administration) is considered skilled even if it can be successfully taught to the patient's caregiver. Patients and caregivers perform many skilled tasks on a daily basis.
- **Unskilled care**—Unskilled care does not require the skills of a trained professional. Activities of daily living and independent ADLs

are unskilled tasks, as are applying prescription cream to a rash and administering oral medications.

Primary Functions of Medicare-Certified Agencies

The principal function of the home health agency is to provide physician-ordered skilled nursing or other therapeutic services to homebound patients on a part-time, intermittent, or visiting basis. Home health agency care can be preventive, diagnostic, therapeutic, rehabilitative, or long term. Each case must be assessed to determine the complexity of care needed to prevent deterioration of the patient's condition and unnecessary hospitalization, and to identify the type and extent of education or direct care required. Once the comprehensive assessment is completed, the physician establishes a treatment plan or plan of care with the assistance of the registered nurse or therapist case manager.

Home health care orders generally cover the following categories:

- Skilled observation and assessment of a condition
- Evaluation and management of a complex care plan
- Teaching and training activities
- Direct care services
- Services provided by professionals

The professional nursing services offered by a home health agency include the following:

- Evaluating and reevaluating patient needs
- Developing and implementing the plan of care
- Providing direct nursing services, treatments, and preventive proce dures: medication administra tion, insulin administration, injections, infusions, vascular access device care, wound care, tube feedings, catheter insertion, nasopharyngeal and tracheal aspiration, ostomy care, oxygen administration, veni puncture, rehabilitation nursing care, nutrition monitoring, spiritual support, pain and symptom management, and terminal and comfort care
- Observing for signs and symptoms, problems, and progression or regression and reporting all to the attending physician
- Educating, supervising, and counseling the patient, family, or caregiver about nursing care and related problems
- Supervising and training other nursing personnel (aides)

The duties of home health agency skilled physical therapists include the following:

- Evaluating and reevaluating patients and their therapy needs (tests are conducted to establish baseline data for functional impairment and abilities, and to aid in development of the care plan)
- Providing direct treatments to relieve pain, develop or restore function, and maintain maximum performance
- Using equipment such as ultraviolet light, diathermy devices, ultrasonographic devices, whirlpool and contrast baths, moist packs, and other durable medical equipment (e.g., walkers, braces, and wheelchairs)
- Educating the patient, family, or caregiver in the care and use of durable medical equipment and therapy modalities
- Instructing other health team personnel, including nurses, aides, the patient, family, and caregivers, in the therapy program

The duties of home health agency skilled speech therapists include the following:

- Evaluating and reevaluating the patient for speech, hearing, and language disorders

- Identifying, recommending, or providing appropriate speech and hearing services
- Instructing other health team personnel, including aides and caregivers, in the therapy program
- Helping families to develop communication techniques (i.e., communication boards, signaling)

The duties of home health agency occupational therapists include the following:

- Evaluating and reevaluating the patient's level of functional impairment and ability to perform self-care, including activities of daily living
- Instructing other health team personnel, including nurses, aides, and caregivers, in the therapy program

The duties of home health agency medical social workers include the following:

- Helping the health care team to understand the social and emotional factors related to the patient's health and care
- Assessing social and emotional factors affecting compliance with the plan of care
- Assessing the caregiver's capacity and potential, including but not limited to ability to cope with the problems of daily living, acceptance of the illness or injury or its impact, role reversal, sexual problems, stress, anger, or frustration, and making the necessary referrals to ensure that the patient receives the appropriate treatments
- Helping the caregiver to secure or utilize the services of other community agencies as needs are identified
- Helping the patient or caregiver to submit paperwork for alternative funding.

The duties of home health agency home health aides include:

- Helping the patient with all aspects of personal or custodial care
- Performing incidental household services essential to the patient's health care (e.g., bed making, laundering, preparation of light meals, shopping)
- Assisting with administration of medications that ordinarily are self-administered
- Helping the patient perform exercises as outlined by therapists
- Reporting changes in the patient's condition to the supervising professional nurse

The website of the Centers for Medicare & Medicaid Services (CMS; formerly the Health Care Financing Administration) is a useful resource for information on Medicare coverage and regulations. For key information on Medicare see the Centers for Medicare and Medicaid and Medicare websites, refer to the following:

www.cms.hhs.gov/—Main CMS website

www.access.gpo.gov/su_docs/—Regulatory and other information

www.medicare.gov/Coverage/Home.asp—Medicare website for coverage questions

IMPACT OF GOVERNMENTAL CHANGE ON HOME HEALTH CARE

Not only has the home health industry been affected by the overriding health care crisis in America, but during the past several years the industry has experienced a dramatic and at times devastating overhaul by the federal government. Home health agencies were created after the enactment of the Medicare program in 1965 and remained relatively unknown to most consumers and many physicians for many years. Spending on home health care was just a small portion of the federal budget. Payments for home health care were disbursed according to a cost-based, fee-for-service model for each visit made within the six basic disciplines designated by the Medicare administration. During the 1990s, changing demographics, an aging population, and a broadening of Medicare coverage of home health services resulted in significant expansion of this once-small industry into the fastest growing component of health care. Attention turned to home health care expenditures, and a number of investigations by the Office of Inspector General (OIG) of the Department of Health and Human Services revealed overutilization of services, fraudulent billing, and abuse of the benefit in some parts of the country. Operation Restore Trust (ORT) hit the industry hard with federal surveys and ultimately resulted in the closure of over 3000 home health agencies nationally. The Balanced Budget Act (BBA) of 1997 brought more changes, including tightened interpretation of regulations, such as removal of venipuncture from the list of skilled services. This change affected many homebound patients who otherwise did not have access to laboratory services for monitoring blood levels of medications. The BBA also set in motion the final stages of introduction of a planned prospective payment system (PPS), which had been under research for nearly 10 years. The interim payment system wreaked havoc on most agencies for a brief period prior to the introduction of PPS, which finally eliminated fee-for-service reimbursements as of October 1, 2000.

Now home health agencies must operate in a new frontier, much like managed care organizations or hospitals using the diagnosis-related group system. The health care crisis ultimately hit the home health industry with PPS, a version of managed care to control costs and conserve resources. Payment is made prospectively now, and agencies face the challenge of providing adequate and appropriate home health services with limited dollars per episode of care. Leaders in home care see case management as the key to survival, and the case management model is emerging as the primary model of care delivery. "Whereas managed care is a system of cost-containment programs, case management is a process of care delivery sometimes used within the managed care system."[4]

PPS and the Outcome and Assessment Information Set

The PPS methodology was based on audited cost reports of home health agencies, standardized for case mix and wage variances. One huge change for home health agencies was the development of the Outcome and Assessment Information Set (OASIS) project, which was part of the Outcome-Based Quality Improvement initiative within the PPS environment. OASIS is a comprehensive assessment tool used to collect data about the clinical and functional status of patients and ultimately to determine payment amounts.

The new OASIS tool, comprised of 97 assessment questions, was written into regulation via the Medicare conditions of participation, and its use became a requirement for all Medicare-certified agencies in April 1999. OASIS is the property of the Center for Health Services and Policy Research, in Denver, Colorado, and was developed for the CMS. For a full copy of the OASIS forms and links to the Medicare site for the OASIS implementation manual, see the website www.cms.hhs.gov/oasis/oasisdat.htm. Also see the following website for OASIS regulations: www.cms.hhs.gov/oasis/hhregs.asp.

The OASIS questions cover areas such as social, demographic, and environmental attributes; available support systems; functional and health status; and service utilization by home health care patients. The data collected must be entered into software designed for OASIS and then transmitted regularly to the state and federal governments. The cost of implementing this system was significant for home health agencies, and the Balanced Budget Refinement Act brought only minimal relief in the form of a $10 payment for every new beneficiary.

By October 1, 2000, every agency in the country had transitioned to the new PPS. The data collected by the agency are converted into a score based on the clinical, functional, and service dimensions of care. Services required by the patient are projected based on the scores assigned to the patient's level of required services or the home health resource group into which the patient is classified. These scores are converted into case-mix weights and ultimately into dollar amounts. Payment is based on a 60-day episode of care. Fifty percent of the payment is forwarded to the agency shortly after admission to care. The remaining amount, modified by any adjustments based on changes in the patient's condition, is paid at the end of the episode with the final claim. Reassessment OASIS data are collected at defined intervals during the episode and again at discharge or transfer from the agency. The goal of PPS is to measure the intensity of care and services required by each patient and to translate it into a payment level.

Significant changes in a patient's condition are considered in payment adjustments, as are the presence of wounds; orthopedic, neurologic, and diabetic conditions; and the need for intensive therapy services. The primary and secondary diagnoses must be carefully selected to reflect the majority of services needed for an episode of care and then must be correctly coded according to professional coding standards (*International Classification of Diseases, Ninth Revision* [ICD-9]).

Payment is based on ICD-9 codes and OASIS scores. As mentioned earlier, initial payment is made at the start of the 60-day episode of care—50% of the estimated case-mix-adjusted payment, including planned therapy. Final payment occurs at the end of the episode—50% of the actual case-mix-adjusted episode payment. Adjustments reflect actual therapy received, low-utilization payment adjustments, partial episodic payments, and adjustments for significant changes in condition. Outlier payments are made for unusual costs, with the total amount not to exceed 5% of the basic payment. Outlier payments are modeled after those in the hospital PPS. For more information on home health and PPS, see the following:

www.onlinestore.cch.com/default.asp?Session ID=&Cat=338 WBID={5993FF68-FCOC-11D6-A915-00508BE3712D}—Commerce Clearing House (CCH)

www.nahc.org/NAHC/LegReg/01bp/legpri. html—National Association of Home Care

www.cms.hhs.gov/providers/hhapps/ hhfact.asp—CMS website

Due to the many changes and the resulting complete overhaul of the Medicare home health reimbursement structure, the CMS now has data to compare agency utilization of services, associated costs, and community practice differences across the country. Agencies must now focus on care delivery models of managed care to control costs and conserve resources.

FINANCIAL IMPACT

Home health agencies were forced to reorganize and revise their operations, processes, forms, and systems. Much organizational restructuring and downsizing occurred, along with buyouts, acquisitions, and mergers. Small proprietary agencies were forced to close or be acquired by larger systems to survive the catastrophic changes. OASIS required agencies to purchase new software and computer systems, for the first time in some cases. Data entry clerks are needed as well as additional resources for quality assurance (QA) staff to monitor compilation and transmission of the very detailed data reports and oversee error corrections. QA staff also must conduct internal studies of adverse event outcomes, which are generated through OASIS data and are used by the state to prioritize agencies for survey and to investigate worrisome quality trends. The government has also mandated the creation of corporate compliance programs to monitor internal compliance with regulations. These requirements have been very costly.

The latest threat to home health agencies, which came in September 2000, was the establishment of "immediate jeopardy" guidelines by the CMS. A finding (by a state surveyor) of immediate jeopardy puts a provider on a fast track of 23 days for termination of the Medicare provider agreement and probable agency closure. See Transmittal 19 at the CMS website (www.cms.hhs.gov/manuals/) for additional information on manuals, transmittals, and other memoranda.

Agencies with a history of high utilization of Medicare benefits, about 15% of which were in southern states, felt a significant negative effect, whereas those in regions that used fewer services were predicted to have a more favorable experience with PPS. Nonetheless, all agencies were faced with cash-flow problems due to the 50% initial payment change.

The PPS law also specifies that all home health services listed in 1861(m) of the Social Security act are subject to consolidated billing requirements and bundled into the home health agency charges while the patient is under the home health plan of care. The only exception to the bundling rule is for durable medical equipment (DME) that might be needed for the home care plan. This means that therapy services in an outpatient clinic cannot be billed directly to Medicare while the patient is under the home health plan of care, so agencies must establish contracts with outpatient providers. However, physi-cian services or nurse practitioner services are not included. Medical supplies, both routine and nonroutine, are also subject to the consolidated billing requirements.

Impact on Referrals and Operations

Clearly home health agencies have been under fire and have been the focus of increased scrutiny by the government through OIG investigations and ORT, and through the BBA, OASIS, PPS, and the restriction on venipuncture services. Home health agencies must now more closely screen and evaluate all referrals and admissions for appropriateness to comply with the numerous regulatory requirements of federal and state agencies, accreditation organizations, and the fiscal intermediaries who pay the claims. Case managers and discharge planners may find that agencies that previously welcomed any and all referrals are now more the intake gates closely guarding.

Provision of medical supplies, such as wound care supplies, must also be arranged or contracted by the home health agency. Discharge planners now must be aware of the various contractual agreements that exist for each agency when arranging for home care supplies and may not be able to refer patients to companies they dealt with in the past.

Impact on Home Health Case Managers

Home health case managers have had to convert from a fee-for-service mindset to a mindset of managed and coordinated care. Now, more than ever, the case manager in home health must be organized and efficient, and must assume a role of leadership and collaboration with the home health team and the patient in the development of a goal-directed plan of care. This role in managing and coordinating care extends to other segments of the continuum of care when the home health patient must be transferred to acute-care, SNF, or custodial care settings. It is important that the home health case manager foster collaborative relationships with case managers at other levels of care.

Historically, home health case managers, especially those who were able to function independently and autonomously, achieved high levels of satisfaction in their work. Home health case managers have been increasingly burdened with paperwork, and the industry has suffered the exit of some long-term home care staff, who have departed for other settings or have left their chosen discipline altogether. Recruitment of qualified home care staff for far fewer agencies has become a problem.

Another difficulty agencies now face is that of measuring productivity in the PPS model. Traditionally requirements for nursing staff visits were based on number of visits and were set at 5 to 6 visits per day to cover expenses. Many home care leaders are questioning this approach and are looking for new ways to measure productivity, now that providing incentives based on number of visits is not cost effective. The challenge is to provide the right mix of services and supplies to patients while ensuring that underutilization does not occur. How outcomes will be used to measure staff and organizational performance is now the big question.

Referral Coordination

Before referring a patient to a home health agency, case managers must consider the following variables:

- Attitudes of the patient, family, or caregiver toward home care
- Availability, ability, and willingness of the patient, family, or caregiver to participate in the care
- Adequacy and suitability of the agency personnel to manage care at a given level of complexity
- Comparative benefits of home care and care in an extended-care,

subacute-care, skilled nursing, or intermediate-care facility (in terms of cost and skilled care capabilities)
- Likelihood that the patient's medical, nursing, and social needs can be met adequately at home
- Availability of a home setting
- Adequacy of physical facilities in the home to support proper care
- Adequacy of the home structural and electrical systems to handle all equipment needed

As previously stated, Medicare and many health care payers require that home health agency care meet certain criteria. Case managers will find that agencies insist on receiving backup clinical documentation to support the referral because state surveyors now expect to see these data in the home health medical record. The criteria for home health care services are as follows:

- They must be provided in accordance with written physician orders and a written treatment plan.
- They must be provided by or supervised by a licensed professional (nurse or therapist).
- They must relate directly and specifically to a treatment regimen.
- They must be reasonable and medically necessary.
- They must meet standards of practice and be safe and effective for the treatment of the particular condition.

Home health agencies are required to have on file the patient's clinical history and physical examination report, discharge summaries, or progress notes that can provide support or justification for needed home care services. Case managers who consistently provide the necessary information with a referral establish good rapport with agency staff and develop reliable agency and personnel resources to assist them with patient placement and timely discharge planning.

In addition to offering intermittent skilled services, many home health agencies also provide "registry" or private duty nurses for patients who require care by hourly, shift, or live-in registered nurses; licensed vocational or practical nurses; certified home health aides; homemaker aides; and companions.

Case managers must know the various agencies, their capabilities, and the health care payer's policy on home benefits. Collaboration between case managers in the hospital and those in home care is the key to the development of a high-quality and cost-effective plan of care. At times case managers may have to seek an extra-contractual waiver when a certain combination of cost-effective staffing is found to be adequate to provide the required level of patient care but is excluded or limited by the patient's health care policy. For example, many policies cover only the cost of a registered nurse and not the cost of a home health aide, even though use of the aide might be more cost effective.

Development of the Plan of Care: Duration of Treatment

The frequency, type, and duration of the skilled services provided depend on multiple case variables. In most cases, skilled services are goal directed and have a predictable end point. Services are no longer considered medically necessary or appropriate for reimbursement when the following conditions occur:

- Documentation indicates that the patient or caregiver can safely and effectively perform the skilled service without direct supervision.
- Documentation reveals no significant change in the patient's status and it appears that none is expected, no significant change has occurred in the therapeutic regimen, or there has been no indication of deterioration in the patient's condition for at

least the last several weeks. The patient's care has become custodial.

- Services consist solely of observation and assessment of the patient.
- Services are ordered by a physician without any designation of skilled care.
- The patient has reached a plateau at which no continued improvement or restorative potential can reasonably be predicted.

There are common exceptions to these guidelines. Patients who receive care for the maintenance of Foley catheters, feeding tubes, and vascular access devices are usually covered as long as the patient is homebound and unable to go to a clinic to receive the services.

Case managers in home health agencies are chiefly responsible for coordinating the various services and communicating with other team members and the physician. Most agencies conduct formal weekly or biweekly case conferences for this purpose, but care planning, collaboration, and coordination frequently occur "on the fly" or informally.

Federal regulations and most state regulations mandate that quarterly or biannual utilization review of home care services be conducted within the quality management program of a Medicare-certified and state-licensed agency. These reviews must be multidisciplinary and must determine if the services provided by each discipline are adequate, appropriate, timely, and safe.

Documentation of Home Care Services

To support coverage by the health care payer, home health agency documentation of services must include information on the following, at a minimum:

- Diagnosis and all existing conditions that are relevant to the care plan
- Level of need, frequency of visits, and category of personnel required (e.g., special care, special dressings

or supplies, laboratory testing, observation, education, long- and short-term goals)

- Any changes in condition, communications to the doctor, related physician's orders, and changes in the care plan
- Responses to treatments and recommendations for changes in the care plan
- Referrals and coordination with other community agencies and resources
- Medications, including type, frequency, and any side effects
- Any special diet, hydration, instruction of patient or caregiver, and patient's response
- Rehabilitation potential, home exercise program
- Psychosocial, emotional, or social problems
- All instruction given and patient and caregiver response to teaching
- Communication and collaboration between personnel in different specialties

Medicare-certified agencies are required to complete OASIS assessment for all patients 18 years of age or older. Information in this assessment can be valuable to the case manager because it measures the patient's functional status and ability to perform activities of daily living. The complete OASIS users' manual can be found on the CMS website at www.cms.hhs.gov/oasis/default.asp.

BARRIERS TO HOME CARE

Major barriers to establishing home care are the lack of a caregiver, financial limitations, and limited community resources to support this level of care. Patient safety in the home is a chief concern and is common to many of the following barriers:

- There is no home (landlord restrictions are common for renters) or the home is structurally or electrically unfit to accommodate equipment.
- The patient or family does not accept a home care plan.
- The home environment is inadequate (e.g., lack of water, heat, air conditioning, electricity, refrigeration, or telephone; lack of cleanliness; lack of space for special equipment). If patients are physically dependent on medical equipment, they are often advised to purchase backup generators or batteries to ensure functioning of the equipment in case of power outages.
- The home care plan is inadequate in terms of staffing, specialties of the personnel, or the ability or willingness of the agency to hire and train necessary staff.
- The patient, family, or caregiver is unable or unwilling to learn care techniques.
- The caregiver has physical or mental limitations.
- The home situation is abusive.
- A physician is unavailable or unwilling to assume responsibility for the patient's care.
- Transportation to the nearest resources is unavailable.
- No local agencies or resources are available to provide the required level of care. In rural areas, deliveries of supplies may occur infrequently, and so these items may have to be ordered in bulk quantities and well in advance of running out of needed items.
- An agency is available, but staffing is limited and available nurses do not have necessary specialty training.
- A conservatorship must be established prior to moving the patient to the care setting, or the conservatorship proceedings have been started but the patient cannot be moved

until a temporary or final conservator is appointed.

- The physician refuses to approve a transfer.
- Cultural, ethnic, perceptual, or language factors preclude or delay a move.
- Problems are encountered in teaching care procedures and relate to patient or caregiver issues such as (1) lack of readiness caused by emotions, perceptions, stress, or role reversal; (2) inability to read and comprehend instructions; (3) visual impairment; (4) altered coping ability.

SUMMARY

Home health agencies are among the most frequently utilized postacute-care providers. Despite the impact of the changes that have occurred since passage of the BBA, agencies are beginning to thrive again, and new agencies are springing up to meet the ever-increasing demand for home care services. These agencies provide services for patients who are homebound and require continued skilled care. In addition, many technology-dependent patients need hourly private duty nursing.

When hourly private duty nursing is required, the number of hours of care is case specific, but for many patients a minimum of 8 hours of care per day is necessary to allow the primary caregiver time to sleep. It is wise to seek or approve hourly care in increments, lest blanket approval establish the expectation that this level of care will be a long-term service. Because many health care payers limit home care benefits, the extracontractual process may be used as a last resort, especially if private duty nursing is required.

Within home health agencies, case managers assess, plan, implement, evaluate, coordinate care, and communicate with and refer to community resources, DME companies, infusion companies, and physicians. Case managers oversee the plan of care throughout an episode or multiple episodes. They interface with insurance case managers and acute-care discharge planners, SNFs, and board-and-care facilities.

Historically, case management in home care has proven to be a satisfactory career choice for many professionals who enjoy working autonomously. Despite the enormous changes wrought on the industry, these health care professionals continue to derive satisfaction from working with patients in a home setting to achieve the best functional independence and health status possible.

Chapter Exercises

1. List three eligibility criteria a patient must meet to qualify for Medicare coverage of home health services.
2. Name five examples of skilled nursing care in the home setting.
3. Describe the referral options for a 61-year-old uninsured patient with multiple chronic health problems who lives alone in an unsafe home environment, is demented, and was admitted to the hospital for failure to thrive. She has been receiving total parenteral nutrition (TPN) but is beginning to take by mouth food; however, she requires assistance with feeding and with all activities of daily living. The TPN will be discontinued in a few days. The social worker and business office are unable to locate any next of kin.

Suggested Websites and Resources

www.cms.hhs.gov/providers/hha/—CMS website for Medicare conditions of participation for home health agencies *www.cms.hhs.gov/providers/*—CMS website for Medicare conditions of participation for all providers

www.medicare.gov/publications/pubs/pdf/hh. pdf—Medicare publications

www.cms.hhs.gov/—Main CMS website

www.access.gpo.gov/su_docs/—U.S. Government Printing office and the official federal government information at your fingertips

www.medicare.gov/Coverage/Home.asp—Medicare website for coverage questions

www.cms.hhs.gov/oasis/default.asp—CMS website on OASIS

www.cms.hhs.gov/oasis/hhregs.asp—CMS website on OASIS regulations

www.cms.hhs.gov/providers/hhapps/hhfact. asp—CMS PPS website

www.cms.hhs.gov/manuals/—CMS website for manuals, transmittals, and memoranda

REFERENCES

1. Humphrey CJ, Milone-Nuzzo P: *Orientation to home care nursing,* Gaithersburg, Md, 1996, Aspen.
2. Health Care Financing Administration: *Home health agency manual,* Pub No 11, *Coverage of services, Rev 277,* Baltimore, Md, The Administration, available on-line at www.cms.hhs.gov/manuals/pm_trans/ R293HHA.pdf.
3. Marrelli TM: *Handbook of home health standards and documentation guidelines for reimbursement,* ed 4, St Louis, 2001, Mosby.
4. Cesta TG, Hussien AT, Fink LF: *The case manager's survival guide: winning strategies for practice,* St Louis, 1998, Mosby.

BIBLIOGRAPHY

Center for Health Services and Policy Research: *OASIS-B1, 8/00,* Denver, August 2000, The Center.

Hilgendorf PM: Profile of the successful home health case manager, *Nursing Management* 27(10):32Q-32V, 1996.

Powell SK: *Case management: a practical guide to success in managed care,* ed 2, Baltimore, 2000, Lippincott Williams & Wilkins.

Hospice and the Transition to End-of-Life Care

Brad Stuart, MD

OBJECTIVES

- To understand the evolution of hospice in the United States and methods of patient referral
- To learn physiologic criteria of hospice eligibility for heart failure, emphysema, and other noncancer diagnoses
- To consider the role of case management in the transition from active treatment to end-of-life care

In the United States today, death is the last taboo. Studies show that Americans are more willing to talk about sex and drug use with their children than to discuss end-of-life care with their parents. According to a 1999 survey, more than 80% of respondents believe it is extremely important to make sure that dying patients' wishes are respected. However, only about 15% of adults in the United States have completed an advance directive. In addition, most people are unaware of important resources for care at the end of life. Eighty percent had never heard the term *hospice*, and of those who were familiar with it, only 2% associated it with pain control and only 7% knew that hospice provides support for dying patients and their families.

Many barriers prevent open discussion of death and dying in our society. We are a "can-do, fix-it" culture, and our health care system reflects these values. We are impatient with uncertainty. We value mastery but are often afraid of mystery; spiritual issues surrounding death are minimized, even though the potential for growth can be profound. As providers, we may equate the death of a patient with incompetence or failure. We may lack training in assessment of the emotional and spiritual needs of our patients. We may sacrifice our own personal needs, including the need to process our own grief and loss issues, for the sake of professionalism and productivity. All of these attitudes preclude confronting issues at the end of life in an open and productive manner.

Patients and families are often reluctant to consider death an acceptable outcome of medical care, and providers may conspire with them in fostering false hope for a cure when survival is unlikely. The growth of these attitudes has been encouraged by the success of public health interventions such as widespread sanitation practices and risk factor modification and also by accelerating progress in surgery, pharmaceuticals, and medical technology. For example, antibiotics, available only for the last half of the twentieth century, were the first effective intervention against acute infections, which before that time had been the primary cause of death in all of human history. Only recently have we regarded the reversibility of disease as a given and considered death as a violation of the imperative to cure.

Two demographic trends have supported this new cultural bias toward the treatment imperative and away from the naturalness of dying. First, life expectancy has increased and will continue to do so for the foreseeable future. In 1940, a woman aged 65 years could expect to live 13 more years. By the year 2000, this additional life expectancy had risen to 19 years, and by 2040 it will reach 21 years. Second, the period of morbidity or chronic illness that many people experience before death has been reduced. From the mid-1980s to the mid-1990s, health-related quality of life improved more for those older than 85 years than for those of any other age group. Americans are living longer and healthier lives than at any time in the past. These trends have been widely publicized and reinforced through the media in many ways, from news features through direct-to-consumer pharmaceutical advertising. The compression of morbidity against an ever-receding time of mortality has convinced many Americans that dying is optional, or at least, according to one humorist, meant only for underachievers.

On the other hand, the aging of the population, the stubborn refusal of chronic illness to submit to acute-care practices, and the growing awareness of health care cost inflation and the urgent need to contain it have finally forced providers to take dying into account. Despite its traditional reluctance to accept death, the U.S. health care system has begun to accept the necessity of confronting this enemy and, if not embracing

it, at least negotiating a truce. A new interest in both the clinical and cultural aspects of the end of life has emerged.

Care at the end of life is emerging as a new focus of attention in medical treatment, academic investigation, and policy-making. Numerous demographic and sociologic trends, as well as several well-publicized research reports, have converged to produce this effect:

- Data showing that Medicare spends approximately one quarter of its annual budget on the fewer than 5% of its enrollees who die during that year
- Multiple studies demonstrating the inadequacy of pain and symptom management throughout the health care system across all treatment settings, particularly in the dying, but in patients at other stages of disease as well
- The 1995 SUPPORT study,[1] which documented widespread shortcomings in the treatment of seriously ill and dying patients in academic medical centers
- The Institute of Medicine's 1997 report, "Approaching Death: Improving Care at the End of life,"[2] which criticized institutional and professional attitudes and practices concerned with care of the dying
- The growth of managed care, which has stimulated accelerating interest in end-of-life care as a value-adding and cost-saving measure

New ethical and moral questions have arisen from the collision between medicine's expanding technologic capabilities and the need to control costs. Most patients and families feel entitled to life-extending care, and no attempt to ration health care in the United States has yet succeeded. Medicare expenditures are more than six times higher each year for patients who die than for those who survive. Managed care, particularly in the Medicare health maintenance organization setting, has just begun to confront the task of sorting out what kind of care seriously ill patients need from what they might demand, regardless of its utility or futility. Case management is increasingly used in managed Medicare to target patients who are high utilizers.

The highest utilizers, however, are often patients near the end of life. Many of these patients and their families want "everything done" and have trouble letting go. Often their stubborn insistence on aggressive care is grounded in ignorance about alternatives to hospitalization. Their providers may believe that once options for cure have run out, nothing more can be done. However, intensive care and support are available for most patients with late-stage chronic illness in the form of hospice and palliative care. It is important for case managers to understand how hospice works and how to create better access to hospice enrollment for patients with end-stage illness. In addition, case managers should understand their own crucial role in helping patients with late-stage chronic illness make the transition to end-of-life care.

APPROPRIATE UTILIZATION OF HOSPICE

Hospice is a team-oriented approach to medical care, pain and symptom management, and emotional and spiritual support expressly tailored to a patient's needs and wishes. Support is extended as well to the patient's caregivers and family, defined as the people that the patient prefers to have close by. Hospice's focus is on caring, not curing. Its services are provided mostly in patient's homes but also in freestanding hospice units and skilled nursing, residential care, and other long-term care facilities.

Of approximately 2.4 million deaths in the United States in 1999, more than 600,000, or 29%, occurred in hospice. The number of patients enrolled in hospice each year is growing at an annual rate of more than 20%. Ninety-six percent of hospice patient days were provided at home. General inpatient care, which may be provided at an inpatient hospice facility or in contracted hospital beds for patients with intractable pain or inadequate care giving at home, accounted for 3% of days. Respite care, which is usually provided for patients with overburdened caregivers, was provided for 0.3% of patient days, and the same amount went to continuous care, in which staff are provided in the home on a 24-hour basis for up to five days at a time. Medicare was the payment source for 82% of patient days; 5% was paid by Medicaid, and 10%, by private insurance.

Hospice should be considered as an adjunct to case management for any patient whose life expectancy is 6 months or less. Frequently, patients who experience clinical decline near the end of life, as well as their families and caregivers, have accelerating needs that are difficult to satisfy through case management alone. Hospice provides intensive services at a time when patients and families may suffer if usual medical care is continued. Life-sustaining treatment can be increasingly burdensome and expensive under these circumstances.

Financial considerations at the end of life are important to patients, families, and payers. Almost one third of families with a chronically ill member spend their entire life savings on medical care and associated costs. Hospice can help relieve the financial, as well as the medical, psychosocial, and spiritual, burdens of care at the end of life. Access to the hospice benefit substantially reduces out-of-pocket expenses incurred by most patients near the end of life. Services available without charge to Medicare recipients include the following:

- Physician services for medical direction of patient care
- Regular home visits by registered nurses and licensed practical nurses

- Home health aides for services such as dressing and bathing
- Social work and counseling
- Drugs for pain and symptom management
- Durable medical equipment such as hospital beds and commodes
- Medical supplies such as dressings, catheters, and incontinence supplies
- Volunteer support to assist patients, caregivers, and families
- Physical, speech, and occupational therapy
- Nutritional and dietary counseling

Typically, a loved one serves as the patient's primary caregiver in the home, and this individual or another helps make decisions if the patient becomes incompetent. Hospice staff are required to be available 24 hours a day, 7 days a week. If continuous care is required, it may be provided for short periods. Many hospices will accept patients who live alone, but as death approaches and care needs increase, privately hired caregivers or placement in long-term care facilities may be necessary.

Hospice also decreases Medicare and health plan costs, primarily by preventing unnecessary hospitalizations at the end of life. A 1995 study showed that for every dollar spent on hospice, $1.52 was saved in Medicare Part A and B expenditures. Savings per patient in the last month of life averaged $3192. Case managers should develop relationships with hospice admission coordinators, team supervisors, and nurses to more effectively utilize hospice to increase quality of care and contain costs.

Although the number of hospice referrals is increasing rapidly, patients are referred late in life. The median length of stay in 1999 was only 29 days, and almost one third of new enrollees died within 7 days. Late hospice referrals are unfortunate, because suffering may not be relieved and resources may be wasted. Patients should be referred to hospice early enough that they and their families can benefit fully from its services. A period of at least 2 months' enrollment before death is optimal so that pain and other symptoms can be controlled, advance planning can be accomplished, caregiver support can be arranged, the dying process can be managed, and healthy grieving and bereavement can be facilitated. Late referrals to hospice leave insufficient time to establish the quality of relationship necessary to accomplish these goals.

If a case manager is in doubt, it is better to refer patients to hospice earlier rather than later. Hospice programs will inform providers if a potential enrollee does not appear terminal; Medicare regulations forbid them to enroll patients who are likely to survive longer than 6 months. Any provider may refer a patient to hospice, or a family member may choose to call the agency. Many hospice programs provide consultative visits at home or in the hospital to evaluate both medical and emotional readiness before the actual hospice enrollment process takes place.

Regulations require that potential hospice enrollees be eligible for Medicare Part A. In addition, a certificate of terminal illness must be signed by both the attending physician and the hospice medical director, stating that the patient has less than 6 months' life expectancy, assuming the disease runs its normal course. Hospice enrollees waive standard Medicare benefits for treatment of their terminal illness, although they may continue to receive standard Medicare benefits for treatment of conditions unrelated to the terminal diagnosis.

Enrollees are initially certified for a first 3-month benefit period. Recertification for a second 3-month period is permissible if the patient still appears to be terminal. If patients survive longer than 6 months, they may be recertified for an indefinite series of additional 2-month benefit periods as long as clinical decline continues. Patients whose condition stabilizes or improves for an extended length of time after hospice enrollment must be discharged, but they may be readmitted when their clinical status again declines.

HOSPICE HISTORY: CANCER CARE AND PAIN CONTROL

The first hospice program in the United States opened in Connecticut in 1974 and was funded by a grant from the National Cancer Institute. The characteristics and needs of patients with cancer dictated how hospice was to evolve. Because cancer tends to cause consistent anorexia, cachexia, and fatigue in its late stages, it was relatively easy to determine when patients with cancer were about to die. This led to defining hospice eligibility as terminal illness, or 6 months' life expectancy. Also, it was recognized that standard oncology practice often ignored the emotional, psychosocial, and spiritual needs of patients and their families. Through an interdisciplinary team approach, hospice developed the first holistic approach to patient care in the United States.

Pain management became another hallmark of hospice. Because approximately two thirds of patients with cancer eventually experience pain so severe that it becomes disabling and because cancer pain often increases in intensity as patients near the end of life, hospice became adept at using morphine and other opioids in large doses that had previously been considered lethal. Cancer pain was found to be preventable through regular opioid dosing. Opioid requirements over a 24-hour period were found to be actually lower with this preventive approach than when analgesics were administered only in response to patients' complaints of pain.

These two pillars of hospice, care of the terminally ill with scrupulous attention to pain management, were institutionalized when Congress passed legislation in 1983 creating the Medicare Hospice Benefit. This reimbursement stream enabled hospice to grow from a fringe phenomenon into a comprehensive approach to care at the end of life. Hospice's full integration into the medical system is still evolving but will accelerate as the focus of care continues to shift from the hospital inpatient environment to the outpatient sector, and further, into patient's homes.

Hospice has been used for increasing numbers of patients with cancer. Sixty percent of U.S. cancer deaths now occur in hospice. Patients with cancer become eligible for hospice when definitive treatment (i.e., surgery, chemotherapy, and radiation therapy) fails to control the disease. Many hospice programs will not accept patients who are still receiving disease-modifying therapy; however, many will pay for palliative chemotherapy and radiation, as well as for ancillary treatments such as blood transfusions and administration of erythropoietin. Treatment for conditions not related to the terminal diagnosis may be provided and billed outside of hospice.

Pain and Symptom Management

Although comprehensive treatment of pain management is beyond the scope of this chapter, appropriate use of analgesics should be mentioned because many patients with cancer require them before they become terminal. Unfortunately, cancer pain management is inadequate for up to two thirds of patients in the United States.[3] Many health care professionals are inadequately trained in analgesic therapy or are unwilling to treat pain effectively. Reinforcing this tendency are widespread regulatory and law enforcement practices that incentivize providers to ignore pain rather than to treat it aggressively. In most cases, particularly those involving severe cancer pain, successful treatment requires the administration of opioid analgesics.

Several artificial barriers to opioid prescribing are important to note. Fears of addiction are unfounded; of 12,000 patients with cancer in one large study, only six were found to show signs of true addiction. Fear of respiratory depression is also inappropriate; morphine and other opioid analgesics are safe and effective even for patients in whom they were formerly thought to be contraindicated (e.g., those with lung cancer and obstructive lung disease). Finally, fear of prosecution for opioid prescribing is overemphasized; regulatory scrutiny is unusual if these medications are given for appropriate indications in patients with cancer. Several states have enacted severe pain laws that remove concerns about provider liability in these cases. In fact, in light of recent litigation in which a physician was found guilty of elder abuse for failing to prescribe opioids for patients with cancer and severe pain, prosecution for undertreatment of pain may now be a more legitimate fear than prosecution for overprescribing opioids.

Morphine is the most studied, most frequently used, and least expensive opioid analgesic. Usually, patients begin receiving morphine sulfate immediate-release in forms such as oral morphine solution (Roxanol) or tablets every 4 hours around the clock and are then switched to slow-release preparations (e.g., MS Contin, Oramorph SR, and others) every 12 hours, with morphine sulfate immediate-release given for breakthrough pain. Morphine has no ceiling dose; it should be titrated upward until pain is controlled or toxic effects occur. The most common mistake in cancer pain management is the assumption that if pain persists during administration of morphine, the drug is ineffective. Instead, the morphine dose should be increased until pain is controlled or until symptoms of toxicity occur.

Other oral opioids include oxycodone (OxyFast, OxyContin, and others), hydromorphone (Dilaudid), and methadone, which unlike other opioids is active against neuropathic pain but may accumu-

late to toxic levels over time because its half-life is longer than its duration of action. Transdermal fentanyl (Duragesic) is useful for patients who cannot swallow. Combinations of weaker opioids with acetaminophen (Vicodin, Tylenol with codeine, and others) should be replaced with morphine or other pure opioids in cases in which pain is severe to safeguard against toxic effects of acetaminophen. Meperidine (Demerol) should be avoided because of a neurotoxic metabolite, as should partial opioid agonists such as pentazocine (Talwin). Opioids can also be administered sublingually, rectally, and by means of subcutaneous or intravenous infusion; but studies show that oral opioids are effective in more than 85% of even the worst cases of cancer pain. In rare cases, intrathecal infusions are necessary.

Adjunctive nonopioid analgesics should also be used whenever possible, because they are opioid-sparing. Nonsteroidal anti-inflammatory drugs should be given in most cases of painful bone metastases unless they are contraindicated because of a history of peptic ulcer or gastrointestinal bleeding. Anticonvulsants, tricyclic antidepressants, and other drug classes must be considered for neuropathic pain, because it is only partially responsive to opioids.

Symptoms other than pain may also be managed with oral or sublingual medication. Dyspnea responds well to morphine, which may be safely administered if it is started in low doses and titrated upward slowly. Nausea and vomiting can be treated with sublingual haloperidol (Haldol) in low doses, as well as oral metoclopramide (Reglan). Agitation or delirium often results from overmedication or drug interactions; once these are ruled out, haloperidol or other neuroleptics can help calm both patients and caregivers. For agitation that may occur close to death, barbiturates such as pentobarbital (Nembutal) or secobarbital (Seconal) may be compounded for administration by means of a suppository or transdermal gel.

NONCANCER DISEASE: A NEW FRONTIER

One of the major reasons that patients are referred late to hospice is prognostic uncertainty. It is often difficult for clinicians to know an individual's prognosis precisely enough to determine when the illness is terminal. Prognostic uncertainty is especially challenging in cases of noncancer disease. The clear signs of end-stage disease often seen in cancer are frequently chronic or absent in end-stage heart, lung, and other noncancer illnesses. This may account for the fact that although more than 50% of patients with cancer now die in hospice, only about 15% of patients with terminal illnesses other than cancer do.

Hospice can provide intensive care in the home setting for the terminal phase of many chronic illnesses that are usually treated in the hospital because they are perceived as being too difficult for family and caregivers to cope with. In fact, the intensive symptom management, caregiver support, and family counseling provided by hospice may make death at home preferable to hospital treatment in these cases. Examples of these conditions include terminal hemorrhage of esophageal varices in patients with end-stage liver disease or death from amyotrophic lateral sclerosis (ALS), when hospice counseling and treatment may help prevent tracheostomy and mechanical ventilation.

As an aid in determining when hospice referral is appropriate, the National Hospice and Palliative Care Organization drafted guidelines in 1996 for noncancer diagnoses.[4] Although these criteria have not been found to correlate precisely with 6-month prognosis in individual cases, they have been adapted for use as local medical review policies by the U.S. Centers for Medicare & Medicaid Services (CMS;

formerly the Health Care Financing Administration). These local medical review policies have become federal eligibility criteria for hospice for patients with noncancer diagnoses. However, it is important to know that patients do not need to meet these criteria exactly to qualify for hospice enrollment. The primary determinant of hospice eligibility is a life expectancy of 6 months, as judged by the clinician and supported by the hospice medical director.

GENERAL CRITERIA OF HOSPICE ELIGIBILITY

All patients referred to hospice must have a condition that is both terminal and progressive. The patient or family should have been informed of this, and treatment goals should be consistent with relief of symptoms rather than cure of underlying disease. Clinical progression of disease may be documented by notes from a physician, case manager, or nurse assessment; results of laboratory or radiologic studies; and/or hospitalization or emergency department use. Many patients qualify for hospice because of diminished functional status; this disability should be recent rather than simply chronic and should amount to a Karnofsky Performance Status of less than 50% or dependence in at least three of six activities of daily living. Unintentional weight loss of more than 10% over 6 months is also a helpful determinant of hospice eligibility. In cases in which it is difficult to determine whether patients are declining rapidly enough for hospice referral, it is often useful to ask patients or family members how well the patient was functioning one month and three months before the current evaluation. The rate of clinical decline can then be estimated.

Hospice enrollment requires a terminal *condition*, not a terminal *diagnosis*. Patients do not need to conform to a disease-specific local medical review policy to qualify for hospice. For instance, elderly patients who experience irreversible clinical decline may be referred to hospice even if they do not have a dominant diagnosis. Any patient who fits the general criteria outlined previously may be considered for hospice referral.

Diagnosis-specific criteria follow. Again, these are cues for hospice referral rather than inviolable criteria for eligibility; many patients within weeks or months of death do not necessarily exhibit these signs and symptoms. Clinical judgment is important.

DIAGNOSIS-SPECIFIC CRITERIA

End-Stage Heart Disease

Patients with end-stage heart disease most commonly present with systolic heart failure, which results from left ventricular enlargement. However, an increasing proportion of elderly patients with heart failure have preserved systolic function, also known as *diastolic dysfunction*, with small left ventricular size but recurrent episodes of "flash" pulmonary edema. Both subsets of patients with heart failure can respond well to morphine, which lowers sympathetic tone and systemic oxygen consumption. Patients with systolic heart failure qualify for hospice when they have dyspnea at rest or with minimal exertion (New York Heart Association functional class IV) despite optimal treatment with diuretics, angiotensin-converting-enzyme inhibitors, and more recently, β-adrenergic blockers. These patients usually have left ventricular ejection fractions of 20% or less as determined by echocardiogram or coronary artery catheterization. Any patient who no longer responds to inotropic infusions (usually milrinone or dobutamine) is a hospice candidate.

Patients who have disabling angina at rest that is refractory to treatment with β-blockers and nitrates and who are not candidates for coronary revascularization are also eligible for hospice. Other factors that may trigger hospice admission for patients with end-stage heart disease are refractory supraventricular or ventricular arrhythmias, a history of cardiac arrest and resuscitation, recurrent syncope, cardiogenic brain embolism, or concomitant heart failure and acquired immunodeficiency syndrome (AIDS).

End-Stage Lung Disease

Patients with obstructive disease (e.g., emphysema or chronic bronchitis) and restrictive disease (e.g., pulmonary fibrosis or interstitial pneumonia) are eligible if they have disabling dyspnea at rest that is poorly responsive to bronchodilators. Most are oxygen-dependent. Patients with obstructive disease usually have a forced expiratory volume in 1 second of less than 30% of predicted value after bronchodilator administration. Most hospice-eligible patients will have been hospitalized, many on multiple occasions, and some will have undergone endotracheal intubation and mechanical ventilation. Cor pulmonale, or right-sided heart failure caused by lung disease, is common in this population. Hypoxemia at rest during administration of supplemental oxygen, with oxygen saturation of less than 88% or Po_2 less than 55 mm Hg, is common, as is hypercapnia with Pco_2 greater than 50 mm Hg. Tachycardia at rest, with heart rate greater than 100 beats/min in a patient with known severe chronic obstructive pulmonary disease, is also a helpful finding for determining hospice eligibility.

Dementia

Determining prognosis in dementia is challenging, because death results from comorbid conditions rather than the process of dementia itself. Patients with dementia so advanced that cognitive function is largely absent can survive for years if they receive devoted and meticulous care. Appropriateness for hospice is therefore determined both by severity of dementia and the presence of medical complications. In terms of severity, patients usually have difficulty with ambulation. Patients with dementia who can still ambulate without assistance are rarely terminal unless they have significant comorbid disease. On the other hand, loss of ambulatory status, particularly rapid progression to bedridden status, often indicates increased risk of mortality. In addition, these patients usually cannot carry on a meaningful conversation because of cognitive deficits. Common complications of dementia include aspiration pneumonia, particularly if the patient is bedridden, and sepsis caused by pulmonary or urinary tract infection or fever that is recurrent after antibiotic treatment even if the source of infection is unknown. Multiple stage 3 to 4 nonhealing decubitus ulcers may also be seen. Nutritional factors are also helpful indicators: dysphagia or refusal to eat, resulting in the inability to maintain adequate intake of food and fluids, or progressive weight loss with or without hypoalbuminemia (serum albumin level ≤ 2.5 g/dl) may also prompt referral to hospice.

Human Immunodeficiency Virus and Acquired Immunodeficiency Syndrome

The advent of highly active antiretroviral therapy (HAART) initially resulted in a decrease in mortality associated with human immunodeficiency virus (HIV) infection and AIDS, as well as a change in attitudes among both patients and providers as AIDS appeared to become a chronic rather than a terminal illness. Hospice referrals of patients with HIV infection dropped dramatically. Recently, however, hospice enrollments of patients with HIV and AIDS are again increasing as resistance to HAART develops over time and because some patients choose not to adhere to complex or toxic drug regimens.

Patients with HIV/AIDS are appropriate candidates for hospice when their CD4+ counts decrease below 25 cells/μL, or when HIV RNA viral loads rise above 100,000 copies/ml, whether or not they are receiving antiviral therapy. Functional status has usually decreased significantly, and opportunistic diseases are usually present such as malignancies including solid tumors, lymphoma, especially of the central nervous system, and Kaposi's sarcoma; progressive multifocal leukoencephalopathy; severe wasting, with loss of 33% or more of lean body mass; organ failure, including heart, renal, and liver failure; and advanced AIDS-related dementia. Hospice programs must determine whether to pay for antiviral, antibiotic, prophylactic, and other therapies; and policies vary by agency. Unless clinical status is declining rapidly, it may not be appropriate to consider hospice for patients who are still committed to HAART.

End-Stage Liver Disease

Cirrhosis is the final common pathway for most of the illnesses that result in liver failure, including alcoholism, hepatitis, some autoimmune diseases, and cryptogenic cases. Laboratory indicators of severely impaired liver function include prolongation of prothrombin time more than five seconds over control value, or international normalized ratio greater than 1.5 in the absence of warfarin sodium (Coumadin), and serum albumin level less than 2.5 mg/dl. Other liver enzyme abnormalities such as elevation of serum aspartate aminotransferase levels do not reflect underlying liver function. Instead, they indicate transient elevations in enzyme levels secondary to acute hepatocellular necrosis, but because the liver has the capacity to regenerate, these abnormalities are not sufficient to determine that the patient is terminal.

Clinical problems commonly encountered in patients who are candidates for hospice referral include ascites refractory to sodium restriction and diuretics, as well as related syndromes such as spontaneous bacterial peritonitis and hepatorenal syndrome, hepatic encephalopathy refractory to dietary protein restriction and lactulose, and recurrent variceal bleeding. Factors that further increase mortality include progressive malnutrition or muscle wasting, active alcoholism, hepatocellular carcinoma, and active hepatitis B or C.

End-Stage Renal Disease

Any patient with end-stage renal disease undergoing dialysis who elects to discontinue it should be considered for hospice referral. Most patients with end-stage renal disease die within 1 to 2 weeks after dialysis is stopped, but some who began dialysis while they still had residual renal function may live longer. Hospice can help control symptoms of progressive uremia in these patients and can also assist families in coping with the uncertainty of when death will occur.

Whether patients are discontinuing dialysis or are appropriate dialysis candidates but refuse the procedure, the primary laboratory indicator of critical renal impairment is a serum creatinine level greater than 8.0 mg/dl or greater than 6.0 mg/dl in patients with diabetes. This corresponds to a creatinine clearance of approximately 10 ml/min for patients of Medicare age who are of average body weight. Patients with diabetes who have a creatinine clearance of 15 ml/min or less are appropriate candidates for hospice. The blood urea nitrogen level should not by itself be considered as an indicator for hospice referral, because significant elevations can be observed as a result of prerenal azotemia caused by dehydration or other transient causes. Clinical indicators of severe renal failure include oliguria with urine output less than 400 ml in 24 hours; uremic syndrome, consisting chiefly of confusion, restlessness or obtundation, nausea and vomiting, and generalized pruritus; hyperkalemia, with a serum potassium level greater than 7.0 mg/dl; and intractable fluid overload.

Stroke and Coma

Hospice referral is appropriate for patients who have had an acute thromboembolic or hemorrhagic stroke if patients have severe deficits in function that have not improved after several days of supportive care. Coma that persists longer than 3 days after a stroke strongly predicts early mortality. Among patients with any four of the following signs after a stroke, the mortality rate is 97% by two months: abnormal brain stem response; absent verbal response; absent withdrawal response to pain; serum creatinine level greater than 1.5 mg/dl; or age greater than 70 years. Dysphagia severe enough to significantly limit intake of food or fluids should prompt hospice referral if tube feedings are refused.

Dramatic recovery is possible after an acute stroke. After several weeks or months have passed, however, maximal benefit will have been achieved through rehabilitation. After this time, the effects of stroke are chronic. Patients with chronic stroke effects should be referred to hospice if functional status is declining, if severe poststroke dementia is present, or if nutritional status and oral intake are poor (or if tube feedings are deliberately reduced by caregivers or family who are legal surrogate decision makers). As in cases of dementia, the onset of medical complications such as aspiration pneumonia, sepsis, or intractable decubitus ulcers should also prompt hospice referral.

Amyotrophic Lateral Sclerosis and Other Neurologic Disorders

ALS tends to progress in a linear fashion over time. Therefore its course is relatively predictable in comparison with other noncancer diseases. Patients with ALS that has progressed to advanced stages within a year after symptoms first appeared usually continue to experience rapid disease progression and are therefore appropriate candidates for hospice referral. The two factors affected by ALS that are critical for survival are the ability to breathe, which is a function of chest wall and diaphragmatic muscle strength, and the ability to swallow, which is affected by progressive dysmotility of the first third of the esophagus. Both of these structures are composed of skeletal muscle, which is innervated by motor nerves projecting from spinal tracts affected by ALS. Patients who have dysphagia and refuse feeding tubes or patients with feeding tubes who elect to discontinue artificial nutrition and hydration because of other disabilities related to ALS may be referred to hospice. Similarly, patients whose breathing becomes critically impaired, measured by forced vital capacity of less than 30% of predicted value or the development of severe dyspnea at rest, are appropriate candidates for hospice referral. Many of these patients receive bilevel positive airway pressure (BiPAP) therapy, but because BiPAP therapy requires coordinated movements of the glottis even in sleep to prevent ventilation of the esophagus, it eventually becomes ineffective in ALS. Once this happens, death follows quickly unless the patient is ventilated mechanically. Patients should be referred before this occurs so that treatment of dyspnea and anxiety can be accomplished and counseling to prevent tracheostomy can begin.

Other neurologic and neuromuscular degenerative diseases are also amenable to hospice intervention. Chief among these are Parkinson's disease, multiple sclerosis, Huntington's disease, and rarer degenerative disorders such as progressive supranuclear palsy. In Parkinson's disease, referrals to hospice are appropriate when patients lose the ability to ambulate; tremor by itself is not a terminal condition even when it is severe. The terminal phase of most other neurologic diseases is signaled by progressive disability, the development of dependence in activities of daily living, nutritional deficits, and comorbid complications.

MANAGING THE TRANSITION TO END-OF-LIFE CARE

Any patient who is entering the end stages of chronic illness and who is no longer responding adequately to disease-modifying or life-sustaining treatment or who wants this treatment withheld or discontinued should be referred to hospice. However, not all of these patients will make the transition from active treatment to hospice care. Several regulatory and attitudinal factors may limit access to hospice in these cases:

- A patient's illness must be terminal to qualify for hospice. Those who have a high likelihood of survival beyond 6 months, those who do not want to abandon curative treatment in favor of palliative care, and those whose physicians will not sign the certificate of terminal illness may not enroll.
- Prognostic uncertainty delays many enrollments because providers cannot determine when the patient's condition has progressed from advanced chronic illness to terminal status. Unpredictable clinical downturns are the rule in these cases, and a patient's condition may progress from stable to dying only days or weeks before death. This is a primary cause of late hospice referrals.
- Psychologic, social, and cultural denial of awareness about death causes many patients, families, and physicians to resist a diagnosis of terminal illness and to refuse to consider hospice as a treatment option.
- To qualify for hospice, patients must choose to forego usual (i.e., life-

sustaining) treatment in exchange for the assurance of comfort care. Many patients and families are not ready to make this difficult choice and therefore decline hospice until very late in the disease trajectory.

- Many patients, particularly those with noncancer diagnoses, continue to respond to treatment until death is imminent. Although cure is not possible in many of these cases, the treatment imperative often remains strong because definitive treatment never appears completely futile.
- Patients whose conditions are stabilized for more than one or two months must be discharged from hospice and be returned to usual care. An indeterminate number of such patients die before they can reenroll.

These factors all tend to push hospice to the end of the disease trajectory or to make it unavailable for many patients with chronic illness. In the U.S. health care system, a wide gap separates acute medical treatment from end-of-life care. Patients with chronic illness usually are treated immediately for any exacerbation, often enduring multiple rehospitalizations. At the other end of the spectrum lies hospice, which is often underutilized. No mechanism yet exists to bridge this gap; therefore, the risk of overtreatment for patients with end-stage illness is high.

Case managers are positioned to act as transition managers for many patients with advanced chronic illness. Transition management can bridge the gap between acute and end-of-life care through systematic application of patient and family education and advance care planning. Although a comprehensive discussion of transition management is beyond the scope of this chapter, some of the skills and attitudes necessary for its practice follow:

- The experience necessary to judge when chronic illness is reaching its end stages
- The flexibility to know when to pursue immediate treatment if disease is reversible, and comfort care when it is not (often both approaches must be used simultaneously)
- A broad knowledge of the palliative management of pain and other symptoms and the expertise and courage to apply it aggressively when necessary
- Sensitivity and assertiveness in communications with patients and families concerning disease process and prognosis
- The patience and persistence necessary to pursue the advance planning process as it evolves through the disease trajectory so that patient and family preferences for care can be ascertained and actualized

NOTES ON ADVANCE CARE PLANNING

A fundamental mistake is to assume advance care planning is accomplished once the patient or a surrogate decision maker signs an advance directive. These documents are often merely "snapshots" of patient and family attitudes and preferences about end-of-life management at one point in time. They may be executed before the patient is ill enough to understand from firsthand experience his or her illness and its treatment. On the other hand, they may be signed when the patient is near death, without benefit of full discussion about treatment options. Studies show that advance directives are ineffective in determining treatment in more than 80% of cases, because they are not specific enough to apply to current clinical situations at the time of hospitalization or because they are not available at the site of care.

Advance care planning should be an ongoing, real-time process that takes into account the evolution of the disease and the patient's and family's responses, both emotional and rational, to advancing illness and its treatment. Preferences for care often change once certain modes of care are experienced, and changes in these preferences may be unpredictable. For example, patients with end-stage emphysema who have never experienced endotracheal intubation and mechanical ventilation have differing responses after they undergo this procedure. When contemplating whether they would like to repeat this experience, some will refuse it because they suffered through the experience, whereas others will accept it because it offers a few minutes more of life. These values and preferences can only be captured if patients are followed up carefully through multiple disease exacerbations.

Another fallacy is to assume that a do not resuscitate (DNR) order always prevents unwanted aggressive care. DNR orders only take precedence after cardiopulmonary arrest. Many patients with DNR orders and end-stage chronic illness undergo emergency hospital treatment with each exacerbation, because emergency personnel are trained to apply full resuscitative measures if patients are at all responsive. Some first responders will withhold such measures as intubation if patients are hospice enrollees. However, thorough advance care planning entails discussion and documentation of preferences for or against specific resuscitation measures, preferably with a standardized approach that includes documents that can both cue the discussion and record preferences for or against specified interventions. Finally, a do not transport order may be more effective than a DNR order in preventing use of unwanted emergency treatment measures for patients who want to stay at home to die.

SUMMARY

End-of-life care, and particularly hospice, should be viewed as an important resource by case managers. Improvements in quality of life, pain and symptom management, caregiver and family support, and cost containment are all possible when hospice and palliative care are utilized. However, it is often difficult to know when a patient's illness is terminal, and other barriers to optimal utilization of hospice exist. The clinical guidelines for noncancer diagnoses listed in this chapter may be helpful, and hospice and palliative care providers can be consulted for help in determining hospice eligibility and in facilitating enrollment.

Transition management helps patients with late-stage chronic illness to bridge the gap between immediate life-sustaining treatment and end-of-life care. The transition management role will become increasingly important as the health care system comes to grips with aging and chronic illness. Case managers are well positioned to provide transition management. Specific reimbursement for long-term care case management may become available after the conclusion of the Medicare Coordinated Care Demonstration project, currently underway.

Chapter Exercises

1. In a group discuss the evolution of hospice in the United States and methods of referral.
2. In a group discuss typical criteria of referral for diagnoses that are noncancer related and why these patients need hospice support no differently than patients with cancer.
3. In a group discuss the role of the case manager and the contributions one can make as patients and families enter the end-of-life cycle.

Suggested Websites and Resources

National Hospice and Palliative Care Organization—*www.nhpco.org*

Hospice Association of America—
www.hospice-america.org
Hospice Patients' Bill of Rights—
www.hospice-america.org

REFERENCES

1. The SUPPORT Principal Investigators: A controlled trial to improve care for seriously ill hospitalized patients, *JAMA* 274:1591-8, 1995.
2. Field M, Cassel C, editors: *Approaching death: improving care at the end of life*, Washington, DC, 1997, National Academy Press.
3. Cleeland CS, Gonin R, Hatfield AK et al: Pain and its treatment in outpatients with metastatic cancer, *N Engl J Med* 330:592-596, 1994.
4. Stuart B, Alexander C, Aranella C, et al, for the Standards and Accreditation Committee, Medical Guidelines Task Force: *Medical guidelines for determining prognosis in selected non-cancer diseases*, Alexandria, Va, 1996, National Hospice and Palliative Care Organization. Copies may be obtained by calling the National Hospice and Palliative Care Organization (NHPCO) at 800-646-6460. The document includes worksheets for each diagnostic group. These are useful for determining when patients are appropriate candidates for hospice referral. They may also be copied and given to physicians or other providers who would benefit from this aid for determining hospice eligibility.

Emergency Department Nurse Case Manager

Marsha L. Scribner, RN, MSN, CPUR

OBJECTIVES

- To understand the goals of the emergency department (ED) case manager
- To learn the primary functions of the ED case manager
- To learn the characteristics of ED case management that set it apart from other types of case management
- To understand why is it necessary for the ED case management program to be both vertically and horizontally integrated within the system
- To understand which high-risk patients are seen in the ED
- To learn which types of services are available for frequent ED users
- To learn what the Emergency Medical Treatment and Active Labor Act is and to understand how it affects the intervention process
- To understand the critical pathway and how is it implemented in the ED
- To understand how determinations for admissions are reviewed for appropriateness
- To learn the expected barriers for the new ED case manager

The search for cost savings in today's financially tight health care delivery system has led health care organizations to unique and often previously unrecognized methods of cost containment. Today, more and more health care organizations are joining the search and are integrating previously independent health care processes to achieve quality outcomes and to improve resource use. This need has prompted the creation of innovative programs and case management strategies that are proving effective in providing not only better service but also better-quality indicators for quarterly outcome reports. One arena in which the attempt to ensure high quality, cost-effectiveness, service implementation, and appropriateness of care comes face to face with the managed care dilemma is the ED. The use of a case manager in the ED setting provides a point of entry for intervention and implementation of an appropriate level of care in a collaborative process with the patient, family, caregiver, ED and hospital staff, and community resource networks.

Because utilization management is a broad process and reaches into the system interdepartmentally as well as into the community, ED case management can be viewed as a gatekeeping tool to improve utilization of patient services and assure appropriate inpatient admissions. Effective case management in the ED has a significant positive financial impact on the health care system as a whole and provides good patient outcomes in today's health care delivery market. The objectives of this chapter are primarily to explore the role of the ED case manager and to gain insight into the functions performed by this individual.

GOALS

One of the primary expectations of any managed care system is that specific goals concerning utilization of resources will be met and that measurable outcomes will be produced that show successful goal attainment. The benefits derived from implementing a case management program in the ED are similar to those gained when such a program is put in place elsewhere in the health care system. The old adage of providing the right patient with the right care at the right time supplies the framework for ED case management. A clear understanding of the ED case manager's purpose while in the ED is essential. Thus, assessing patients identified as at risk, implementing services, monitoring utilization of previous services, ensuring that the patient is or will be in the most appropriate level of care, and using the most appropriate health care resources at the right time and cost while the patient is in the ED allows the earliest possible initiation of treatment. Issues relevant to the patient under assessment are addressed, documented, and resolved in a consistent and timely manner. Outcomes are improved, and patient satisfaction remains at a high level.

In general, goals are aimed at improving patient services by providing more opportunities to identify issues and problems, introducing better ways to measure the success of interventions, and producing more clearly defined outcomes as a basis for reducing unnecessary admissions and promoting placements at the appropriate level of care.

FUNCTIONS

Although all ED case management programs utilize the case manager as a gatekeeper, the actual processes embraced by each program differ from one ED to another. Thus the roles and responsibilities of the ED case manager vary among EDs. Because few precedents currently exist for ED case management program innovation, there is no uniformity in program design or implementation.[1-3] ED case management models are new and still evolving. They remain dependent on previous case management models that target the inpatient population or the community-based population.[4] The uniqueness of the ED creates a need for case management interventions that are specific to its fast-paced environment. The ED patient is neither an inpatient nor a community-based patient. The ED patient is a transitional patient, with both community support needs and medical service needs that can lead to admission or discharge. The ED case manager must have one foot planted squarely in the inpatient world and the other in the outpatient world. Decisions about utilization of medical resources must be made within narrow time frames and within the context of cost and quality of care. Figure 24-1 shows the interaction and exchange that must occur to achieve reliable care coordination and maintain quality standards. This model provides a theoretical framework for ED case management and offers insight into the importance of the integrating internal and external resources in both a vertical and a horizontal manner. The coordination and integration of provider services plays a substantial role in quality improvement and cost containment. This model guides the

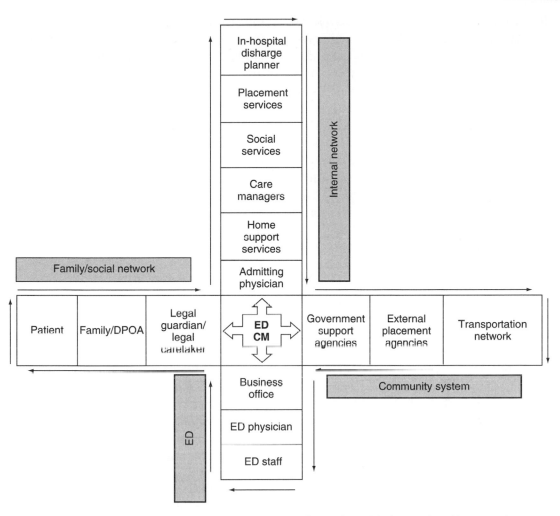

Figure 24-1 Emergency department case management *(ED CM)* model of vertical and horizontal integration. *DPOA*, Durable power of attorney.

ED case manager by focusing on the resources that are integral to the process of achieving patient-centered outcomes within short time frames.

That managed care companies and health care facilities are in the business of staying in business is a given fact. Thus, the first basic function of the ED case manager is to provide outcomes that show cost savings to these health care institutions. "Every act, every decision, every deliberation of management has as its first dimension an economic dimension."[5] The second basic function is to collaborate productively with other health care partners to produce positive results. During a busy day in the ED, many forces come into play that set limits on what can be accomplished. An example of this is the scenario in which a physician requests an ambulance to transport a patient back to a board-and-care facility. Is this a poor utilization of resources? What are the forces involved? Does the patient have funds to pay privately for transportation? Will the board-and-care facility provide the transportation? Can a gurney van be arranged within the hour so that the patient does not tie up an ED bed? These forces set the limits on what can be accomplished. They do not direct the final outcome. It is through the ED case manager's actions—working collaboratively, discovering the forces, and then creating new forces—that positive outcomes occur. The third basic function is to collaborate with the patient to reensure positive outcomes. This implies that the patient has abilities and limitations that require attention and case management. The fourth basic function is to balance present with future needs. The ED case manager must consider not only the immediate needs of the ED visit but also the long-term future needs for patient safety. It is the successful integration of these four basic functions into the ED case manager's role and responsibilities that determine the success or failure of any ED case management program model.

FIELDS

Wheatley[6] wrote about field theory and described how organizational systems are influenced by many fields. She mentions the need to imagine organizational spaces as fields, with employees as waves of energy, spreading out in regions of the organization. If one has ever spent a few hours in an ED, one will begin to sense the presence of dynamic leadership fields. The staff can be viewed as energy beacons, each flashing with power and energy and each having the capacity for leadership at any given moment. In some the leadership beacons are blinking brightly, while in others the beacons shine at a normal candle power—for now! Soon, the rush hour is on and all the leadership beacons are glowing. Everyone is a star! The energy that is generated fills the ED with tension, anticipation, and force. Out of chaos comes clarity of purpose. Ideas are generated, and plans are made, challenged, and remade. The ED physician's field gates open and energy is expelled into the next overlapping field—the patient's field, the staff's field, the business office's field, the organization's field,

or the case manager's field. These fields do not arise in a vacuum. Each leadership field can be created only through collaboration and exchange of ideas. Each patient is showered with charged information. Then the broadcasters of the knowledge, care, and treatment rekindle their beacons, and the process of field regeneration starts again.

ROLES AND DUTIES

Just what does the ED case manager do? What is in the job description, and what are the tools needed to complete an 8- to 12-hour day providing case management in the ED? What comprises the ED case manager's dynamic field of leadership? The various roles listed in Box 24-1 provide a clue, since they are roles that are fused into the knowledge base comprising the dynamic field of the ED case manager. The information that the case manager can provide on any given day at any given hour to whomever requests it is the key to creating the outcome. This knowledge base is created by, regenerated by, and synchronized with the roles that make up the position of case manager as a whole.

Box 24-2 lists the people and agencies in the ED case manager's collaborative partnership network. These comprise the

---

BOX 24-1
Roles of a Case Manager

- Reviewer
- Clinician
- Consultant
- Discharge planner
- Risk manager
- Advisor
- Negotiator
- Collaborator
- Advocate
- Teacher
- Facilitator
- Social worker
- Program manager

occurs in most ED case management programs.

THE HIGH-RISK PATIENT

Patients become high risk when either their medical needs or their social needs overwhelm their ability to maintain self-care. The first step in assisting these patients is identifying them. While risk assessments can be beneficial when they are completed in the physician's office, time constraints in the ED allow only for the use of written guidelines. These guidelines are developed to mesh with the specific ED case manager's roles and duties, so some high-risk indicators used in one program may not be used in another. Some ED patients are considered high risk if they are 65 years of age, are at risk of developing life-threatening illness, and/or are living alone. Others are considered high risk if they are alcohol or drug abusers and are unable to provide food and shelter for themselves. Box 24-3 provides a list of high-risk indicators that would be used in the ED by most case managers.

FREQUENT USERS

A frequent user of an ED is simply a patient who comes into the ED with either urgent-emergent or nonurgent needs at a rate higher than that in the standards set by that particular hospital. An example of frequent use would be three times in 3 months or six times in 1 year. Another example of a frequent-use criterion is two or more admissions, two or more ED visits, or five or more home health visits within 1 year. Whether or not the patient has insurance is not the issue. The question is primarily whether overutilization of nonurgent ED services has occurred and whether alternative medical or nonmedical services can be obtained in lieu of a visit to the ED. Identifying these nonurgent overutilizers is significant only if

---

BOX 24-2
Dynamic Leadership Fields

- Admitting physician
- ED physician
- Financial counselor
- Social worker or mental health counselor
- Minister or grief counselor
- ED primary care nurse
- Hospital bedside nurse
- Hospital nursing supervisor
- Conservator or legal guardian
- Clinic or physician's office nurse
- Skilled nursing facility placement team
- Home health department
- Home infusion services
- Pharmacy
- Disease care manager
- DME department
- ED technician
- ED clerical support staff
- Admitting office
- Transportation network personnel
- Translation services
- Legal counselors
- Entitlement program offices
- Clinical pathways and care maps
- Board-and-care and assisted-living placement agencies
- Government agencies and social service protective agencies
- Security, police, and sheriff's departments
- Family, friends, neighbors, landlord
- Local shelters and food banks
- Hospital clothes closet staff
- Hospital business office
- Managed care utilization review and case management department

DME, Durable medical equipment; *ED*, emergency department.

---

many fields that interact with the ED case manager on an ongoing basis. "We cannot hope to influence any situation without the respect for the complex network of people who contribute to our organizations."[6]

Table 24-1 shows a grid for specialty roles A through F. For each role are listed the duties that a particular ED case manager performs. The role of each individual case manager differs from that of the others, but all have some duties in common. This is an example of the role blending that

TABLE 24-1
A Comparison of Emergency Department Case Manager Duties

	Role A	Role B	Role C	Role D	Role E	Role F
Specialties						
Advanced practice nurse (MSN)				X	X	
Social worker (MSW)			X			
Discharge planner (BSN)	X	X			X	
Certified case management nurse						X
Duties						
Identifies high-risk patient	X	X	X		X	
Reviews and makes recommendations for in-hospital/ observation admissions or outpatient services for all ED patients with non–life-threatening illnesses						X
Has social worker support in the ED for placements and linkages to lower levels of care						X
Creates care plans for all ED patients						X
Home safety evaluation	X	X	X		X	
Functional ADL assessment	X		X		X	
Caregiver support assessment	X	X	X		X	
Interview with caregiver/family	X	X	X		X	
Placement	X	X	X			
SNF	X	X	X			
Board-and-care/residential care	X	X	X			
Shelter	X		X			
Alternative housing	X		X			
Transportation determination	X	X	X			
Performs utilization review	X	X			X	
Requests preauthorization		X			X	
Observation	X	X			X	
Tracks observation patients		X				
Inpatient admissions	X	X			X	
Applies review criteria	X	X			X	
InterQual criteria (InterQual certification)	X				X	
Milliman Care Guidelines	X	X			X	
Starts discharge plan	X		X		X	
Expedites clinical pathway	X	X			X	
Develops ED care map				X		
Ensures quality of care	X	X	X		X	
Tracks quality issues		X				
Provides grief counseling	X		X		X	
Provides AIDS counseling					X	
Acts as ED project manager				X		
Repatriation to network facility	X				X	
HMO/IPA	X				X	
ED transfers	X				X	
Network to network	X					
Network to nonnetwork	X					
Physician consultation	X				X	
From SNF	X				X	
Back to SNF	X				X	
Provides patient education	X	X				
Frequent ED use	X	X				
Home care needs	X	X			X	
Home health/hospice	X	X			X	
DME	X	X			X	

Continued

TABLE 24-1
A Comparison of Emergency Department Case Manager Duties—cont'd

	Role A	Role B	Role C	Role D	Role E	Role F
Caregiver support	X	X	X		X	
Nutrition program	X	X	X		X	
Warfarin (Coumadin) therapy program	X	X				
Home infusion therapy program	X	X				
Medical care coverage	X	X	X		X	
Eligibility/benefits	X	X	X		X	
Program for medically indigent	X	X	X		X	
Medicaid	X	X	X		X	
Member services	X	X	X		X	
Medicare/CMS	X	X	X		X	
Letters of coverage denial	X	X	X			
Provides follow-up	X	X	X		X	
Schedules follow-up medical appointments					X	
Makes next-day follow-up telephone call		X			X	
Makes same-day callbacks					X	
Abnormal lab test results/radiographs					X	
Makes care manager referral	X	X	X		X	
Refers to social services	X	X	X		X	
Abuse/neglect			X			
Domestic violence			X			
Family dysfunction			X			
Alcohol/drug abuse			X			
Mental illness			X			

ADL, Activities of daily living; *AIDS,* acquired immunodeficiency syndrome; *BSN,* Bachelor of Science in Nursing; *CMS,* Centers for Medicare & Medicaid Services; *DME,* durable medical equipment; *ED,* emergency department; *HMO,* health maintenance organization; *IPA,* independent practice association; *MSN,* Master of Science in Nursing; *MSW,* Master of Social Work; *SNF,* skilled nursing facility.

BOX 24-3
Patient Characteristics Indicating High Risk

- Utilizes emergency department for all health care needs
- Is unable to meet health care needs
- Has poor or no caregiver support network
- Has difficulty with ambulation
- Experienced a recent change in mental status
- Needs custodial skilled nursing home care
- Abuses alcohol
- Has behavior problems
- Has difficulty performing activities of daily living
- Needs conservatorship
- Is mentally incompetent
- Lives alone
- Shows indications of abuse, neglect, or financial exploitation
- Unable to pay bills, insurance copayments, etc.

alternative resources have been put in place, the patient agrees to use them. and the patient complies with this agreement.

The blame for overutilization of ED services for nonurgent needs cannot always be put squarely on the patient. Many of these patients are directed to the ED by their managed care toll-free call center or by their clinic or primary care provider, or come because they have no other resource to turn to for their medical needs. Table 24-2 shows who these patients are and from where they come.

Many studies have been done on measures to prevent nonurgent use of the ED and to link resources for the homeless, the poor, the socially isolated, those lacking insurance entitlements, and those who have drug or alcohol problems.[7,8] Studies conducted by the Civilian Health and

TABLE 24-2
Frequent Emergency Department User Profile

Type of User	Referred by Call Center	Referred by Clinic/PCP Office	Does Not Know Where Else to Go for Care	Brought by Family	Sent by SNF Physician	Sent by Board-and-Care Operator	Patient Called 911	Other Called 911	Sent by Home Health/Hospice Nurse
Frail elderly from home	X	X		X		X	X	X	X
Resident of skilled nursing facility	X			X	X			X	
Chronically ill patient	X	X		X		X	X		X
Patient with chronic pain	X	X		X			X	X	X
Patient with cardiac arrhythmia	X	X		X			X		X
Noncompliant diabetic	X	X	X	X					X
Noncompliant asthmatic	X	X	X	X					X
Person in a mental health crisis	X	X	X	X		X			
Alcohol abuser			X				X	X	
Uninsured person			X				X	X	
Homeless person			X				X	X	
Drug-seeking person	X	X		X					
Patient unable or unwilling to make PCP appointments	X			X			X	X	
Non–English-speaking person	X	X		X				X	

PCP, Primary care physician; *SNF,* skilled nursing facility.

Medical Program of the Uniformed Services, now TRICARE, and their elderly population have been conducted in an attempt to decrease their nonurgent ED usage and frequent hospital admissions.[9-11] An interesting study in which ED patients completed a self-classification asking them to rate their symptoms as emergent, urgent, or nonurgent yielded surprising results. It found that "a small but clinically significant percent of the ED patients who self-classify their symptoms or presentations as nonurgent actually have a medical condition warranting admission to the hospital."[12] These studies have told the experts what is or is not working to decrease nonurgent usage and why. Table 24-3 lists some of the published solutions that have proved successful and some that have failed.

EMERGENCY MEDICAL TREATMENT AND ACTIVE LABOR ACT

In 1986, the Emergency Medical Treatment and Active Labor Act (EMTALA) was enacted, primarily in response to concerns that some EDs were turning away indigent and uninsured patients who came seeking treatment.[13] Some of these patients were being sent out or transferred to other local hospital EDs before the patient's condition was stabilized and before an accepting physician was found. This practice is commonly called "patient dumping," and such behavior is now prohibited under EMTALA regulations. Because EMTALA was passed as part of the Comprehensive Omnibus Budget Reconciliation Act (COBRA) of 1986, it is sometimes referred to as the COBRA law. Since the passage of EMTALA, all EDs must complete a medical screening examination on any patient seeking medical treatment in its ED, whether or not that patient has the ability to pay or provides evidence of medical insurance coverage. When patients are to be transferred to preferred provider network hospitals for treatment, their condition is first stabilized, and then transfer arrangements are completed through a doctor-to-doctor collaboration. Both parties must be in agreement and that the patient can be safely transferred by ambulance. The ED case manager becomes involved in patient transfers when there is a need to transfer a patient to a preferred provider network hospital. The case manager may also

TABLE 24-3
Results of Various Programs to Decrease ED Visits by Frequent Users

Program Action Rate	Percent Success
Improvement of access to outpatient care[11]	40%
Letter-writing campaign to frequent ED users[11]	33%
Levy of substantial ED visit copayments[17]	30%
Use of multidisciplinary case management without community advocacy[18]	5%
Development of individualized ED patient care plans[18]	5%
Introduction of capitated chronic care program for frail seniors[10]	43%
Use of LCSW case management for homeless, alcohol or drug users[8]	35%
Use of multidisciplinary care plan meetings and community advocacy[19]	35%
On-site ED case management interventions[20]	18%
Use of disease management for asthma and COPD[21]	76%
Initiation of social work case intervention program for the frail elderly[22]	No data
Establishment of primary care physician as gatekeeper for all nonurgent ED requests[23]	35%

LCSW, Licensed clinical social worker; *ED*, emergency department; *COPD*, chronic obstructive pulmonary disease.

become involved in assisting with an "appropriate transfer" if a need exists for medical or psychiatric treatment that can only be provided at a facility with specialized capabilities, such as a neonatal intensive care unit or a burn unit.

EMTALA defines an *appropriate* transfer as a transfer to another facility when the patient's condition has not yet been stabilized but the medical benefits of the transfer outweigh the medical risks of the transfer. If, on the other hand, the patient has been stabilized and there is only a need for transfer to a provider network hospital, the transfer is permitted and is not restricted by the statute. EMTALA does not prohibit an inquiry into availability of medical insurance or ability to pay; it does state that there must be no delay in examination or treatment to obtain this information. For the ED case manager, timing is everything. Medical coverage must be determined before an admitting physician is contacted but not before the medical examination has commenced or the patient has been stabilized. The case manager works in collaboration with the business office to obtain medical insurance determinations and identify coverage idiosyncrasies. The case manager acts as a facilitator once the ED physician determines that the patient can safely be transferred to a network facility by contacting the facility and requesting a bed for admission. The case manager also makes the initial call to the network primary care physician and facilitates the physician-to-physician discussion concerning the emergent care received and the need for transfer to a network hospital. These activities all occur within the strict guidelines set forth in the EMTALA statutes.

CRITICAL PATHWAYS AND CARE MAPS

The concept of a continuum of care justifies the need for nursing case management. Defining what the continuum of care actually is and what it allows the nurse case manager to do sets the role and responsibilities of that particular case manager. In the ED the continuum of care extends from the patient's home into the ED. From the ED it can proceed in many directions: admission, placement in another facility, home health care, outpatient follow-up, durable medical equipment, or back home. Because contact with the patient occurs within short time frames, however, the ED case manager's focus is considered episodic. That does not mean that there is no continuum within the emergency care process; it simply means that case management interventions are completed within the workday.

Some EDs have elected to use critical pathways or care maps. These pathways define the coordination of ED care over a continuum of 0 to 12 hours for specific high-risk complaints such as chest pain, asthma, or chronic obstructive pulmonary disease (COPD). They include a time frame for ED case management assessment and intervention. A critical pathway starts when the patient is first assessed by the ED nurse and continues until the patient is admitted, transferred, or discharged. The ED case manager can provide some interventions, such as family interviews and calls to the patient's care facility, at any time along the continuum of care but must wait until the patient has been medically evaluated and stabilized before actually interviewing the patient. Critical pathways for inpatient admissions are available in the ED and are employed by the admitting physician to save time, provide outcomes data, and expedite care through the use of a coordinated plan of action. Examples of inpatient critical pathways are those for ruling out myocardial infarction and for managing COPD, pediatric asthma, pneumonia, and congestive heart failure. Some ED case managers provide input into the development of ED critical pathways and some monitor use of these critical pathways for compliance and variances. A variance occurs when there is a deviation from the pathway. A positive variance may be that patient care was delivered within a shorter time than designated on the pathway. A negative variance may be a delay in receiving services such as radiography, laboratory testing, or consultations. Implementation of ED critical pathways has dramatically shortened the length of time that some patients spend in the ED.[14] "With the cost of ED visits continually rising, patient acuity levels increasing, and resources declining, expedient, coordinated, multidisciplinary action is crucial in giving total quality care to each patient."[15]

UTILIZATION REVIEW IN THE ED

The case management process extends beyond discharge planning for patients identified as needing coordination of comprehensive or multifaceted services across the continuum of care. ED case managers may provide utilization review for all admissions to observation and inpatient levels of care, or only for inpatient admissions of high-risk patients who may have complex discharge needs. The process of utilization review is the same as that for telephone review except that the reviewer is face to face with the admitting physician. This can be problematic if there is a difference of opinion as to the required level of care. Most utilization review programs have policies and procedures for handling conflicting decisions, and these may include participation of a medical advisor for final review determinations. Various screening tools are used to aid in the utilization review process. The InterQual criteria and Milliman Care Guidelines are two such tools. The ED case manager will need to become certified by InterQual before applying InterQual review criteria to a case for admission.

Before the actual admission, the patient's ED chart, as well as the admitting physician's orders and progress notes, is reviewed. This is termed an assessment of medical necessity and evaluation of appropriateness for the requested level of care. If possible, the patient is interviewed and the family is consulted to identify discharge needs. If the requested admission has been denied by the utilization review medical director, then the ED case manager must inform the admitting physician and the patient of this adverse determination. The patient receives a denial letter from the ED case manager and is informed of the reason for the denial and the process for appeal.

"The case managers also reduce ED admissions by finding alternatives to decrease inappropriate or social admissions. This method includes coordinating home health care and procuring home medical equipment before the patient's discharge from the ED."[16] A survey found that 75.6% of ED case managers screen for medical necessity of inpatient admission for observation once it is ordered by the admitting physician.[2] Not surprisingly, cost savings are significant when patients can be given services at a lower level of care, such as through placement in a skilled nursing facility or provision of home health services.

BARRIERS

Many new ED case managers come up against fundamental medical paradigms when initiating a new program in the ED. The ED culture and attitudes are based on certain concepts that appear at first glance to be counter to the case management process. Listed below are some of the barriers that have been found to inhibit the effectiveness of new ED case management programs.

- The ED staff does not understood the need for an ED case management nurse. The case manager is known as the person who "likes to talk to old people" or the social worker who "helps the drunks and crazies."

- The ED physicians feel threatened when the case manager reviews charts and asks questions. Basically, the physicians lack a good understanding of the role and responsibilities of the case manager.
- The case manager's actions and/or nonactions come under question by the ED staff. For example: No one seems to understand why the case manager needs to be in the patient's room talking to the patient. There is a sense that the case manager is in the way and hinders the ability of the ED nurses to care quickly for the patient.
- Basic philosophical differences are seen in care models that lead to misunderstandings. The model of the ED staff and physicians is a medical model. The case management model focuses on the empirical value of health care services and the business value of concrete accountability.
- ED staff and physicians are not concerned about cost savings or payer sources but about providing quality medical care and abiding by the EMTALA regulations.
- The ED physicians are slow to make referrals to case management, and when they do some requests are for clerical assistance. This indicates unclear perceptions of the duties and roles of the ED case manager on the part of the ED physicians.

SUMMARY

Emergency case management values the relationships between care giving and advocacy. It provides the entry point for interventions that cascade into other dynamic learning fields within the system.

It provides the best processes for multidisciplinary collaboration and organization of services in an environment of time pressure and chaos. In preparing for this dynamic role one cannot overlook the importance of the patient's place in the continuum of care. The patient's satisfaction with the whole process, from entry into emergency medical care to discharge, is based on perceptions and on expectations that are met or not met. Patient advocacy is inherent in the basic concepts that guide the nursing profession. That we as nurses care is not enough any longer; the needs and expectations go far beyond that. Patients need and are demanding more from the health care system, as can be seen from the fact that they are appearing at the doorstep of EDs all across the country with nonurgent medical needs. So what are the needs that the health care system can address? Patients are not simply requesting but are demanding that the health care system achieve maximal quality, manage costs, and provide appropriate accessibility. When one of these demands is not met sufficiently, patients will look for alternatives in accessing health care. Can the ED case manager make a difference in this trend? The challenge is all too real, and attempts are being made to answer this challenge as case managers work in advocacy roles to promote better access to care and influence organizational systems to use their own dynamic learning fields as sources of change. It's a jungle!

We're getting a patient in room 5 in 20 minutes, but don't stop what else your doing. Multitask, and juggle.
My neighbor just arrived, the firemen brought her in by ambulance.
Della, her name is Della. They call her Room 5. I need to find the connections.
Where is Room 5's family? What happened?
Someone is yelling obscenities in room 10, and A baby is screaming.
The Captain has taken charge and

Room 5 is surrounded by a flash of power and
energy.
The field-gates open, a life is being saved.
A call is made, a referral is completed.
Salve is placed on the baby's wound
Please talk to the mother.
Look in on Room 21, he's old and may need
help with . . .
something
everything
caring
love

Marsha Scribner, MSN, RN

Chapter Exercises

1. List the primary goal of good ED case
   management.
2. List the four basic functions of the ED
   case manager.
3. List at least three characteristics that
   distinguish ED case management from
   general medical/surgical case management.
4. Give an overview of your perception of
   why both vertical and horizontal integration are important to the success of
   an ED case management program.
5. List at least five areas of high-risk
   patients who should be seen by an ED
   case manager before discharge.
6. List at least four services that are
   available for frequent users of ED services.
7. Go to the EMTALA website and
   research the law, and discuss whether
   EMTALA law is followed as intended
   by your local ED.
8. If your hospital uses pathways, discuss
   how it is implemented in your local
   ED.
9. Follow a case from ED to admission
   and determine whether a review
   against national guidelines was conducted to determine appropriateness
   for admission.
10. List at least four barriers to effective ED
    case management services.

Suggested Websites and Resources

www.medlaw.com/lawtoc.htm—EMTALA law
www.pnhp.org/Press/1996/emergency.html—
  Physicians for a National Health
  Program website and a Harvard study
  on ER usage
www.acep.org/—American College of
  Emergency Physicians
www.cdc.gov/nchs/SSBR/024tab.htm—
  Centers for Disease Control and
  Prevention website on ER usage
www.drugabusestatistics.samhsa.gov/—Office
  of Applied Studies website on drug
  abuse

REFERENCES

1. Veenema TG: The ten most frequently asked ques
   tions about case management in the emergency
   department, *J Emerg Nursing* 20(4):289-292, 1994.
2. Niemi K: Tracking patients, tracking costs, *Nurse
   Manager* 30(1):47-48, 1999.
3. Hospital breaks new ground with ED discharge
   planning, *Hospital Peer Review* 21(10):135-137,
   1996.
4. Cohen EL, Cesta TG: *Nursing case management: from
   essentials to advanced practice applications,* ed 3,
   St Louis, 2001, Mosby.
5. Drucker PF: *The practice of management,* Harper
   Business Edition, New York, 1993, HarperCollins.
6. Wheatley MJ: *Leadership and the new science,* San
   Francisco, 1994, Berrett-Koehler.
7. Baker D, Stevens C, Brook R: Regular source of
   ambulatory care and medical care utilization by
   patients presenting to a public hospital emergency
   department, *JAMA* 271:1909-1912, 1994.
8. Orkin RL, Boccellari A, Azocar F et al: The effects of
   clinical case management on hospital service use
   among frequent users, *Am J Emerg Med* 18(5):603-
   608, 2000.
9. Sund J, Sveningson L: Case management in an integrated delivery system, *Nurse Management* 29(6):
   24-25, 1998.
10. Initiative cuts ED visits, hospital admissions,
    Hospital Case Management 9(4):59-61, 2001.
11. Kravitz R, Zwanziger J, Hosek S et al: Effect of a large
    managed care program on emergency department
    use: results from the CHAMPUS Reform Initiative
    evaluation, *Ann Emerg Med* 31(6):741-748, 1998.
12. Caterino JM, Holliman CJ, Kunselman AR:
    Underestimation of case severity by emergency
    department patients: implications for managed
    care, *Am J Emerg Med* 18(3):254-256, 2000.
13. Miller GL: *A resource for current information about the
    Federal Emergency Medical Treatment and Active Labor
    Act, also known as COBRA or the Patient Anti-*

Dumping Law, available on-line at www.uplaw.net (link: Emergency Care—EMTALA Implementation and Enforcement Issues [PDF format]), accessed 2001.

14. Pins CL, Swanson ME: A suburban community emergency department's adaptation of case management, *J Emerg Nursing* 19(6):503-509, 1993.

15. Nelson MS: Critical pathways in the emergency department, *J Emerg Nursing* 19(2):110-114, 1993.

16. Conn AD, Shimkus GV, Inbornone R: Leadership dimension—eyeing the ED's open door: how case managers can reduce unnecessary admissions, *Dimensions in Critical Care Nursing* 19(2):35-36, 2000.

17. O'Grady KF, Manning WG, Newhouse JP et al: The impact of cost sharing on emergency department use, *N Engl J Med* 313:484-490, 1985.

18. Spillane LL, Lumb EW, Cobaugh DJ: Frequent users of the emergency department: can we intervene? *Acad Emerg Med* 4(6):574-580, 1997.

19. Pope D, Fernandes CM, Bouthillette F et al: Frequent users of the emergency department: a program to improve and reduce visits, *Can Med Assoc J* 162(7):1017-1020, 2000.

20. Warner M: *SAC frequent ED patient tracking (quarterly report),* Sacramento, Calif, April 2001, Kaiser Permanente Medical Center—Sacramento Area Campus, Submitted to the UM Committee.

21. Federwisch, n.d.

22. Public sector contracting report: Repeated ER visits, admissions of frail seniors signal need for social management, *Monthly Guide to Medicare and Medicaid Managed Care* 5(2): 21-24, 1999.

23. Hurley RE, Freund DA, Taylor DE: Gatekeeping the emergency department: impact of a Medicaid primary management program, *Health Care Management Review* 14(2):63-71, 1989.

BIBLIOGRAPHY

Adler RB: *Communicating at work,* ed 3, New York, 1989, Random House.

Bower KA, Falk CD: Case management as a response to quality, cost, and access imperatives. In Cohen EL, editor: *Case management in the 21st century,* St Louis, 1996, Mosby.

Clough J: Risk identification: management versus avoidance. In Cohen EL: *Case management in the 21st century,* St Louis, 1996, Mosby.

Cohen EL, Cesta TG: *Nursing case management: from concept to evaluation,* ed 2, St Louis, 1997, Mosby.

Cohen EL, De Back V: *The outcomes mandate: case management in health care today,* St Louis, 1999, Mosby.

Hurley RE, Freund DA, Taylor DE: Gatekeeping the emergency department: impact of a Medicaid primary management program, *Health Care Management Review* 14(2):63-71, 1989.

Murer CG, Brick LL: *The case management sourcebook,* New York, 1997, McGraw-Hill.

Repeated ER visits, admissions of frail seniors signal need for social management, *Public Sect Contract Rep* 5(2):21-24, 1999.

Senge PM, Kleiner A, Roberts C et al: *The fifth discipline fieldbook: strategies and tools for building a learning organization,* New York, 1994, Currency-Doubleday.

Walsh KM: ED case managers: one large teaching hospital's experience, *J Emerg Nursing* 25:17-20, 1999.

Whitehill C: A model of emergency case management: developing overall strategies and outcomes. In Cohen EL, Cesta TG, editors: *Nursing case management from essentials to advanced practice application,* ed 3, St Louis, 2001, Mosby, pp 173-184.

Quality, Credentialing, and Audits

CHAPTER
25

Introduction to Quality, Credentialing, and Audits

Peggy A. Rossi, BSN, MPA, CCM, CPUR

OBJECTIVES

- To identify the key differences between quality management and quality improvement
- To describe two key agencies that oversee quality in the health care industry
- To describe why benchmarking is important
- To describe why credentialing is important
- To describe the four elements of Quality Improvement System for Managed Care (QISMC)
- To describe why it is important to have processes in place to audit internal operations and test staff on a regular basis

Quality in health care is everyone's business. It is no longer sufficient for organizations to establish quality programs just to meet the mandates and requirements for regulators, purchasers, or accreditation bodies. Quality is defined as a planned, systematic, organization-wide approach to the measurement, assessment, and improvement of an organization's performance, thereby continually improving the quality of patient care and services provided.[1] If quality is to be the dominant factor in an organization, a continuous quality improvement (CQI) process must be in place. CQI is defined by the Joint Commission on Accreditation of Healthcare Organizations (JCAHO) as a means and management process or approach to the continuous study and improvement of the processes of providing health care services to meet the needs of individuals and groups.[1] In essence, CQI can be divided into three aspects[1]:

1. **Measurable quality**—This can be defined objectively as compliance with or adherence to standards. It is assumed that quality can be adequately, if not completely, measured once health care professionals define the standards of care under which they can comfortably work.

2. **Appreciative quality**—This is the comprehension and appraisal of excellence beyond minimal standards and criteria, requiring the sometimes even unarticulated judgments of skilled, experienced practitioners and sensitive, caring persons.

3. **Perceptive quality**—This is that degree of excellence that is perceived by the recipient or the observer of care rather than by the provider of care.

QUALITY ASSURANCE VERSUS QUALITY IMPROVEMENT

Although quality assurance (QA) for health care changed in 1992 when the JCAHO, in its accreditation manual for hospitals, announced its adoption of new standards designed to reorient multiple entities of health care providers to CQI, the concepts and practices of quality improvement (QI) were in actuality introduced into U.S. industry by W. E. Deming and Joseph Juran in the 1980s.[1]

Traditional quality programs historically used the QA approach as they performed and monitored activities. Unfortunately, this activity was done in varying degrees and resulted in varied effectiveness. In recent years, the focus and commitment to quality has changed. The emphasis is now on QI, and more importantly, continuous improvement in processes, as well as immediate and sustained outcomes.

One of the most difficult transitions that health care professionals have had to struggle with over the last few years has been the shift from QA to QI. In general, QA focuses on reducing errors and meeting standards set up by the provider organization or external licensing and other regulatory bodies, and provider-defined outcomes are used as the measurement tools. Unfortunately, QA works episodically and retrospectively and is used to track morbidity and mortality statistics or in response to identified problems while focusing on statistical outliers to determine accountability once errors have occurred. QA activities are also used when clinical status is measured. Measures of clinical status are often the hard data used to determine the efficiency and efficacy of care.

QI, on the other hand, focuses prospectively on improving processes even without the identification of a problem, meeting the needs of customers, and measuring customer-defined outcomes. QI works continuously and proactively and involves all employees in the activities of systems evaluation and system change. Such an approach can be used to not only improve the quality of care for the majority of customers but also to decrease the number of outliers along the way. Customers can be internal or external users of health care.[2]

Use of a QI approach assumes that most people want to perform well and will improve when the advantage is clearly shown. This is by far more fair to all stakeholders in the process than the retrospective QA practices of the past. Use of before-the-fact measures to provide accountability to the system constitutes a sort of accounting control that attempts to prevent suboptimal use of resources. The use of valid and reliable outcomes measurement tools, along with administrative controls, which use feedback to make adjustments and prevent mistakes in the future, has the potential to effect rapid changes in the quality of service delivery.[2]

The Demand for Quality

The larger purchasers of health care who are primary drivers for changes in health care remain very concerned about the rising costs of health care. As a result, they are demanding proof that the quality of care received is the best possible for the dollars spent. They want positive outcomes maximized and adverse effects minimized. The demand for quality in managed care is based on five factors or forces. First and foremost is cost containment and its potential negative impact on quality. This is the single most powerful force behind the current demand for medical quality controls. Because health care organizations have developed their policies and procedures, provider contracts, health care delivery systems, and reimbursement methods with the intent to gain profits through cost containment, patient care has been placed at risk. Thus consumers approach health care in an atmosphere of fear and apprehension about the quality of health care they will receive. Consequently, health care purchasers, payers, regulators, and many patients now expect definitive information about the value, in terms of both cost and quality, of the services purchased or received.

A second force is the increased public awareness of the wide range of quality services available within the U.S. health care system. The U.S. health care system is under constant scrutiny, and patients today expect and demand more of their physicians than in the past. Because of the media and other factors, patients in today's health care system approach their physicians with distrust because they are more conscious of the fact that physicians' financial motivations may be in conflict with their own expectations of service and care.

Competition within the health care system market is the third force. Unlike hospitals, which have had quality programs in place for years, managed care organizations (MCOs) have not. Historically, MCOs relied on price and reputation to sell their products. Only in the last few years, as purchasers and regulators have placed demands on them, have MCOs developed or paid attention to quality as a force that drives competition. Because data that focus on quality are now available, consumers and health care purchasers can be more informed and ultimately more satisfied.

The fourth force is the control of the U.S. health care system by contracts and service relationships, which creates a highly integrated delivery system and market. Because of the many types and numbers of service vendors and subdelegations, responsibility for quality controls may be less than clear. Thus MCOs must develop sophisticated organizational strategies and techniques to survive, report, and at the same time meet the challenges of quality control for the services they provide.

Finally, despite the belief that quality of medical care is directly related to expenditures, this is not true. The transition from a cost-based reimbursement system to one of prospective payment has heightened the perceived conflict between quality and cost. Because quality is driven by external demands, this conflict is further heightened and it creates tension between increasing demands for well-documented quality of care and the economic reality of restricting increases in the cost of providing care.

Basically, quality for health care organizations has 10 dimensions. These dimensions provide the framework for a well-balanced, integrated quality, cost, and risk perspective program. They are the same dimensions evaluated by organizations such as the JCAHO and the National Committee for Quality Assurance (NCQA). The 10 dimensions are as follows[1]:

1. Appropriateness of care and the correct use of resources
2. Availability of services to meet needs and ease of obtaining health care
3. Competency of practitioners and staff and the degree to which practitioners and staff adhere to professional or organizational standards of care
4. Continuity and coordination of care among all professionals and across the continuum of care
5. Effectiveness of care—the degree to which care is provided in the correct manner and the degree to which desired outcomes are reached
6. Efficacy of care and the power of a procedure or treatment to improve health status
7. Efficiency of care and the relationship between outcomes and the resources used to deliver health care

8. Respect and caring and the degree to which the patient is involved in his or her own health care decisions and to which those providing services do so with sensitivity and respect for the patient's needs, expectations, and individual differences

9. Safety and the degree to which the health care intervention minimizes risks of adverse outcomes for both the patient and provider

10. Timeliness of care and the degree to which needed care is provided to the patient at the most beneficial or necessary time

Commitment to Quality

Quality is no longer just a buzzword. The quality programs of today for health care organizations must be action plans that define quality goals and motivate employees to achieve them. Commitment to quality starts at the senior management level and must become a top priority for all persons within an organization.

For a quality program to work, senior management must ensure that the culture and climate of the organization is ready for the aggressive approach quality requires as programs are implemented, monitored, and then sustained. For quality to work, four essential elements must be in place[3]:

1. Agreement on what quality is and how it should be monitored (e.g., consensus statement about which measurable aspects of quality [e.g., clinical outcomes, patient satisfaction, appropriateness of care] will be monitored and which monitoring methods will be used [e.g., patient satisfaction survey, physician profiles])

2. A shared perception that management and professional staff are serious about dealing with quality problems (i.e., longstanding quality problems are identified and management and staff take an active role in correcting the problems rather than looking the other way)

3. Open, honest, and constructive communication (i.e., provider climate must discourage finger pointing and blame and facilitate cooperative approaches to performance improvement)

4. Enough of the right staff (i.e., there must be enough staff in the quality department to allow performance analysis rather than mere compliance with regulatory, accreditation, or purchaser demands)

In addition to a QI approach to work, leadership and planning will be critical for integrating existing activities with the new improved activities if a systematic and organization-wide approach is to be successful. Basically, to reach goals, one must plan, test, act on, and check effectiveness. The JCAHO has developed a 10-step monitoring and evaluation approach for determining the success of QI. This approach is now used by many accrediting agencies as they survey organizations during the accreditation process. The 10 steps are as follows:

1. Assign responsibility
2. Define the scope of care and services
3. Identify important aspects of care and services
4. Identify indicators
5. Establish a means to trigger assessments
6. Collect and organize data
7. Initiate evaluation
8. Take actions to improve care and services
9. Assess effectiveness of actions and ensure that improvement is maintained
10. Communicate results to relevant individuals and groups

Employees, as well as management, must be involved in all aspects of the quality processes. Equally as important, they must have an understanding of who the customers are and the importance of internal customers, as well as the many external customers, to an organization. The major goal of QI is to have both categories 100% satisfied. Well-defined corporate values and a supportive corporate culture are two essential ingredients for any QI or enhancement activities an organization undertakes to reach goals.

The quality enhancement process in health care must identify customers and meet their requirements and expectations by adhering to and maintaining standards of professional performance. In the health care arena, providers and organizations must be concerned with meeting the requirements of both internal and external customers, as well as professional standards.

Who are the external and internal customers? External customers of health care are the health care purchasers, patients, physicians, and third-party payers. If external customers are dissatisfied, each entity can easily take its business elsewhere. Internal customers are employees and departments who depend on one another in the daily operations of the organization. Turf issues or threats of unionization are two primary manifestations of dissatisfaction among internal customers.

After the customers and their requirements are identified, the next step is identification of the professionals who will be involved and definition of professional standards. Professional standards generally take three forms: structure, process, and outcomes. Customer requirements and professional standards are then further defined in terms of indicators. Indicators are measurable variables related to customer requirements and professional standards. A standard itself may serve as an indicator if it can be stated in measurable terms. Outcome indicators are often used as proxies for measurement of structure and process.[3]

OUTCOMES

Quality in the health care field has a long tradition of being measured in terms of morbidity and mortality statistics. Both morbidity and mortality are affected by patient characteristics such as age, severity of principal diagnosis, severity and extent of comorbidities, functional status, socioeconomic status, and even patients' attitudes toward interventions. More recently, a third quality measure, clinical status, has been added. Clinical status measures include objective biochemical, physiologic, anatomic, and histologic indicators of disease, such as presenting signs or the results of laboratory tests and x-ray examinations. Such measures have traditionally been the hard data from which efficiency and efficacy of care have been judged, and they are the indices that physicians have been trained and socialized to use in guiding and evaluating care.[2]

Unfortunately, the old QA approach used to measure health care relied on provider-defined outcomes of care, or in essence, statistical outliers such as morbidity, mortality, and clinical endpoints. With QA, all studies and implemented approaches for improvement were always conducted retrospectively. In contrast, QI is an immediate and continual process, which can be used even when there are no identified problematic areas. QI also incorporates a user- or customer-defined outcome approach and tools (e.g., patient satisfaction with cost of care, functional health, feelings of well-being, and health-related quality of life). Through the use of user-defined health outcome tools, the QI program can often take a simplistic approach and a QI effort can be achieved.

Evaluation of the effects of patient characteristics, nursing or case management interventions, and the health care system in general requires the identification of measurable patient outcomes. Patient outcomes are dependent on not only a patient's interaction with the health care system but also, in many cases, on what happens when the patient is or is not compliant with the directions for self-care and management.

In all health care organizations, conclusions about quality management are based on statistical significance of the outcomes and variations from expected performance levels as determined by the team or peer group when there is a significant difference between actual performance and the predetermined measure or expected outcome or when repeated data collection demonstrates a pattern in contrast to the expected one or a trend over time. Conclusions about data are reached when unexpected patterns of care or clinical competence related to structure, process, or outcome are identified; when attention is focused on high-priority issues for important processes in care or service; when differences in patterns of care or clinical competence between groups or subgroups are identified; and when the range of acceptable variations in patterns of care or clinical competence is clarified.

Outcomes in health care are often divided into the following categories:

- Clinical
- Physical/physiologic
- Psychologic/psychosocial
- Integrative
- Evaluative
- Hospital clinical outcomes

Because consumers and providers of health care have been concerned, with good reason, about the extent to which cost concerns are trumping quality concerns, the National Coalition of Health Care used the International Communications Research group to conduct a telephonic poll of 1011 households to query the public about quality of care and outcomes. The results are as follows[4]:

- Eight of 10 Americans believe the quality of medical care is being compromised in the interest of profit.

- Seventy-nine percent of Americans believe quality care is unaffordable for average Americans.
- Seventy-four percent of Americans believe hospitals cut corners to save money.
- Eighty percent of Americans believe that health insurers often compromise quality to save money.
- Only 4% of the respondents expressed confidence that the health care system would take care of them, and only 15% had complete confidence in hospital care.

Patient outcomes are influenced by a number of patient-specific characteristics, as well as organizational factors. Also, because outcomes are shared by all disciplines, it is important to identify outcomes attributable to a specific discipline to establish effectiveness and assign accountability. It is necessary to delineate the accountability of each provider, as well as that of the health care team as a whole, to manage and measure quality. It is also important to identify the intermediate outcomes that influence the health and satisfaction of patients, the achievement of which may be the primary responsibility of one discipline.

Because patients receive care in a variety of settings and because the U.S. health care system is highly integrated, it is important to establish intermediate outcomes, since only intermediate outcomes may be achieved in any given setting before the patient is transferred to another setting. Intermediate outcomes that facilitate or hinder the achievement of end outcomes, such as improved health status, must be measured to examine their effect on end outcomes and to determine how organizational structures and care delivery processes affect the achievement of these intermediate outcomes. Many of the discipline-specific outcomes will be intermediate rather than end outcomes. If the discipline most concerned with the outcome has not identified the need to measure the outcome, important outcomes may be missing from critical pathways, diagnosis-specific measures, and other measures used to evaluate health care effectiveness.

Intermediate outcomes include measures that assess patients' knowledge, attitudes, and behaviors and measures of the effects of nursing interventions directed at assisting patients in modifying behaviors to improve health status. If nursing does not measure these outcomes, the effectiveness of nursing interventions cannot be assessed, and the data needed to analyze the effects of changes in knowledge, attitude, and behavior on health status may be missing, since other disciplines do not routinely measure these outcomes. In addition to identification of the disciplines responsible for specific outcomes, any measures used should be standardized and validated. If the nursing profession is to become a full participant in clinical evaluation, it is essential that patient outcomes influenced by nursing care be measured in conjunction with outcomes important to other disciplines and, ultimately, to patients.[4]

Case managers should routinely investigate the extent to which high-priority outcomes reflect a commitment to quality-of-life concerns. Quality-of-life experts continually remind us that quality-of-life judgments are multidimensional and subjectively incorporate physiologic, mental, social, and spiritual functioning. The subjectivity of quality-of-life issues necessitates flexibility in designing plans of care. Sadly, the current health care system is structured to meet the needs of hypothetical statistical persons, and this works for most people but not for those who may be considered outliers.[4]

Unless the parties responsible for ensuring outcomes achievement are designated and held accountable, outcomes will often exist only on paper. One of the key responsibilities of case managers as they work with patients is to ensure the right

providers are working within the system for the same type of outcomes. This often entails clarifying who is responsible for what and then developing mechanisms to measure accountability. All too frequently, no one individual assumes the coordinator role.

Although *quality* has been a buzzword for years, reporting on quality activities remains a challenge. Most health care organizations evaluate quality on the basis of data they collect on cost of care, utilization of resources, and member satisfaction.

DATA

Depending on its objectives, its particular licensure and accreditation standards, or various internal or external demands for information, the organization must collect information and analyze it for use in making decisions that will result in improvements. Much of the information collected by the organization will not only be required by the regulators and accrediting bodies but also by large health care purchasers and as a tool for contract negotiation. More importantly, it will be used to validate success, and ultimately, survival in the health care marketplace.

Data collection is a discipline that starts by identifying or assessing what information is really needed, whether it is collectable, and which entity or department is best suited to be accountable for the actual collection. As one starts the process of data collection, it is important to identify the population, prevalence, or topic to be studied. Once this is done, one must then determine what percentage of the issue or population will be studied (100% or a sampling) to capture the data needed. If sampling is used, one must then determine whether the sample size will be selected based on nonprobability or probability sampling. Nonprobability sampling can be broken down into three techniques: convenience (use of data most readily available), quota (e.g., 10%), and purposive (e.g., cases selected because they demonstrate a desired characteristic and can be measured against specific, predetermined criteria). Probability sampling can also be broken down into three techniques: simple random (e.g., selecting every case in a defined population), stratified random (e.g., sampling patients receiving intravenous therapy at home by diagnosis, type of solution, or with or without complications), or systematic random (e.g., randomly selecting the first case and then every nth case thereafter).

If sampling is used, a sample size should be no less than 30 or no less than 5% of the expected population. The following are guidelines to use as cases are selected:

- If the cases to be studied are greater than 600 per quarter, at least 5% of the cases must be studied.
- If the cases to be studied are less than 600 per quarter, at least 30 cases must be studied.
- If the total number of cases per quarter is less than 30, 100% of the cases must be studied.

Data can be collected in a variety of ways, but in most cases, collection will be prospective, concurrent, or retrospective or will be done though a variety of focused studies. When a data collection tool is developed, it should be kept simple, the elements necessary to monitor the specified issue or indicator should be included, and electronic scanning should be considered because it increases accuracy and saves time compared with a manual tally process. During development, it is important to test the tool to ensure that it is capturing the data desired; and as this is done, one must consider whether the tool will have the ability to do the following:

- Measure what it is supposed to measure (validity)
- Measure in a reproducible way what it is supposed to measure (reliability)

- Select all cases in the category by using the variables being examined (sensitivity)
- Differentiate between the cases wanted and those similar but not in the desired category (specificity)
- Be used easily and provide results that can be easily understood (usability)
- Capture and measure the needed information (recordability)

Tools commonly used to collect the data are worksheets, check sheets, surveys, interviews, and administrative data reviews downloaded from the electronic management information system used by the organization.

Collection methods for capturing data can be real-time, prospective, concurrent, or retrospective. Data sources that might used to conduct an audit or study include daily logs, financial reports, surveys, medical information systems reports, medical records or on-line clinical data, reviews of actual processes as they occur (observations or interviews), referrals from staff, encounter forms, incident reports or other occurrence reports, and results of planned studies or other data summaries. Data can further be monitored or captured through the use of variance reporting, utilization review, the appeals process, peer review, case-specific reviews, or benchmarking.

Once the data are collected, they must be analyzed and summarized. Use of summarized data allows meaningful interpretation and formulation of accurate conclusions regarding the issue studied. In some cases the data will serve as a tool for trending to determine the type, cause, or extent of a problem or to determine the type and results of best practices.

BENCHMARKING

Benchmarking is a tool and a formal measurement process used to compare specific organizational data collection methods with those of other organizations whose collection methods are considered to be best practices. In health care, quality management activities are increasing dependent on accepted national standards of care and practice guidelines. These standards are then used as benchmarks as an organization develops performance measures and indicators; they are also used as the impetus for action and improvement for care.

As an organization starts to identify the need for benchmarking, one must know the operation, the leaders and competitors, and the best practices that can be copied or modified and incorporated into existing operations. The ultimate goal is to gain and sustain superiority in the marketplace. As one starts the process of benchmarking, it is important to define the following[1]:

- What is most critical to success?
- What areas are causing the most trouble?
- What are the major deliverables for the area?
- What products are provided to patients/customers?
- What factors are responsible for patient/customer satisfaction?
- What problems have been identified in the operation?
- Where are the competitive pressures felt?
- What performance measures are being tackled?
- What are the major cost components?

When benchmarking is used in managed care, an organization that participates in a referenced database as it compares clinical, financial, and operational data has an opportunity to identify and respond to best practices. Such data will be helpful as the organization approaches contracting with providers. Of equal importance is that purchasers be confident that the organization is using the data to improve outcomes. Thus most organizations have incentives to use benchmark data when they want to identify opportunities for improvement; predict quality, price, and outcome for their services; develop effective and credible practice guidelines and influence physician practice patterns; and increase an understanding of processes, costs, and utilization patterns. It is through the use of benchmark data that best practices are identified.

COMPONENTS OF EXCELLENCE

The JCAHO no longer requires an annual evaluation of an organization's quality management program. However, the JCAHO does evaluate the performance improvement standards and processes of planning, design, measurement, assessment, and improvement and ensures that these standards are used to provide evidence that an organization's performance improvement activities are effective. On the other hand, organizations that use NCQA for accreditation are required to have their QI program descriptions evaluated annually and updated as necessary. For both accreditation organizations, quality management activities must demonstrate the following components for excellence[1]:

- Valid, reliable data and other information about important functions and associated processes of care and services are used for surveys or as tools when improvement is needed.
- Collaboration for continuous improvement in organizational performance by all appropriate leaders, medical staff, departments and services, cross-functional teams, and committees is evident.
- Timely assessment of data to identify significant variations in processes and outcomes, both desirable and those used to validate best practices, is evident.

- Identification and prioritization of quality initiatives, performance measures, variances, and other opportunities to improve care and services are evident.
- Thorough assessment of patterns, trends, sentinel events, and any identified problems is evident.
- Appropriate tested improvement actions plans for all prioritized activities are evident.
- Validated effectiveness of actions and strategies implemented to improve care and processes are evident, and when they are implemented, there is evidence that the changes have been sustained.
- Proven maintenance of quality performance improvement gains is evident.
- Communication of clear information across and within all appropriate departments and services and within the organization as a whole is evident.
- Complete documentation and follow-up are present.
- Supportive quality management structure and systems are evident, as is information management.
- Support and involvement of key leaders are evident.
- Integration with all other pertinent activities, including utilization management, risk management, and safety practices, is evident.
- Ongoing quality education efforts are evident throughout the organization.

HEALTH PLAN EMPLOYER DATA AND INFORMATION SET

Health Plan Employer Data and Information Set (HEDIS) is a core set of health plan performance measures initially released by the NCQA in 1993, which has been updated on a regular basis since. The goal of the NCQA through the use of HEDIS is to improve the quality of patient care through partnerships with managed care plans, employer/purchasers, consumers, and the public sector (Medicare and Medicaid).

Basically, HEDIS is used by health plans to standardize measurement and reporting of performance information for specific populations and in specific areas such as effectiveness of care, access and availability of care, satisfaction with the experience of care, health plan stability, use of services, cost of care, informed health care choices, and health plan descriptive information.

Two primary methods are used to capture the data: administrative (information from claims encounters and membership data from each applicable population to be surveyed are used) and hybrid (411 cases as determined by administrative data or medical records for each applicable population or a combination of administrative data and survey data is used).

Two tools used by health care purchasers, consultants, and policy makers are report cards and NCQA's Quality Compass reports. From the data collected for HEDIS, many health plans now produce what are called *report cards*. These report cards show how the organization did in specific areas (e.g., providing members with preventive care and services or member satisfaction with care). In addition to report cards, many health plans also participate in NCQA's Quality Compass. The Quality Compass consists of data from a national database of comparable performance and accreditation information about health plans and is an excellent source of information for making contract decisions, setting performance improvement directions and priorities, and other actions. An in-depth list of requirements related to HEDIS and the Quality Compass can be found on the NCQA's website at www.ncqa.org.

QUALITY IMPROVEMENT SYSTEM FOR MANAGED CARE

As indicated earlier in this text, the Quality Improvement System for Managed Care (QISMC) is a very complex system for measuring QI, and its standards and guidelines are important tools used by the Centers for Medicare & Medicaid Services (CMS) for both Medicare and Medicaid programs. As a result, states have implemented the QA provisions required by the Balanced Budget Act of 1997 and then as further amended by the Balanced Budget Refinement Act of 1999. QISMC is a process used by CMS to monitor the quality of services provided by MCOs for either their enrolled Medicaid or Medicare beneficiaries.

QISMC is a rigid and demanding quality monitoring system that is divided into four domains, each requiring specific standards to be met. QISMC's standards and guidelines are intended to achieve four major goals:

1. To clarify the responsibilities of both CMS and individual states in promoting quality as value-based purchasers of services for vulnerable populations
2. To promote opportunities for partnership among all entities involved with QI efforts (i.e., CMS and individual states, as well as other public and private entities)
3. To develop a coordinated quality oversight system for Medicaid and Medicare with the intent of reducing duplicate or conflicting efforts while sending a uniform message on quality to organizations and consumers
4. To ensure effective use of available quality measurement and improvement tools, as well as the flexibility to incorporate new techniques or processes

For full information on QISMC see CMS's website at www.cms.hhs.gov.

ACCREDITATION, CREDENTIALING, AND CERTIFICATION

Accreditation

In today's health care arena, all health care organizations, regardless of the type of services provided or clients served, are under continual scrutiny. This scrutiny can originate from a variety of entities including consumer groups and regulatory and public agencies. If organizations receive federal funding, they are under even closer scrutiny and are constantly being audited or surveyed by a variety of agencies.

Although an organization must be licensed to do business, accreditation and licensure are two entirely different processes. Licensure is the *mandatory act* of granting and receiving approval to conduct business in a state, and for most health care organizations that provide direct care to patients (e.g., hospitals, long-term care agencies, skilled nursing facilities), licenses are granted by the state's department of health services. In contrast, if the entity is an MCO, it is licensed or certified by the Department of Insurance, Department of Corporations, or in California, the Department of Managed Health Care. Before a license is granted, the organization is subjected to a survey that ensures its operations and any entity that provides services for its clients will be in compliance with state and federal laws and regulations.

Once licensed, many health care organizations seek a *voluntary stamp of approval* through application for accreditation. Accreditation is not a condition of licensure, but licensure is a condition for accreditation. If the organization receives federal funding for any of its clients, accreditation is a necessary component of doing business. Accreditation is believed by many health care organizations, purchasers, and public entities to be the gold stamp of approval, indicating that the organization offers quality services to clients.

Although there are a multitude of accrediting bodies, all have been developed with the purpose of responding to external demands for accountability. The type of accreditation sought will depend on the type of clients served. For example, the two most prominent accrediting bodies are as follows:

1. The JCAHO was established in 1951, has expanded through the years, and now has 10 accreditation programs for facility-type services.

2. The NCQA, which is the primary accrediting body for MCOs and health maintenance organizations, was formed in 1979 by the Group Health Association of America and the American Managed Care Review Association. The Group Health Association of America is now the American Association of Health Plans. The NCQA works with MCOs, health care purchasers (large employers), state regulators, and consumers to develop standards and performance measures that can effectively evaluate the structure and function of medical and quality management systems to ensure that organizations meet established quality standards.

The following is not an all-inclusive list, but other accrediting bodies include:

- The American Accreditation Health Care Commission/Utilization Review Accreditation Commission is a voluntary accreditation body for private utilization management organizations, preferred provider organizations, and workers' compensation programs. Many states now require this type of accreditation for specific organizations, and more details can be found in the managed care section of this text.
- Accreditation Association for Ambulatory Health Care (AAAHC).

- The Commission for Accreditation of Rehabilitation Facilities accredits rehabilitation centers and is currently working with the National Adult Day Care Services Association on accreditation for adult day care centers.
- The Medical Quality Commission is a separate organization associated with the American Medical Group Association, which accredits prepaid group practices.
- The Community Health Accreditation Program, a subsidiary of the National League of Nursing, accredits home care and community health care organizations.
- The American Association of Blood Banks sets standards for blood banks and transfusion services.
- The Commission on Office Laboratory Accreditation accredits office-based laboratories.
- The American College of Radiology accredits radiation oncology and mammography services.
- The Commission on Cancer accredits cancer programs in hospitals.
- The Council on Accreditation accredits outpatient mental health and residential care centers and alcohol and substance abuse treatment centers.
- The College of American Pathologists accredits clinical laboratories.
- The American Accreditation Program Inc. is the leading organization for preferred provider organizations.

The JACHO offers 10 separate programs for accreditation:

1. Hospital accreditation
2. Accreditation of behavioral health care
3. Accreditation of long-term care
4. Accreditation of ambulatory care
5. Accreditation of home health care
6. Accreditation of health care networks

7. Accreditation for pathology and clinical laboratory services, which is a separate program to meet Clinical Laboratory Improvement Amendments requirements
8. Accreditation of long-term care pharmacies
9. Accreditation of preferred provider organizations
10. Accreditation of managed behavioral health care

For NCQA accreditation, eligible organizations must have been in business for a minimum of 18 months and must provide comprehensive health care services to enrolled members through a defined benefit package in both ambulatory and inpatient settings. Additionally, they must have an active quality management system and have access to essential clinical information about their members because the NCQA surveys the following areas during an accreditation site visit:

- Quality management and improvement
- Utilization management
- Credentialing and recredentialing
- Member rights and responsibilities
- Preventive health services
- Medical records

The NCQA also has accreditation programs that allow an MCO to have separate accreditations in the following areas:

- Managed care
- Managed behavioral health
- Credentialing
- Certification of physician organizations

Although the names for accreditation might be different for each entity, most accreditation bodies use one or more of the following means to assess compliance with their applicable standards for the final awarding of accreditation. The areas reviewed often include the following:

- Documents that validate compliance (program description, work plan, policies, and procedures)

- On-site observation and interviews of staff by surveyors
- Examples of standard implementation processes
- Medical records
- Assessment of services systems

As a final act in the accreditation process, the accrediting agency uses the following scores to reflect an organization's compliance with the standards; and, although each of the agencies uses different criteria and methods for making accreditation determinations, these agencies use similar scoring and final accreditation determinations.

JCAHO

Areas are scored as follows:

- Substantial compliance
- Significant compliance
- Partial compliance
- Minimal compliance
- Noncompliance
- Not applicable

Final accreditation determination:

- Accreditation with commendation
- Accreditation without a type I recommendation
- Accreditation with a type I recommendation
- Provisional accreditation
- Conditional accreditation
- Preliminary nonaccreditation
- Not accredited

NCQA

Areas are scored as follows:

- Full compliance
- Significant compliance
- Partial compliance
- Minimal compliance
- Noncompliance
- Not applicable

Final accreditation determination:

- Full accreditation
- One-year accreditation
- Provisional accreditation
- Denial of accreditation status

- Deferral of accreditation status (delay in consideration pending additional information)
- For most accreditation agencies, accreditation is granted for one to three years.

Credentialing

Licensure by individual states ensures and conveys to the public that an individual health care provider has completed basic education for his or her profession and has passed a knowledge-based examination and thus possesses a minimum level of competency to practice and has not committed any criminal acts. Credentialing is a process used by many health care organizations to further validate and ensure that their staff members have the appropriate qualifications to provide the level of care for which they were hired or contracted (e.g., verification of licensure, Drug Enforcement Agency certification, graduation from medical school and residency program, board certification). Certification is the process of validating that the professional has the expertise, experience, and a knowledge base beyond the basic level of practice.

Certification

Although there are many types of certifications for case management, the National Case Management Task Force in 1992 set out to standardize case management services. The result of this task force was the appointment of the Commission of Certification of Insurance Rehabilitation Specialists, now known as the *Commission for Disability Management Specialists*, to develop a certification program designed specifically for case managers. The program was developed by using the criteria developed by the National Task Force, and the final certification program became known as the *Certified Case Manager (CCM)*.

Since 1992, the number of additional certifications of case managers has grown, and the certification process covers

providers with special interests as their fields have expanded to include case management services. As a result of the growth of case management and the successes seen in the management of health care quality, efficacy, and costs, case management can now be found in almost every conceivable health care setting. As the types of case management services have grown, so have the varieties of case management. Some of the many types of case management certifications include the following:

- American Board of Quality Assurance and Utilization Review Physicians (ABQAURP)
- Certified Case Manager (CCM)
- Certified Disability Management Specialist (CDMS)
- Care Manager Certified (CMC)
- Certified Managed Care Nurse (CMCN)
- Certified Occupational Health Nurse–Case Manager (COHN-CM)
- Certified Professional Disability Management (CPDM)
- Certified Professional in Healthcare Quality (CPHQ)
- Certified Professional in Utilization Review (CPUR)
- Certified Rehabilitation Registered Nurse (CRRN)
- Certified Rehabilitation Nurse–Advanced (CRRN-A)
- Certified Nursing Case Manager (RN, CM)

Questions about these certifications can be directed to the National Association for Certifying Agencies (NACA), a division of the National Organization for Competency Assurance (NOCA). Its website is www.noca.org/.

Certification is a highly individual and personal choice. However, certification, like accreditation, sets the individual apart from others and is considered by many to be the gold standard. In addition to the certification processes for individuals, over the past several years, an accreditation process for case management organizations has been developed.

Accreditation of a case management unit assists in standardizing case management practices by measuring the programs against consistent benchmarks. Thus just as certification is important to an individual, accreditation is important to the unit or organization providing the case management services.

For more information on accreditation of case management organizations, please see American Accreditation Health-Care Commission/URAC website at www.urac.org or the Commission for Accreditation of Rehabilitation Facilities, the Rehabilitation Accreditation Commission website at: www.Carf.org.

AUDITS

Audits are reviews conducted by governmental agencies and accrediting organizations to determine a health care organization's compliance with statutory and regulatory mandates or standards developed by the respective accrediting organization. Audits or reviews are can be conducted by a variety of state and federal entities such as the Department of Health and Human Services, The CMS, JACHO, NCQA, the Office of Inspector General (OIG), and any number of large auditing firms hired by large purchasers of health care to audit the MCOs that serve the bulk of their employees.

As organizations prepare for either accreditation surveys or audits by the many players in health care, it is important to understand why audits are performed and what is evaluated during site surveys. Before any audit or survey, most organizations are given ample time (e.g., 12 months' advance warning) to assemble the documents and files that will be reviewed. However, if the organization is not in compliance, the auditing agency can make unannounced surveys or visits at any time.

Therefore it is best to remain in compliance with all appropriate standards and to keep documents in order at all times.

In most cases, the documents reviewed are very similar, and there are many similarities between categories of review for the various auditing entities, even though the tools vary. For example, quality of care, patient rights and responsibilities, financial integrity, documentation and record keeping, utilization management, and appeals and grievances are among the typical sections in a review tool. In most cases, the following documents must be current and in order:

- Program description and work plan
- Job descriptions
- Organizational chart
- Policies and procedures
- Minutes of committee meetings
- Survey reports and findings and any actions taken when opportunities for improvement were identified
- Results of any studies undertaken and any actions taken when opportunities for improvement were identified
- Actual member files, denial letters, or other communication, which may be reviewed to ensure timeliness standards are met; and for case management, the case management plan, actions taken for the case, and the types of services and referrals made for the member
- Training manuals and documents, as well as interrater reliability testing results and actions taken when opportunities for improvement were identified
- Data reports
- Financial reports
- Credentialing files or personnel files

In addition to the review of any documents, the auditors or surveyors may interview key members of the staff. An interview, called *an entrance interview*, is also conducted at the start of the process;

and at the close of the audit or survey, the auditors will conduct a summation conference or exit interview during which a brief description of findings will be presented. Written findings are submitted to the organization within approximately four to six weeks of the actual site survey or audit.

Internal Audits

Regardless of whether an organization is surveyed or audited by outsiders, it is important in case management and utilization management to have processes in place by which staff can be audited on a regular basis for their performance. These audits should be in addition to any inter-rater testing of staff that validates consistency in case determinations or case actions.

These internal audits can be performed by using a predeveloped checklist that validates expected case events will and did occur, and if not, provides supporting documentation as to the reason. Internal audits are also an excellent way to assist with the ongoing education of staff and to capture events that require additional education as they happen.

■ SUMMARY

The current crisis in the U.S. health care system stems from many factors, but in part it is due to the lack of confidence health care consumers have in the conventional approaches historically used for QA. The situation calls for quality management strategies that are consistent with the complexities of today's health care organizations and thus the shift from a QA retrospective approach to a prospective QI process.

With the emphasis on quality comes an emphasis on data collection. Much of the data collected for the organization will be required not only by the regulators and accrediting bodies but also by large health care purchasers and as a tool when con-

tracts are negotiated. More importantly, data can be used to validate success, and ultimately, survival in the health care marketplace.

In addition to proof of organizations' worth through studies and the production of data, large health care purchasers, government bodies, and consumers seek organizations that have received a *voluntary stamp of approval* through application for accreditation. Accreditation is not a condition of licensure, but licensure is a condition for accreditation. If an organization receives federal funding for any of its clients, it must be accredited as a condition of doing business. Accreditation is believed by many health care organizations, purchasers, and public entities to be the gold stamp of approval, meaning that the organization offers quality services to clients.

As important as accreditation is to an organization, so is certification for health care professionals. Certification, if received from the right organization, like accreditation, can be a stamp of approval that the individual has the expertise and knowledge to perform at an advanced level of practice.

Because health care organizations are continually under scrutiny, every department and unit must be prepared at all times for an audit or survey, regardless of whether it is planned or unannounced. For case managers, this means keeping charts current and accurate and documenting the steps taken and the reasons for taking them.

Chapter Exercises

1. Describe the key differences between quality management and quality improvement.
2. List the two key agencies that oversee quality in the healthcare industry.
3. Describe in your own words why it is important to use benchmarks as data are presented for use.

4. Describe in your own words why you feel credentialing is important and what it means to you.
5. List the four elements of QISMC.
6. In a group setting discuss the importance of audits and why it is important to conduct internal audits as well as to test the staff on at least an annual basis.

Suggested Websites and Resources

www.ncqa.org—NCQA
www.jacho.org—JCAHO
www.carf.org— Commission for Accreditation of Rehabilitation Facilities
www.urac.org—URAC
www.chapinc.org—Community Health Accreditation Program
www.cola.org—Commission on Office Laboratory Accreditation
www.cmsa.org—CMSA
www.allhealthnet.com/Nursing/Specialty+Cer tifications+Board—Nursing specialties
www.cphq-hqcb.org—Healthcare Quality Certification Board
www.cdec1.com—Commission on Health Care Certification (CHCC)
www.cdms.org—Certification of Disability Management Specialists
www.abqaurp.org—American Board of Quality Assurance and Utilization Review Physicians (ABQAURP)
www.urac.org—American Healthcare Commission/Utilization Review Accreditation Commission (URAC)
www.nbccc.org—National Board for Certification in Continuity of Care

www.ccmcertification.org—Commission for Case Manager Certification
www.cfcm.com—Center for Case Management Administrator, Certified
www.AIOCM.com—American Institute of Outcomes Case Management
www.rehabnurse.org—Commission on Rehabilitation Counselor Certification
www.crccertification.com—Association of Rehabilitation Nurses
www.NursingWorld.org—American Nurses Credentialing Center

REFERENCES

1. Brown JA: *The healthcare quality handbook: a professional resource and study guide*, Pasadena, Calif, 1998, Managed Care Consultants.
2. Newell M: *Using nursing case management to improve health outcomes*, Gaithersburg, Md, 1996, Aspen.
3. Boland P: *Making managed healthcare work: a practical guide to strategies and solutions*, Gaithersburg, Md, 1993, Aspen.
4. Cohen EL, De Back V: *The outcomes mandate: case management in health care today*, St Louis, 1999, Mosby.

BIBLIOGRAPHY

American Nurses Association: *CHN communique (Council of Community Health Nursing)*, Washington, DC, 1991, The Association.
DMSA standards of practice, *Case Manager* 5 (1):59-71, 1994.
James G: *Making managed care work: strategies for local market dominance*, Chicago, 1997, Irwin Professional Publishing.
Kirk R: *Managing outcomes, process, and cost in a managed care environment*, Gaithersburg, Md, 1997, Aspen.
Kongstvedt PR: *The managed care handbook*, Gaithersburg, Md, 1993, Aspen.
Powell SK: *Nursing case management: a practical guide to success in managed care*, Philadelphia, 1996, Lippincott-Raven.

Quality Management for Case Managers

Anne P. Foster, RN, MSN, CPHQ

OBJECTIVES

- To state three indicators that measure the quality and utilization of resources
- To list three types of standards applicable to case managers
- To identify two ways of breaking down barriers to achieve the goals of low utilization and high quality

VALUE OF CASE MANAGEMENT

Case managers play a critical role in the provision of quality care. They accomplish this goal in both direct and indirect ways. Case managers have a direct influence on the safety and comfort of patients in any setting. Through excellent communication skills and knowledge of resources, case managers can enhance confidence in the health care system, which will result in patient satisfaction.

Case managers have an indirect influence on improving the quality of care by pinpointing system problems that affect efficiency, identifying omissions such as failure to implement the physician's orders, and promoting an interdisciplinary approach in care planning. Case managers identify threats to optimal wellness as part of their assessment, monitoring, and observational responsibilities.

A discharge or transfer care plan that is well thought out, well implemented, and well monitored can prepare the patient and his or her family or significant others for success at the next level of care. Readmission is an measure of quality that should be tracked in every health care setting. Causes of readmission should be analyzed and trends identified, so that reasons related to the patient, the health system, and the delivery of care are identified as opportunities to improve in the future.

GUIDELINES IN CASE MANAGEMENT

Case managers have an important role in any setting in upholding organizational practices. These most frequently take the form of policies and procedures. Often they are approved clinical pathways or are referred to as critical pathways or care maps. These standardized multidisciplinary tools are used to identify care processes and monitor the patient's progress toward expected outcomes. The clinical pathways do the following:

- Address the multidisciplinary aspects of care management

- Facilitate communication
- Improve coordination
- Increase efficiency
- Provide predictability
- Furnish a means of determining variance
- Improve the quality of care

The role of the case manager can be to initiate the development of clinical pathways, monitor compliance, and/or provide variance reports based on the monitoring efforts. The tracking of variances is often part of a quality improvement evaluation process whose results will be reported to the appropriate clinical committees.

Evidence-based guidelines are similar to clinical pathways. These tools may look like clinical pathways, but they are based exclusively on research and clinical trials. The conclusions from these studies provide the path to follow. Case managers may participate in the research activity but usually are involved in the implementing the guidelines and monitoring their use.

Disease management is a clinical management process that provides guidelines across the continuum of care from primary prevention to ongoing long-term maintenance for individuals with chronic health conditions. Disease management programs are an integrated system of implemented interventions, measurements, and refinements designed to optimize clinical and economic outcomes for a specific chronic disease by doing the following:

- Facilitating proper diagnosis
- Maximizing clinical effectiveness
- Eliminating ineffective diagnostic and therapeutic procedures
- Maximizing the efficiency of care delivery
- Maximizing self-management skills to ensure improved outcomes as a whole

Features that differentiate a disease management program from a clinical pathway include the following:

- A disease management program focuses on the continuum of a disease, not just on acute episodes.
- It is population based.
- It incorporates standardized treatment-based plans and guidelines.
- It calls for regular follow-up.
- It requires meticulous record keeping (usually on computer).
- It is patient centered.
- It is multidisciplinary.
- It has measurable results and is data driven.
- It is proactive and prevention oriented, and provides early intervention.
- It uses a clinical practice improvement approach.

The goal of disease management programs is to minimize exacerbation of disease and decrease hospital admissions and emergency department visits. Case managers contribute to the success of disease management programs by following the established guidelines in performing their work.

Clinical pathways, whether evidence based data or not, and disease management programs enhance quality and reduce unnecessary costs associated with variance from guidelines and unhealthy practices.

CHALLENGES OF ORGANIZATIONAL CASE MANAGEMENT STANDARDS VERSUS CASE MANAGEMENT STANDARDS OF PRACTICE

A standard is an established rule, according to *Webster's Dictionary*. Standards are requirements set by several entities, including professional, accrediting, licensing, and employing organizations, and the courts. As the basis for professional licensing, the nursing practice act in each state determines the scope of allowable practice and the parameters of practice; these are therefore considered standards. The Case

Management Society of America, an international nonprofit professional organization founded in 1990, developed the Standards of Practice for Case Management. These standards provide a framework for defining case management roles in a variety of settings and specialties. They are a working tool for the development, administration, and evaluation of case management services. The Commission for Case Manager Certification developed the Scope of Practice for Case Managers as a representation of professional opinions regarding what constitutes appropriate delivery of effective case management services. The following are some clarifying points:

- Case management is an advanced practice of an already established professional identity (e.g., registered nurse, licensed social worker). Thus, each case manager's professional scope of practice applies. The scope of practice for case management therefore includes the following:
  - The case manager's professional scope of practice
  - The employer's governing policies and procedures
  - The Case Management Society of America's Standards of Practice for Case Management
  - Case managers are expected to operate within their individual scope of practice.
  - It is considered unethical for case managers to operate outside the limits of their individual scope of practice.

Each employing organization, whether a health plan, hospital, or home health agency, has its own standards. These take the form of policies, procedures, and job descriptions. They are based on other applicable sets of standards such as those of the Joint Commission on Accreditation of Healthcare Organizations (JCAHO), the National Committee for Quality Assurance (NCQA), and state and regional licensing boards.

The courts of law establish standards of care or practice by using the principle of the "reasonable and prudent" person. When there is no clear standard applicable to an issue in a case, the court may ask, "What would a reasonable and prudent professional do in this instance?" The use of expert witnesses, those with an educational and experiential background similar to that of the accused in a lawsuit, is the most common method of applying the principle of the reasonable and prudent person. It should be noted that negligence to follow established standards is not an excuse not to follow them.

CASE MANAGER ACCOUNTABILITY

Case managers, like all health care employees or contractors, are accountable for their performance. JCAHO has set the standard that the specific duties to be performed must be defined for each individual position. The competencies required of case managers form the basis of the job description and all evaluations, which are referred to as competency-based performance evaluations. The competencies required for case management are determined by each organization but most likely will include competencies under the broad headings shown in Table 26-1, which also provides examples of measurable components of these competencies.

Case managers must have the ability to evaluate a situation and make recommendations to the physician and payer that are based on the best interests of the patient. Cost considerations in arranging contracted services and limitations of benefits are included in this evaluation. A fine line is frequently walked between limiting cost and maintaining quality. However, poor quality costs the most!

TABLE 26-1	
Competencies for Case Managers	
Competency Area	**Measurable Component**
Management of patient care	Effectively plans care with an interdisciplinary approach
Position-specific functions	Provides accurate information to payers
Patient safety	Identifies high-risk situations for patient population
Age-specific care requirements	Assesses for potential and actual skin breakdown
Pain management	Monitors for physiologic and behavioral signs of pain
Performance improvement	Demonstrates performance improvement
Fiscal management	Identifies cost-saving opportunities that do not compromise quality of care
Compliance	Follows the code of conduct
Organization-wide essential functions	Demonstrates behavior conducive to positive guest relations

HEALTH CARE PERFORMANCE PRESSURES AND PROCESSES

Several external events have affected case managers and the quality of their work. These events are implementation of the prospective payment system (PPS), nationwide nurse staffing shortages, and higher expectations from patients. Faced with more restrictive payment systems and staffing shortages, often without allowable contractor fill-ins, the case manager must work harder to balance the demands to maximize reimbursement and the higher expectations from patients, which results in more time-consuming interviews.

The implementation of PPS in the United States in 1983 began the era of federal payment limitations to health care organizations. The system was first implemented for acute-care institutions, and the reimbursement for these institutions as well as for home health agencies and skilled nursing facilities is now determined by the acuteness of the patient's care needs as noted on a document transmitted to the fiscal intermediary. PPS, however, has created an opportunity for case management. In the days of cost-based reimbursement, little motivation existed for organizations to hire nurses to oversee spending because the money was coming back without question.

CUSTOMER SATISFACTION AND THE REASON FOR MEASURING IT

The customers of the case manager should be identified, and customer satisfaction with the case manager's performance measured. These customers include patients, families and significant others, physicians, clinical professionals, payers, and externally involved personnel (e.g., police).

For the organization, the case manager's relationship with each of these categories of customer is critical to conducting business both internally and externally. Case managers must have the special traits of good listening skills, a collaborative attitude, and good clinical knowledge to succeed. For the aforementioned customers to feel satisfied, the case manager must communicate in a way that is informative, is not directive, and is not perceived as threatening.

As part of a performance improvement (or quality management) process, the customers are asked a series of questions and the results are then examined for trends and analyzed by a member of the performance improvement staff. This information should be used to improve the customer satisfaction results by putting in place an action plan.

Customer satisfaction is critical for maintaining business and developing new opportunities. Case managers are in a special position because they are in frequent contact with external community customers, and they must create a positive image through their competence and caring.

MEASUREMENT OF UTILIZATION AND COSTS

How do we know if we are successful? If we did not decide where we want to be, any result will be satisfactory. The squeeze on the health care dollar is obvious when a review of the bottom line is conducted. Case managers play a critical role in saving dollars through review of resource usage. The objective measurement of specific indicators that are defined for the given setting and that show how case management influences resource utilization is important in evaluating overall organization-wide goals as well as in assessing the performance of the individual case manager. Table 26-2 offers suggested utilization indicators for different health care settings.

The choice of which data to measure must be made by those who know what information is most important to obtain and who have the means to collect these data. The time period for which data will be collected, the methods of determining the sample, who will review the data, and when and where the data will be presented must be determined.

The following are examples of indicators used at many acute-care hospitals:

- Average length of stay (by payer, unit, physician, department)
- Cost per day (with breakdown of ancillary charges)
- Denials of days and stays (by payer, unit, physician)
- Readmission rate (by payer, unit, physician, case manager, type of discharge)

DATA AS THE DRIVER

Continuous quality improvement (CQI) is the health care term that is analogous to the term *total quality management* (TQM) coined by Dr. W. Edwards Deming in 1970. Dr. Deming helped the Japanese become more efficient and effective after World War II. His famous 14 points (Box 26-1) describe the concept of TQM, which has been widely adopted in the United States under the name CQI. In addition to these 14 points, using visual tools to display data and working in teams are considered cornerstones of this concept.[1]

The CQI philosophy centers on processes and considers processes rather than people to be responsible for variances in performance. The goal is for everyone to

---

TABLE 26-2
Utilization Indicators

Setting	Indicator
Acute-care hospital	Length of stay, ancillary costs/day, readmission rate
Skilled nursing facility	Length of stay, ancillary costs/day
Home health care	Number of visits when patient is not at skilled level
Rehabilitation	Number of patients who fail to achieve rehabilitation goals
Hospice	Number of patients who qualify for but are not receiving services
Ambulatory care clinics	Number of encounters for ambulatory care, including number of no-shows per patient

BOX 26-1
Fourteen Points of Total Quality Management

1. Develop constancy of purpose.
2. Incorporate the new philosophy.
3. End reliance on mass inspection.
4. Improve the system on a constant basis.
5. Knock down barriers.
6. Eliminate fear.
7. Knock down interdepartmental barriers.
8. Get rid of slogans, exhortations, and targets.
9. Refuse to use work standards, quotas, and numerical goals.
10. Use modern supervision methods.
11. Offer on-the-job training.
12. Begin self-improvement programs.
13. Refuse to award business on the basis of price alone.
14. Elicit help from all teammates to accomplish these goals.

Data from Walton M: *The Deming management method*, New York, 1986, Putnam Publishing.

try every day to perform his or her job better, not merely to try to attain the minimal level of competence that will satisfy standards. Teams are needed to analyze processes for future improvement. Team members should be selected based on their experience, expertise, or frequent use of the process involved. The creation of teams is a very useful method to accomplish tasks that are complex, need a long-lasting solution, have sufficient time for completion, and/or require input from a variety of viewpoints. Teams may not be the best problem-solving mechanism when time is critical, the outcome is predetermined, or an individual decision is appropriate.

The improvement cycle that is followed by teams or other reviewers is Plan, Do, Check, and Act, which can be defined as follows:

Plan
- Define the problem including listing goals or outcomes.
- Describe the current process; a literature search and an internal evaluation may be performed.
- Create a flowchart that visually shows the steps of the process under review and facilitates achieving a common view.

Do
- Carry out the plan with a pilot project, data collection, and education.
- Use tools such as histograms, check sheets, and surveys to display the data collected.

Check
- Evaluate the outcome and process results using comparative and baseline data.
- Use helpful tools such as force field analysis to identify driving and resisting forces.

Act
- Implement changes at the right speed, possibly in stages.
- Communicate outcomes.
- Use helpful tools such as the fishbone diagram, which identifies the root cause of a problem.

"In God we trust. All others must use data." The author of this aphorism is unknown, but it is considered a credo for statisticians.

Tools (charts) are used to help members of a group, team, or committee understand what the data are saying. The following tools, displayed *adjacent to* the discussion group, are the most commonly used tools for information display:

Cause-and-effect diagrams
- A cause-and-effect diagram is used to explore and display all of the possible causes of a specific problem or condition. It is also known as a fishbone diagram because of its shape, or an Ishikawa diagram, after its originator, Kaoru Ishikawa (Figure 26-1). The benefits of this type of diagram are as follows:
  - The creation process is educational and spurs discussion.

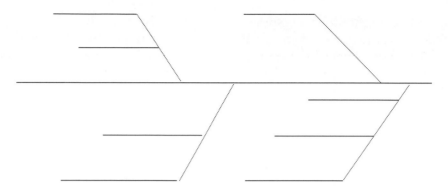

Figure 26-1 Cause-and-effect diagram.

- The diagram helps groups (teams) focus on the issue at hand.
- Its use results in an active search for the cause.
- Data usually are collected to construct the diagram.
- It demonstrates the level of understanding. The more complex the diagram, the more sophisticated the workers' knowledge of the process.
- It has widespread use for problem solving.

Flowcharts

- A flowchart is used to display pictorially how all the steps of a process are related to each other (Figure 26-2). Drawing a flowchart of a process helps a team make the first step in improving a process. The flowchart uses standard symbols to represent the types of processing and steps to take. Use of a flowchart will bring everyone to the same understanding of what the process is.

Pareto charts

- The Pareto principle is defined by J. M. Juran, a colleague of Deming, as the "phenomenon whereby, in any population that contributes to a common effect, a relative few of the contributors account for

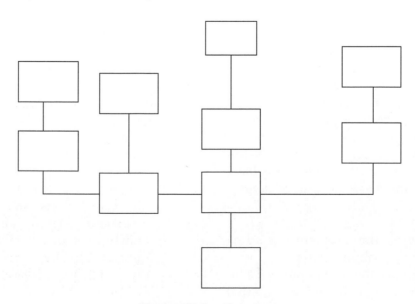

Figure 26-2 Flow chart.

the bulk of the effect."[1] Sometimes this principle is described as the 80/20 rule; that is, 80% of the impact is due to 20% of the problems. A commonly used bar graphic technique, construction of a Pareto chart, helps determine priorities (Figure 26-3). The data are displayed from most frequent problem to least frequent problem. This arrangement assists in prioritizing types of errors and weeding out trivial or unrelated problems.

Run charts

- A run chart displays data over a period of time so that trends can be identified (Figure 26-4).

Histograms

- A histogram measures how frequently an event occurs, usually against a reference time frame (Figure 26-5).

Scatter diagrams

- A scatter diagram is a method of charting the relationship between two variables (Figure 26-6). This type of chart shows the data

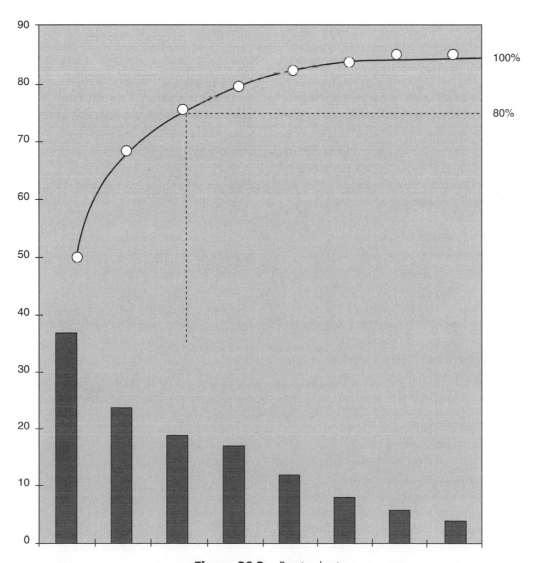

Figure 26-3   Pareto chart.

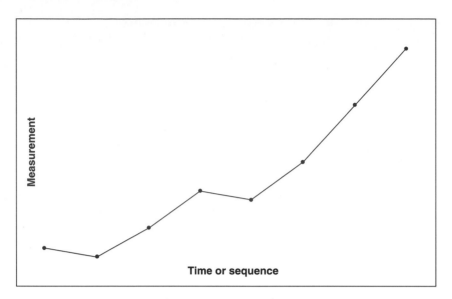

Figure 26-4 Run chart.

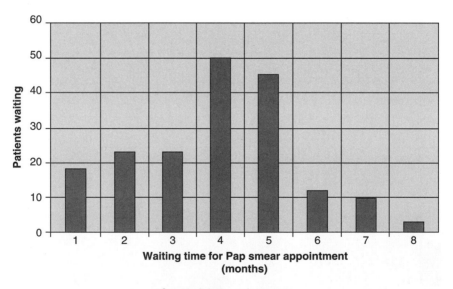

Figure 26-5 Histogram.

points as dots with no lines connecting them. When the data are
analyzed, the eyes are drawn to the
part of the graph that has the most
dots. The variable representing the
"cause" is graphed on the horizontal axis and that representing the
"effect" on the vertical axis.

Control charts

- A control chart is a continuing
  guide to constant improvement
  (Figure 26-7). It is similar to a run
  chart with statistically determined
  upper and lower limits drawn on
  either side of the process average.
  The data, well displayed, can

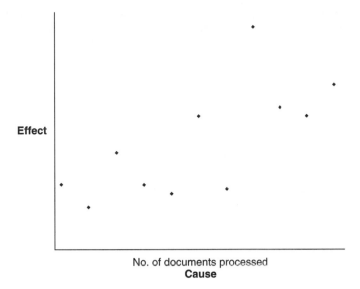

Figure 26-6   Scatter diagram.

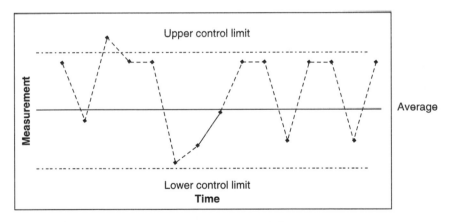

Figure 26-7   Control chart.

demonstrate the following to an organization:

- How it is doing
- How it compares with other organizations (e.g., benchmarking)
- Which processes are working and which are not
- What are the risks to the well-being of the organization
- Which goals are being achieved and which are not

Case managers may be in a position to present data to a group. Often the data, or what they reveal, may be surprising to some of the participants. It is a good idea first to present any politically sensitive data to the supervisor and lead physician, when applicable.

IDENTIFICATION OF BARRIERS AND OBSTACLES

There is a nationwide shortage of nurses in the workforce. This carries over to the case management field. Often case managers carry such high patient loads that only the bare minimum can be accomplished.

Frequently case managers are requested to collect data related to quality indicators while they are performing their usual functions. This may create a conflict, as case managers can barely complete their utilization and discharge planning functions. Barriers related to case managers' performance of quality management activities include lack of time, poor education regarding the task, and a belief that the data will not show anything meaningful. Case managers are in a position to help their institutions improve systems because they can identify factors that delay care and service. They should be provided with a mechanism for forwarding information on variances to the right source so that improvements can be made. The following are examples of barriers confronting case managers:

- System issues
- Resource containment
- Underdevelopment or lack of processes
- Personnel issues
- Physicians
- Caregivers
- Families and patients
- Difficulty of collecting objective information
- Waste of resources
- Disruption of quality care
- Time required to work toward solutions

BENCHMARKING, TARGETS, AND VARIANCES

Benchmarking is the comparison of actual practice to a best practice. A best practice is considered the best possible practice or the best in its class. It is achieved by one entity but may not be possible for all due to internal and external variations. The practice is closely linked to performance, as measured by indicators such as average length of stay or managed care bed days.

Benchmarking, or best practice comparisons, is used to compare internal findings with those in the market or nation.

Comparison of performance with that of competitors or colleagues, or best practices creates an objective view of how the organization is doing.

Such a comparison enables the organization to view its improvements against the performance of others with a proven track record. Benchmarking provides a point of reference from which measured evaluations can be made. These data confirm excellence and set the pace while helping managers set realistic targets. A target is often the value of some performance indicator that the organization believes it can reach in a defined period of time. This differs from the benchmark number, which if not the target, is considered achievable for that specific time frame.

There are two types of benchmarking. Internal benchmarking compares services in similar departments or compares functional areas to one another. External benchmarking compares results in the organization with state, regional, or national results.

Benchmarked data have value to an organization through the reporting structure. When quality and cost information is presented to committees, the participants, especially medical staff members, find it interesting and motivating to be told the benchmark for a given indicator. It is important to the organization's leadership to know how the organization stands in comparison to competitors.

Using benchmarks with care is critical. Benchmarking generally gives the most positive results in setting short- and long-term goals. When an inapplicable best practice is used, however, frustration can result. The expression "Compare oranges to oranges, not apples to oranges" has application here.

OUTCOME MEASUREMENT

Outcome measurement is the process of identifying desired end states and designing systems and processes to achieve them. Important outcomes applicable to case management are those relating to the achievement of clinical, quality, cost, and revenue goals. The challenge is not only to select outcomes applicable to the given line of business, but also to design measurement systems so that the data can be turned into meaningful information. It is important to decide whether a process monitor is also needed to evaluate the particular care issue or whether outcome measurement alone is sufficient. The processes and structures also need review. Outcome research is the study of outcomes in health care using precise data collection to learn new truths. The goal of outcome measurement conducted to support improvement is to evaluate current practices and create changes to achieve better patient care. The target audience is often quality improvement teams in health care organizations.

ACCREDITATION OF ORGANIZATIONS

Accreditation surveys cost money both in fees to the reviewing organizations and in outlays for the staff required internally or externally to assist with preparation of the survey. Accreditation is considered voluntary. But is it truly? Many managed care contracts (with health maintenance organizations [HMOs]) are contingent upon accreditation of the provider organization. The Centers for Medicare & Medicaid Services (CMS), formerly the Health Care Financing Administration, accepts JCAHO accreditation rather than conducting its own reviews for certification. However, the CMS reserves the right to conduct validation and other surveys based on information received or random selection. Consumers are becoming increasingly more aware of accreditation as the "Good Housekeeping seal" for health care organizations.

The JCAHO evaluates and accredits nearly 18,000 health care organizations and programs in the United States. It is an independent, not-for-profit organization that is the nation's predominate standards-setting and accrediting body in health care. On-site surveys are conducted at least every 3 years. Laboratories must be surveyed every 2 years. Formed in 1951, the JCAHO has developed professionally based standards and evaluates the compliance of the following types of health care organization with these standards:

- General, psychiatric, children's, and rehabilitation hospitals
- Health care networks, including integrated delivery networks, HMOs, and preferred provider organizations
- Home care organizations, including those that provide home health services, personal care and support services, home infusion and other pharmacy services, durable medical equipment services, and hospice services
- Nursing homes and other long-term care facilities, including subacute-care programs and dementia programs
- Assisted-living facilities that provide or coordinate personal services
- Behavioral health care organizations, including those that provide mental health and addiction services, and services to persons with developmental disabilities
- Ambulatory care providers, including outpatient surgical facilities, rehabilitation centers, infusion centers, group practices, and others
- Clinical laboratories

JCAHO's standards address the organization's level of performance in key functional areas, such as patient rights, patient treatment, performance improvement, and infection control. ORYX was initiated in February 1997 to integrate the use of outcomes and other performance measurement data into the accreditation process. When the program was implemented, each facility chose a measurement system from among those provided by the list of JCAHO-approved vendors; the vendor then took the data from the accredited facility, formatted it, and sent it to JCAHO. Sets of core performance measures are used. The four initial core measurement areas for hospitals are as follows:

1. Acute myocardial infarction
2. Heart failure
3. Community-acquired pneumonia
4. Pregnancy and related conditions

The NCQA is an independent, non-profit watchdog organization whose mission is to improve health care quality. The NCQA evaluates quality using three different methods:

1. Accreditation (based on a rigorous on-site review of key clinical and administrative processes)
2. The Health Plan Employer Data and Information Set (HEDIS; a tool used to measure performance in areas such as immunization and mammography)
3. Member satisfaction survey

Although participation in NCQA accreditation and certification programs is voluntary, more than half the nation's HMOs currently participate. Nearly 90% of all health plans measure their performance using HEDIS. Individuals and corporate leaders consider HEDIS data in choosing health plans for themselves and their employees. As of this writing, the current version is HEDIS 3.0, which includes the following set of reporting measurement categories:

- Effectiveness of care (e.g., advising smokers to quit, administering flu shots, administering beta-blockers after heart attack)
- Access to and availability of care (e.g., appointment access, telephone access, availability of primary care providers)
- Satisfaction with the experience of care (e.g., annual member health

survey, descriptive information in survey)
- Health plan stability (e.g., member disenrollment rates, physician turnover, performance indicators)
- Use of service (e.g., rate of well-child visits in the first 15 months of life and adolescent well-care visits)
- Cost of care (e.g., high-occurrence and high-cost diagnosis-related groups, rate trends)
- Informed health care choices (e.g., language translation services, new member orientation and education)
- Health plan descriptive information (e.g., board certification and residency completion, provider compensation)
- Testing set (e.g., number of people in the plan who smoke, number receiving chlamydia screening)

One of the issues confronting integrated delivery systems and other types of combined organizations is the variation in standards established by different accrediting or certifying organizations. Yet each has a similar goal. These standards vary enough that the organization may need to perform different studies or initiate different quality measurement activities. The good news is a beginning trend among organizations to coordinate efforts and collaborate to develop one performance measure that will be accepted by all accrediting bodies for assessing a similar outcome or goal.

In 1998, the Performance Measurement Coordinating Council (PMCC) was developed by the American Medical Association (a partnership of physicians and their professional associations dedicated to promoting the art and science of medicine and improvement of public health), the JCAHO, and the NCQA (previously defined) with this same goal of developing a single integrated set of standards. Although the PMCC was discontinued, the organizations agreed to continue their joint efforts to work together on condition-specific measurement sets. In April 2001, the first common set of evidence-based measures for evaluating performance in health care was developed for diabetes care.

ROLE OF THE CASE MANAGER IN ACCREDITATION

Case managers must be aware of applicable standards. The JCAHO standards contain a chapter entitled "Continuum of Care," which deals with discharge planning and the linking of levels of care within an organization. Each organization must have a utilization management and discharge planning process. The NCQA sets standards for the review of utilization indicators for resource consumption. Therefore, case managers must follow the standards applicable in their individual setting.

COMPLIANCE PROGRAMS AND THE HEALTH INSURANCE PORTABILITY AND ACCOUNTABILITY ACT

The benefits of a corporate compliance program to an organization are many and include the following:

- It causes the organization to examine itself.
- It creates a code of conduct.
- It results in a more intelligent and lenient government response if questionable activity is identified.
- It prevents the imposition of a government-created compliance plan.
- It assists the organization in monitoring critical aspects of safe and ethical practice.

Compliance Program Components

The seven elements of a compliance program are as follows:

1. Designation of a compliance officer and other appropriate bodies, such as a compliance committee. It is important that the compliance officer and program report directly to the chief executive officer.
2. Development and distribution of written standards of conduct, as well as written policies and procedures that promote commitment to compliance and address specific areas of potential fraud (e.g., billing, coding).
3. Development and implementation of regular, effective education and training programs for all affected employees.
4. Maintenance of a process to receive complaints, such as a hotline, and the adoption of procedures to protect anonymity of complainants.
5. Development of a system to respond to allegations of improper or illegal activities and the initiation of appropriate disciplinary actions against employees who have violated internal compliance policies, regulations, or federal health care program requirements.
6. Use of audits and/or other evaluation techniques to monitor compliance and to assist in addressing identified problem areas.
7. Investigation and remediation of identified system problems and the development of policies addressing the discharge or retention of sanctioned individuals.

The Health Insurance Portability and Accountability Act (HIPAA) of 1996 is a federal regulation that has been partially implemented, as of this writing. The following are three major areas of focus:

- Portability of health insurance coverage between employer group health plans, including elimination of an exemption for a preexisting condition (implemented)
- Measures for preventing fraud and abuse in health care (implemented)

- Provisions for administrative simplification, including the following:

Transactions codes	October 2002
Privacy	April 14, 2003
Security	Expected to be fall of 2003

Portability has helped many workers to retain health insurance when they start a new job, rather than becoming uninsured. *Fraud* is a deliberate deception perpetrated for unlawful or unfair gain—an incident or practice that intentionally deceives or misrepresents claims against the federal health care programs. *Abuse* is taking advantage of a weakness in the organization. The findings of fraud and abuse have been remarkable. The government initially spent $1 million and found $1 billion in fraud within the first year. Operation Restore Trust, a project to eliminate fraud and abuse started in 1995, found $23 in overpayments for every $1 of legitimate reimbursement. HIPAA allowed for additional funding and expansion of these efforts. The Balanced Budget Act of 1997 also supported another step-up of efforts. The False Claims Act allowed whistleblowers who initiated successful lawsuits in fraud and abuse cases to receive up to 30% of the funds recovered by the government.

Administrative simplification portions of HIPAA involve transaction codes, privacy, and security. *Transaction codes* will become uniform for quicker data preparation and better understanding of what is being transmitted. *Privacy* provisions concern the disclosure of "protected health information" (PHI), which is individually identifiable health information that is transmitted or maintained, in any form or medium, by an entity covered under HIPAA. The organizations affected include health care providers, health plans, employers, and health care clearinghouses. It is critical to perform an assessment of the organization to identify what is PHI and to teach its employees to not divulge this information except to someone who needs to know it. Administrative simplification requires appointing a privacy officer, training staff in the correct handling of PHI, implementing sanction policies, establishing methods to monitor processes to ensure enforcement, and documenting overall compliance with the pertinent regulations. The *security* component of administrative simplification requires institution of procedures to guard the integrity, confidentiality, and availability of data. Safeguards are both physical (protecting records in a locked area) and technical (preventing unauthorized computer access).

The case manager's role in HIPAA compliance centers on privacy and security. Case managers transmit PHI verbally, in writing, via telephone, and by facsimile. Measures must be taken to identify the reason for the communication and the security of the transmission. Such studies might include validation studies in which one validates that fax machines are sending documents to the correct location. In these studies documents are faxed to commonly used numbers with a request that the recipient resend the document to indicate whether the intended recipient received the document. Case managers should never leave PHI documents unattended.

SUMMARY

Many definitions, perceptions, and processes are being used in health care today as organizations attempt to measure and report their quality activities. Over the past few decades health care organizations have used a variety of processes to measure their quality assurance programs. As such, they have used a series of programs that monitor and evaluate their activities, all with varying degrees and varying effectiveness. More recently, many quality programs are now called *quality improvement programs*, in which the emphasis is on a continuous quality improvement process that measure outcomes.

As indicated in this chapter, case managers play a critical role in the provision of quality care, and this is accomplished through both direct and indirect ways. Direct ways are what case managers use to influence their patients to make the right decisions. This is accomplished using excellent communication skills and resource knowledge, with the end result being increased patient satisfaction. Indirect ways are when the case manager identifies system problems that affect service efficiency.

Quality, to be effective, must be a system-wide process that touches every aspect of care and services provided. Once areas of concern are identified, studies and their outcomes will play a vital part as any corrective actions are developed and implemented.

Chapter Exercises

1. Describe how causes of readmission should be handled.
2. Discuss the uses of the following data display charts: control chart, histogram, and Pareto chart.
3. Define *protected health information*, and list examples of what it includes.

Suggested Websites and Resources

Accreditation

www.jcaho.org
www.ncqa.org

Outcomes Management:

www.hightidepress.com
www.outcomesmanagement.com/
www.pbhi.com/Providers_public/Practitioner Manual/GeneralManual/PractMan_ C00.asp

Case Management Practice

www.ccmcertification.org

Compliance

www.cms.hhs.gov—Centers for Medicare & Medicaid Services
www.oig.hhs.gov/—Health and Human Services, Office of Inspector General
www.hhs.gov/ocr/hipaa—Specific site for interpretation of HIPAA, Office of Civil Rights

REFERENCE

1. Walton M: *The Deming management method*, New York, 1986, Putnam.

BIBLIOGRAPHY

California Managed Healthcare Quality Coalition: *Annual conference materials*, Pasadena, Calif, February 2001, The Coalition.
California Managed Healthcare Quality Coalition: *Utilization management quarterly tools*, Pasadena, Calif, 2001, The Coalition.
Coleman CE, Joseph AH: *HIPAA self-assessment and planning, a guide to the privacy and security standards*, ed 2, Marblehead, Mass, 2001, Opus Communications.
National Association for Healthcare Quality: *Annual educational conference materials*, Glenview, Ill, September 1999, The Association.
Quality Management Program: *Learning tree university extension*, Chatsworth, Calif, 2001, The Program.

The Importance of Credentialing

Gary S. Wolfe, RN, CCM

OBJECTIVES

- To discuss why credentialing is important not only for an individual but also for an organization
- To identify one key document that is the basis for credentialing
- To list at least two types of credentialing for case management

Credentialing in health care is a broad subject but in essence concerns a person's qualifications to perform specific tasks. Credentialing has long been a topic of conversation, since health care providers deal with human life, and organizations such as hospitals and other health providers as well as payers have a responsibility to members to ensure that the people performing health care tasks are well qualified to do so. Credentialing can be defined as the process of evaluating a person's qualification vis-à-vis the job to be performed. Credentialing plays a significant role in the quality management process for an organization.

DEFINITION OF CASE MANAGEMENT

There has long been discussion in case management about qualifications for case managers. Several factors must be taken into consideration in determining what the qualifications of a case manager should be. The first issue is the definition of case management. The definition speci-

fies what the case manager does for the case management client. One generally accepted definition of case management is that used by the Commission for Case Manager Certification. The commission defines case management as "a collaborative process that accesses, plans, implements, coordinates, monitors, and evaluates the options and services required to meet an individual's health needs, using communication and available resources to promote quality, cost-effective outcomes."[1] After case management is defined, the next issue is the philosophy of case management. A philosophy is a statement of belief setting forth principles that guide the case manager. The Commission for Case Manager Certification has developed the following philosophy:

Case management is not a profession in itself, but an area of practice within one's profession. Its underlying premise is that when an individual reaches the optimum level of wellness and functional capability, everyone benefits: the individuals being served; their support systems; the health care delivery systems; and the various reimbursement sources.

Case management services are a means for achieving client wellness and autonomy through advocacy, communication, education, and identification of service resources, and service facilitation. The case manager helps identify appropriate providers and facilities throughout the continuum of services, while ensuring that available resources are being used in a timely and cost-effective manner to obtain optimum value for both the client and the reimbursement source. Case management services are best offered in a climate that allows direct communication between the case manager, the client and appropriate service personnel, to optimize the outcome for all concerned.[1]

The definition and philosophy may vary depending on the model and practice setting of case management but should generally specify what case management is and how it will be performed. Determining the definition and philosophy is the beginning of the development of a job description, which is an essential item in the credentialing process. Other important documents to take into consideration in the credentialing process are the standards of practice as developed by professional organizations for individuals licensed as health care providers and the scope of practice as set forth by the various state boards of practice. The job description delineates the role, responsibilities, and work of the case manager.

JOB DESCRIPTION

The job description is the source document that is the basis of credentialing. Components of a job description generally include the following:

- Job title
- Supervisor
- Summary of position
- Duties and responsibilities
- Required knowledge
- Functions
- Qualifications, including education, experience, licenses, and certifications

Careful thought should be given to the development of a job description. If the job description is well developed, as it should be, it is used in the recruitment process as well as in the evaluation of performance. Job descriptions are necessary documents, but historically, little time generally has been given to their development. Consequently, organizations do not have good job descriptions. A well-developed job description will assist in the credentialing process and facilitate obtaining good performance from an employee because the employee will know what is expected of him or her. Clear communication about performance expectations is the first step toward achieving good work performance from an employee and forms the basis for credentialing.

The job description should clearly delineate the responsibilities and functions of the case manager. In other words, the job description should outline the case management process. Job descriptions should be written for the generalist case manager as well as the specialist depending on the size of the case management organization and the type of case management, which is based in turn on the definition of case management being used.

The qualifications section of the job description should reflect the required knowledge, duties, and responsibilities. The qualifications section of a job description should reflect the type of credentials, licenses, and certifications as well as the level or years of experience required for a position. Except for worker's compensation case management in certain states, no state regulates or licenses the practice of case management.

Most case manager job descriptions start with a requirement for a license or health care certification such as registered nurse or licensed social worker. Case management builds on that license with specific experience and education. If a clinical case management model is being used, then the case manager's experience should include appropriate clinical experience. Because case management involves coordinating care across the continuum, many case management job descriptions require clinical experience in at least two delivery settings such as a hospital and a home health agency or a long-term care facility. If a case manager is to work in rehabilitation, experience in rehabilitation might be required. When the job description is developed, the clinical experience specified must match the tasks that will be required of the case manager. If the case manager is to be effective, he or she must anticipate events along a disease continuum. Most of this anticipatory knowledge comes from experience. If the case manager is assigned to any of the highly specialized case management programs such as those for preterm infants, diabetic patients, or asthmatic patients, his or her experience should be in the given clinical specialty. If the case manager is to perform general case management tasks, then general experience is acceptable. Chronic disease and disease management programs usually require specialty case managers. Because there are few educational programs to prepare case managers, case management experience may be the only means of confirming knowledge of case management. The organization may require that the case manager have a certain number of years of experience in case management within a certain time period.

In addition to experience, education is important to define in a job description, but the required education must relate to the job to be performed. Because most case managers already have a health care license, they have some basic education. In some instances additional experience may be accepted in lieu of education. The job description should define what is acceptable education. This is usually done by specifying a degree in a particular field, such as a bachelor of science in nursing.

A requirement may be included for a certain amount of continuing education in case management to demonstrate how the person obtained case management skills. The continuing education should have been completed within a certain period of time to demonstrate recent and current knowledge.

If licensure is required, the job description should stipulate that the case manager hold a current license in a particular discipline such as nursing.

The job description may require that the person have a case management certification or obtain case management certification within a certain time after being hired. Many case management certifications exist. See Table 27-1 for a listing of common case management certifications. There are both generalist and specialty case management certifications. Certification is a voluntary process initiated by an individual who wishes to show that he or she has achieved a certain level within a field. Certification is a process of validating the knowledge, skills, and abilities of individual practitioners. Certification is based on predetermined standards, including education, acceptable experience, and an examination, and typically builds on an existing defined health license such as that for registered nurse or licensed clinical social worker. Certification boards are usually governed by independent bodies that define and set standards for certification and administer the certification process. Recertification is based on demonstrating acceptable employment in the field and fulfilling a predetermined number of continuing education requirements, or retaking the examination. Certification is an opportunity for an individual to show that a certain level of expertise has been achieved and that education and experience have been validated through an examination. For the employer or consumer of case management services, certification is a benchmark of quality. If a

TABLE 27-1
Common Case Management Certifications

Certification	Acronym	Specialization	Sponsoring Organization	Contact Information
American Board of Quality Assurance and Utilization Review Physician	ABQAURP	Utilization management for physician and allied health professional	American Board of Quality Assurance and Utilization Review Physicians	American Board of Quality Assurance and Utilization Review Physicians 4890 W. Kennedy Blvd. #260 Tampa, FL 33609
Advanced Certification Continuity of Care	A-CCC	Multidisciplinary discharge planning, case management	National Board for Continuity of Care Certification	National Board for Continuity of Care Certification 1350 Broadway Suit 1705 New York, NY 10018 212-356-0691
Certified Case Manager Certification	CCM	Multidisciplinary case management	Commission for Case Manager	Commission for Case Manager Certification 1835 Rohlwing Rd. Suite D Rolling Meadows, IL 60008 847-818-0292
Certified Disability Management Specialist	CDMS	Disability management, insurance-based rehabilitation, vocational counseling	Certified Disability Management Specialist Commission	Certified Disability Management Specialist Commission 1835 Rohlwing Rd. Suite E Rolling Meadows, IL 60008 847-394-2106
Case Management Administration Certified	CMAC	Case management administration	Center for Case Management	Professional Testing Corporation 1211 Avenue of the Americas New York, NY 10056 212-852-0400

Continued

TABLE 27-1
Common Case Management Certifications—cont'd

Certification	Acronym	Specialization	Sponsoring Organization	Contact Information
Care Manager Certified	CMC	Gerontology, counseling, social work, mental health	National Academy of Certified Care Managers	National Academy of Certified Care Managers 3389 Sheridan St. Suite 170 Hollywood, FL 33021 847-394-2106
Certified Managed Care Nurse	CMCN	Nursing in managed care	American Board of Managed Care Nursing	American Board of Managed Care Nursing 4435 Waterfront Dr. Suite 101 Glen Allen, VA 23060 804-747-9698
Certified Occupational Health Nurse—Case Manager	COHN-CM	Occupational health nursing case management	American Board for Occupational Health Nurses	American Board for Occupational Health Nurses 201 E. Ogden Ave. Suite 114 Hinsdale, IL 60521 630-789-5799
Certified Professional in Healthcare Quality	CPHQ	Quality management, utilization management, risk management	Healthcare Quality Certification Board of the National Association for Healthcare Quality	Healthcare Quality Certification Board National Association for Healthcare Quality P.O. Box 1880 San Gabriel, CA 91778 800-346-4722
Certified Professional Utilization Review	CPUR	Utilization management, case management	InterQual	McKesson HBOC, Inc. 293 Boston Post Rd. West Suite 180 Marlborough, MA 01752 508-651-2600

Certified Rehabilitation Registered Nurse, Certified Rehabilitation Nurse—Advanced	CRRN, CRRN-A	Rehabilitation nursing	Rehabilitation Nursing Certification Board 4700 W Lake Ave. Glenview, IL 60025 800-229-7530
Certified Nursing Case Manager	RN, Cm	Nurse case management	American Nurses Credentialing Center 600 Maryland Ave. SW Suite 100 West Washington, DC 20024 800-284-2378
Certified Rehabilitation Counselor	CRC	Rehabilitation counseling, case management	Commission on Rehabilitation Counselor Certification 1835 Rohlwing Rd. Suite E Rolling Meadows, IL 60008 847-394-2104
Professional, Academy for Healthcare Management; Fellow, Academy for Healthcare Management	PAHM, FAHM	Managed care	Academy for Healthcare Management 2300 Windy Ridge Parkway Suite 600 Atlanta, GA 30339 800-667-3133

person has a certain certification, then one knows what their basic experience and skills are. Since case managers are not regulated in any state, except for some case managers in worker's compensation, certification is an excellent method of validating education and experience.

HARMONIZATION OF CERTIFICATION REQUIREMENTS AND TYPES OF CASE MANAGEMENT SERVICES

The certification required should match the type of case management services being provided. If the case manager is performing generalist tasks, one of the general case management certifications, such as that of certified case manager offered by the Commission for Case Manager Certification may be appropriate. If the person is performing disability case management, certified disability management specialist may be the appropriate certification. There are several clinical certifications that may not be unique to case managers but would be an appropriate certification for a case manager functioning in a specialty case management or disease management program. For example, if the case manager is a registered nurse working in rehabilitation, it may be appropriate for the case manager to be certified in rehabilitation nursing (certified rehabilitation registered nurse); if the case manger is working in a diabetic disease management program, certification as a diabetic educator may be appropriate. Depending on the type of case management being performed, both generalist case management certification and specialty certification may be required.

INDIVIDUALS AND ENTITIES THAT SHOULD BE CREDENTIALED

Who should be credentialed? There are several groups of individuals who should be credentialed. The process is similar for all. All case managers should be not only

certified by their recognized professional association (e.g., CMSA, ANA) but also credentialed by their employing organization or the group that has contracted with them to perform case management. All providers, whether they are within a contracted provider network or are used by a case manager on an individual basis, should also be credentialed. An employing organization has the responsibility to verify that case managers have the required credentials and to document such verification. The source document for credentialing employees is the job description. The job description should list the credentials necessary for that particular position. Copies of licenses and certifications, and an application attesting to employment and education are included as part of the credentialing process. If the case manager is contracted for case management services to a health plan or organization, the requirements that would be spelled out in a job description should be spelled out in the contract or letter of agreement, which serves the same purpose as a job description. The contracting organization would want verification of possession of the required credentials.

Contracted provider networks are credentialed just as are employees of an organization. In most health plans or organized delivery systems, a separate department handles credentialing, and the case management department is notified of those credentialed within the network and the specific credentials that a provider holds. The contract between the provider and the health plan or organized delivery system delineates the qualifications that the provider must meet.

Many times, case managers use a provider outside the network or a very specific type of provider for certain services. Providers of hard-to-find services or those with unique specialties may not be in the normal contracted network, or the case manager may be working outside the normal geographical area. These providers must be credentialed as well. The case manager would set educational, experience, and certification requirements for this provider. If the provider is an organized delivery system, the provider must be licensed to provide such services in the state in which it is operating. For example, if a case manager were contracting with a home health care company, he or she would want to confirm that the company was licensed in that state. An application or some documentation that the provider meets the requirements would have to be obtained. A note documenting that the credentials have been verified should be placed in the case management file.

The credentialing process must be documented. Once the standards are determined, whether for a case manager, a contracted network provider, or a single provider for a unique situation, a file should be created that contains the application and copies of licenses and certifications to demonstrate that possession of the required credentials has been verified. Documentation is an important step in the credentialing process. It is through this documentation process that one confirms that the provider holds the credentials the provider claims to possess.

FREQUENCY OF CREDENTIALING

Credentialing is an ongoing process and should occur at regular intervals. The interval should be set forth in the organization's credentialing standards. The interval is typically annually or every 2 years. If during that time it is felt that the credentials of the provider have changed, the case manager should inquire and reverify the credentials.

Continuing education can be an important component of credentialing, especially in case management. Case managers are expected to have current knowledge of diseases and treatments. With the advances in medical science, continuing

education is really necessary for all health care providers, depending how long ago their basic education was completed. There are various ways to measure continuing education. The job description or contract may specify that a certain number of hours of continuing education must completed in a certain period of time, and it may designate the subject(s) of the continuing education. A record of participation in workshops, attendance at educational conferences, and completion of self-study programs provides some indication of the amount of continuing education obtained. The Internet also has become a major source for continuing education as well as a source of reference material for the health professional.

■ SUMMARY

Credentialing is a necessary and important step in the process of providing health care services. Whether it be credentialing of a case manager, a provider within a network, or a single provider for a unique situation, credentialing is necessary to help ensure quality. The responsible organization must set standards through a job description or contract that spells out what credentials an individual must hold to perform the expected services. Effective credentialing reduces risk and liability.

Chapter Exercises

1. Indicate why credentialing is important and what benefits it offers to individuals and to the organizations they serve.
2. Identify one key document that is basic in indicating what credentials are required for a given job.
3. Name some of the types of credentials many of your colleagues have and conduct a survey to learn on what and how they were tested and what is necessary for recredentialing.

Suggested Websites and Resources

www.urac.org/—American Accreditation Health Care Commission/URAC

www.aaahc.org/—Accreditation Association for Ambulatory Health Care (AAAHC)

www.carf.org/—Commission for Accreditation of Rehabilitation Facilities (CARF)

www.carf.org/CARF/AdultDayServ.htm—CARF website for accreditation of adult day care services

www.nursingworld.org/mods/mod6/ceac4.htm—Community Health Accreditation Program (CHAP), a subsidiary of the National League of Nursing (NLN), which accredits home care and community health care organizations

www.cfcm.com/resources/certification.asp—Center for Case Management

www.cdms.org/—Certification of Disability Management Specialists

www.crccertification.com/—Commission on Rehabilitation Counselor Certification

www.lcpconsultants.com/certs4.html#clcp—Life Care Planning Certification

www.legalnurse.com/—Legal Nursing Certification

www.interqual.com/article.cfm?area=educat&areaID=7&articleID=109—McKesson Health Solutions website for InterQual and Certification Utilization Review Professional (CPUR)

www.cphq.org—Healthcare Quality Certification Board

REFERENCE

1. Case Management Society of America: Case management definition/philosophy, Little Rock, Ark, The Society, available on-line at www.cmsa.org/pdf/DefofCM.pdf.

CHAPTER

28

Audits

Patricia Sweetland Roberts, RN, MS

OBJECTIVES

- To identify the primary rule for a successful audit
- To define the difference between mandatory audits and voluntary audits
- To identify the importance of interdepartmental communication
- To define corrective actions and the importance they have on health care organizations
- To identify the role policies and procedures have on the audit process

The thought of going through an audit may alarm a novice case manager. However, a case manager who understands audits and appreciates its role in the licensing, contracting, funding, accrediting, and marketing of an organization realizes there is no need for intimidation. Audits are reviews conducted by governmental agencies and accrediting organizations to determine a health care organization's compliance with statutory and regulatory mandates or standards developed by the respective accrediting organization. An experienced case manager knows that preparing for an audit is not an event; it is an unending process that requires diligent attention to detail and careful documentation according to established protocols.

In general, audits are either *mandatory reviews* required by law, or *voluntary reviews* requested by an organization for purposes of receiving a "stamp of approval" that may be utilized to demonstrate its level of compliance with accrediting standards. All health care organizations must meet statutory and regulatory requirements. Large employers, state and municipal governments, and other entities that administer benefits for large numbers of employees frequently require organizations to be accredited in order to fulfill their contractual obligations. Therefore, most health care organizations are involved in both regulatory and accrediting audits.

The distinction is clouded between governmental mandates and private accreditation when state laws or regulations require or permit accreditation by an outside organization. In such cases, requirements generally fit in one of three categories:

1. **Mandated**—Accreditation is required in order to become licensed, or continue to be licensed by the state.
2. **Deemed**—Accreditation is optional but exempts the organization from certain licensing requirements.

3. **Required standards**—Accreditation is optional but activities must be conducted in accordance with nationally recognized accrediting organization standards[1]

AUDITING ENTITIES

Who conducts audits? There are a number of agencies and organizations that conduct audits. It is up to the health care organization that will be audited to identify who will be conducting an audit and prepare accordingly for their particular areas of interest. Different auditing entities focus on different aspects of the health care organization's business. These entities are often referred to by acronyms. Their names or acronyms may be included in the written documentation of other governmental or accrediting organizations. Without knowing the names of the organizations or their commonly used acronyms, it may be difficult to understand audit-related materials. Below is a brief description of some major auditing entities.

- **U.S. Department of Health and Human Services (HHS)**—HHS is the principle agency of the federal government responsible for protecting the health of Americans and providing related services. The Department administers a multitude of programs. Among these are two that are significant to the discussion of this chapter on audits.
- **Centers for Medicare & Medicaid Services (CMS)**—CMS, formerly Health Care Financing Administration (HCFA), is the division of HHS that administers the Medicare and Medicaid programs.[2] This is also the division that is responsible for auditing or overseeing auditing functions for Medicare and Medicaid providers and suppliers. Providers, as defined by Medicare, include hospitals, hospices, nursing homes, and home health agencies. Suppliers are entities such as laboratories, clinics, and physical therapy offices that are typically associated with diagnosis and therapy rather than sustained patient care.[3] Medicare + Choice Organizations are also audited by CMS biennially, according to federal requirements.

- **Office of Inspector General (OIG)** —OIG helps "ensure cost-effective health care, improve quality of care, address access to care issues, and reduce the potential for fraud, waste, and abuse. Through audits, evaluations, and inspections, OIG recommends changes in legislation, regulations, and systems to improve health care delivery systems and reduce unnecessary expenses."[4]
- **State Survey Agencies (SAs)**— Survey agencies, such as a State Department of Health or similar department, contract with the CMS to assess compliance with the requirements that providers and suppliers must meet, by federal law, to participate in Medicare and Medicaid programs.[5] The functions that the state agencies perform under contract with CMS are referred to as the certification process.[6]
- **Departments of Insurance (DOI)**— State Departments of Insurance are responsible for protecting the "interests of insurance consumers," according to the National Association of Insurance Commissioners. NAIC is an organization that includes regulators from every state as well as the District of Columbia and four territories of the United States.[7] State Insurance Commissioners issue Certificates of Authority to entities that wish to enter the insurance market in a given state. This necessitates an

extensive application and on-site review process. Possession of such a certificate is also required for any managed care organization that intends to submit a Medicare + Choice application to the CMS.

- **Joint Commission on Accreditation of Healthcare Organizations (JCAHO)**—JCAHO is an independent, not-for-profit organization that has developed standards and has audited health care organizations for compliance with those standards for the past fifty years. JCAHO provides evaluation and accreditation services for hospitals, health care networks, home care organizations, nursing homes, long-term care facilities, assisted-living facilities, behavioral health care facilities, ambulatory care facilities, and clinical laboratories. Hospitals accredited by JCAHO are deemed to meet the requirements of the federal Conditions of Participation regulations based on their JCAHO accreditation.[8] "The mission of the Joint Commission on Accreditation of Healthcare Organizations is to continuously improve the safety and quality of care provided to the public through the provision of health care accreditation and related services that support performance improvement in health care organizations."[9]

- **National Committee for Quality Assurance (NCQA)**—NCQA is an independent accrediting organization established in 1990. It accredits managed care organizations including HMOs, PPOs, and Managed Behavioral Health Care Organizations through on-site review of the care and services delivered by applicant organizations. Both clinical and administrative processes are evaluated during audits conducted by a team that comprises physicians and others with managed care expertise. HEDIS (Health Plan Employer Data and Information Set) standards have also been introduced into the NCQA accreditation process recently.[10]

- **American Accreditation Health-Care Commission (URAC)**—URAC is a nonprofit organization that developed standards for the managed care industry and offers the following 10 accreditation programs:

  1. Case Management Organization
  2. Credential Verification Organization
  3. Health Call Center
  4. Health Network
  5. Health Plan
  6. Health Utilization Management
  7. Health Provider Credentialing
  8. Workers' Compensation Network
  9. Workers' Compensation Utilization Management
  10. External Review

URAC Case Management Standards are designed for organizations that provide case management services either by phone or on-site with public or privately funded benefit programs. The standards cover several categories including: staff structure and organization; staff management and development; information management; quality improvement; oversight of delegated functions; and organizational ethics and complaints.[11]

BASICS OF AN AUDIT

Significant similarities exist in the way auditing entities conduct audits, even though the auditing tool and team composition is unique. Each of these entities is dedicated to determining the organization's compliance with established criteria stated in regulations, standards, or conditions. Understanding the basic steps of an audit makes it easier for a case manager to adjust to the unique auditing methods of various auditing entities (Box 28-1).

Written Notice of Audit

This is actually a misnomer under certain circumstances because health care organizations may voluntarily request application materials to initiate an accrediting process rather than receiving a "written notice." However, audits conducted by governmental agencies are announced through written notices. These notices, which are standard format letters, typically provide specific information regarding the purpose and scope of the audit, dates on which the audit will take place, and the composition and credentials of the audit team. Attachments to the letters indicate what materials and/or data must be submitted prior to a site visit. Finally, the letters provide information regarding the type of documents that will be reviewed on-site and which personnel will be interviewed while the auditors are on-site.

Organizations seeking accreditation must follow application instructions for the respective accrediting body to receive written materials and initiate the audit process. The specific process varies slightly with each organization. Information regarding audits by the accrediting organi-

zations may be accessed via the websites listed at the end of the chapter.

It should be noted that there is an important exception to receiving written notification regarding an audit. Both regulatory agencies and accrediting organizations may make unannounced visits. Such an audit may be precipitated by review of data that indicates a change in the level of compliance with regulations or standards, complaints from the public, failure to produce required reports, fraud, marketing irregularities, financial issues, or other concerns. This underscores the significance of developing, maintaining, and adhering to policies and procedures that support compliance with regulatory mandates and accrediting standards as an ongoing process.

Submission of Required Materials and Data

Submission of materials and data provides the first opportunity during an audit for a health care organization to demonstrate compliance (or ongoing compliance) with regulatory mandates or accrediting standards. This portion of the audit is labor-intensive, detail-oriented, and demanding of interdepartmental cooperation. Preparation of materials may take a few weeks or longer depending on the maturity of the organization and the nature of the audit.

BOX 28-1
Basic Steps of an Audit

1. Written notice of audit
2. Submission of required materials and data
3. Communication between organization and auditors: submission of additional materials
4. On-site review
   - Entrance interview
   - Interviews with employees, patients/members, physicians, and board members
   - Review of documents and data
   - Exit interview
5. Written findings
6. Corrective action plan

In most cases, Information Technology plays a key role in data gathering and report production.

Fulfillment of the requirements for "desk-review materials" is dependent on accurate documentation and appropriate gathering and reporting of data, as mandated by regulation or standard. Written notices and accrediting applications contain specific instructions that must be followed exactly in order to meet requirements. Documentation by case managers has been discussed earlier in the book. The importance of documentation, not just for one case or by one case manager, but for the whole department during the entire period being audited takes on significance as the organization prepares materials for submission to the auditing entity. Therefore, it is important to underscore the statement at the beginning of this chapter that "... preparing for an audit is not an event; it is an unending process that requires diligent attention to detail and careful documentation according to established protocols."

Certain "look-back" periods apply to most audits. For example, during a CMS Medicare + Choice Organization audit (site visit), the M+CO must provide information regarding appeals, claims, membership records, and other information during the six-month period prior to the audit. Therefore, all documentation that has taken place during that period is open to audit. It is customary for auditors to request samples for review, but they may audit any records, according to regulatory and contractual guidelines. The emphasis on timely, accurate, well-organized documentation becomes even more critical when one recognizes that records covering several years must be made available for review by auditors per statutory or regulatory mandates.

The health care organization is best served by responding to written questions, displaying data, presenting information, and collating binders exactly in response to the directions provided in the written notice of audit or application packet. If a case manager is asked to provide information, it should be prepared in the specific format requested and submitted in a timely manner so that the interdepartmental effort will be successful. In other words, "read the directions." It sounds simple, but organizations that overlook this regret it when they are required to repeat their efforts or suffer graver consequences.

Communication Between Organization and Auditors: Submission of Additional Materials

Although the process varies by entity, the primary objective during the "desk review phase" is to determine initial compliance. Upon receipt of written materials and data from the health care organization, a completeness review takes place by the regulatory agency or accrediting organization. In some cases, there is need for communication to clarify contents, request additional information, or select a sample from a "universe" that was submitted as part of the filing. The auditing entity communicates with the organization electronically, by phone, or by mail until any issues regarding the submission have been resolved.

In unusual circumstances, the auditing agency or accrediting organization may inform the health care organization that the materials submitted do not support moving ahead in the typical process. This may be due to lack of administrative and management capacity, failure to meet financial requirements, miscarriage of regulatory or contractual obligations, or other reasons stated by the auditing entity. Such action rarely comes as a surprise to the affected health care organization because the auditing entity will typically have worked with the organization to resolve these issues for quite some time.

On-Site Review

- Entrance interview
- Interviews with employees, patients/members, physicians, and board members
- Review of documents and data
- Exit interview

The on-site portion of the audit allows auditors to confirm findings from review of written materials and to interview employees, patients (members), physicians, board members, and others. It is the auditors' opportunity to see how the organization is actually providing care and services and to determine through personal observation if the clinical and administrative practices comply with stated criteria and are in concert with submitted materials.

Auditors use specific tools to guide their on-site reviews. For example, the National Committee for Quality Assurance (NCQA) uses *Surveyor Guidelines for the Accreditation of MCOs* during visits to accredit managed care organizations, while the CMS uses the *Medicare + Choice Contractor Performance Monitoring System Guide* during monitoring visits to assess compliance with regulatory mandates. Unfortunately, there is no standard measurement for compliance among the various federal and state laws and accrediting standards. Therefore, the case manager must be aware of the criteria for each of the agencies or organizations that audit his or her health care organization.

Significantly, there are many similarities between categories of review for the various auditing entities even though the tools vary. Quality of care, patient rights and responsibilities, financial integrity, documentation and record keeping, utilization management, and appeals and grievances are among the typical sections in a review tool. If not labeled exactly as such, they may be imbedded in another section and included in the audit process.

Audit tools are available to health care organizations prior to audits. Government forms are generally accessible on the Internet at no charge. Accrediting organization tools must be ordered from the respective organization, as indicated in Box 28-2.

Entrance Interview

An introductory meeting, sometimes called an entrance interview, initiates most audits. The sessions include members of the survey team and administrative and management personnel from the health care organization. Auditors introduce themselves and describe the purpose and scope of the audit as well as the agenda. In most cases, the Chief Executive Officer or another senior representative presents an overview of the health care organization and discusses significant changes since the

---

BOX 28-2

Information for Ordering and Accessing Audit Tools

1. Centers for Medicare & Medicaid Services (CMS)
   - Medicare + Choice Contractor Performance Monitoring System Guide: www.cms.hhs.gov. healthplans/monitoring/2001guide.asp.
   - HCFA Program Manuals—State Operations—HCFA Publication 7 (State Survey Agencies)
2. National Committee for Quality Assurance (NCQA): www.ncqa.org
3. Joint Commission on the Accreditation of Healthcare Organizations (JCAHO): www.jcaho.org
4. American Accreditation HealthCare Commission (URAC): www.urac.org

last audit if it is a monitoring (reaccreditation, resurvey) visit. He or she also addresses the strengths of the organization and strategic plans. If it is a new organization, the presentation usually addresses the capacity of the organization including administrative and financial ability to meet all required criteria.

The case manager is commonly an entrance interview participant and must be keenly aware of the information exchanged during the session since the meeting lays the foundation for the entire visit. Each department will have shared responsibility for bringing critical information regarding departmental operations, compliance, strengths, and weaknesses to the CEO's attention as his or her presentation has taken shape in weeks before the visit. Following the CEO's presentation, auditors may pose questions or add critical information to the introductory meeting discussions. Their input affects the manner in which individual interviews are handled later in the visit. In some cases, more depth will be required in responding to certain questions, documentation that was not initially anticipated will be required, or additional persons may be interviewed. An attentive ear during the entrance interview will help the case manager feel more prepared for the individual interview if he or she thinks about what exactly is being said, what the auditors' "hot points" are, and precisely what is being asked of the organization.

The goal is to create and provide a flow of written and verbal information for the auditors from the time they arrive until they leave that substantiates compliance with regulatory mandates or accrediting standards. Each department will have identified critical issues and made them known to the CEO well in advance of the site visit. Responses during individual interviews tie to those critical issues, the exchange of information during the entrance interview, and to specific items in the audit tool. The flow of information must continue from one department to another where operational linkages exist.

By assigning responsibility for each section of the audit tool to specific persons in various departments well in advance of the site visit, strengths and vulnerabilities regarding compliance with regulatory mandates or accrediting standards can be identified. Not only is that information communicated to the CEO for potential inclusion in his or her entrance interview remarks; it is also used to build upon strengths and minimize vulnerabilities in preparing for the site visit. If administration and department managers communicate on a regular basis and appraise each other of critical compliance issues, this effort is less ominous and the opportunity for a successful audit outcome is much greater.

Interviews with Employees, Patients/Members, Physicians, and Board Members

The determination regarding who will be interviewed depends on the type of organization being audited and the scope and nature of the audit. Some audits are narrowly focused, while others are broad. For example, an audit for accreditation of a Case Management Organization would obviously involve interviews with fewer professional disciplines than a JCAHO accreditation survey at a hospital. Based on the scope and nature of the audit, auditors advise the organization about who must be interviewed. Interview times and assignments are known in advance of the site visit so interviewees can be well-prepared.

It must be understood that auditors may interview anyone, within their regulatory and contractual scope, while they are on-site. The organization has only one opportunity to make a first impression with the auditor team. Therefore, in this day of "business casual" dress, a determination must be made regarding what the dress will be while auditors are on-site. The author recommends business attire for *all* employees, whether they anticipate being interviewed or not. This sets the tone for the audit. Business suits, sport coats, dress shirts, and ties are appropriate for men; dresses, skirts, blouses, and jackets are appropriate for women. This excludes clinical settings, of course, in which certain personnel wear uniforms and would continue to do so during an audit.

The physical environment during interviews also contributes to the overall impression of auditors. In addition to mandated requirements for health and safety standards (kitchen cleanliness, patient equipment, fire extinguishers, fire doors, etc.), the individual work environment makes a statement regarding how a health care organization conducts business. Are files in order? What is the condition of offices? Are in-baskets piled with papers? Are confidential materials displayed on bulletin boards? Is the office floor stacked with files? Are computer screens timed-out and secured? With pressures of decreased resources and increased caseloads, it may be difficult to maintain the picture-perfect office, but case management departments need policies and procedures that address confidentiality, documentation, record maintenance and security, electronic transfer of member/patient information, etc. They must strive for compliance on a regular basis and audit their efforts internally. In anticipation of the site visit, an all-out effort to assure compliance with those policies and procedures must take place so that work areas are neat, reflect a professional appearance, and enable the person being interviewed to retrieve information readily. The same level of tidiness and cleanliness is required in public locations of the building.

Preparation for actual interviews, as for the entire audit, is an interdepartmental exercise. Effective, high-quality health care is not delivered by departments that operate in an isolated environment. Communication between utilization management and case management, admissions and clinical units, and marketing and enrollment contributes to excellence in clinical and administrative services. In much the same way, communication between all departments facilitates preparation for successful interviews during the on-site portion of an audit.

Recall again the statement at the beginning of the chapter, "...preparing for an audit is not an event; it is an unending process that requires diligent attention to detail and careful documentation according to established protocols." Preparation for interviews begins long before an audit. It begins with an understanding of the regulatory mandates and accrediting standards and their incorporation in protocols, policies, and procedures. Those policies and procedures must support the regulatory and accrediting requirements for each department *and* demonstrate coordination of processes across department lines. Case managers and their colleagues who are interviewed must be aware of the regulations and standards, describe the policies and procedures that support those mandates, defend case management records according to the policies and procedures, and present data in support of compliance. This means that each representative who will be interviewed must be intimately familiar with factual information regarding regulations, guidelines, policies and procedures, data, and other materials for his or her department and linkages to other departments. This may require months or years of preparation depending on the nature of the audit.

Preparation also includes responding to specific questions in the review tool and providing clear documentation as required by the regulatory or accrediting organization. Fortunately, this process is usually an "open-book test." The auditing entities provide copies of the audit tools they use so the health care organization may prepare for the on-site visit by assigning specific sections of the tool to appropriate departments and personnel within the departments. Coordination of preparation for interviews across department lines is important so that interdepartmental relationships may be described accurately by everyone involved. For example, if utilization management responds to a question regarding how they refer patients to case management, it holds to reason that the case manager would describe the process in the same manner during his or her interview. Policies and procedures for both departments should also support responses from each interview. Further, the policies and procedures must "bridge" from one department to another so that the processes described in the interviews are supported by seamless documents.

Mock interviews conducted by colleagues or an outside consultant are helpful to organizations preparing for on-site reviews. In addition to having knowledge of regulatory mandates, accrediting standards, policies and procedures, and familiarity with important data, it is important to feel comfortable with the interview *process*. Some employees are comfortable in the audit environment, while others are quite intimidated. Practicing with peers helps unravel nerves and make all interviewees come together as a team. Dress rehearsals using the actual audit tool, followed by post-performance critiques, are desirable to make the exercise most realistic. Individual coaching may be offered to those needing extra attention.

Review of Documents and Data

While on-site, auditors review documents and data requested prior to their arrival. Those materials must be organized and collated by the health care organization according to auditing entity directions. In the absence of specific directions, the documents should be labeled similar to the

audit tool for ease of information retrieval. Review of the materials takes place by auditors in a secure, private room reserved for their use with ample space for laptop computers and telephones.

In addition to the materials requested prior to the visit, auditors routinely review an extensive number of additional documents to ensure a thorough assessment of compliance. The exact nature and number of documents is dependent on the type of audit. Box 28-3 includes typical documents that may be under scrutiny. Audit tools provide clear direction regarding which documents should be available for review for each auditing entity.

Individual department representatives and Information Technology staff should remain available to supplement materials at the request of the survey team. In some cases, this may require forwarding information after the on-site review if it is not accessible while the auditors are visiting the organization. However, every attempt should be made to fulfill requests while auditors are on-site.

Auditors utilize different audit tools, as discussed earlier. However, it is typical for all survey teams to make use of some type of survey grid that identifies regulations, standards, or conditions. The grid also includes a column for "Met" or "Not Met" or a numerical value to indicate whether the health care organization has complied with the specific item or element on the grid. This grid is used to assess the level of compliance documented through the review as well as during interviews. Each element receives a rating or score.

Exit Interview

Auditing entities conduct a meeting at the conclusion of the on-site visit to communicate with representatives of the health care organization in a group setting. The amount of information shared at the meeting (summation or exit conference) varies. According to the CMS State Operations

tors, their organizations, or external reviewers before a final decision is made regarding licensing, contracting, or accrediting status. Participants should not expect final decisions to be announced at the exit interview and should not be disappointed or dismayed by lack of information.

Administrators and managers who have participated in interviews and those who are accountable for follow-up actions should participate in the exit conference. It is a mistake to take the communication lightly even if detailed information is not shared. If the auditors request additional documentation during the exit interview, it should be prepared and forwarded to them posthaste so that it contributes favorably to the audit outcome. Further, those who are accountable for action should review all recommendations made during the entire audit and assure that the recommendations are appropriately considered for inclusion in policies and procedures, forms, letters, other documents, and training. A postexit conference during which managers and administrative staff debrief and discuss follow-up processes and responsibilities serves this purpose well.

Written Findings

Licensing determinations, levels of accreditation (or the decision to deny accreditation altogether), the ability to gain contracts with the government, or recommendations to certify an organization as meeting Conditions of Participation are among the most critical types of written findings. Millions of dollars and the ability of an organization to develop, continue, or expand a line of business or product are frequently at stake. Therefore, all of the effort that goes into the "...unending process that requires diligent attention to detail and careful documentation according to established protocols" is well worth it.

Auditing entities follow different processes after an on-site visit before issuing final written findings. Some issue

Manual, the purpose of an exit conference is to "informally communicate preliminary survey team findings and provide an opportunity for the interchange of information, especially if there are differences of opinion."[12] Final findings are not typically shared with the organization during the meeting. NCQA conducts a "summation conference" at the conclusion of an accrediting visit. During that conference, preliminary findings are summarized but a determination regarding compliance with NCQA standards is not made, nor are conclusions drawn regarding accreditation status.[13] These are typical of meetings held at the conclusion of on-site visits for most audits.

At the conclusion of the on-site visit, work remains to be completed by the audi-

interim or preliminary findings and allow the health care organization to comment on factual errors, while others request additional information prior to completing the final report. Certain accrediting organizations use experts to conduct an external review to assure nonpartial judgment regarding compliance with standards before issuing the written report. Review of findings by persons other than those who conducted the on-site review provides some measure of objectivity and consistency across the region, state, or country.

Written findings generally summarize the purpose of the on-site audit and the basis on which the review was conducted. For example, a letter from CMS indicates, "[Name of organization] meets eligibility requirements for a Medicare + Choice (M+C) coordinated care plan contract under Sections 1851–1859 of the Social Security Act (SSA) and the federal regulations at 42 CFR 422.501. CMS has based this finding on a review of your application...and the on-site review."[14] Such a letter is sent to an organization that has sought a contract with CMS to offer an M+C product and has achieved that goal. A state department assessing compliance of a managed care organization with state regulations likewise identifies the dates of an audit, the name of the act (law), and the section(s) in accordance with which an audit was conducted. Accrediting organizations reference specific standards or conditions.

A governmental final report may be issued pending acceptance of a corrective action plan (CAP) or upon agreement that certain corrective actions will be completed after the written findings have been issued. If standards were identified by an accrediting organization as insufficient or unsatisfactory, the report may stipulate specific timeframes for their correction or the findings may affect future decisions. Whatever the exact process for notification and content, written findings are exceed-

ingly important to initial or continuing operations of the health care organization and must be taken seriously.

Corrective Action Plan

A corrective action plan is a mandated written response to deficiencies identified by auditors. The plan addresses specific findings and details the manner in which they will be corrected. Requirements for corrective action plans vary by auditing entity and the type of organization audited. The term *corrective action* is used in this chapter in a generic manner because accrediting organizations generally refer to corrective actions by other terms. However, all auditing entities routinely require health care organizations to respond to deficiencies in a prescribed manner and within a specific timeframe. Written findings also routinely require precise descriptions of the actions that will be taken to assure full compliance with regulations or standards. Auditors have the authority to accept or deny an action plan.

Examples of Findings Requiring Corrective Action Plans

Examples of findings requiring corrective action plans include, but are not limited to, the need for improvements in the following areas:

- Interdepartmental communication
- Professional training
- Documentation
- Procedures regarding advance directives
- Adherence to patient rights and responsibilities
- Adherence to patient restraint regulations
- Data gathering, reporting, and analysis
- Credentialing processes
- Documentation
- Adherence to marketing guidelines

The manner in which the organization responds in the corrective action depends on the nature of the finding. An organization may be required to develop a plan regarding how it will correct specific operational issues. That may necessitate writing or rewriting policies and procedures or the assurance that a department or multiple departments will abide by new or existing practices. Obviously, the policies and procedures must comply with regulations and standards. This requires vigilance regarding changes in regulations and standards. In some cases, additional oversight and internal program auditing may be required. At other times, the corrective action may be related to the maintenance of the physical plant, employee and public safety issues, human resource concerns, or a multitude of other issues pertaining to clinical and administrative management of the health care organization. This explains why preparation and follow-up to an audit must be an interdepartmental effort and be supported by senior management to ensure coordination and follow-up.

Corrective actions are highly significant to the organization's relationship with the regulatory agency or accrediting organization and to its continued business success. Failure to take completion of corrective actions seriously and to follow through on the execution of plans may result in punitive damages including fines, or failure to obtain or maintain a license, contract, or accreditation. The ability to market or enroll members in managed care plans may also be suspended, thereby causing significant financial hardship for the affected organization.

Ramifications of failed corrective action plans are stated in regulations and written documents from auditing organizations. Individuals within the health care organization must be assigned responsibility to develop and coordinate plans and communicate effectively with the auditing entity until the deficiencies are fully satisfied. This important activity must receive attention from senior management to be successful.

It must be remembered, once again, that "preparing for an audit is not an event; it is an unending process that requires diligent attention to detail and careful documentation according to established protocols." Corrective action plans prepared for one audit need to be considered in anticipation of consecutive audits *and during interim periods.* Auditors determine compliance with corrective action plans during subsequent audits. Therefore, improvements made by organizations as a result of a corrective action plan should be fully incorporated in organizational operations and routinely audited for compliance. Case managers are critical to this effort. They must abide by regulatory mandates and accrediting standards that have been institutionalized through policies and procedures. Those documents must incorporate changes necessitated by CAPs.

AUDIT FOCUS

Due to lack of standardization between federal, state, and accrediting entities that conduct audits, there is no single source that defines what is required during an audit. However, a case manager may become familiar with the mandates of auditing entities that pertain to his or her organization. Key information about their audit processes is also available with a small amount of research. Such research will allow the case manager to focus only on audits particular to his or her organization rather than being overwhelmed by trying to retain information about all auditing entities for all lines of business and all products.

First, it is necessary to know what line(s) of business and what product(s) are audited, or will be audited for his or her organization. If Medicaid is the only line of business being audited, for example, that will limit the number and types of auditing entities involved. The same is true, of course, for Medicare or commercial. If the health care organization is "straight-Medicare," that is, only involved in providing Medicare services, it stands to reason that it will be audited only for the Medicare line of business.

In established health care facilities and organizations with multiple lines of business, the compliance officer, quality improvement department, regulatory affairs department, governmental affairs department, or business development department are typical sources of information regarding what entities conduct audits. It is not unusual for liaison with auditing entities to be handled by different departments such as quality improvement handling NCQA relationships and governmental affairs handling CMS communication. Therefore, it may take communication with more than one department to gather information regarding auditing relationships. In smaller or newly formed organizations, the search obviously involves fewer people but may require more effort on the part of the case manager. The end result will be identification of the entity responsible for conducting the audit(s).

After identifying the line of business, product, and agency or organization responsible for conducting the audit(s), the case manager must determine which programs or modules have been or will be accredited. These terms apply to accrediting agencies. For example, URAC (American Accreditation HealthCare Commission) has separate accreditation programs, as described earlier in this chapter, including case management organization standards, health utilization management standards, health plan standards, and others.[11] Identification of such modules may further narrow the focus of information that the case manager must understand.

After narrowing the focus, the case manager is able to avail himself or herself of regulatory mandates, accreditation standards, and audit tools that apply specifi-

cally to the audit(s) that will be conducted in his or her organization. Such materials may be available in-house, via the Internet, or through the auditing entity. The information is invaluable to the case manager and his or her understanding of what is expected by the auditing entity. By studying the materials and communicating with representatives at the agencies or organizations, the case manager will be able to focus clearly on the audits specific to his or her organization and contribute to successful audit outcomes.

POLICIES AND PROCEDURES AS A FOUNDATION

As an organization prepares for an audit, the ongoing development, implementation, review, and revision of policies and procedures is critical. Demonstration of adherence to the policies and procedures is also imperative. All auditing entities require the existence of sound policies and procedures that support compliance with respective regulations or standards.

Written policies and procedures must be developed based on federal laws and regulations, state laws and regulations, accrediting conditions and standards, and the organization mission statement. The foundation for policies and procedures should follow the order diagrammed below with federal laws and regulations forming the base. The reason for this is that all organizations that receive Medicare, Medicaid, and other federal funding must abide by federal laws and regulations. Generally, if state law is stricter, that law applies. However, federal law may preempt state laws in some important areas that apply to policies and procedures. Therefore, look to the federal law and regulations first in building policies and procedures and continue through the levels of authority. The final, and very important step, rests with the organization's mission statement. Consideration for the core values, behavior patterns, and organizational vision will contribute to effective policies and procedures within a department and across departmental lines.

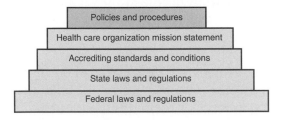

There are three major considerations regarding policies and procedures that are significant to audits:

1. If the case management department fails to take regulatory and accrediting mandates into consideration when developing policies and procedures, compliance with the mandates will very likely fall short during audits.

2. If the department fails to take its relationship with other departments into consideration when developing policies and procedures, the auditors will readily identify a "silo mentality" during an audit. The "silo mentality" is one in which departments operate independently, lack effective interdepartmental communication, and do not coordinate operations effectively. It is also an environment in which full compliance is rarely achieved.

3. If the department fails to apply the *most restrictive* regulation or standard, it leaves itself vulnerable to less than favorable findings. For example, if a care plan must be established within fewer hours to meet an accrediting standard than a regulatory mandate, apply the accrediting standard in the department policies and procedures. That way, the department is assured of meeting or exceeding both the regu-

latory and accrediting requirements in the policy and procedure.

In order to avoid pitfalls, a prescribed policy and procedure process must take place initially and at least annually. The process provides for review of regulatory requirements and assessment of accrediting standards to assure that the policies and procedures meet changes in criteria. It is essential to make the exercise an interdepartmental effort so that linkages between departments are established and remain intact on a continuing basis.

INTERNAL AUDITS

Much like keeping an automobile maintained, it is important to keep a health care organization prepared between audits, whether the organization is a hospital, long-term care facility, health plan, or any other organization that is audited by a regulatory or accrediting agency or organization. Internal audits offer one of the best ways to maintain preparedness for audits by regulatory or accrediting entities. Many well-managed organizations have departments dedicated to conducting internal program audits and educating various departments regarding audit processes and content. Others depend on consultants to assist them with mock site visits in anticipation of a regularly scheduled audit.

An internal audit may involve one department or several departments simultaneously. It entails a thorough review of policies and procedures, training manuals, records, contracts, letters, forms, and other written documentation as well as interviews with department personnel and a walk through of the physical plant. Typically, the internal auditor makes use of the same auditing tools as the regulatory or accrediting entity would during an actual audit and schedules an internal audit at least quarterly. The author recommends scoring internal audits so that measurable change may be shared with management and resources may be allocated when desirable changes fail to take place.

Preparation for the internal audit necessitates review of the audit tool and assignment of each section so that employees accept responsibility for responding verbally to specific sections of the tool and gathering or developing documentation that substantiates compliance with particular sections.

The internal auditor or consultant is able to gain significant insight into the level of compliance via the internal audit process. By educating and coaching staff regarding regulatory and accrediting mandates, he or she seeks to maintain or improve the level of compliance. Policies and procedures may be changed, professional education may be initiated or focused on problem areas, continued assessment and coaching may take place, influence of management may be invoked, or disciplinary action may be imposed if improvement is not evidenced. The goal is to identify problem areas and strive to meet or exceed mandated criteria on an ongoing basis.

AUDIT PREPARATION

Once again, reflect on the statement regarding preparation for an audit. "An experienced case manager knows that preparing for an audit is not an event; it is an unending process that requires diligent attention to detail and careful documentation according to established protocols." This is true. It is also true that there is a period between receipt of written notice of an audit and the conclusion of the audit process when an inordinate amount of energy, attention to detail, and team effort is required to achieve a successful audit outcome. Successful audits do not take place without sustained dedication to compliance and a burst of energy and detail-oriented teamwork in the short term. Preparing for audits is hard work. It

takes organizational focus, leadership, and an analytical approach.

Key to successful audit preparation is leadership by a dedicated employee or consultant who understands the audit process, has a working relationship with the auditing entity, excellent written and verbal skills, and the ability to bring people together under stressful circumstances. An organization that wishes to have a successful audit outcome should not shortchange itself by trying to "add on" audit management to someone who has other full-time responsibilities. The risks are far too great.

Many health care organizations have procedures in place to guide audit preparation upon receipt of written notice. Procedures may be customized to a specific auditing agency or organization. That customization is guided to a great extent by the attachments to the written notice described earlier in this chapter. However, those attachments generally describe *what* must be submitted and in *what* timeframe. It is left to the health care organization to determine *how* a multitude of tasks will be accomplished in a relatively short period of time. All departments, including case management, must be familiar with the procedures for audit preparation in order to meet the expectations of the audit team and achieve the goals of the organization.

Assignment of responsibility for each item in the audit tool is an essential part of preparing for any audit. Sometimes one person assumes sole responsibility, and other times a small group with a lead person is assigned the role. Timeframes, deliverables, and the format in which materials will be submitted are also determined so that the organization is able to work in concert. Frequent status meetings take place to assess progress and confer among teams and individuals.

In addition to preparation of written materials, reporting of data, and submission of samples that must take place prior to the on-site review, the organization must also prepare employees, board members, physicians, and others for interviews. As described earlier in the chapter, some may feel quite comfortable in the interview environment while others do not. It is not unusual to find that certain members of the team know their business in great detail but do not interview well. Therefore, practice and coaching is required to bring everyone to a certain level of confidence in both content and delivery. It is important that representatives who are both *knowledgeable and accountable* and can speak *on behalf of the organization* be interviewed. Each must be reminded that it is incumbent upon the auditors to *ask the questions,* while employees should *limit their responses to the questions asked.* This should be rehearsed during audit preparation.

There are also certain considerations regarding who will be interviewed from "outside" the organization. Will it be a physician or hospital administrator contracted with an HMO? Is he or she willing to be interviewed and well-prepared? Is a hospital board member out of town/state? How will his or her interviews tie in with the CEO's? Will "outside" interviewees want to know what "typical" interview questions might be? The person designated as the audit leader or coordinator is responsible for responding to questions and helping everyone feel as comfortable as possible. Conduct of a mock site visit also falls within the realm of the audit leader or a consultant. "Outside" interviewees frequently benefit from participating in such an exercise.

Preparation, display, and collation of materials are also an important part of preparing for an audit. Written notices and application materials provide clear direction regarding what must be submitted for presite visit review (presurvey, desk-review) *and* on-site review. Additional materials may be agreed upon during either phase of the review or may be requested following the on-site review or as part of a corrective action plan (CAP). If the health care organization reads the directions and responds carefully to the instructions provided by the auditing entity, it minimizes the need for repeating work or submitting additional information at a later date. Consideration for the manner in which information is presented also makes it easier for both the auditors and the health care organization to locate materials during the on-site visit.

The author recommends that organizations label and tab binders in a consistent manner so that auditors may find materials quickly and easily. Headings for different sections should also be similar and both a table of contents and index should be used to assist the auditors search for specific items. In addition, "Notes to Reviewers" should be used for items that may be confusing to the reviewers. The notes are used to explain why something unusual is included or how a particular document is arranged. Each of these recommendations, of course, must be balanced against the directions included in the written notice and attachments. However, the organization should always ask, "How can I make it most convenient for the auditors to find and review the materials—and therefore contribute to a positive audit outcome?"

Because many of the documents submitted as part of the presurvey process are critical to support compliance, they are also helpful during on-site interviews. Therefore, the organization's effort contributes to their ability to respond readily to auditor's questions during the on-site portion of the audit. If the materials are well-organized for the auditors, they will also be well-organized for the employees who will be interviewed. This means the organization will have accomplished good organizational planning well in advance of the on-site portion of the audit.

GAME TIME—THE ON-SITE VISIT

At the beginning of the chapter, various segments of an on-site visit were discussed. But a visit by auditors involves far more than segments of a process. The energy and dedication involved in a successful visit is difficult to describe, just as the electricity in the air on the first day is hard to put into words.

Early on the first day there are concerns about how the auditors will ask questions, and how employees, patients, doctors, and other "outside" parties will respond. There are butterflies, even among seasoned employees, about whether preparations have been adequate and if they've gathered the appropriate data and other supportive materials. What about policies and procedures? Are they up-to-date with the most recent regulations and standards? Has routine equipment maintenance taken place? Is the physical plant in tip-top shape? Is all documentation correct and timely? Are files in order? Thoughts such as these float through the minds of participants even though they've checked regulations, standards, and audit tools and have conducted internal audits so many times. Why? Because they are striving for compliance and a successful audit outcome.

And then, if the organization is well-disciplined and coached, like any other team, when the entrance interview begins they go out and do the best they can individually and as members of a team. Any nervous energy is focused into the task at hand. They remember, "preparing for an audit is not an event; it is an unending process that requires diligent attention to detail and careful documentation according to established protocols." They have given that diligent attention consistently and have not been complacent since the last audit. They have documented appropriately; gathered, reported, and analyzed data; communicated across departmental lines; developed, revised, and adhered to policies and procedures; followed other administrative and managerial guidelines; and prepared themselves as well as they possibly could for the audit. The interviews provide one more opportunity to demonstrate their level of compliance.

■ SUMMARY

The goal is to demonstrate compliance with regulations or standards, maximize the organization's strengths and minimize its weaknesses, have a successful audit, and learn how to do it *better* next time. This is part of the cycle of audits. The skills and experience that participants take from each audit simply fold into the flow of future audits. They wait for the arrival of the written report that guides them to the next step in the flow. Each time, they remember the cardinal rule of successful audits: an audit is not an event.

Chapter Exercises

1. What is the cardinal rule for successful audits?
2. What is the difference between mandatory audits and voluntary audits?
3. What is the importance of interdepartmental communication?
4. What are corrective actions and what importance do they have to the health care organization?
5. What role do policies and procedures play in an audit?

Suggested Websites and Resources

www.cms.hhs.gov—Centers for Medicare & Medicaid Services
www.ncqa.org—National Committee for Quality Assurance
www.urac.org—American Accreditation HealthCare Commission

www.jcaho.org—Joint Commission on Accreditation of Healthcare Organizations

www.dhhs.gov/progorg/oig/modcomp/index. htm—Department of Health and Human Services Office of Inspector General site that provides compliance program guidance

www.dhhs.gov/progorg/oig/new.html— Department of Health and Human Services Office of Inspector General site that provides a list of "What's New?"

www.mcareol.com—Managed Care On-Line site that provides managed care data files, news, publications, and tools. Some information available to the public; extensive information available by subscription

www.mediregs.com—Mediregs site that provides direct access to federal laws, regulations, manuals, operational policy letters, and other documents; available by subscription only

REFERENCES

1. American Accreditation HealthCare Commission: *URAC government relations—states that recognize URAC/ American Accreditation HealthCare Commission Accreditation,* June 2000, available on-line at www.urac.org/programs/govtrelationsstates.htm.
2. U.S. Department of Health and Human Services: *HHS: what we do,* 2001, available on-line at www.hhs.gov/news/press/2001pres/01fsprofile.html.
3. Health Care Financing Administration: *HCFA program manuals—state operations* (HCFA Pub 7), Section 1000, Sept 1, 2001, available on-line at www.mediregs.com/cgi-bin/hc_pm.
4. U.S. Department of Health and Human Services: *The orange book—program and management improvement recommendations,* 2000, Office of Inspector General, available on-line at www.os.dhhs.gov/org.
5. Section 1864 of the Social Security Act [42 U.S.C. 1395 aa], available on-line at www.ssa.gov/OP_Home/ssact/comp-ssa.htm.
6. Health Care Financing Administration: *HCFA program manuals—state operations* (HCFA Pub 7), Section 1010, Sept 1, 2001, available on-line at www.mediregs.com/cgi-bin/hc_pm.
7. National Association of Insurance Commissioners: *The NAIC—a tradition of consumer protection,* 1994–2000, available on-line at www.naic.org/1misc/aboutnaic/about/about01.htm.
8. Rules and regulations, Medicare and Medicaid programs; hospital conditions of participation: patients' rights; interim final rule, *Federal Register* 64(127):36070, July 12, 1999.
9. Joint Commission on Accreditation of Healthcare Organizations, *Facts,* 2001, available on-line at www.jcaho.org/aboutjc/facts.html.
10. National Committee for Quality Assurance, *NCQA timeline,* 2001, available on-line at www.ncqa.org/about/timeline.htm.
11. American Accreditation HealthCare Commission: *Overview of URAC accreditation programs and standards,* Aug 30, 2001, available on-line at www.urac.org/summaries.htm.
12. Health Care Financing Administration: *HCFA program manuals—state operations* (HCFA Pub 7), Section 2724, Sept 1, 2001, available on-line at www.mediregs.com/cgi-bin/hc_pm.
13. National Committee for Quality Assurance: *Section 2: evaluation process, 2000 surveyor guidelines for the accreditation of MCOs,* Washington, DC, 1999, The Committee.
14. Centers for Medicare & Medicaid Services: *M+C coordinated care plan contract approval notification letter,* Washington, DC, 2001, The Centers.

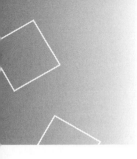

Index